Pancreatic Cancer

M. D. ANDERSON SOLID TUMOR ONCOLOGY SERIES

Series Editor: Raphael E. Pollock, M.D., Ph.D.

PUBLISHED VOLUMES

Liver Cancer
Edited by STEVEN A. CURLEY, M.D.

Breast Cancer
Edited by S. EVA SINGLETARY, M.D.

Pancreatic Cancer
Edited by DOUGLAS B. EVANS, M.D., PETER W.T. PISTERS, M.D.,
and JAMES L. ABBRUZZESE, M.D.

Andrew M. Lowy • Steven D. Leach
Philip A. Philip
Editors

Pancreatic Cancer

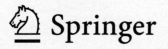 Springer

Editors
Andrew M. Lowy
University of California
San Diego
La Jolla, CA
USA

Steven D. Leach
Johns Hopkins University
    School of Medicine
Baltimore, MD
USA

Philip A. Philip
Wayne State University
Detroit, MI
USA

Series Editor
Raphael E. Pollock
University of Texas
M.D. Anderson Cancer Center
Houston, TX
USA

ISBN: 978-0-387-69250-0   e-ISBN: 978-0-387-69252-4
DOI: 10.1007/978-0-387-69252-4

Library of Congress Control Number: 2007934646

Printed on acid-free paper

9 8 7 6 5 4 3 2 1

springer.com

Preface

This volume of the M.D. Anderson Solid Tumor Oncology Series details the significant developments in the field of pancreatic cancer research, diagnosis, and treatment that have occurred in the past 5 years. The authors represent a diverse group of experts who have endeavored to provide a historical perspective on pancreatic cancer care, combined with a practical evaluation of available data, to allow clinicians to assimilate these facts into their treatment algorithms. While progress on the clinical front has been slower than desired, the ability to perform large-scale clinical trials in both the adjuvant and advanced disease settings has improved dramatically.

We have seen the development of the first mouse models that accurately recapitulate features of the human disease, tools that will enable pancreatic cancer researchers to ask new important questions aimed at early detection, biology, and therapy. An increased understanding of pancreatic cancer genetics and biology along with the rapid advancement of high throughput screening has led to the development of an unprecedented number of novel therapies for pancreatic cancer in preclinical and early phase clinical trials. The convergence of these events gives new hope that major advances in pancreatic cancer therapy will be realized during our lifetime.

We greatly appreciate the exceptional contributions of the authors, each of which reflects their commitment to the field of pancreatic cancer research and treatment.

Andrew M. Lowy, M.D.
University of California, San Diego,
Moores Cancer Center, La Jolla, California

Contents

Contributors

Judith Abrams, PhD
Karmanos Cancer Institute, Wayne State University, Detroit, Michigan, USA

N. Volkan Adsay, MD
Emory University Hospitals, Department of Pathology, Atlanta, Georgia, USA

Solomon Afelik, PhD
Barbara Davis Center for Childhood Diabetes, University of Colorado, HSC,
Denver, Colorado, USA

Syed A. Ahmad, MD
University of Cincinnati, Barrett Cancer Center, Cincinnati, Ohio, USA

Steven R. Alberts, MD
Mayo Clinic College of Medicine, Division of Medical Oncology, Rochester,
Minnesota, USA

Waddah B. Al-Refaie, MD
The University of Texas M. D. Anderson Cancer Center, Houston, Texas, USA

Deniz Altinel, MD
Emory University Hospital, Atlanta, Georgia, USA

Asfar S. Azmi, PhD
Karmanos Cancer Institute, Wayne State University School of Medicine,
Detroit, Michigan, USA

Johanna C. Bendell, MD
Duke University Medical Center, Division of Medical Oncology, Department
of Medicine, Durham, North Carolina, USA

Edgar Ben-Josef, MD
University of Michigan, Department of Radiation Oncology, Ann Arbor,
Michigan, USA

Andrew V. Biankin, BMedSc, MB, BS, PhD
Garvan Institute of Medical Research, and Bankstown Hospital, Sydney,
NSW, Australia

Daniel D. Billadeau, MD
Mayo Clinic, Division of Oncology Research, Rochester, Minnesota, USA

A. William Blackstock, MD
Wake Forest University, Department of Radiation Oncology, Winston-Salem,
North Carolina, USA

Genevieve M. Boland, MD, PhD
Massachusetts General Hospital, Department of Surgery, Boston,
Massachusetts, USA

Michael Bouvet, MD
University of California, San Diego and Moores Cancer Center, La Jolla,
California, USA

William R. Brugge, MD
Massachusetts General Hospital, Boston, Massachusetts, USA

Kieran A. Brune, BS, The Sol Goldman Pancreatic Cancer Research Center
and the John Hopkins Medical Institutions, Baltimore, Maryland, USA

Eric S. Calhoun, PhD
John Hopkins University School of Medicine, Baltimore, Maryland, USA

Jared Cassiano, MS
University of Utah, Department of Human Genetics, Salt Lake City, Utah, USA

Carlos Fernandez-del Castillo, MD
Massachusetts General Hospital, Harvard Medical School, Boston,
Massachusetts, USA

Kyuran Ann Choe, MD
University of Cincinnati College of Medicine, Cincinnati, Ohio, USA

Peter H. Cosman, BA, MBBS, PhD, FRACS
Garvan Institute of Medical Research, Sydney, and Bankstown Hospital,
Bankstown, Sydney, Austria

Christopher H. Crane, MD
The University of Texas M. D. Anderson Cancer Center, Radiation Oncology
Department, Houston, Texas, USA

Stefano Crippa, MD
Massachusetts General Hospital, Harvard Medical School, Boston,
Massachusetts, USA

Brian G. Czito, MD
Duke University Medical Center, Department of Radiation Oncology,
Durham, North Carolina, USA

Jean-Paul De La O, BA
University of Utah, Department of Human Genetics, Salt Lake City, Utah, USA

Sameer P. Desai, MD
University of Michigan, Division of Hematology-Oncology, Ann Arbor,
Michigan, USA

Jeffrey A. Drebin, MD, PhD
University of Pennsylvania School of Medicine, Philadelphia, Pennsylvania, USA

Bassel El-Rayes, MD
Karmanos Cancer Center, Wayne State University, Detroit, Michigan, USA

Michael B. Farnell, MD
Mayo Clinic College of Surgery, Rochester, Minnesota, USA

Mariano Fernandez, MD
University of Cincinnati College of Medicine, Cincinnati, Ohio, USA

Noriyoshi Fukushima, MD
University of Tokyo, Tokyo, Japan

Michael C. Garofalo, MD
University of Maryland School of Medicine, Radiation Oncology Department,
Baltimore, Maryland, USA

Michael Goggins, MD
The Sol Goldman Pancreatic Cancer Research Center and the John Hopkins
Medical Institutions, Baltimore, Maryland, USA

Julia B. Greer, MD, MPH
University of Pittsburgh Medical Center, Division of Gastroenterology,
Hepatology and Nutrition, Pittsburgh, Pennsylvania, USA

Paul J. Grippo, PhD
Robert H. Lurie Comprehensive Cancer Center, Feinberg School of Medicine,
Northwestern University, Chicago, Illinois, USA

David G. Heidt, MD
University of Michigan Medical School, Department of Surgery, Ann Arbor,
Michigan, USA

Lance Heilbrun, PhD
Karmanos Cancer Institute, Wayne State University, Detroit, Michigan, USA

Sunil R. Hingorani, MD, PhD
Fred Hutchinson Cancer Research Center, University of Washington School
of Medicine, Seattle, Washington, USA

Ralph H. Hruban, MD
The Sol Goldman Pancreatic Cancer Research Center and the John Hopkins
Medical Institutions, Baltimore, Maryland, USA

Elizabeth M. Jaffee, MD
The Sidney Kimmel Comprehensive Cancer Center, John Hopkins University
School of Medicine, Baltimore, Maryland, USA

Jan Jensen, PhD
Barbara Davis Center for Childhood Diabetes, University of Colorado, HSC,
Denver, Colorado, USA

Ahmed O. Kaseb, MD
The University of Texas M. D. Anderson Cancer Center, Houston, Texas, USA

Matthew H. Katz, MD
The University of Texas M. D. Anderson Cancer Center, Houston, Texas, USA

James G. Kench, BSc (Med)
Garvan Institute of Medical Research, Sydney, and Institute of Clinical Pathology
and Medical Research, Westmead, Australia

Scott E. Kern, MD
The Sidney Kimmel Comprehensive Cancer Center, John Hopkins University
School of Medicine, Baltimore, Maryland, USA

George P. Kim, MD
Mayo Clinic College of Medicine, Division of Hematology-Oncology,
Jacksonville, Florida, USA

Alison Klein, PhD
The Sidney Kimmel Comprehensive Cancer Center, John Hopkins University
School of Medicine, Baltimore, Maryland, USA

Dan Laheru, MD
The Sidney Kimmel Comprehensive Cancer Center, John Hopkins University
School of Medicine, Baltimore, Maryland, USA

Dung Le, MD
The Sidney Kimmel Comprehensive Cancer Center, John Hopkins University
School of Medicine, Baltimore, Maryland, USA

Steven D. Leach, MD
John Hopkins University School of Medicine, Baltimore, Maryland, USA

Jeffrey E. Lee, MD
The University of Texas M. D. Anderson Cancer Center, Houston, Texas, USA

Yiwei Li, PhD
Karmanos Cancer Institute, Wayne State University School of Medicine,
Detroit, Michigan, USA

Kaye M. Reid Lombardo, MD
Mayo Clinic College of Medicine, Rochester, Minnesota, USA

Andrew M. Lowy, MD
University of California, San Diego and Moores Cancer Center, La Jolla,
California, USA

David M. Lubman, PhD
University of Michigan Medical School, Departments of Surgery and Chemistry,
Ann Arbor, Michigan, USA

Anirban Maitra, MBBS
The Sol Goldman Pancreatic Cancer Research Center and the John Hopkins
Medical Institutions, Baltimore, Maryland, USA

Adhip P.N. Majumdar, PhD, DSc
John D. Dingell VA Medical Center, Detroit, Michigan, USA

Laleh G. Melstrom, MD
Northwestern University, Feinberg School of Medicine, Chicago, Illinois, USA

Nipun B. Merchant, MD
Vanderbilt University School of Medicine, Nashville, Tennessee, USA

Neil D. Merrett, MBBS
Bankstown Hospital, Bankstown, Sydney, Australia

David Misek, PhD
University of Michigan Medical School, Department of Surgery, Ann Arbor,
Michigan, USA

Mussop Mohammad , BSc
Wayne State University School of Medicine, Internal Medicine, Detroit,
Michigan, USA

Ramzi M. Mohammad, PhD
Wayne State University School of Medicine, Internal Medicine, Detroit,
Michigan, USA

Abdool R. Moossa, MD
Department of Surgery, University of California, San Diego, , San Diego,
California, USA

L. Charles Murtaugh, PhD
University of Utah, Department of Human Genetics, Salt Lake City, Utah, USA

Attila Nakeeb, MD
Indiana University School of Medicine, Indianapolis, Indiana, USA

Haydee Ojeda-Fournier, MD
University of California, San Diego and Moores Cancer Center, La Jolla,
California, USA

Alexander A. Parikh, MD
Vanderbilt University School of Medicine, Nashville, Tennessee, USA

Bhaumik B. Patel, MD
John D. Dingell VA Medical Center, Detroit, Michigan, USA

Rebecca P. Petersen, MD, MSc, Duke University Medical Center, Department
of Surgery, Durham, North Carolina, USA

Philip A. Philip, MD, PhD
Karmanos Cancer Institute, Wayne State University, Detroit, Michigan, USA

Jane Pruemer, Pharm.D, BCOP
James L. Winkle College of Pharmacy, University of Cincinnati, Barrett Cancer
Center, Cincinnati, Ohio, USA

William F. Regine, MD
University of Maryland School of Medicine, Department of Radiation Oncology,
Baltimore, Maryland, USA

Andrew S. Resnick, MD
University of Pennsylvania School of Medicine, Philadelphia, Pennsylvania, USA

Michelle Rockey, PhD, BCOP
University Hospital, Cincinnati, Ohio, USA

Fazlul H. Sarkar, PhD
Karmanos Cancer Institute, Wayne State University School of Medicine, Detroit,
Michigan, USA

Michael G. Sarr, MD
Mayo Clinic College of Medicine, Rochester, Minnesota, USA

Nathan Schmulewitz, MD
University of Cincinnati, Division of Gastroenterology, Cincinnati, Ohio, USA

Thomas Schnelldorfer, MD
Mayo Clinic College of Medicine, Rochester, Minnesota, USA

L. Andrew Shirley, MD
Thomas Jefferson University, Philadelphia, Pennsylvania, USA

Diane M. Simeone, MD
University of Michigan Medical School, Departments of Surgery and Molecular
and Integrative Physiology, Ann Arbor, Michigan, USA

Aaron C. Spalding, MD, PhD
University of Michigan, Department of Radiation Oncology, Ann Arbor,
Michigan, USA

Chris H. Takimoto, MD, PhD
University of Texas Health Science Center at San Antonio, South Texas
Accelerated Research Therapeutics, San Antonio, Texas, USA

Kyla Terhuns, MD
Vanderbilt University School of Medicine, Nashville, Tennessee, USA

Sarah P. Thayer, MD, PhD
Massachusetts General Hospital, Department of Surgery, Boston,
Massachusetts, USA

Duangpen Thirabanjasak, MD
Chulalongkorn University, Bangkok, Thailand

Michael John Tisdale, PhD, DSc
School of Life and Health Sciences, Aston University, Birmingham,
United Kingdom

Douglas S. Tyler, MD
Duke University Medical Center, Department of Surgery, Durham,
North Carolina, USA

Andrew L. Warshaw, MD
Massachusetts General Hospital, Harvard Medical School, Boston,
Massachusetts, USA

Stacy Wentworth, MD
Wake Forest University, Department of Radiation Oncology, Winston-Salem,
North Carolina, USA

David C. Whitcomb, MD, PhD
University of Pittsburgh, Departments of Medicine, Cell Biology & Physiology,
and Human Genetics; University of Pittsburgh Medical Center: University
of Pittsburgh Cancer Institute, Pittsburgh, Pennsylvania, USA

Curtis J. Wray, MD
The University of Texas M. D. Anderson Cancer Center, Houston, Texas, USA

Charles J. Yeo, MD
Thomas Jefferson University, Philadelphia, Pennsylvania, USA

Mark M. Zalupski, MD
University of Michigan, Division of Hematology-Oncology, Ann Arbor,
Michigan, USA

Narcis O. Zarnescu, MD
University of Pittsburgh Medical Center, Department of Surgery, Pittsburgh,
Pennsylvania, USA

Section I
Molecular Pathology and Epidemiology

Chapter 1
Spectrum of Human Pancreatic Neoplasia

N. Volkan Adsay, Duangpen Thirabanjasak, and Deniz Altinel

1 Introduction

Classification of pancreatic neoplasia is based on their cellular lineage, i.e which histologic cell type of the pancreas they recapitulate, which is in essence the main determinant of their clinicopathologic and biologic characteristics. Virtually every cell type that exists in the pancreas has been described to have one or more neoplastic counterparts.

Cellular components of the pancreas can be regarded under six categories (*1*) (Fig. 1.1): (1) *acinar* and (2) *ductal*, which together constitute the exocrine component of the organ responsible for the production of digestive enzymes (trypsin, chymotrypsin, lipases, and others) and their transportation to the duodenum, respectively; (3) *islets of Langerhans*, the endocrine component, which is responsible for the production of hormones involved in regulation of glucose and other metabolic activities; (4) *ambiguous cells*, such as centroacinar cells, which are less well characterized; (5) *supportive elements*, which encompass fibrous tissue, vessels, nerves, and other connective tissue elements; and (6) *"potential" cells*, such as stem cells, the existence of which is evidenced based on in vitro studies, but their representatives in normal human pancreata have not yet been clearly identified in histologic sections (*2*).

In the ensuing text, an overview of the clinicopathologic characteristics of pancreatic neoplasia is discussed based on their lineage. Emphasis is given to those that are more common and not covered in the other chapters of this book.

2 Ductal Neoplasms

The ducts, which give rise to the vast majority pancreatic neoplasms, in fact constitute the least sophisticated component of this organ (*3*). They are merely responsible for transportation of acinar products to the ampulla of Vater. It may not be surprising, however, that ducts are more prone to neoplastic transformation, considering that most adult cancers, such as breast, prostate, lung, and colon, arise from

A.M. Lowy et al. (eds.), *Pancreatic Cancer.*
doi: 10.1007/978-0-387-69252-4, © Springer Science+Business Media, LLC 2008

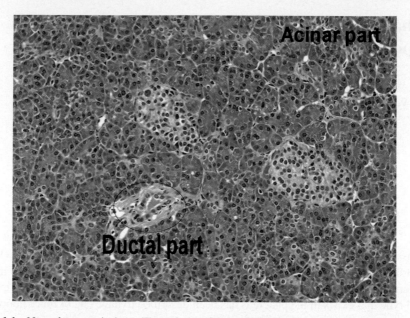

Fig. 1.1 Normal pancreatic tissue. The majority of the epithelial elements in the pancreas are acinar cells, which drain their products into the terminal portion of the ductal system (the centroacinar cells) and then into increasingly larger ducts. In a normal pancreas, the ducts are lined by a single layer of cuboidal epithelial cells without obvious mucin. The third epithelial component, the endocrine elements, are represented as scattered nested clusters of cells within the islets of Langerhans

epithelia with high regenerative capacity and from cell types that have secretory properties and produce mucin-type glycoproteins. Moreover, the ducts are the only component of the pancreas exposed to the outside world (mutagens), and the fact that most pancreatic adenocarcinomas arise in the head of the organ may be related to this phenomenon.

It is also important for cancer researchers to recognize that although ducts give rise to most common neoplasia of the pancreas, they constitute only a very small minority of pancreatic tissue (*1*) (see Fig. 1.1), and thus comparison of "normal" and "malignant" pancreas is *not* a comparison of non-neoplastic versus cancerous ducts, but rather normal acini versus malignant ducts, which is essentially like comparing apples and oranges.

The ductal system begins with the centroacinar unit (see Fig. 1.1), and through intralobar and interlobar ducts, adjoins the main pancreatic duct, eventually opening into the duodenum. Ductal cells produce some amount of mucin, more so in larger ducts, presumably for protection and providing the appropriate milieu for the acinar enzymes.

Findings that characterize ductal differentiation in the pancreas include tubular structures (lumen-forming units; also referred to as glands or ducts), cysts (columnar epithelial-lined cavities), papillae (finger-like projections from an epithelial-lined surface), and mucin formation (which can be intracytoplasmic, luminal, or stromal). Mucin-related glycoproteins and oncoproteins such as MUC1, CA19-9, CEA, and DUPAN are typically detectable by immunohistochemistry in mucinous ductal tumors. Expression of certain subsets of cytokeratin, such as CK19, and mutations in K-ras oncogene or loss of SMAD4/DPC4 are also fairly specific, and are typically lacking in endocrine or acinar tumors with a few exceptions. Rare scattered endocrine cells can be seen in almost any ductal tumor; however, evidence of acinar differentiation such as enzyme activity is exceedingly uncommon.

2.1 Invasive Ductal Adenocarcinoma

Invasive ductal carcinoma, also called pancreatobiliary type adenocarcinoma because of its morphologic and biologic kinship to biliary carcinomas (3), is the most common neoplasm of the pancreas, constituting >85% of pancreatic tumors that come to clinical attention. It is one of the deadliest of all cancers, with a 5-year survival <5%, and it is the fourth leading cause of cancer deaths, with a higher mortality in the United States than prostatic cancer since 2004 (4). It is also responsible for a substantial number of cases with carcinomas of unknown primacy (5), because it is often widely disseminated at the time of diagnosis, and the primary tumor may not be obvious unless carefully investigated. In fact, because of its infiltrative pattern, early dissemination, and rapid fatality, the primary tumor seldom forms a compact lesion that measures more than 5 cm. Along the same lines, only 20% of the cases are deemed resectable at the time of diagnosis (6).

As in other major cancers of epithelial organs, pancreatic adenocarcinoma is most common in the seventh decade (mean age 63), and it is very uncommon in patients younger than 40 years old (6).

The differential diagnosis of pancreas cancer from benign conditions of this organ is a well-known challenge (7–10). At the macroscopic level, it is a scirrhous carcinoma with ill-defined borders that is difficult to distinguish from any benign, scar-forming lesion of this organ; i.e., chronic pancreatitis, in particular autoimmune (9, 11) and paraduodenal types (10). Microscopically, it is often "well differentiated," characterized by well-formed glandular elements that can closely resemble benign ducts (7, 12) and conversely, benign ductal epithelium can show substantial atypia that may mimic adenocarcinoma. Even experts can sometimes have difficulty in making this diagnosis.

Invasive ductal adenocarcinoma has some morphologic characteristics that are fairly unique to this type of cancer. Despite its often well-differentiated glandular pattern (Fig. 1.2), it has tremendous propensity for insidious infiltration. Commonly, individual malignant glands are identified far away from the main tumor, presumably related to their remarkable affinity for perineurial and vascular invasion. *Perineurial* invasion (Fig. 1.3) is identified in close to 80% of the cases, although this figure may prove to be even higher if the entire tumors are examined microscopically. Perineurial invasion is also thought to contribute to back pain, one of the more common symptoms of pancreas cancer. *Vascular* invasion (Fig. 1.4) is also

6

N.V. Adsay et al.

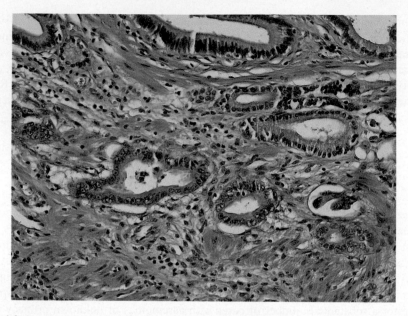

Fig. 1.2 Invasive ductal adenocarcinoma, well differentiated. Widely separated, well-formed glandular units lined by one to two layers of cuboidal cells showing nuclear atypia

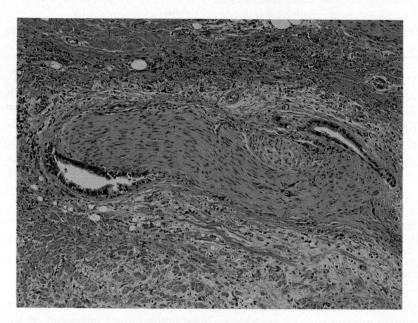

Fig. 1.3 Invasive ductal adenocarcinoma with perineural invasion

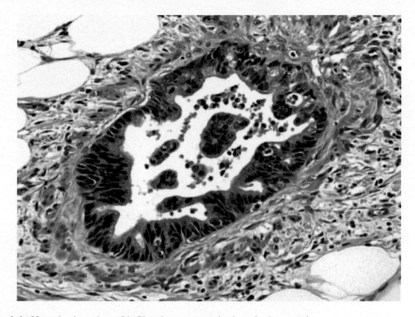

Fig. 1.4 Vascular invasion of infiltrating pancreatic ductal adenocarcinoma

common, and may in fact be responsible for the rapid spread of the carcinoma cells. Interestingly, pancreatic carcinoma cells have an almost unique ability to form exceedingly well-formed glandular elements, even in vascular spaces.

Another aspect of pancreatic ductal adenocarcinoma is the degree of intratumoral heterogeneity seen in this tumor, which is reflected in the frequent mixture of glandular and solid (nonglandular) patterns as well as in the high degree of genetic instability (*13*) documented in these tumors. In recognition of this important aspect of ductal adenocarcinoma, we recently proposed a different grading system involving a score that incorporates the presence of different patterns within the same tumor (*13*). The cells in pancreatic adenocarcinoma are typically cuboidal with variable amount of cytoplasm that contains mucin and mucin-related glycoproteins, and may occasionally demonstrate predominance of a specific organelle creating distinctive patterns such as "foamy-gland" (with swollen, altered mucin), "clear-cell" (abundant glycogen), and "oncocytoid" or "hepatoid" variants with prominent mitochondria or lysosomes, respectively (*3*).

One of the most characteristic features of ductal adenocarcinoma is *desmoplastic stroma* (Fig. 1.5). Perhaps more so than in any other cancers, pancreatic adenocarcinoma is associated with abundant fibroinflammatory changes in the stroma, to a degree that there is often a lot more stromal tissue than invasive carcinoma cells in a given tumor. This dilution phenomenon creates major problems for both diagnosticians and researchers. This is an important pitfall, in particular for studies that utilize "global" arrays, which do not discriminate between the cellular compartments of the specimen; thus the importance of immunohistochemical or in situ hybridization methods in verification.

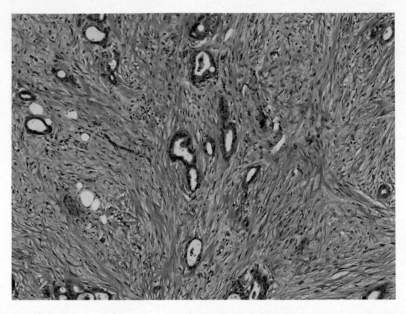

Fig. 1.5 Desmoplasia is the fibroinflammatory reaction of stroma which is often abundant in ductal adenocarcinoma. The tumor consists of well-formed glands surrounded by abundant desmoplastic stroma

2.2   Other Invasive Carcinomas of Ductal Lineage

There are other types of invasive carcinomas in the pancreas that are of ductal lineage but are regarded separately from the conventional ductal adenocarcinomas of this organ (*3*).

Undifferentiated carcinoma (see Fig. 1.6) can be regarded as the least differentiated form of ductal adenocarcinoma (DA) in which characteristic tubule formation is no longer evident or only focal (*14*). These are rare tumors and their demographics do not seem to differ from ordinary DA, except that they may have even more aggressive behavior. Undifferentiated carcinomas include sarcomatoid (spindle cell) carcinoma, anaplastic giant cell carcinoma, and carcinosarcoma. Rarely, the sarcomatoid components of these tumors may show aberrant differentiation, including bone and cartilage formation.

"Undifferentiated carcinoma with osteoclast-like giant cells" (Fig. 1.7) is the name commonly used for a distinctive tumor type characterized by abundant osteoclastic giant cells in the background of a sarcomatoid carcinoma. Recent studies have shown that the osteoclastic (*14, 15*) giant cells are indeed histiocytic in nature (*15*) and thus non-neoplastic; the reasons for this chemotaxis are unknown. The true neoplastic cells in this tumor type are the sarcomatoid cells. An adenocarcinoma component, or in some cases a mucinous cystadenocarcinoma, may be present. They often appear well demarcated, and form a large solitary mass.

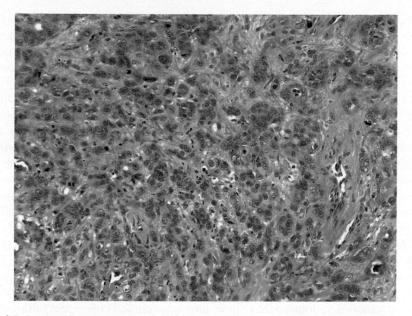

Fig. 1.6 Poorly differentiated carcinoma of pancreas. The cells do not show any duct formation, but instead infiltrate as cords and individual cells

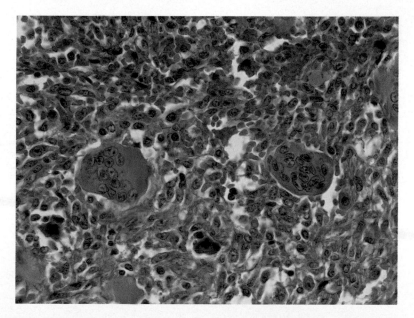

Fig. 1.7 Osteoclastic giant cell sarcoma (undifferentiated carcinoma with osteoclastic giant cells). This tumor contains neoplastic undifferentiated cells that vary from epithelioid to spindled, mixed with varying numbers of non-neoplastic multinucleated osteoclasts of the histiocytic origin

Squamous differentiation is often seen in conventional DAs (i.e., adenosqua-mous carcinoma) (*16*, *17*), but rare pure examples of squamous cell carcinoma without any glandular components may also be seen. They may have variable degrees of keratinization. Squamous cell carcinoma and adenosquamous carcinoma of this region are highly aggressive tumors (*16*, *17*).

Colloid carcinoma (*18*, *19*) (pure mucinous or mucinous noncystic carcinoma) (Fig. 1.8) is characterized by extensive stromal mucin deposition. Some studies have found that tumors composed almost exclusively of this pattern, where the mucin-to-epithelium ratio is very high and most carcinoma cells are floating within the mucin (detached from the stroma), have a different biology with an unusually protracted clinical course (*20*). Colloid carcinomas also tend to be larger and better demarcated than DAs, and their molecular alterations appear to be different. They are often associated with intraductal papillary mucinous neoplasms (see other chapters).

Medullary carcinomas akin to those seen in the gastrointestinal tract associated with microsatellite instability have also been reported in the pancreas (*21*, *22*). Syncytial nodules of large, poorly differentiated epithelioid cells with a pushing pattern of invasion characterize medullary carcinomas. In one study (*21*), a subset of these tumors were found to have more protracted clinical course, but further data are necessary to elucidate the behavior of these rare tumors.

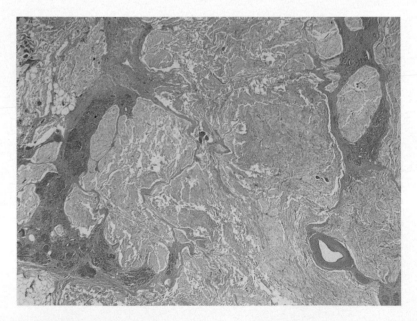

Fig. 1.8 Colloid carcinoma (mucinous noncystic carcinoma). The tumor is composed of large stromal mucin lakes in which are suspended relatively scanty strips and clusters of cells, with only minimal pleomorphism

2.3 Noninvasive Ductal Neoplasia

2.3.1 Pancreatic Intraepithelial Neoplasia

It has been speculated for decades that proliferative lesions in the ducts precede the development of invasive ductal carcinoma (*23, 24*). These proliferations have been referred to under a plethora of terms, including hyperplasia and dysplasia, but are now referred to as pancreatic intraepithelial neoplasia (PanIN) (*25*) (Fig. 1.9) in recognition of their neoplastic nature. PanINs comprise a spectrum of neoplastic transformation ranging from those used to be called mucinous "hypertrophy" or "metaplasia" to frank carcinoma in situ. While PanIN-3 is uncommon and seldom detected in the absence of invasive carcinoma, early PanINs, in particular PanIN-1, are common incidental findings even in normal pancreata (*26*). PanINs are reviewed in detail in other chapters of this book.

2.3.2 Mass-Forming Preinvasive Neoplasia

In the pancreas, there is a group of ductal neoplasms characterized by cyst formation (with or without papillary nodules), and are by nature noninvasive but may be associated with (or progress into) invasive carcinoma. In that, they are similar to

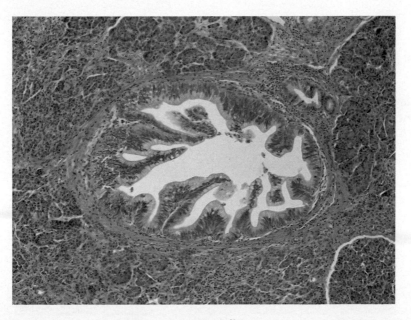

Fig. 1.9 This is an example of pancreatic intraepithelial neoplasia 2 (PanIN 2), which shows tall columnar cells but in addition exhibits full thickness nuclear pseudostratification and mild to moderate nuclear atypia

PanINs; however, in contrast with PanINs, which are incidental/microscopic forms of dysplasia, these tumors form clinically detectable masses before they become invasive (*27*). The tumor types that can be placed under this umbrella category, which we refer to as mass-forming preinvasive neoplasia, are *mucinous cystic neoplasms* (Fig. 1.10), *intraductal papillary mucinous neoplasms,* and *intraductal oncocytic papillary neoplasms* (*28*). These tumors share several characteristics: (1) They are ductal-type tumors. (2) They form cysts lined by mucinous epithelium. (3) They may have papillary nodules, which often connote transformation to higher grade dysplasia. (4) They exhibit a spectrum of neoplastic transformation, ranging from adenoma to carcinoma in situ. (5) Carcinomatous foci maybe haphazardly distributed within the tumor. (6) They act as precursors of invasive carcinoma, and as such they form a distinct pathway of carcinogenesis, akin to adenoma-carcinoma sequence in the gastrointestinal (GI) tract.

These are being encountered with increasing frequency. In some institutions they constitute >10% of pancreatic resections (*29*). An estimated 2% of invasive pancreatic carcinomas arise in association with these tumors. They are potentially curable tumors, but there are controversies regarding their management. It is important to recognize the clinicopathologic characteristics of this group and the differential features of the entities under this category. These tumors are reviewed in detail in other chapters of this book.

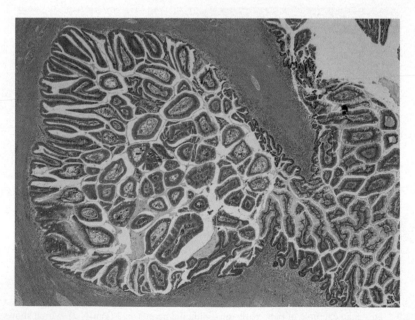

Fig. 1.10 Intraductal papillary mucinous neoplasia (IPMN) is characterized by florid arborizing growth of neoplastic ductal epithelium in papillary architecture

2.4 Serous Ductal Neoplasia

Serous adenomas (*30–32*) (Fig. 1.11) are the only pancreatic tumors of ductal lineage that lack conventional features of mucinous differentiation, possibly recapitulating centroacinar cells. Serous tumors can be considered as the innocent among ductal neoplasia, because unlike their mucinous kindreds they do not show any association with malignancy. They form relatively large masses (mean size, 9 cm; some up to 25 cm), and occur predominantly in elderly women (mean age 63; female/male = 3/1). They tend to be well demarcated. Typically, they are composed of thousands of small cysts, each measuring only millimeters, hence the synonym *microcystic adenoma*. However, rare "macrocystic" and "solid" examples of serous adenomas are also on record. Microcystic serous cystadenomas often have a central stellate scar. The defining microscopic feature is a simple, nonmucinous, cuboidal epithelium that contains intracytoplasmic glycogen, resulting in characteristic clear cytoplasm. Along the same lines, the cyst contents are depleted of the mucin-related glycoproteins and oncoproteins that are typically found in mucinous pancreatic tumors, a feature that may help in the preoperative diagnosis (*33*). Microscopically, these lesions are very similar to the cysts seen in Von-Hippel Lindau disease, and in fact some serous cystadenomas do show VHL gene alterations. Of interest, serous cystadenomas are often reported to coexist or "collide" with other pancreatic neoplasms and with congenital pathologic conditions (*32*).

Malignant serous tumors (serous cystadenocarcinomas) (*34–36*) are exceedingly uncommon, and only the presence of metastases or angioinvasive growth separates

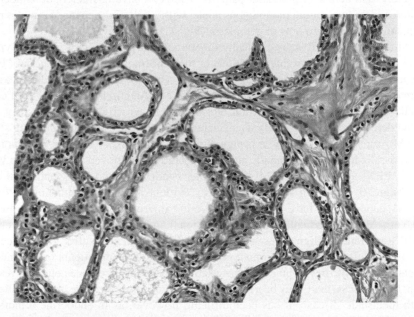

Fig. 1.11 Serous cystic adenoma is characterized by numerous minute cysts and glands that show low cuboidal appearance with clear cytoplasm, intermingling with the proliferated small capillaries

these tumors from their benign counterparts (i.e., the cytological appearance is entirely bland). For practical purposes, serous cystadenomas limited to the pancreas are regarded as uniformly benign (37).

3 Endocrine Neoplasia

Focal endocrine differentiation, especially in the form of scattered cells, is quite common in pancreatic neoplasia of ductal and acinar nature and is of no known biologic significance. It is also mostly disregarded in classification of tumors. The true endocrine tumors of the pancreas are the pancreatic endocrine neoplasms.

3.1 Pancreatic Endocrine Neoplasms

The vast majority of endocrine tumors of the pancreas are well differentiated pancreatic endocrine neoplasms (PENs, previously referred to as islet cell tumors) (13, 38–41). Grossly, PENs are usually solid, circumscribed, and fleshy, although multinodular and sclerotic examples occur. Rarely, cystic degeneration may occur (42– 44), with a central unilocular cyst lined by a cuff of viable tumor. PENs recapitulate the morphologic features of the islet cells by forming nested, gyriform, trabecular, or rarely also acinar or glandular patterns. The cells have characteristic endocrine features including round, monotonous nuclei with a salt-and-pepper chromatin pattern and moderate amounts of cytoplasm (Fig. 1.12).

Almost half of PENs are clinically functional and present with signs or symptoms of inappropriate production of one or more hormones; these functional PENs are named based upon the hormonal syndrome (insulinoma, glucagonoma, gastrinoma, somatostatinoma, VIPoma, and others). Nonfunctional PENs (45, 46) constitute an ever-enlarging proportion of pancreatic endocrine tumors, as they are being detected more commonly as incidental findings on abdominal imaging studies. Most insulinomas follow a benign clinical course, likely because insulinomas are typically highly symptomatic and are detected and removed when they are very small. PENs associated with MEN-1 or other syndromes tend to be multifocal and less aggressive (47). In addition to grossly evident and usually functional PENs, MEN1 patients also have numerous endocrine microadenomas, defined as PENs <0.5 cm. Most sporadically occurring functional and nonfunctional PENs are clinically low-grade malignancies. More than half of patients suffer recurrence or metastasis following resection and a sizeable proportion of patients only come to attention after the development of metastatic disease that precludes curative resection. Nonetheless, there may be a relatively protracted clinical course, even in patients with metastatic disease. It has been difficult, however, as in endocrine tumors of other organs, to determine which PENs are more likely to metastasize (48, 49). Findings that are more commonly associated with more aggressive behavior

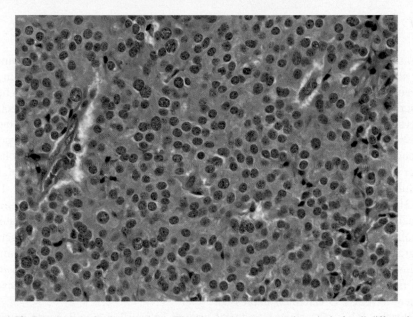

Fig. 1.12 Pancreatic endocrine neoplasm. The histologic appearance is typical of well-differentiated endocrine tumors, with nests and trabeculae of relatively uniform epithelial cells separated by scant fibrovascular stroma. Cytologically, the tumors have the typical "salt-and-pepper" chromatin pattern of endocrine tumors, and mitoses and necrosis are inconspicuous

include size >3 cm, functional PEN other than insulinoma, extrapancreatic or vascular invasion, high mitotic activity, high proliferation index (based on immunohistochemical staining for Ki-67), CK19 expression, and tumor aneuploidy; however, some PENs lacking all of these features may still metastasize. The most recent WHO classification (*50, 51*) separates "well-differentiated pancreatic endocrine tumors" (those lacking metastases) from "well-differentiated pancreatic endocrine carcinomas" (those with metastases) and further predicts "benign" or "malignant" behavior in the former group based on size, mitotic rate, and vascular invasion. Another recent proposal (*52*) divides PENs into low- and intermediate-grade groups based on the mitotic rate (less than or greater than 2 mitoses per 50 high power fields) and necrosis. The two groups exhibit a highly significant difference in prognosis, although no subset is specifically regarded to be utterly benign.

4   Acinar Neoplasia

Acinar differentiation can sometimes be seen as a focal component of endocrine neoplasia. It is also a major component of pancreatoblastoma (see the following). Tumors with predominant or pure acinar differentiation are acinar cell carcinomas. No benign counterpart of these tumors has been clearly documented.

4.1   Acinar Cell Carcinoma

Acinar cell carcinomas (ACCs) (*53–56*) of the pancreas are uncommon, accounting for no more than 1–2% of pancreatic carcinomas (*3*). Most patients are adults in the seventh decade, and there is a male predominance. Pediatric cases have also been described, but are very rare. The presenting symptoms are generally nonspecific. Elevated serum AFP levels are noted in some patients. A minority of patients present with a lipase (enzyme) hypersecretion syndrome characterized by subcutaneous fat necrosis, polyarthralgia, and occasionally eosinophilia. Most cases have liver metastases early in the course of the disease. The tumors are generally highly cellular, lacking the desmoplastic fibrous stroma of ductal adenocarcinomas (Fig. 1.13). The cellular population is monotonous and arranged in solid sheets and nests punctuated by acinar and small glandular spaces. The cytoplasm is moderate to focally abundant and shows eosinophilic granularity in the apical regions, reflecting aggregates of zymogen granules that are highlighted by the immunohistochemical stains for specific enzymes (trypsin, lipase, and chymotrypsin), of which trypsin is the most useful. Mutation in K-ras gene (seen in >90% of ductal carcinomas) is absent in ACCs. B-catenin is expressed.

Rarely, ACCs may show intraductal growth or papillary/papillocystic patterns and mimic intraductal neoplasia (*19*). Some studies suggest a more indolent behavior for these variants. Rare ACCs presenting as cystic lesions are also on record.

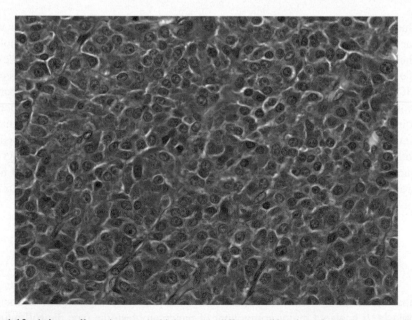

Fig. 1.13 Acinar cell carcinoma. At high power, diffuse proliferation of cells having moderate amounts of amphophilic cytoplasm and basally located nuclei. Prominent nucleoli are also a characteristic feature

Recently, a rare benign cystic lesion of acinar origin (acinar cell cystadenoma; cystic acinar transformation) (57), which is typically an incidental microscopic change, but also rarely may form a clinically detectable mass, has been described.

5 Neoplasms with Multiple Lineage (Mixed Carcinoma and Pancreatoblastoma)

While aberrant differentiation seldom occurs in ductal neoplasia, it is fairly common in nonductal tumors, in particular acinar neoplasia often has a mixed component, usually endocrine, detectable by immunohistochemistry (55). If the latter constitutes >25% of the tumor, it is classified as mixed acinar–endocrine carcinoma, a tumor that appears to be biologically similar to pure acinar cell carcinoma (56, 58, 59). Mixed ductal–endocrine tumors and mixed ductal–acinar tumors are exceedingly rare. Those we have seen had the two components almost in a "collision" and behaved like a ductal carcinoma.

Perhaps the ultimate example of a pancreatic tumor with "polyphenotypic" differentiation is pancreatoblastoma (Fig. 1.14). It is an extremely rare childhood tumor of the pancreas (mean age 4, with a second small peak in thirties) (60–64). Pancreatoblastomas are usually large (7–18 cm). Some cases are

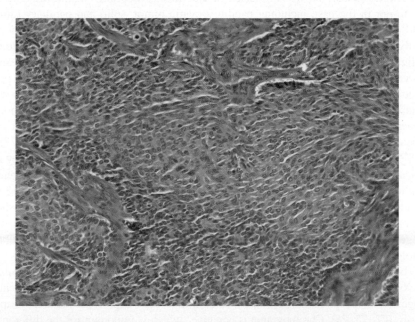

Fig. 1.14 Pancreatoblastoma. Several squamoid corpuscles illustrated here that are composed of spindle to epithelioid cells with abundant cytoplasm and less dense nuclei are characteristics of pancreatoblastoma

associated with elevated serum alpha-fetoprotein levels, and occasional cases are seen in association with Beckwith-Wiedemann (65, 66) or familial adenomatous polyposis coli syndromes (18). Pancreatoblastomas are malignant tumors, with a 5-year survival of about 25%, although children diagnosed before the development of metastases may be curable. Pancreatoblastomas are predominantly acinar neoplasms. Microscopically they have sheets of primitive appearing epithelial cells and acinar formations. A characteristic and peculiar microscopic finding is the squamoid nest, which is a small morular arrangement of squamoid cells (67), specific for this tumor type. Typically pancreatoblastomas exhibit all three lines of pancreatic differentiation, acinar, endocrine and ductal, with acinar elements being the most consistently present (62). Molecular, genetic findings of pancreatoblastomas are different than those of ductal adenocarcinoma (68).

6 Tumors of Uncertain Histogenesis

6.1 Solid-Pseudopapillary Tumor

Solid-pseudopapillary tumor (SPT) is a peculiar neoplasm of unknown origin (69, 70), and its obscure nature is reflected in the various descriptive names assigned to this tumor in the past, including papillary cystic tumor, solid and papillary tumor, solid and cystic tumor, Frantz tumor, and many others (71–74). It is seen predominantly in young women (mean age 25, >80% female) (72, 75–77). It is an indolent malignant neoplasm for which complete resection is curative in most cases. In a small percentage (about 15%), however, metastases are noted, usually either to liver or peritoneum. Metastases are typically present at the time of diagnosis. Even patients with metastases appear to have a protracted clinical course; fatality due to this tumor is exceedingly uncommon. A few highly aggressive SPTs have been reported that appear to exhibit high-grade malignant transformation of a conventional SPT (77).

SPTs are relatively large tumors, with a mean size of 8–10 cm. Although they are typically solid cellular tumors, cystic degeneration is common. Degenerative changes combined with the preservation of the cells around the microvasculature create the pseudopapillary microscopic pattern. The cells are round to oval and often show nuclear grooves. Intracytoplasmic hyaline globules and aggregates of foamy macrophages are characteristic findings (Fig. 1.15). Calcifications may be seen. Overall the histologic picture may closely resemble that of endocrine neoplasia.

The immunophenotype of this tumor is quite distinctive and interesting, but fails to disclose the line of differentiation of the cells. The tumor typically expresses vimentin, progesterone receptors, CD56, and CD10 and, to a lesser degree, keratin and synaptophysin (72, 75, 78). Chromogranin is negative, which is important for the differential diagnosis with PENs. Recently, β-catenin11 and cyclinD1 expression have been found in these tumors, suggesting an alteration in the *wnt* signaling pathway.

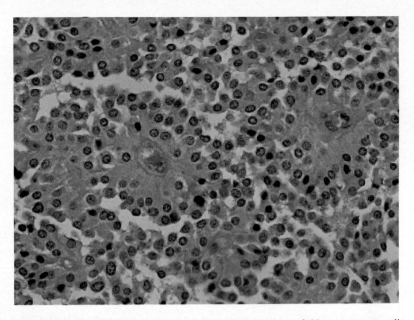

Fig. 1.15 Solid-pseudopapillary tumor. The solid, cellular regions of this tumor surrounding the small vessels, form the extensive pseudopapillary pattern with the cleft-like areas in between those structures

7 Miscellaneous Cystic Pancreatic Lesions

In addition to pseudocysts, cystic and intraductal mucinous neoplasms and serous cystic tumors, there are other uncommon cystic lesions in the pancreas (*76, 79, 80*).

Lymphoepithelial cysts (LECs) (*81*) are usually peripancreatic rather than intrapancreatic, and they occur predominantly in adult men (mean age 52, M/F = 3/1). Unlike their salivary gland counterparts, pancreatic LECs do not show associations with autoimmune syndromes, HIV, or malignancies such as lymphoma. They may occur in any part of the pancreas, and may be unilocular or multilocular. They are characterized by variably keratinized squamous lined cysts immediately surrounded by a rim of lymphoid tissue, some with lymphoid follicles and a capsule. The cyst contents may extravasate into the cyst wall and cause an inflammatory reaction, including granulomas. LEC-like epidermoid cystic tumors may evolve in intrapancreatic accessory spleens. *Dermoid cysts* (*81*) are similar to LECs but lack the lymphoid tissue and show skin adnexal elements, including sebaceous glands. *Lymphangiomas* (*82*) are seen in young women (mean age 29, M/F = 1/3) and form endothelial-lined cysts surrounded by a rim of lymphoid tissue. *Squamoid cyst of pancreatic* ducts (Fig. 1.16) is a recently described entity that is probably reactive in nature but may produce high CEA levels (*80*). *Congenital cysts* and *intestinal duplications* may also form cystic lesions in the

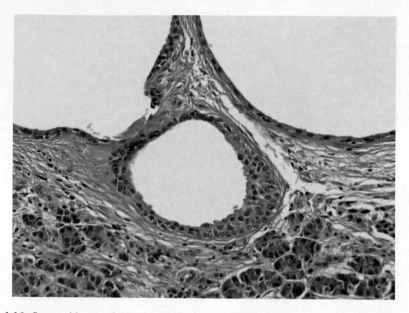

Fig. 1.16 Squamoid cyst of pancreas. Benign cystic lesion with notably high CEA level. The cysts can be either uniloculated or multiloculated, lined by squamous metaplastic epithelial cells usually containing concentrated concretion within the lumen

vicinity of the pancreas and periampullary region. These may have variable lining including respiratory type, intestinal, squamous, or transitional.

8   Pseudotumors

As discussed in the ductal adenocarcinoma section, benign chronic inflammatory and fibrosing conditions of the pancreas may be difficult to distinguish from carcinomas, both clinically and pathologically. Chronic pancreatitis of any etiology, including alcoholic, obstructive, or even those with granulomatous inflammation such as mycobacterial infection, may lead to segmental fibrosis and a tumorous mass (8, 83). There are, however, certain subtypes of chronic pancreatitis that are especially prone to form pseudotumors and mimic carcinomas, as discussed in the following.

Lymphoplasmacytic sclerosing pancreatitis (LPSP; also referred to as *autoimmune* or duct-centric pancreatitis) (11, 83–85) is often misdiagnosed as carcinoma. LPSP is typically seen in patients in the fourth to sixth decades. High serum IgG4 levels are very helpful in the preoperative diagnosis of LPSP. LPSP may be associated with other autoimmune disorders such as Sjögren's syndrome and ulcerative colitis as well as with components of the multifocal fibrosclerosis syndrome (retroperitoneal and mediastinal fibrosis, Riedel's thyroiditis, inflammatory pseudotumor of the orbit, and sclerosing cholangitis). Microscopically, dense periductal lymphoplasmacytic infiltrates, interstitial fibrosis with abundant myofibroblasts arranged in a storiform pattern, and obliterative venulitis are characteristic.

Some forms of *anatomic* pancreatitis (i.e., pancreatic fibroinflammatory masses associated with anatomic or functional variations of the ducts and periampullary structures) also commonly form pseudotumors. Some of these appear to be centered around the minor papilla. Affected patients are predominantly men in their forties with a history of alcohol abuse. In some cases, the fibroinflammatory process is in the region between common bile duct, duodenum, and pancreas (so-called *groove pancreatitis*) (*86*). In others cystic change in the duodenal wall is prominent (*paraduodenal wall cyst* or *cystic dystrophy of the duodenum*) (*86–88*). Microscopically, these lesions have a dense myofibroblastic proliferation within which lobules of pancreatic tissue are scattered, with cystic ducts containing inspissated enzymatic secretions. Extravasated ductal contents may elicit a cellular stromal reaction as well as inflammation. These cases are referred to as paraduodenal pancreatitis (*10*).

Some developmental abnormalities may also lead to pseudotumors. Recently, a *solid and cystic hamartoma* and a *cellular hamartoma* (*89*) have been reported to present as a pancreatic tumors in adults.

Lipomatous hypertrophy (*66*) of the pancreas may also lead to a mass that can be mistaken as carcinoma. *Adenomyomatous hyperplasia* (*90*) of the ampulla, a common finding in the general population reported in 40% of autopsies, has also been implicated as the cause of biliary obstruction mimicking a periampullary carcinoma.

9 Mesenchymal Tumors

Primary mesenchymal tumors of the pancreas are exceedingly uncommon (*91, 92*); however, those from neighboring sites may secondarily involve the pancreas. Especially gastrointestinal stromal tumors and retroperitoneal sarcomas may appear to be centered in the pancreas. A variety of benign mesenchymal tumors, including fibromatosis (desmoid tumor), solitary fibrous tumor, schwannoma, and several others have been reported in the pancreas. Primary sarcomas include primitive neuroectodermal tumor, synovial sarcoma, desmoplastic small round cell tumor (*93*), leiomyosarcoma, and malignant fibrous histiocytoma, all of which are largely documented in single case reports.

10 Secondary Tumors

It is not too uncommon for a widely metastatic malignant neoplasm to involve the pancreas; however, the majority of these are clinically undetected lesions identified only at autopsy (*3, 94–96*). Autopsy studies have shown that most secondary

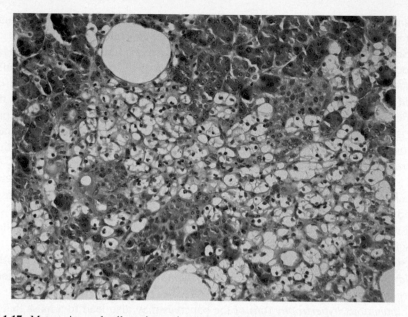

Fig. 1.17 Metastatic renal cell carcinoma in pancreas. Note the infiltrative tumor cells with clear cytoplasm, intermixing with the surrounding benign pancreatic tissue.

tumors involving the pancreas are of pulmonary origin, followed by gastrointestinal carcinomas.

There are, however, a few metastatic tumors that are prone to involve the pancreas in the absence of other metastatic foci, mimicking a primary carcinoma. Lymphomas and renal cell carcinomas (Fig. 1.17) appear to be the most common tumor types responsible for such cases. Renal cell carcinomas in particular are known to form polypoid ampullary nodules, or even to grow within the ducts.

References

1. Klimstra DS. Pancreas. In: Sternberg SS (ed.) Histology for pathologists. New York, Lippincott-Raven, 1997.
2. Vyas P AA, Sarkar F, Leach S, et al. In search of stem cell in pancreatic ducts: the nature of round, non-ductal appearing cells in human pancreatic ducts. Mod Pathol 2003, 16(1):287A.
3. Klimstra DS, Adsay N. Benign and malignant tumors of the pancreas. In: Odze R, Goldblum JR, Crawford JM (eds.) Surgical pathology of the GI tract, liver, biliary tract and pancreas. Philadelphia, Saunders, 2004.
4. Jemal A, Siegel R, Ward E, et al. Cancer statistics, CA Cancer J Clin 2006, 56:106–130.
5. Pavlidis N, Briasoulis E, Hainsworth J, et al. Diagnostic and therapeutic management of cancer of an unknown primary. Eur J Cancer 2003, 39:1990–2005.
6. Evans DB, Willet CG. Cancer of the pancreas. In: DeVita VT, Rosenberg SA (eds.) Cancer principle and practice of oncology. Philadelphia, Lippincott Williams & Wilkins, 2001, 1126–1161.
7. Adsay NV, Bandyopadhyay S, Basturk O, et al. Chronic pancreatitis or pancreatic ductal adenocarcinoma? Semin Diagn Pathol 2004, 21:268–276.

8. Adsay NV, Basturk O, Klimstra DS, et al. Pancreatic pseudotumors: non-neoplastic solid lesions of the pancreas that clinically mimic pancreas cancer. Semin Diagn Pathol 2004, 21:260–267.
9. Adsay NV, Basturk O, Thirabanjasak D. Diagnostic features and differential diagnosis of autoimmune pancreatitis. Semin Diagn Pathol 2005, 22:309–317.
10. Adsay NV, Zamboni G. Paraduodenal pancreatitis: a clinico-pathologically distinct entity unifying "cystic dystrophy of heterotopic pancreas", "para-duodenal wall cyst", and "groove pancreatitis". Semin Diagn Pathol 2004, 21:247–254.
11. Zamboni G, Luttges J, Capelli P, et al. Histopathological features of diagnostic and clinical relevance in autoimmune pancreatitis: a study on 53 resection specimens and 9 biopsy specimens. Virchows Arch 2004, 445:552–563.
12. Adsay V, Logani S, Sarkar F, et al. Foamy gland pattern of pancreatic ductal adenocarcinoma: a deceptively benign-appearing variant. Am J Surg Pathol 2000, 24:493–504.
13. Hernandez LV, Mishra G, Forsmark C, et al. Role of endoscopic ultrasound (EUS) and EUS-guided fine needle aspiration in the diagnosis and treatment of cystic lesions of the pancreas. Pancreas 2002, 25:222–228.
14. Hoorens A, Prenzel K, Lemoine NR, et al. Undifferentiated carcinoma of the pancreas: analysis of intermediate filament profile and Ki-ras mutations provides evidence of a ductal origin. J Pathol 1998, 185:53–60.
15. Westra WH, Sturm P, Drillenburg P, et al. K-ras oncogene mutations in osteoclast-like giant cell tumors of the pancreas and liver: genetic evidence to support origin from the duct epithelium. Am J Surg Pathol 1998, 22:1247–1254.
16. Adsay V, Sarkar, F, Vaitkevicius V, et al. Squamous cell and adenosquamous carcinomas of the pancreas: a clinicopathologic analysis of 11 cases. Mod Pathol 2000, 13(1):179A.
17. Kardon D, Thompson LD, Przygodzki RM, et al. Adenosquamous carcinoma of the pancreas: a clinicopathologic series of 25 cases. Mod Pathol 2001, 14(5):443–451.
18. Adsay NV, Pierson C, Sarkar F, et al. Colloid (mucinous noncystic) carcinoma of the pancreas. Am J Surg Pathol 2001, 25:26–42.
19. Seidel G, Zahurak M, Iacobuzio-Donahue C, et al. Almost all infiltrating colloid carcinomas of the pancreas and periampullary region arise from in situ papillary neoplasms: a study of 39 cases. Am J Surg Pathol 2002, 26:56–63.
20. Adsay NV, Merati K, Nassar H, et al. Pathogenesis of colloid (pure mucinous) carcinoma of exocrine organs: coupling of gel-forming mucin (MUC2) production with altered cell polarity and abnormal cell-stroma interaction may be the key factor in the morphogenesis and indolent behavior of colloid carcinoma in the breast and pancreas. Am J Surg Pathol 2003, 27:571–578.
21. Goggins M, Offerhaus GJ, Hilgers W, et al. Pancreatic adenocarcinomas with DNA replication errors (RER+) are associated with wild-type K-ras and characteristic histopathology. Poor differentiation, a syncytial growth pattern, and pushing borders suggest RER+. Am J Pathol 1998, 152:1501–1507.
22. Wilentz RE, Goggins M, Redston M, et al. Genetic, immunohistochemical, and clinical features of medullary carcinoma of the pancreas: a newly described and characterized entity. Am J Pathol 2000, 156:1641–1651.
23. Kloppel G, Bommer G, Ruckert K, et al. Intraductal proliferation in the pancreas and its relationship to human and experimental carcinogenesis. Virchows Arch A Pathol Anat Histol 1980, 387:221–233.
24. Sommers SC, Murphy SA, Warren S. Pancreatic duct hyperplasia and cancer. Gastroenterology 1954, 27:629–640.
25. Hruban RH, Adsay NV, Albores-Saavedra J, et al. Pancreatic intraepithelial neoplasia: a new nomenclature and classification system for pancreatic duct lesions. Am J Surg Pathol 2001, 25:579–586.
26. Andea A, Sarkar F, Adsay VN. Clinicopathological correlates of pancreatic intraepithelial neoplasia: a comparative analysis of 82 cases with and 152 cases without pancreatic ductal adenocarcinoma. Mod Pathol 2003, 16:996–1006.
27. Longnecker DS, Adsay NV, Fernandez-del Castillo C, et al. Histopathological diagnosis of pancreatic intraepithelial neoplasia and intraductal papillary-mucinous neoplasms: interobserver agreement. Pancreas 2005, 31:344–349.

28. Adsay NV, Merati K, Andea A, et al. The dichotomy in the preinvasive neoplasia to invasive carcinoma sequence in the pancreas: differential expression of MUC1 and MUC2 supports the existence of two separate pathways of carcinogenesis. Mod Pathol 2002, 15:1087–1095.
29. Tanaka M, Chari S, Adsay V, et al. International consensus guidelines for management of intraductal papillary mucinous neoplasms and mucinous cystic neoplasms of the pancreas. Pancreatology 2006, 6:17–32.
30. Adsay NV, Klimstra DS, Compton CC. Cystic lesions of the pancreas. Introduction. Semin Diagn Pathol 2000, 17:1–6.
31. Bassi C, Salvia R, Molinari E, et al. Management of 100 consecutive cases of pancreatic serous cystadenoma: wait for symptoms and see at imaging or vice versa? World J Surg 2003, 27:319–323.
32. Compton CC. Serous cystic tumors of the pancreas. Semin Diagn Pathol 2000, 17:43–55.
33. Brugge WR, Lewandrowski K, Lee-Lewandrowski E, et al. Diagnosis of pancreatic cystic neoplasms: a report of the cooperative pancreatic cyst study. Gastroenterology 2004, 126:1330–1336.
34. Matsumoto T, Hirano S, Yada K, et al. Malignant serous cystic neoplasm of the pancreas: report of a case and review of the literature. J Clin Gastroenterol 2005, 39:253–256.
35. Shintaku M, Arimoto A, Sakita N. Serous cystadenocarcinoma of the pancreas. Pathol Int 2005, 55:436–439.
36. Strobel O, Z'Graggen K, Schmitz-Winnenthal FH, et al. Risk of malignancy in serous cystic neoplasms of the pancreas. Digestion 2003, 68:24–33.
37. Balcom JHT, Keck T, Warshaw AL, et al. Telomerase activity in periampullary tumors correlates with aggressive malignancy. Ann Surg 2001, 234:344–350; discussion 50–51.
38. Heitz PU, Oberholzer M. Electron microscopy as a tool in the diagnosis of endocrine tumors. Pathol Res Pract 1984, 178:427–430.
39. Lam KY, Lo CY. Pancreatic endocrine tumour: a 22-year clinico-pathological experience with morphological, immunohistochemical observation and a review of the literature. Eur J Surg Oncol 1997, 23:36–42.
40. Solcia E, Capella C, Riva C, et al. The morphology and neuroendocrine profile of pancreatic epithelial VIPomas and extrapancreatic, VIP-producing, neurogenic tumors. Ann N Y Acad Sci 1988, 527:508–517.
41. Thompson GB, van Heerden JA, Grant CS, et al. Islet cell carcinomas of the pancreas: a twenty-year experience. Surgery 1988, 104:1011–1017.
42. Adsay NV, Klimstra DS. Cystic forms of typically solid pancreatic tumors. Semin Diagn Pathol 2000, 17:81–88.
43. Iacono C, Serio G, Fugazzola C, et al. Cystic islet cell tumors of the pancreas. A clinico-pathological report of two nonfunctioning cases and review of the literature. Int J Pancreatol 1992, 11:199–208.
44. Ligneau B, Lombard-Bohas C, Partensky C, et al. Cystic endocrine tumors of the pancreas: clinical, radiologic, and histopathologic features in 13 cases. Am J Surg Pathol 2001, 25:752–760.
45. Hochwald S, Conlon K, Brenann M. Nonfunctioning pancreatic islet cell tumors. In: Doherty GM, Skogseid B (eds.) Surgical endocrinology. Philadelphia, Lippincott Williams & Wilkins, 2001, pp 361–373.
46. La Rosa S, Sessa F, Capella C, et al. Prognostic criteria in nonfunctioning pancreatic endocrine tumours. Virchows Arch 1996, 429(6):323–333.
47. Donow C, Pipeleers-Marichal M, Schroder S, et al. Surgical pathology of gastrinoma. Site, size, multicentricity, association with multiple endocrine neoplasia type 1, and malignancy. Cancer 1991, 68:1329–1334.
48. Bertelli E, Regoli M, Bastianini A. Endocrine tissue associated with the pancreatic ductal system: a light and electron microscopic study of the adult rat pancreas with special reference to a new endocrine arrangement. Anat Rec 1994, 239:371–378.
49. Pelosi G, Bresaola E, Bogina G, et al. Endocrine tumors of the pancreas: Ki-67 immunoreactivity on paraffin sections is an independent predictor for malignancy: a comparative study with proliferating-cell nuclear antigen and progesterone receptor protein immunostaining, mitotic index, and other clinicopathologic variables. Hum Pathol 1996, 27:1124–1134.

50. Kloppel GHR, Longnecker DS, Adler G, et al. Tumours of exocrine pancreas. In: Hsa LA (ed.) World Health Organization classification of tumours: pathology and genetis tumours of the digestive system. Lyon, France, IARC Press 2000, pp 219–251.
51. Solcia E, Capella C, Klöppel G (eds.) Tumors of the pancreas. Washington, DC, American Registry of Pathology, 1997, pp 145–209.
52. Hochwald SN, Zee S, Conlon KC, et al. Prognostic factors in pancreatic endocrine neoplasms: an analysis of 136 cases with a proposal for low-grade and intermediate-grade groups. J Clin Oncol 2002, 20:2633–2642.
53. Holen KD, Klimstra DS, Hummer A, et al. Clinical characteristics and outcomes from an institutional series of acinar cell carcinoma of the pancreas and related tumors. J Clin Oncol 2002, 20:4673–4678.
54. Hoorens A, Lemoine NR, McLellan E, et al. Pancreatic acinar cell carcinoma. An analysis of cell lineage markers, p53 expression, and Ki-ras mutation. Am J Pathol 1993, 143:685–698.
55. Klimstra DS, Heffess CS, Oertel JE, et al. Acinar cell carcinoma of the pancreas. A clinico-pathologic study of 28 cases. Am J Surg Pathol 1992, 16:815–837.
56. Ohike N, Kosmahl M, Kloppel G. Mixed acinar-endocrine carcinoma of the pancreas. A clinico-pathological study and comparison with acinar-cell carcinoma. Virchows Arch 2004, 445:231–235.
57. Zamboni G, Terris B, Scarpa A, et al. Acinar cell cystadenoma of the pancreas: a new entity? Am J Surg Pathol 2002, 26:698–704.
58. Klimstra DS, Rosai J, Heffess CS. Mixed acinar-endocrine carcinomas of the pancreas. Am J Surg Pathol 1994, 18:765–778.
59. Ulich T, Cheng L, Lewin KJ. Acinar-endocrine cell tumor of the pancreas. Report of a pancreatic tumor containing both zymogen and neuroendocrine granules. Cancer 1982, 50:2099–2105.
60. Dhebri AR, Connor S, Campbell F, et al. Diagnosis, treatment and outcome of pancreatoblastoma. Pancreatology 2004, 4:441–451; discussion 52–53.
61. Horie A, Haratake J, Jimi A, et al. Pancreatoblastoma in Japan, with differential diagnosis from papillary cystic tumor (ductuloacinar adenoma) of the pancreas. Acta Pathol Jpn 1987, 37:47–63.
62. Klimstra DS, Wenig BM, Adair CF, et al. Pancreatoblastoma. A clinicopathologic study and review of the literature. Am J Surg Pathol 1995, 19:1371–1389.
63. Palosaari D, Clayton F, Seaman J. Pancreatoblastoma in an adult. Arch Pathol Lab Med 1986, 110:650–652.
64. Shorter NA, Glick RD, Klimstra DS, et al. Malignant pancreatic tumors in childhood and adolescence: The Memorial Sloan-Kettering experience, 1967 to present. J Pediatr Surg 2002, 37:887–892.
65. Drut R, Jones MC. Congenital pancreatoblastoma in Beckwith-Wiedemann syndrome: an emerging association. Pediatr Pathol 1988, 8:331–339.
66. Kerr N, Fukuzawa R, Reeve AE, et al. Beckwith-Wiedemann syndrome, pancreatoblastoma, and the wnt signaling pathway. Am J Pathol 2002, 160(4):1541–1542.
67. Nishimata S, Kato K, Tanaka M, et al. Expression pattern of keratin subclasses in pancreatoblastoma with special emphasis on squamoid corpuscles. Pathol Int 2005, 55:297–302.
68. Cao D, Maitra A, Saavedra JA, et al. Expression of novel markers of pancreatic ductal adenocarcinoma in pancreatic nonductal neoplasms: additional evidence of different genetic pathways. Mod Pathol 2005, 18:752–761.
69. Kissane JM. Carcinoma of the exocrine pancreas: pathologic aspects. J Surg Oncol 1975, 7:167–174.
70. Kissane JM. Pancreatoblastoma and solid and cystic papillary tumor: two tumors related to pancreatic ontogeny. Semin Diagn Pathol 1994, 11:152–164.
71. Kloppel G, Morohoshi T, John HD, et al. Solid and cystic acinar cell tumour of the pancreas. A tumour in young women with favourable prognosis. Virchows Arch A Pathol Anat Histol 1981, 392:171–183.
72. Kosmahl M, Seada LS, Janig U, et al. Solid-pseudopapillary tumor of the pancreas: its origin revisited. Virchows Arch 2000, 436:473–480.

73. Pettinato G, Manivel JC, Ravetto C, et al. Papillary cystic tumor of the pancreas. A clinico-pathologic study of 20 cases with cytologic, immunohistochemical, ultrastructural, and flow cytometric observations, and a review of the literature. Am J Clin Pathol 1992, 98:478–488.
74. Stommer P, Kraus J, Stolte M, et al. Solid and cystic pancreatic tumors. Clinical, histochemical, and electron microscopic features in ten cases. Cancer 1991, 67:1635–1641.
75. Klimstra DS, Wenig BM, Heffess CS. Solid-pseudopapillary tumor of the pancreas: a typically cystic carcinoma of low malignant potential. Semin Diagn Pathol 2000, 17:66–80.
76. Papavramidis T, Papavramidis S. Solid pseudopapillary tumors of the pancreas: review of 718 patients reported in English literature. J Am Coll Surg 2005, 200:965–972.
77. Tang LH, Aydin H, Brennan MF, et al. Clinically aggressive solid pseudopapillary tumors of the pancreas: a report of two cases with components of undifferentiated carcinoma and a comparative clinicopathologic analysis of 34 conventional cases. Am J Surg Pathol 2005, 29:512–519.
78. Ladanyi M, Mulay S, Arseneau J, et al. Estrogen and progesterone receptor determination in the papillary cystic neoplasm of the pancreas. With immunohistochemical and ultrastructural observations. Cancer 1987, 60:1604–1611.
79. Kosmahl M, Pauser U, Peters K, et al. Cystic neoplasms of the pancreas and tumor-like lesions with cystic features: a review of 418 cases and a classification proposal. Virchows Arch 2004, 445:168–178.
80. Othman M, Basturk O, Groisman G, et al. Squamoid cyst of pancreatic ducts: a distinct type of cystic lesion in the pancreas. Am J Surg Pathol 2007, 31:291–297.
81. Adsay NV, Hasteh F, Cheng JD, et al. Lymphoepithelial cysts of the pancreas: a report of 12 cases and a review of the literature. Mod Pathol 2002, 15:492–501.
82. Paal E, Thompson LD, Heffess CS. A clinicopathologic and immunohistochemical study of ten pancreatic lymphangiomas and a review of the literature. Cancer 1998, 82:2150–2158.
83. Kloppel G, Maillet B. Chronic pancreatitis: evolution of the disease. Hepatogastroenterology 1991, 38:408–412.
84. Klimstra DS, Adsay NV. Lymphoplasmacytic sclerosing (autoimmune) pancreatitis. Semin Diagn Pathol 2004, 21:237–246.
85. Suriawanata A, Cubukcu-Dimopula O, Weber S, et al. Histopathology of lymphoplasmacytic sclerosing pancreatitis. Mod Pathol 2002, 15:294A.
86. Stolte M, Weiss W, Volkholz H, et al. A special form of segmental pancreatitis: "groove pancreatitis". Hepatogastroenterology 1982, 29:198–208.
87. Cohn JA, Neoptolemos JP, Feng J, et al. Increased risk of idiopathic chronic pancreatitis in cystic fibrosis carriers. Hum Mutat 2005, 26:303–307.
88. Procacci C, Graziani R, Zamboni G, et al. Cystic dystrophy of the duodenal wall: radiologic findings. Radiology 1997, 205:741–747.
89. Pauser U, Kosmahl M, Sipos B, et al. (Mesenchymal tumors of the pancreas. Surprising, but not uncommon). Pathologe 2005, 26:52–58.
90. Handra-Luca A, Terris B, Couvelard A, et al. Adenomyoma and adenomyomatous hyperplasia of the Vaterian system: clinical, pathological, and new immunohistochemical features of 13 cases. Mod Pathol 2003, 16(6):530–536.
91. Khanani F, Kilinc N, Nassar H, et al. Mesenchymal lesions involving the pancreas. Modern Pathology 2003, 16(1):279A.
92. Lüttges J, Pierre E, Zamboni G, et al. Malignant non-epithelial tumors of the pancreas. Pathologie 1997, 18(3):233–237.
93. Bismar TA, Basturk O, Gerald WL, et al. Desmoplastic small cell tumor in the pancreas. Am J Surg Pathol 2004, 28:808–812.
94. Ferrozzi F, Bova D, Campodonico F, et al. Pancreatic metastases: CT assessment. Eur Radiol 1997, 7:241–245.
95. Opocher E, Galeotti F, Spina GP, et al. (Diagnosis of secondary tumors of the pancreas. Analysis of 13 cases). Minerva Med 1982, 73:577–581.
96. Roland CF, van Heerden JA. Nonpancreatic primary tumors with metastasis to the pancreas. Surg Gynecol Obstet 1989, 168:345–347.

Chapter 2
Molecular Genetics of Pancreatic Cancer

Eric S. Calhoun and Scott E. Kern

1 Introduction

In cancer, genome stability is compromised. Ductal adenocarcinoma of the pancreas is no exception. Considerable progress in the identification and characterization of somatic and/or germline genetic alterations has provided the mechanistic foundations of this genetically complex disease. Numerous alterations, including chromosomal copy-number gains, amplifications and homozygous deletions, loss of heterozygosity (LOH) with and without copy number reduction, and balanced and unbalanced structural re-arrangements, are commonly observed (1–4). Gross chromosomal changes are often complemented by smaller, more subtle alterations affecting the open reading frames of proto-oncogenes, tumor suppressors, and genome caretaker genes (5–8). Continued evaluation of these and additional yet-unidentified genetic alterations should translate into rational diagnostic and treatment strategies.

This chapter describes the spectrum and frequency of genetic alterations observed in ductal adenocarcinomas of the pancreas, as organized by the underlying presence of two, largely mutually exclusive, types of genome instability: chromosomal instability (CIN) and microsatellite instability (MIN). This distinction is justified, as each tumor type exhibits unique histologic and molecular characteristics (9).

2 Chromosomal Instability

The vast majority of pancreatic cancers (97%) have CIN, characterized by numerous chromosomal copy-number gains and losses, amplifications and homozygous deletions, translocations, and inversions. At first glance, these alterations appear random. Careful examination of overlapping genomic alterations has, however, revealed the recurrent targeting of select genes for disruption. The spectrum of altered genes, as well as the types of alterations, makes each pancreatic tumor rather distinctive.

A.M. Lowy et al. (eds.), *Pancreatic Cancer*.
doi: 10.1007/978-0-387-69252-4, © Springer Science + Business Media, LLC 2008

2.1   Required Genetic Mutations

Disruptions of at least two genes in pancreatic cancer are nearly universal. The first, K-ras (12p12.1), is an oncogene. A GTP-binding and hydrolyzing enzyme, the K-ras protein functions as a second messenger in growth factor receptor signaling pathways that stimulate the transition through the G1 phase of the cell division cycle. This activity is dependent upon bound GTP, remaining active as long as the nucleotide remains unhydrolyzed. Somatic mutations affecting the GTP-binding pocket can disrupt the ability of K-ras to hydrolyze GTP, rendering the protein constitutively active. Mutations of the codons Gly12, Gly13, or Gln61 are commonly associated with constitutively active K-ras, although recurrent alterations in Ala146 in colorectal cancers suggest additional hotspots may exist (*10, 11*).

Ninety-five percent of pancreatic cancers harbor activating mutations in K-ras, representing the highest fraction of any tumor type (*12, 13*). The COSMIC (Catalogue of Somatic Mutations In Cancer) database lists the most common alteration in pancreatic cancer as the Gly12Asp substitution, accounting for ~50% of all pancreatic cancer cases, whereas total alterations in Gly12 account for ~99% of all mutations (*14*). The paucity of Gly13 mutations is unusual in that significantly higher frequencies are noted in other cancers (e.g., colorectal cancer: Gly13Asp, 15.8%; total Gly13 mutations, 17.3%). Conversely, Gly12Arg substitutions are commonly observed in pancreatic cancer (11.6%), whereas they occur infrequently in colorectal cases (1.0%). The underlying reasons for these tumor-specific mutational preferences are unknown.

The second (virtually required) disruption in pancreatic cancer involves CDKN2A (p16, 9p21.3), one of the most frequently altered genes in cancer. A classical tumor-suppressor, p16 regulates cell cycle progression by inhibiting cyclinD-CDK4/6, the kinase complex responsible for initiating the G1/S phase transition. Inherited alterations in p16 cause FAMMM (familial atypical multiple mole melanoma), a syndrome characterized by numerous dysplastic nevi having atypical shape, color and/or size, a propensity for developing melanoma and a distinct risk of pancreatic cancer (nearly a 20-fold increased risk) (*15–18*).

The incidence of p16 alterations in sporadic pancreatic cancer is dramatic, with inactivation of this gene occurring in 98% of cases. Unlike K-ras activation, however, gene disruption (i.e., inactivation) occurs through multiple mechanisms including nearly half by homozygous deletion, more than a third by intragenic mutations with LOH, and the remainder by epigenetic promoter silencing (*19, 20*).

2.2   Frequently Mutated Genes

Genes mutated at a frequency >25% suggest they provide a supportive (i.e., selective advantage) role in the development of cancer. The implication that they are not required, however, suggests that other mutations might occasionally substitute for the more common alterations in these genes. Three examples of genes in this category include SMAD4 (18q21.1), TP53 (p53, 17p13.1), and NCOA3 (AIB1, 20q12), and for each there is limited evidence of substitute gene targets (*21, 22*).

Inactivation of SMAD4 occurs in approximately 45% (30% by homozygous deletion) of pancreatic cancers, but less frequently in other cancer types (*23–26*). Functional characterization has shown that the SMAD4 tumor-suppressor protein is TGFβ-responsive, translocating to the nucleus (with Smads 2 and 3) after TGFβ or activin receptor stimulation to activate expression of genes mediating growth inhibition. Missense mutations in this gene impair protein stability, among other functional defects (*27–29*).

Another frequently mutated gene in pancreatic cancer, and one of the most frequently altered genes in all cancer types, is TP53 (p53, 17p13.1). The tumor-suppressive properties of p53 lie in its ability to transcriptionally activate target genes in response to cellular stresses such as DNA damage. TP53 blocks G1/S and G2/M transitions by increasing p21WAF1/CIP1 and SFN (14-3-3 sigma) expression, and induces programmed cell death in experimental settings (*30–32*). Inactivating mutations occur in 70% of pancreatic tumors, with most affecting the ability of the protein to bind to DNA and activate gene transcription (*33, 34*). Unlike other tumor suppressors, however, homozygous deletions affecting p53 occur very rarely; most mutations are missense mutations. The reason for this remains unknown, but the gene dense region at 17p13.1 may inhibit the formation of homozygous deletions as they would provide a selective disadvantage to cells experiencing the loss of multiple genes.

NCOA3 (AIB1, 20q12) enhances the transcriptional activity of a number of steroid nuclear receptors and is the rate limiting step in estrogen-mediated growth signaling. High-level amplification of this gene has been reported in ~10% of breast cancer tissues and four of nine pancreatic cancer cell lines (*35, 36*). In archival tissues, copy-number gains were observed in >37% of pancreatic cancers (*37*). The observance of such high frequencies of AIB1 gains and amplifications in pancreatic cancer was surprising as pancreatic ductal tissues are not normally controlled by endocrine stimulation. Some of these authors suggest that such an amplification "may indicate that estrogen receptor mediated transcriptional activation confers a growth advantage" to these cells. The clinical relevance of these findings remain to be determined, however, as pancreatic cancers have not yet been shown to have hormone dependence.

2.3   Low-Frequency Mutations

Despite very little variation in clinical outcome, pancreatic tumors have heterogeneous mutational backgrounds that give each tumor a unique molecular signature. Each genetic mutation, occurring in <25% of tumors, may define a distinct subclass of pancreatic tumors with unique molecular properties. Rational treatment strategies attempt to exploit these tumor-specific properties.

2.3.1   Genes Involved in the G1/S Cell Cycle Checkpoint

Many mutations in pancreatic cancer are found in genes whose functions are linked to the control of the cell cycle. The retinoblastoma protein, RB1 (pRb, 13q14.2), acts as the central control point for regulating cell cycle commitment (*38, 39*). When cells are not stimulated to divide by growth factors, pRb inhibits E2F transcriptional activity, thereby restricting progression into S-phase. Upon growth factor stimulation, pRb releases E2F, allowing for the expression of S-phase critical genes. Many different tumors commonly inactivate pRb, however, only rare mutations (<6%) are reported in pancreatic cancer (*40*).

The inactivation of pRb is accomplished by a complex consisting of a regulatory cyclin and a kinase. One member of this complex is CCND1 (Cyclin D1, 11q13.3), working with either cyclin-dependent kinase 4 or 6 to phosphorylate and inactivate pRb. Infrequent Cyclin D1 amplification is reported for several tumor types (*41–43*), such as 2.5% of head and neck squamous cell carcinomas and 0.5–1.5% of colorectal cancers (>10 gene copies), however, the extent of Cyclin D1 amplification is less clear for pancreatic cancer. Using Southern analysis, Gansauge et al. reported 25% (7/28) of pancreatic cancers to have Cyclin D1 amplification (*44*). Each case was additionally reported to have increased expression of Cyclin D1 protein.

Such a high frequency of amplification is questioned by Schutte et al., who found no evidence of amplification in 26 pancreatic cancers (at approximate sensitivity six copies or greater) or Huang et al. (greater than fivefold) in 20 pancreatic cancers and 18 cell lines (*20, 40*). Using SNP arrays, Calhoun et al. found only a single case (*n* = 24) of Cyclin D1 amplification (*2*). After eliminating overlapping samples analyzed by the studies of Schutte et al. and Calhoun et al., only 2.4% (1/42) had Cyclin D1 amplification. The discrepancies in frequencies between these studies are not readily explained.

Another cyclin, CCNE1 (Cyclin E1, 19q12), combines with Cdk2 to phosphorylate several substrates important for G1/S transition and DNA replicative activities (*45–48*). Representing a "point of no return," cells expressing Cyclin E1 become committed to undergoing DNA replication and subsequently mitosis (*49*).

Cyclin E1 was found to be amplified in various tissues including colon adenocarcinoma (1.2%), metastatic, ductal carcinoma of the breast (2.6%), serous carcinoma of the ovary (8%), and adenocarcinoma of the stomach (13.9%) (*50*). In total, 23 instances (1.8%) of Cyclin E1 amplification were reported in various types of tumors. Using immunohistochemistry, Cyclin E1 was found to be overexpressed in ~6% of pancreatic cancers, with gene amplification (two separate cell lines) and mutational inactivation of FBXW7 (the E3 ubiquitin ligase responsible for Cyclin E1 degradation) identified as possible mechanisms for the increased expression (*51*).

2.3.2   Genes Involved in Double-Strand–DNA Break Repair

An additional class of genes mutated in pancreatic cancer is involved in the repair of DNA interstrand crosslinks and double-strand breaks. Collectively, genes involved in

DNA repair are known as genome-maintenance genes or "caretakers" with a primary role in maintaining the sequence integrity of the genome (8, 52). Germline inheritance of an inactive allele often leads to a predisposition to cancer.

BRCA2 (FANCD1, 13q12.3), which participates with Rad51 and BRCA1 to prevent and/or repair DNA double-strand breaks through homologous recombination, is one example of this type of gene (53, 54). Inherited, inactive alleles (such as the common 6174delT truncating mutation) confer an increased risk for developing ovarian and breast cancers as well as a 3.5- to 20-fold increased risk of developing pancreatic cancer (55).

The mutational frequency of BRCA2 was investigated by Goggins et al. BRCA2 was homozygously inactivated in 7% (3/41) of unselected pancreatic cancers (56). All mutations were derived from germline inheritance: Two samples were confirmed with a matched normal tissue, whereas the third, a 6174delT Ashkenazi Jewish founder mutation, was assumed to be inherited. Inactivation of BRCA2 was found to occur late in precursor lesions of the pancreas (57). Only one case of sporadic pancreatic cancer due to the somatic inactivation of both BRCA2 alleles in pancreatic cancer is yet reported (58).

In 2002, Howlett et al. determined that the Fanconi anemia (FA) complementation-group D1 defect was due to biallelic, truncating mutations in BRCA2 (59). This finding linked Brca2 and other FA proteins into a common DNA damage-responsive pathway. Most FA proteins (Fanc A, B, C, E, F, G, L and M) bind to form a heteromeric, E3 ubiquitin ligase complex which monoubiquitinates and activates FANCD2. After translocating to the nucleus, mUb-Fancd2 colocalizes with Brca1, Brca2, and Rad51 to focal areas of DNA damage during S-phase (59, 60).

Due to the known involvement of BRCA2, other FA genes were subsequently examined for somatic alterations in pancreatic cancer. These studies were largely negative, except for occasional mutations found in FANCC (9q22.3) and FANCG (9p13), arising somatically as well as through germline inheritance (61, 62).

2.3.3 Miscellaneous Gene Mutations

An eclectic set of mutations has been identified in pancreatic cancer. However, the functions of most genes cannot be easily cataloged in classical tumor-promoting pathways (i.e., cell cycle G1/S regulation, maintenance of genome integrity, apoptosis). In some instances, a gene's cellular function may not yet be assigned; therefore, the impact of its alteration in cancer is not known. Despite our lack of understanding, the repeated presence of clonal alterations arising during carcinogenesis suggests that these genes may play an important role in the development of individual cancers. Examples are discussed briefly in the following.

Phosphorylated residues on ERBB2 (HER-2/NEU, 17q11.2-12) serve as docking sites for a number of signal transducers that initiate signaling cascades leading to cell proliferation, differentiation, migration, adhesion, resistance to apoptosis, among other effects (63, 64). Overexpression of ERBB2 in pancreatic cancer was first reported by Hall et al. (65), verified by others (66–69), and associated with amplification in varying degrees (67, 70, 71).

AKT2 (19q13.1-13.2) encodes a serine/threonine protein kinase identified as a homolog of the v-akt oncogene and is activated, along with AKT1, in response to the binding of growth factors such PDGF (72–75). The functional differences between AKT1 and AKT2 activation in cellular signaling pathways important to pancreatic cancer remain to be determined, however. AKT2 is amplified in pancreatic cancer at a frequency of 11% (3/28) to 20% (7/35), suggesting this gene may indeed be important in pancreatic cancer development (76, 77).

The MYB (c-myb, 6q23-24) oncogene has been shown to induce the expression of many genes that regulate proliferation, differentiation, and apoptosis; however, its precise role in cancer remains obscure as normal tissues often express this protein at high levels (78). Examples of MYB amplification have been reported in 29% (5/17) of hereditary BRCA1 breast cancer samples, in 2% (2/100) of sporadic breast cancers as well as in 4–6% of pancreatic cancer cell lines and primary tissues (2, 79, 80).

DCC (deleted in colorectal carcinoma, 18q21.1-21.2) was suggested to play a role as a candidate tumor suppressor gene due to its rare homozygous deletion in colorectal carcinomas and 6% (7/115) of pancreatic carcinomas (25, 81, 82). The common disruption of a neighboring tumor suppressor (SMAD4) and the paucity of intragenic mutations have shed doubt, however, on the role this gene plays in pancreatic cancer.

Inherited mutations in the serine/threonine protein kinase, STK11 (LKB1, 19p13.3), cause Peutz-Jeghers syndrome (83). This rare, autosomal dominant disorder is characterized by hamartomatous polyps of the intestine (predominately in the small intestine), ink-black, spotty pigmentation surrounding the lips, and a dramatically elevated risk of developing many types of cancer. Between the ages of 15 and 64, affected individuals have a 93% cumulative incidence of cancer with a 36% specific incidence of pancreatic cancer (84). The rate of sporadic inactivation of STK11 in pancreatic cancer was reported at 5% (85).

Intragenic mutations and homozygous deletions in MAP2K4 (MKK4, 17p11.2) occur in up to 4% of pancreatic cancers (86–88). This stress-activated protein kinase-cascade pathway member demonstrates both growth control and apoptotic functions. Paradoxically, however, MKK4 has been shown to play a metastasis-suppressing role in an experimental somatic-cell gene knockout model, implying the background mutational environment and other variables may influence the development of a MKK4-null state in pancreatic cancer (89).

The EGFR (7p12) mutation delE746-A750, previously characterized as an activating EGFR mutation in non-small cell lung cancer, was found to occur in 3.6% (2/55) of pancreatic cancers (90). An earlier study failed to find mutations in the kinase domain (exons 18–24) in 92 pancreatic cancer xenografts and nine pancreatic cancer cell lines (91). The involvement of EGFR mutations in pancreatic cancer appears infrequent, but due to the clinical sensitivity of this specific mutation to small molecule inhibitors, further evaluation of this gene's involvement in pancreatic cancer may be warranted (92).

Additional genes, with mutations involving only one or two cases, are reported and listed in Table 2.1. Along with those discussed above, these genes are not frequent players in the development of pancreatic cancer but may be important in the

Table 2.1 Gene mutational frequencies in pancreatic cancer

	Gene	Sporadic	References
CIN	K-ras	95%	*12, 13*
	CDKN2A	98%[a]	*15, 19, 20*
	TP53	70%	*33*
	SMAD4	45%	*23, 101*
	NCOA3	37–44%	*36, 37*
	RB1	<6%[b]	*40*
	ERBB2	<27%	*67, 70, 71*
	AKT2	11–20%	*76, 77*
	CCNE1	<6%[b]	*2*
	DCC	6%	*25, 82*
	STK11	5%	*85*
	MYB	4–6%	*2, 80*
	MAP2K4	2–4%	*87, 88, 101*
	EGFR	0–4%	*90, 91*
	CCND1	0–25%	*2, 20, 40*
	ACVR1B	2%	*101, 102*
	BRCA2	7%[c]	*56, 58*
	FANCC	2%	*61, 62*
	FANCG	1%	*61, 62*
	GUCY2F	3%	*103*
	NTRK3	2%	*103*
	FBXW7	1%	*2*
	ALK5	1%	*21*
	TGFBR2	1%	*21*
MIN	MLH1	100%	*104*
	TGFBR2	100%	*21*
	ACVR2A	100%	*100*
	BRAF	66%	*2*

[a]14% inactivated through promoter methylation. [b]Maximum estimate based upon immunohistochemistry data. [c]Nearly all BRCA2 mutations are inherited, even in unselected cases.

development of individual tumors. The ability to characterize the entire background mutational signature of individual tumors will help to characterize the role each of these plays in pancreatic cancer.

3 Microsatellite Instability

MIN tumors (~3% of pancreatic neoplasms) classically have near-diploid genomes exhibiting very few aberrant chromosomes or altered chromosome ploidy. Instead, MIN tumors have replication errors in primary sequences, especially simple repetitive sequences known as microsatellites (*93*). Mutations or transcriptional silencing in either MSH2 (2p21), MLH1 (3p22.3), or MSH6 (2p16) have been shown to cause this "replication error-positive" phenotype, with the highest prevalence occurring in colorectal cancers (*94–98*). Defects in the MSH2 (31%) and MLH1 (33%) are responsible for the majority of HNPCC cases with mismatch repair gene deficiencies (*99*).

Due to the underlying type of genomic instability, frequent insertions and/or deletions in large mononucleotide tracts (usually 8 or more in length) contained within gene coding sequences are often seen. TGFBR2 (3p24.1) and ACVR2A (2q22.3-23.1) are two such genes that were found to be mutated in all MSI pancreatic tumors examined (3/3) (*21, 100*).

Providing further evidence that MSI and CIN tumors evolve through distinct mechanisms, MSI pancreatic tumors are K-ras wild-type (*51*). Activating mutations in BRAF (7q34, a serine/threonine kinase immediately downstream of K-ras signaling) occur in 33% (3/9) of K-ras wild-type tumors and may complement the lack of K-ras mutations. Intriguingly, these mutations (V599E) were not located within a mononucleotide track, even though two of the samples were known to have microsatellite instability. Exactly why BRAF mutations (versus more traditional K-ras alterations) are selected for in this context remains unknown. Examination of K-ras-mutant tumors failed to identify co-existent BRAF mutations, suggesting they may be mutually exclusive alterations in tumors.

4   Negative Observations in Pancreatic Cancer

Negative Observations in Genetic Oncology (www.path.jhu.edu/NOGO) and the Catalogue Of Somatic Mutations In Cancer (www.sanger.ac.uk/genetics/CGP/cosmic) websites detail negative mutational data that can be used by researchers to identify genes that have (or have not) already been investigated for somatic alterations in specific tissues. Such efforts may help maximize the efficiency of mutation detection screens by decreasing the time and cost spent on redundant investigations.

5   Future Perspectives

Cancers of the pancreas, as well as most other types of neoplasms, are very complex genetically. The ability to characterize all of the genetic alterations in an individual tumor remains theoretically possible, but in reality, unattainable due to the high economic and time commitment costs required using current technologies. Significant strides have been made in chip-based technologies that now permit highly detailed maps of gains and losses across an entire genome to be made, including the identification of novel amplifications and homozygous deletions previously missed due to technical resolution. Such studies now permit a more focused and efficient approach for identifying and characterizing the frequencies of mutational targets in larger panels of pancreatic tumors. Without a single-nucleotide-level resolution, however, arrays will ultimately prove inadequate to describe the mutational background signature of individual tumors. Whole-genome sequencing may one day help catalogue the entire spectrum and characteristics of somatic and germline alterations and enable investigators to fully understand the genetic aspects of cancer.

References

1. Mitelman F, Mertens F, Johansson B. Prevalence estimates of recurrent balanced cytogenetic aberrations and gene fusions in unselected patients with neoplastic disorders. Genes Chromosomes Cancer 2005, 43:350–366.
2. Calhoun ES, Hucl T, Gallmeier E, et al. Identifying allelic loss and homozygous deletions in pancreatic cancer without matched normals using high-density single-nucleotide polymorphism arrays. Cancer Res 2006, 66:7920–7928.
3. Karhu R, Mahlamaki E, Kallioniemi A. Pancreatic adenocarcinoma—genetic portrait from chromosomes to microarrays. Genes Chromosomes Cancer 2006, 45:721–730.
4. Hahn SA, Kern SE. Molecular genetics of exocrine pancreatic neoplasms. Surg Clin North Am 1995, 75:857–869.
5. Bishop JM. Molecular themes in oncogenesis. Cell 1991, 64:235–248.
6. Hunter T. Cooperation between oncogenes. Cell 1991, 64:249–270.
7. Weinberg RA. Tumor suppressor genes. Science 1991, 254:1138–1146.
8. Kinzler KW, Vogelstein B. Cancer-susceptibility genes. Gatekeepers and caretakers. Nature 1997, 386:761, 763.
9. Yamamoto H, Itoh F, Nakamura H, et al. Genetic and clinical features of human pancreatic ductal adenocarcinomas with widespread microsatellite instability. Cancer Res 2001, 61:3139–3144.
10. Ellis CA, Clark G. The importance of being K-Ras. Cell Signal 2000, 12:425–434.
11. Edkins S, O'Meara S, Parker A, et al. Recurrent KRAS Codon 146 Mutations in Human Colorectal Cancer. Cancer Biol Ther 2006, 5:928–932.
12. Smit VT, Boot AJ, Smits AM, et al. KRAS codon 12 mutations occur very frequently in pancreatic adenocarcinomas. Nucleic Acids Res 1988, 16:7773–7782.
13. Almoguera C, Shibata D, Forrester K, et al. Most human carcinomas of the exocrine pancreas contain mutant c-K-ras genes. Cell 1988, 53:549–554.
14. Bamford S, Dawson E, Forbes S, et al. The COSMIC (Catalogue of Somatic Mutations in Cancer) database and website. Br J Cancer 2004, 91:355–358.
15. Czajkowski R, Placek W, Drewa G, et al. FAMMM syndrome: pathogenesis and management. Dermatol Surg 2004, 30:291–296.
16. Hussussian CJ, Struewing JP, Goldstein AM, et al. Germline p16 mutations in familial melanoma. Nat Genet 1994, 8:15–21.
17. Kamb A, Shattuck-Eidens D, Eeles R, et al. Analysis of the p16 gene (CDKN2) as a candidate for the chromosome 9p melanoma susceptibility locus. Nat Genet 1994, 8:23–26.
18. Vasen HF, Gruis NA, Frants RR, et al. Risk of developing pancreatic cancer in families with familial atypical multiple mole melanoma associated with a specific 19 deletion of p16 (p16-Leiden). Int J Cancer 2000, 87:809–811.
19. Caldas C, Hahn SA, da Costa LT, et al. Frequent somatic mutations and homozygous deletions of the p16 (MTS1) gene in pancreatic adenocarcinoma. Nat Genet 1994, 8:27–32.
20. Schutte M, Hruban RH, Geradts J, et al. Abrogation of the Rb/p16 tumor-suppressive pathway in virtually all pancreatic carcinomas. Cancer Res 1997, 57:3126–130.
21. Goggins M, Shekher M, Turnacioglu K, et al. Genetic alterations of the transforming growth factor beta receptor genes in pancreatic and biliary adenocarcinomas. Cancer Res 1998, 58:5329–5332.

22. Kern SE, Hruban RH, Hidalgo M, et al. An introduction to pancreatic adenocarcinoma genetics, pathology and therapy. Cancer Biol Ther 2002, 1:607–613.
23. Hahn SA, Schutte M, Hoque AT, et al. DPC4, a candidate tumor suppressor gene at human chromosome 18q21.1. Science 1996, 271:350–353.
24. Schutte M, Hruban RH, Hedrick L, et al. DPC4 gene in various tumor types. Cancer Res 1996, 56:2527–2530.
25. Thiagalingam S, Lengauer C, Leach FS, et al. Evaluation of candidate tumour suppressor genes on chromosome 18 in colorectal cancers. Nat Genet 1996, 13:343–346.
26. Miyaki M, Kuroki T. Role of Smad4 (DPC4) inactivation in human cancer. Biochem Biophys Res Commun 2003, 306:799–804.
27. Iacobuzio-Donahue CA, Song J, Parmiagiani G, et al. Missense mutations of MADH4: characterization of the mutational hot spot and functional consequences in human tumors. Clin Cancer Res 2004, 10:1597–1604.
28. De Bosscher K, Hill CS, Nicolas FJ. Molecular and functional consequences of Smad4 C-terminal missense mutations in colorectal tumour cells. Biochem J 2004, 379:209–216.
29. Dai JL, Turnacioglu KK, Schutte M, et al. Dpc4 transcriptional activation and dysfunction in cancer cells. Cancer Res 1998, 58:4592–4597.
30. Bates S, Ryan KM, Phillips AC, et al. Cell cycle arrest and DNA endoreduplication following p21Waf1/Cip1 expression. Oncogene 1998, 17:1691–1703.
31. Chan TA, Hermeking H, Lengauer C, et al. 14-3-3Sigma is required to prevent mitotic catastrophe after DNA damage. Nature 1999, 401:616–620.
32. Yonish-Rouach E, Resnitzky D, Lotem J, et al. Wild-type p53 induces apoptosis of myeloid leukaemic cells that is inhibited by interleukin-6. Nature 1991, 352:345–347.
33. Redston MS, Caldas C, Seymour AB, et al. p53 mutations in pancreatic carcinoma and evidence of common involvement of homocopolymer tracts in DNA microdeletions. Cancer Res 1994, 54:3025–3033.
34. Kern SE, Pietenpol JA, Thiagalingam S, et al. Oncogenic forms of p53 inhibit p53-regulated gene expression. Science 1992, 256:827–830.
35. Anzick SL, Kononen J, Walker RL, et al. AIB1, a steroid receptor coactivator amplified in breast and ovarian cancer. Science 1997, 277:965–968.
36. Ghadimi BM, Schrock E, Walker RL, et al. Specific chromosomal aberrations and amplification of the AIB1 nuclear receptor coactivator gene in pancreatic carcinomas. Am J Pathol 1999, 154:525–536.
37. Henke RT, Haddad BR, Kim SE, et al. Overexpression of the nuclear receptor coactivator AIB1 (SRC-3) during progression of pancreatic adenocarcinoma. Clin Cancer Res 2004, 10:6134–6142.
38. Felsani A, Mileo AM, Paggi MG. Retinoblastoma family proteins as key targets of the small DNA virus oncoproteins. Oncogene 2006, 25:5277–5285.
39. Macaluso M, Montanari M, Giordano A. Rb family proteins as modulators of gene expression and new aspects regarding the interaction with chromatin remodeling enzymes. Oncogene 2006, 25:5263–5267.
40. Huang L, Lang D, Geradts J, et al. Molecular and immunochemical analyses of RB1 and cyclin D1 in human ductal pancreatic carcinomas and cell lines. Mol Carcinog 1996, 15:85–95.
41. Sabbir MG, Dasgupta S, Roy A, et al. Genetic alterations (amplification and rearrangement) of D-type cyclins loci in head and neck squamous cell carcinoma of Indian patients: prognostic significance and clinical implications. Diagn Mol Pathol 2006, 15:7–16.
42. Myo K, Uzawa N, Miyamoto R, et al. Cyclin D1 gene numerical aberration is a predictive marker for occult cervical lymph node metastasis in TNM Stage I and II squamous cell carcinoma of the oral cavity. Cancer 2005, 104:2709–2716.
43. Al-Kuraya K, Novotny H, Bavi PP, et al. HER2, TOP2A, CCND1, EGFR, and C-MYC oncogene amplification in colorectal cancer. J Clin Pathol 2006.
44. Gansauge S, Gansauge F, Ramadani M, et al. Overexpression of cyclin D1 in human pancreatic carcinoma is associated with poor prognosis. Cancer Res 1997, 57:1634–1637.

45. Ma T, Van Tine BA, Wei Y, et al. Cell cycle-regulated phosphorylation of p220(NPAT) by cyclin E/Cdk2 in Cajal bodies promotes histone gene transcription. Genes Dev 2000, 14:2298–2313.
46. Zhao J, Kennedy BK, Lawrence BD, et al. NPAT links cyclin E-Cdk2 to the regulation of replication-dependent histone gene transcription. Genes Dev 2000, 14:2283–2297.
47. Okuda M, Horn HF, Tarapore P, et al. Nucleophosmin/B23 is a target of CDK2/cyclin E in centrosome duplication. Cell 2000, 103:127–140.
48. Tokuyama Y, Horn HF, Kawamura K, et al. Specific phosphorylation of nucleophosmin on Thr(199) by cyclin-dependent kinase 2-cyclin E and its role in centrosome duplication. J Biol Chem 2001, 276:21529–21537.
49. Moroy T, Geisen C. Cyclin E. Int J Biochem Cell Biol 2004, 36:1424–1439.
50. Schraml P, Bucher C, Bissig H, et al. Cyclin E overexpression and amplification in human tumours. J Pathol 2003, 200:375–382.
51. Calhoun ES, Jones JB, Ashfaq R, et al. BRAF and FBXW7 (CDC4, FBW7, AGO, SEL10) mutations in distinct subsets of pancreatic cancer: potential therapeutic targets. Am J Pathol 2003, 163:1255–1260.
52. Vogelstein B, Kinzler KW. Cancer genes and the pathways they control. Nat Med 2004, 10:789–799.
53. Chen J, Silver DP, Walpita D, et al. Stable interaction between the products of the BRCA1 and BRCA2 tumor suppressor genes in mitotic and meiotic cells. Mol Cell 1998, 2:317–328.
54. Xia F, Taghian DG, DeFrank JS, et al. Deficiency of human BRCA2 leads to impaired homologous recombination but maintains normal nonhomologous end joining. Proc Natl Acad Sci U S A 2001, 98:8644–8649.
55. Jaffee EM, Hruban RH, Canto M, et al. Focus on pancreas cancer. Cancer Cell 2002, 2:25–28.
56. Goggins M, Schutte M, Lu J, et al. Germline BRCA2 gene mutations in patients with apparently sporadic pancreatic carcinomas. Cancer Res 1996, 56:5360–5364.
57. Goggins M, Hruban RH, Kern SE. BRCA2 is inactivated late in the development of pancreatic intraepithelial neoplasia: evidence and implications. Am J Pathol 2000, 156:1767–1771.
58. Schutte M, da Costa LT, Hahn SA, et al. Identification by representational difference analysis of a homozygous deletion in pancreatic carcinoma that lies within the BRCA2 region. Proc Natl Acad Sci U S A 1995, 92:5950–5954.
59. Howlett NG, Taniguchi T, Olson S, et al. Biallelic inactivation of BRCA2 in Fanconi anemia. Science 2002, 297:606–609.
60. Garcia-Higuera I, Taniguchi T, Ganesan S, et al. Interaction of the Fanconi anemia proteins and BRCA1 in a common pathway. Mol Cell 2001, 7:249–262.
61. van der Heijden MS, Yeo CJ, Hruban RH, et al. Fanconi anemia gene mutations in young-onset pancreatic cancer. Cancer Res 2003, 63:2585–2588.
62. Couch FJ, Johnson MR, Rabe K, et al. Germ line Fanconi anemia complementation group C mutations and pancreatic cancer. Cancer Res 2005, 65:383–386.
63. Olayioye MA, Neve RM, Lane HA, et al. The ErbB signaling network: receptor heterodimerization in development and cancer. Embo J 2000, 19:3159–3167.
64. Yarden Y, Sliwkowski MX. Untangling the ErbB signalling network. Nat Rev Mol Cell Biol 2001, 2:127–137.
65. Hall PA, Hughes CM, Staddon SL, et al. The c-erb B-2 proto-oncogene in human pancreatic cancer. J Pathol 1990, 161:195–200.
66. Williams TM, Weiner DB, Greene MI, et al. Expression of c-erbB-2 in human pancreatic adenocarcinomas. Pathobiology 1991, 59:46–52.
67. Yamanaka Y, Friess H, Kobrin MS, et al. Overexpression of HER2/neu oncogene in human pancreatic carcinoma. Hum Pathol 1993, 24:1127–1134.
68. Lei S, Appert HE, Nakata B, et al. Overexpression of HER2/neu oncogene in pancreatic cancer correlates with shortened survival. Int J Pancreatol 1995, 17:15–21.

69. Day JD, Digiuseppe JA, Yeo C, et al. Immunohistochemical evaluation of HER-2/neu expression in pancreatic adenocarcinoma and pancreatic intraepithelial neoplasms. Hum Pathol 1996, 27:119–124.
70. Safran H, Steinhoff M, Mangray S, et al. Overexpression of the HER-2/neu oncogene in pancreatic adenocarcinoma. Am J Clin Oncol 2001, 24:496–499.
71. Hermanova M, Lukas Z, Nenutil R, et al. Amplification and overexpression of HER-2/neu in invasive ductal carcinomas of the pancreas and pancreatic intraepithelial neoplasms and the relationship to the expression of p21(WAF1/CIP1). Neoplasma 2004, 51:77–83.
72. Franke TF, Yang SI, Chan TO, et al. The protein kinase encoded by the Akt proto-oncogene is a target of the PDGF-activated phosphatidylinositol 3-kinase. Cell 1995, 81:727–736.
73. Staal SP. Molecular cloning of the akt oncogene and its human homologues AKT1 and AKT2: amplification of AKT1 in a primary human gastric adenocarcinoma. Proc Natl Acad Sci U S A 1987, 84:5034–5037.
74. Cheng JQ, Godwin AK, Bellacosa A, et al. AKT2, a putative oncogene encoding a member of a subfamily of protein-serine/threonine kinases, is amplified in human ovarian carcinomas. Proc Natl Acad Sci U S A 1992, 89:9267–9271.
75. Bellacosa A, Testa JR, Staal SP, et al. A retroviral oncogene, akt, encoding a serine-threonine kinase containing an SH2-like region. Science 1991, 254:274–277.
76. Cheng JQ, Ruggeri B, Klein WM, et al. Amplification of AKT2 in human pancreatic cells and inhibition of AKT2 expression and tumorigenicity by antisense RNA. Proc Natl Acad Sci U S A 1996, 93:3636–3641.
77. Ruggeri BA, Huang L, Wood M, et al. Amplification and overexpression of the AKT2 oncogene in a subset of human pancreatic ductal adenocarcinomas. Mol Carcinog 1998, 21:81–86.
78. Lutwyche JK, Keough RA, Hunter J, et al. DNA binding-independent transcriptional activation of the vascular endothelial growth factor gene (VEGF) by the Myb oncoprotein. Biochem Biophys Res Commun 2006, 344:1300–1307.
79. Kauraniemi P, Hedenfalk I, Persson K, et al. MYB oncogene amplification in hereditary BRCA1 breast cancer. Cancer Res 2000, 60:5323–5328.
80. Wallrapp C, Muller-Pillasch F, Solinas-Toldo S, et al. Characterization of a high copy number amplification at 6q24 in pancreatic cancer identifies c-myb as a candidate oncogene. Cancer Res 1997, 57:3135–3139.
81. Fearon ER, Cho KR, Nigro JM, et al. Identification of a chromosome 18q gene that is altered in colorectal cancers. Science 1990, 247:49–56.
82. Hilgers W, Song JJ, Haye M, et al. Homozygous deletions inactivate DCC, but not MADH4/DPC4/SMAD4, in a subset of pancreatic and biliary cancers. Genes Chromosomes Cancer 2000, 27:353–357.
83. McGarrity TJ, Amos C. Peutz-Jeghers syndrome: clinicopathology and molecular alterations. Cell Mol Life Sci 2006, 63:2135–2144.
84. Giardiello FM, Brensinger JD, Tersmette AC, et al. Very high risk of cancer in familial Peutz-Jeghers syndrome. Gastroenterology 2000, 119:1447–1453.
85. Su GH, Hruban RH, Bansal RK, et al. Germline and somatic mutations of the STK11/LKB1 Peutz-Jeghers gene in pancreatic and biliary cancers. Am J Pathol 1999, 154:1835–1840.
86. Teng DH, Perry WL, 3rd, Hogan JK, et al. Human mitogen-activated protein kinase kinase 4 as a candidate tumor suppressor. Cancer Res 1997, 57:4177–4182.
87. Su GH, Hilgers W, Shekher MC, et al. Alterations in pancreatic, biliary, and breast carcinomas support MKK4 as a genetically targeted tumor suppressor gene. Cancer Res 1998, 58:2339–2342.
88. Xin W, Yun KJ, Ricci F, et al. MAP2K4/MKK4 expression in pancreatic cancer: genetic validation of immunohistochemistry and relationship to disease course. Clin Cancer Res 2004, 10:8516–8520.
89. Cunningham SC, Gallmeier E, Hucl T, et al. Targeted deletion of MKK4 in cancer cells: a detrimental phenotype manifests as decreased experimental metastasis and suggests a counterweight to the evolution of tumor-suppressor loss. Cancer Res 2006, 66:5560–5564.

90. Kwak EL, Jankowski J, Thayer SP, et al. Epidermal growth factor receptor kinase domain mutations in esophageal and pancreatic adenocarcinomas. Clin Cancer Res 2006, 12:4283–4287.
91. Calhoun ES, Kern SE. No EGFR mutations identified in pancreatic cancer. NOGO 2004, 8:3.
92. Bild AH, Potti A, Nevins JR. Linking oncogenic pathways with therapeutic opportunities. Nat Rev Cancer 2006, 6:735–741.
93. Eshleman JR, Markowitz SD. Mismatch repair defects in human carcinogenesis. Hum Mol Genet 1996, 5 Spec No:1489–1494.
94. Leach FS, Nicolaides NC, Papadopoulos N, et al. Mutations of a mutS homolog in hereditary nonpolyposis colorectal cancer. Cell 1993, 75:1215–1225.
95. Bronner CE, Baker SM, Morrison PT, et al. Mutation in the DNA mismatch repair gene homologue hMLH1 is associated with hereditary non-polyposis colon cancer. Nature 1994, 368:258–261.
96. Papadopoulos N, Nicolaides NC, Wei YF, et al. Mutation of a mutL homolog in hereditary colon cancer. Science 1994, 263:1625–1629.
97. Akiyama Y, Sato H, Yamada T, et al. Germ-line mutation of the hMSH6/GTBP gene in an atypical hereditary nonpolyposis colorectal cancer kindred. Cancer Res 1997, 57:3920–3923.
98. Miyaki M, Konishi M, Tanaka K, et al. Germline mutation of MSH6 as the cause of hereditary nonpolyposis colorectal cancer. Nat Genet 1997, 17:271–272.
99. Liu B, Parsons R, Papadopoulos N, et al. Analysis of mismatch repair genes in hereditary non-polyposis colorectal cancer patients. Nat Med 1996, 2:169–174.
100. Hempen PM, Zhang L, Bansal RK, et al. Evidence of selection for clones having genetic inactivation of the activin A type II receptor (ACVR2) gene in gastrointestinal cancers. Cancer Res 2003, 63:994–999.
101. Murphy KM, Brune KA, Griffin C, et al. Evaluation of candidate genes MAP2K4, MADH4, ACVR1B, and BRCA2 in familial pancreatic cancer: deleterious BRCA2 mutations in 17%. Cancer Res 2002, 62:3789–3793.
102. Su GH, Bansal R, Murphy KM, et al. ACVR1B (ALK4, activin receptor type 1B) gene mutations in pancreatic carcinoma. Proc Natl Acad Sci U S A 2001, 98:3254–3257.
103. Wood LD, Calhoun ES, Silliman N, et al. Somatic mutations of GUCY2F, EPHA3, and NTRK3 in human cancers. Hum Mutat 2006, 27:1060–1061.
104. Wilentz RE, Goggins M, Redston M, et al. Genetic, immunohistochemical, and clinical features of medullary carcinoma of the pancreas: a newly described and characterized entity. Am J Pathol 2000, 156:1641–1651.

Chapter 3
Pancreatic Intraepithelial Neoplasia

**Ralph H. Hruban, Kieran Brune, Noriyoshi Fukushima,
and Anirban Maitra**

1   Introduction

Most pancreatic cancers are not diagnosed until after the cancer has spread to other
organs and is no longer curable. As a result, the death rate for pancreatic cancer in
this country (34,290/year) is approximately equal to the incidence rate (37,680/
year) (*1*). By contrast, many patients survive the diagnosis of breast cancer, and half
of the decline in breast cancer mortality in the last quarter of a century has come
from improved early detection (*2*). We believe that early detection of preinvasive
lesions is the greatest hope for curing pancreatic neoplasia. This chapter discusses
pancreatic intraepithelial neoplasia (PanIN), the most common precursor lesion in
the pancreas (*3*).

2   Morphology of PanINs

Although the PanIN nomenclature is a relatively recent development, the lesions
now recognized as PanINs were, in fact, described over 100 years ago (*4*). In 1905
the Dutch physician von S.P.L. Hulst described lesions characterized by enlargement
of the cells as well as the architectural formation of papillae ("Hypertrophie der
Zellen . . . relative reine päpilare Wucherung") with a morphologic appearance
between that of normal pancreatic ducts and invasive cancer ("Zwischenformen")
(*4*). These lesions are now called *pancreatic intraepithelial neoplasia*, recognizing
that they are noninvasive intraepithelial neoplasms (*5, 6*). PanINs are defined as
microscopic papillary or flat, noninvasive intraepithelial neoplasms arising in the
smaller pancreatic ducts (*6*). PanIN lesions have been classified into three grades,
one of which is subdivided into A and B subcategories (*5–7*). PanIN-1A is a flat
epithelial lesion composed of columnar cells, with basally located uniform round
to oval uniform nuclei (Fig. 3.1) (*5–7*). The cells can contain abundant mucin and
the nuclei are well oriented relative to the basement membrane. Molecular analyses
suggest that many lesions with this morphology are neoplastic, some may be non-
neoplastic, and the addition of the modifier "L" for lesion (PanIN-1A/L) is therefore

A.M. Lowy et al. (eds.), *Pancreatic Cancer.*
doi: 10.1007/978-0-387-69252-4, © Springer Science+Business Media, LLC 2008

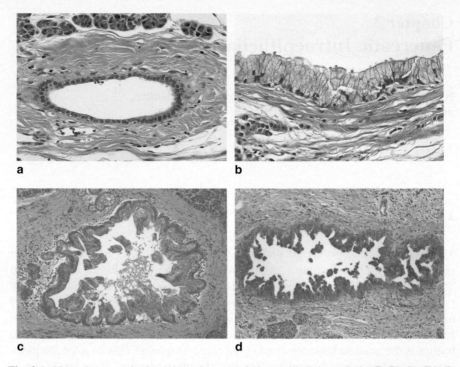

Fig. 3.1 Normal pancreatic duct (**A**) and pancreatic intraepithelial neoplasia (**B–D**). PanIN1-B (**A**), PanIN-2 (**C**), and PanIN-3 (**D**) are characterized by increasing degrees of architectural and nuclear atypia

perfectly acceptable (5–7). PanIN-1B is papillary, but is otherwise morphologically identical to PanIN-1A (5–7). Most PanIN-2 lesions are papillary, and PanIN-2 lesions, by definition, have some nuclear abnormalities, including some loss of polarity, nuclear crowding, enlarged nuclei, pseudostratification, and hyperchromasia (see Fig. 3.1) (5–7). Mitoses are rare in PanIN-2 lesions, and when present are basal and morphologically normal (5–7). PanIN-3 lesions show significant architectural and cytological atypia (see Fig. 3.1) (5–7). PanIN-3 lesions can show cribiforming, the budding off of clusters of cells, and luminal necrosis (5–7). Cytologically the nuclei are enlarged, hyperchromatic and show a loss of orientation such that they are no longer oriented perpendicular to the basement membrane, and the nuclear to cytoplasmic ratio is increased (5–8). Nucleoli are prominent, and mitoses may be luminal or atypical (5–7).

Recently, Brune et al. and Detlefsen et al. have described distinctive changes in the pancreatic parenchyma that are often associated with PanIN lesions (9, 10). The normal pancrtic parenchyma is free of inflammation and scarring, and is composed of lobules of uniform acinar cells surrounding a central duct. The acinar cells have abundant apical cytoplasm and form barely perceptible lumina (10). Some PanIN lesions are associated with atrophic changes in this acinar parenchyma (Fig. 3.2) (9,

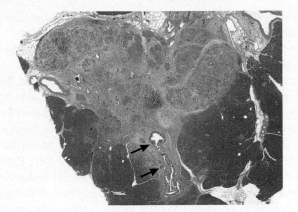

Fig. 3.2 Lobulocentric atrophy associated with a PanIN lesion *(arrows)*

10). This atrophy can range from subtle dilatation of acinar lumina and loss of granularity in the acinar cells, to marked acinar dropout producing lobular units composed almost entirely of islets of Langerhans embedded in scar tissue (*10*). The remarkable thing about the parenchymal atrophy associated with PanIN lesions is that it is dramatically lobulocentric, involving only the lobule harboring the PanIN lesion (*10*). The morphology of the lobulocentric atrophy suggests that it may be caused by local obstruction of the small pancreatic ducts from the PanIN lesions, or by the premature activation of trypsin in the small pancreatic ducts (*10*).

Regardless of its etiology, the lobulocentric parenchymal atrophy associated with PanIN lesions is important because, as discussed later, some foci of lobulocentric parenchymal atrophy are large enough to be detected with currently available imaging modalities (*10*).

3   Who Gets PanINs and How Common Are They?

A number of autopsy studies have examined the prevalence of PanINs in the population and in patients with an invasive adenocarcinoma of the pancreas (*11–15*). For example, Cubilla and Fitzgerald, examined 327 pancreata and compared the prevalence of duct lesions in patients with pancreatic cancer ($n = 227$) to controls without pancreatic cancer ($n = 100$) (*12*). Papillary duct lesions, presumably representing PanIN-2, were three times more common in the pancreata with an invasive cancer than they were in the controls, and 20% of the pancreata with an invasive carcinoma had associated carcinoma in situ (PanIN-3) compared to 0% of the controls (*11*). Kozuka et al., in a larger autopsy-based series, also found that all grades of PanIN were more common in pancreata with an invasive carcinoma than they were in pancreata without an invasive cancer (*12*). In addition, Kozuka et al.

reported that PanINs are more common in the head of the gland than in the tail, and that the prevalence of PanINs increases with age (*12*). Remarkably, 34% of patients over the age of 50 had at least one PanIN, making PanINs one of the most common neoplasms in the human body (*12*).

Chronic pancreatitis, particularly familial chronic pancreatitis, has been shown to be a risk factor for pancreatic cancer, and PanINs have also been studied in pancreata with chronic pancreatitis (*16*). Volkholz et al. identified PanIN lesions in 40% of 280 pancreata with chronic pancreatitis (*17*). Most of these were low-grade (PanIN-1 and -2) lesions (*17*). More recently, Rosty et al. identified PanINs in 74 of 122 (60%) of pancreata with chronic pancreatitis; 7.4% were PanIN-2 and 1.5% were PanIN-3 (*18*). Similarly, Andea et al. reported PanIN lesions in 60% of pancreata with chronic pancreatitis, with 4% of the pancreata showing PanIN-3 (*13*). Thus, PanINs appear to be more common in pancreata with chronic pancreatitis than they are in the general population, but only rarely do these PanIN lesions reach the level of PanIN-3 (*13*).

PanINs have also been reported in association with other peri-ampullary neoplasms (*19, 20*). Agoff et al. studied five resected ampullary adenomas and 17 resected ampullary carcinomas and found PanIN lesions in all cases (*19*). Remarkably, high-grade PanIN lesions were found in 40% of the pancreata, and in some instances these high-grade PanIN lesions extended to the pancreatic parenchymal margin of resection (*19*). Similarly, Stelow et al. carefully examined all pancreata surgically resected at the University of Virginia from June 1, 1991 to March 1, 2005; and PanIN lesions were found in three of three pancreata resected for acinar cell carcinoma, 17 of 18 pancreata resected for a mucinous cystic neoplasm, 16 of 24 pancreata resected for a well-differentiated pancreatic endocrine neoplasm, 10 of 12 pancreata with serous cystic neoplasms, and in two of three pancreata resected for a solid-pseudopapillary neoplasm (*20*).

From these various studies, one can conclude that PanINs are remarkably common neoplasms, that they increase with age, that they are more common in pancreata with chronic pancreatitis, and that they are most prevalent in pancreata with an invasive adenocarcinoma.

4 Molecular Alterations Found in PanINs

A variety of molecular abnormalities have been identified in PanIN lesions. Some of these alterations occur relatively "early" (in PanIN-1 lesions), whereas others occur only in severely dysplastic lesions (PanIN-3 lesions).

Activating point mutations in codon 12 of the K-ras2 oncogene are one of the most common genetic alterations in pancreatic neoplasia, found in >90% of invasive ductal adenocarcinomas of the pancreas, and K-ras gene mutations are common and early events in PanINs (*14, 21–25*). K-ras2 gene mutations have been reported in about a third of PanIN-1 lesions, in approximately half of PanIN-2 lesions, and in 70-90% of PanIN-3 lesions (*14, 21–26*).

p16/CDKN2A gene inactivation is also very common in invasive adenocarcinoma of the pancreas (*27, 28*). Forty percent of invasive adenocarcinomas have homozygous deletions inactivating both alleles of the gene, another 40% have an intragenic mutation coupled with loss of the remaining wild-type allele, and in 15% of the cancers *p16/CDKN2A* is inactivated by promoter methylation (*28*). Inactivation of the *p16/CDKN2A* gene also appears to be a relatively early event in pancreatic neoplasia (*23, 29*). For example, Wilentz et al., using immunohistochemical labeling for the *p16/CDKN2A* gene product, showed that 30% of PanIN-1A lesions, 55% of PanIN-1B and PanIN-2 lesions, and 71% of PanIN-3 lesions had loss of expression of the *p16/CDKN2A* gene product (*26, 29*). Loss of the *p16/CDKN2A* is less common in PanINs studied from pancreata with chronic pancreatitis than it is in PanINs from pancreata with an associated invasive adenocarcinoma (*18*). Aberrant methylation of the *p16/CDKN2A* promoter has been reported in 12% of PanIN-1A lesions, in 4.5% of PanIN-2 lesions, and in 21.4% of PanIN-3 lesions (*30*). At the genetic level, loss of heterozygosity at the *p16/CDKN2A* gene locus on chromosome 9p21 has been reported in PanINs, as has homozygous deletion of the *p16/CDKN2A* gene locus (*31–34*). For example, the *MTAP* gene resides adjacent to the *p16/CDKN2A* gene on chromosome 9p21. Immunolabeling for both p16 and MTAP protein expression can therefore be used to evaluate tissues for *p16/CDKN2A* homozygous deletions, and Hustinx et al. reported concordant loss of p16 and MTAP expression in 8% of PanINs (*33*). Thus, *p16/CDKN2A* gene inactivation, be it by homozygous deletion, promoter methylation or mutation, appears to be an early to intermediate event in PanIN development.

Both *TP53* and *SMAD4/DPC4* gene inactivation appear to be relatively late events in the development of pancreatic neoplasia (*34*). *TP53* and *SMAD4/DPC4* gene inactivation both appear to occur at the PanIN-3/invasive carcinoma level (*32, 34–38*). For example, immunolabeling for the dpc4 protein has been shown to be a good surrogate marker of *SMAD4/DPC4* gene inactivation, and all PanIN-1 and -2 lesions studied by Wilentz et al. showed intact (normal) dpc4 expression, whereas 31% of PanIN-3 lesions showed loss of dpc4 expression indicative of inactivation of the *SMAD4/DPC4* gene (*38*).

Molecular analyses such as those described have therefore helped to identify which genes are targeted in PanIN lesions and the relative sequence of events. They have also been used to demonstrate significant genetic divergence among PanIN lesions (*31*). The development of PanIN lesions is not an orderly progression in which genetic alterations proceed in a preordained sequence. Instead, the genetic events need not occur in a particular order, and there is significant genetic divergence of multiple subclones within a single pancreas (*31*).

Telomere shortening is an early and ubiquitous event in PanIN formation (*39*). Van Heek et al. examined telomere length in a large series of well-characterized PanINs using an in situ hybridization technique, and found significantly reduced telomere signals indicative of shortened telomeres in 96% of the PanINs examined (*39*). Even 91% of PanIN-1A lesions showed significantly reduced telomere lengths (*39*). Telomeres prevent the ends of chromosomes from sticking together and protect against chromosomal breakage-fusion-bridge cycles in dividing cells (*39*).

As noted by van Heek et al., a critical shortening of telomere length in PanINs predisposes these lesions to accumulate progressive genetic abnormalities such as the homozygous deletions and losses of heterozygosity described in the preceding (*39*).

5 Animal Models

An understanding of the genetic alterations in human PanINs and in invasive adeno-carcinomas of the pancreas has formed the basis for the development of genetically engineered mouse models of pancreatic cancer (*40*). As noted, activating point mutations in codon 12 of the K-ras*2* oncogene are an early and common event in the development of pancreatic neoplasia (*23, 25*). S. Hingorani et al. used this observation as a basis on which to build the first successful mouse model of pancreatic cancer (*41*). They directed endogenous expression of mutant K-ras to progenitor cells of the pancreas, and over time some of these mice developed infil-trating ductal adenocarcinomas of the pancreas (*41*). Remarkably, these mice devel-oped ductal lesions that recapitulated the full spectrum of human pancreatic intraepithelial neoplasia (*41*). These lesions, designated mPanIN for mouse PanIN, add to the growing body of evidence that infiltrating adenocarcinomas of the pancreas can arise from histologically well-defined precursor lesions (mPanIN in the mouse, PanIN in humans) (*41*). The speed at which pancreatic cancer develops is accelerated when these mice are crossed with other mice in which the *TP53* or *p16/ink4a* genes are inactivated (*42–44*). These latter models help define the role that inactivation of these tumor suppressor genes play in the development of pancreatic cancer.

Importantly, the creation of genetically engineered mouse models of pancreatic cancer that recapitulate the human disease, down to the development of precursor lesions, provides a wonderful opportunity to study the biology of precursor lesions, and to develop novel early detection methods. For example, Hingorani et al. were able to identify a proteomic serum signature associated with the development of mPanINs (*41*).

6 Gene Expression Studies

A better understanding of the spectrum of genes expressed in PanINs will provide insight into the biology of early pancreatic neoplasia as well as potential new markers for early disease. Gene expression studies of PanIN lesions can be divided into two broad groups-global gene expression analyses and analyses of selected markers.

A variety of techniques have been employed to analyze gene expression patterns in PanINs at the global level (*45–47*). These include serial analysis of gene expres-sion (SAGE), whole-genome oligonucleotide microarrays, and cDNA microarrays

(*45–47*). Prasad et al. used cDNA microarrays to identify 49 genes that were differentially expressed in early PanIN lesions (PanIN-1) (*45*). The genes overexpressed in PanINs included foregut markers such as MUC6, KLF4, pepsinogen and TFF1, and Prasad et al. hypothesized that the expression of these foregut genes may be a manifestation of Hedgehog signaling (*45*). Other genes that have been identified as overexpressed in PanIN lesions in these global studies of gene expression include MUC5AC, S-100P, claudin 1, and claudin 10 (*46, 47*).

The expression of a spectrum of selected markers has been examined in PanIN lesions primarily using immunohistochemical labeling. A great deal of effort has gone into characterizing the patterns of mucin expression in PanINs, and most PanINs have been found to express MUC1, MUC4, MUC5AC, and MUC6, but not MUC2 (*48, 49*). The expression of MUC4 increases with increasing degrees of dysplasia (*50*). For example, MUC4 labeling was observed in 17% of PanIN-1 lesions, 36% of PanIN-2 lesions, 85% of PanIN-3 lesions, and 89% of invasive ductal adenocarcinomas (*50*). These data support the concept of a progression from low-grade PanIN to high-grade PanIN to invasive adenocarcinoma (*50*). In addition, the pattern of mucin expression observed in PanINs (MUC1 positive, MUC2 negative) is distinct from that seen in intestinal-type intraductal papillary mucinous neoplasms (IPMN, MUC1 negative, MUC2 positive), suggesting two distinct pathways to invasive cancer in the pancreas-a PanIN to invasive ductal adenocarcinoma pathway, and an intestinal type IPMN to invasive colloid carcinoma pathway (*48*).

Other proteins of interest that have been shown to be overexpressed in PanINs relative to normal ductal cells include CEACAM6 and cyclooxygenase 2 (*51, 52*). Maitra et al. used tissue microarrays to define the patterns of expression of a large panel of genes in PanINs and found that MUC5 and prostate stem cell antigen expression occurred early, cyclin D1 expression was an intermediate event, and MUC1, mesothelin, and 14-3-3 sigma expression were late changes (*53*). These analyses help define markers for the early detection of pancreatic cancer as well as targets for chemopreventive therapy.

7   Clinical Implications

Clinical follow-up of patients with PanINs has shown that these lesions can progress to invasive adenocarcinoma over time (*54, 55*). Brat et al. reported three patients who developed an infiltrating ductal adenocarcinoma in their residual pancreas after partial pancreatectomy revealed high-grade PanINs (*54*). From these clinical observations, and the weight of the molecular and histologic data presented earlier, it is clear that the identification and treatment of PanIN lesions represents an opportunity to cure pancreatic neoplasia. However, the challenge is, how can we identify PanINs clinically?

Although it is clear that a simple noninvasive inexpensive highly sensitive and specific blood test for PanINs would be the ideal early detection test, no such blood test yet exists.

Until the time when a blood test is developed we will have to rely on existing tech-nologies, such as endoscopic ultrasound (EUS). Canto et al. and Brentnall et al. have shown that EUS can be a safe and effective method to screen asymptomatic individuals at high risk for developing pancreatic cancer because of their family history (6, 56–58). Most recently, Canto et al. screened 78 asymptomatic individuals with the Peutz-Jeghers syndrome or with a strong family history of pancreatic cancer using a combi-nation of computed tomography and EUS (58). Eight of these asymptomatic patients (10% yield of screening) were found to have pancreatic neoplasia including six with an intraductal papillary mucinous neoplasm (IPMN), one with an IPMN that the patient elected to have followed and that progressed to an invasive carcinoma, and one with multifocal PanINs (58). Of note, the lobulocentric atrophy associated with PanIN lesions was detectable by EUS in patients with multifocal disease (10). Lobulocentric atrophy produces chronic pancreatitis-like changes on EUS, including echogenic foci, echogenic strands, lobularity, duct irregularities, dilated main duct, and an echogenic main duct (10). These results demonstrate that a high-risk population can be screened using technologies available today.

8   Current Challenges

As the resolution of pancreatic imaging improves we will be able to detect smaller and smaller lesions. This, unfortunately, is a double-edged sword. On the one hand, improvements in resolution will make it possible to identify the subtle changes associated with PanINs, such as lobulocentric atrophy, and maybe even PanINs themselves. On the other hand, it is clear that many healthy individuals harbor subtle changes in their pancreas that have no clinical significance. For example, Spinelli et al. examined 24,039 scans of the pancreas (computed tomography or magnetic resonance imaging) and found that 290 of the patients (1.2%) had a pancreatic cyst (59). With cysts this common in the general population, the challenge is to distinguish between harmless changes, and changes indicative of a significant precursor lesion (60, 61). To date, there is no definitive answer. Some studies have reported that patients with even small cysts of the pancreas have a 22.5-fold increased risk of developing pancreatic cancer (60), whereas others have suggested that the malignancy risk for cysts up to 3 cm approximates the risk of mortality from surgical resection (61). Clearly, better imaging and more data are needed before definitive statements can be made on what to do with small lesions in the pancreas.

9   Long-Term Goals

Our ultimate goal is to identify and treat curable pancreatic intraepithelial neoplasia before it has the chance to progress to an incurable invasive adenocarcinoma (62). PanINs may be identified through improved imaging, through novel molecular markers, or through new proteomic markers. Although the current treatment is surgical resection, surgical resection of the pancreas can have significant morbidity and even some mortality. The ultimate goal would therefore be to develop novel therapies that nonsurgically ablate PanINs.

References

1. Jemal A, Siegel R, Ward E, et al. Cancer Statistics, CA A Cancer Journal for Clinicians 2008, 58:71–96.
2. Berry DA, Cronin KA, Plevritis SK, et al. Effect of screening and adjuvant therapy on mortality from breast cancer. N Engl J Med 2005, 353(17):1784–1792.
3. Maitra A, Fukushima N, Takaori K, et al. Precursors to invasive pancreatic cancer. Adv Anat Pathol 2005, 12(2):81–91.
4. Hulst SPL. Zur kenntnis der Genese des Adenokarzinoms und Karzinoms des Pankreas. Virchows Arch (B) 1905, 180:288–316.
5. Hruban RH, Adsay NV, Albores-Saavedra J, et al. Pancreatic intraepithelial neoplasia: a new nomenclature and classification system for pancreatic duct lesions. Am J Surg Pathol 2001, 25(5):579–586.
6. Hruban RH, Takaori K, Klimstra DS, et al. An illustrated consensus on the classification of pancreatic intraepithelial neoplasia and intraductal papillary mucinous neoplasms. Am J Surg Pathol 2004, 28(8):977–987.
7. Hruban RH, Klimstra DS, Pitman MB. Atlas of tumor pathology. Tumors of the pancreas, 4th ed. Washington, DC: Armed Forces Institute of Pathology, 2007.
8. Furukawa T, Chiba R, Kobari M, et al. Varying grades of epithelial atypia in the pancreatic ducts of humans. Classification based on morphometry and multilvariate analysis and correlated with positive reactions of carcinoembryonic antigen. Arch Pathol Lab Med 1994, 118:227–234.
9. Detlefsen S, Sipos B, Feyerabend B, et al. Pancreatic fibrosis associated with age and ductal papillary hyperplasia. Virchows Arch 2005, 447(5):800–805.
10. Brune KA, Abe T, Canto MI, et al. Multifocal neoplastic precursor lesions associated with lobular atrophy of the pancreas in patients having a strong family history of pancreatic cancer. Am J Surg Pathol 2006, 30(9):1067–1076.
11. Cubilla AL, Fitzgerald PJ. Morphological lesions associated with human primary invasive nonendocrine pancreas cancer. Cancer Res 1976, 36:2690–2698.
12. Kozuka S, Sassa R, Taki T, et al. Relation of pancreatic duct hyperplasia to carcinoma. Cancer 1979, 43:1418–1428.
13. Andea A, Sarkar F, Adsay NV. Clinicopathological correlates of pancreatic intraepithelial neoplasia: a comparative analysis of 82 cases with and 152 cases without pancreatic ductal adenocarcinoma. Mod Pathol 2003, 16(10):996–1006.
14. Lüttges J, Reinecke-Lüthge A, Mollmann B, et al. Duct changes and K-ras mutations in the disease-free pancreas: analysis of type, age relation and spatial distribution. Virchows Arch 1999, 435(5):461–468.
15. Kimura W, Nagai H, Kuroda A, et al. Analysis of small cystic lesions of the pancreas. Int J Pancreatol 1995, 18(3):197–206.
16. Lowenfels AB, Maisonneuve EP, Dimagno YE, et al. Hereditary pancreatitis and the risk of pancreatic cancer. International Hereditary Pancreatitis Study Group. J Natl Cancer Inst 1997, 89(6):442–446.
17. Volkholz H, Stolte M, Becker V. Epithelial dysplasias in chronic pancreatitis. Virchows Arch A Pathol Anat Histopathol 1982, 396:331–349.
18. Rosty C, Geradts J, Sato N, et al. p16 Inactivation in pancreatic intraepithelial neoplasias (PanINs) arising in patients with chronic pancreatitis. Am J Surg Pathol 2003, 27(12):1495–1501.

19. Agoff SN, Crispin DA, Bronner MP, et al. Neoplasms of the ampulla of Vater with concurrent pancreatic intraductal neoplasia: a histological and molecular study. Mod Pathol 2001, 14(3):139–146.
20. Stelow EB, Adams RB, Moskaluk CA. The prevalence of pancreatic Intraepithelial neoplasia in pancreata with uncommon types of primary neoplasms. Am J Surg Pathol 2006, 30(1):36–41.
21. Yanagisawa A, Ohtake K, Ohashi K, et al. Frequent c-Ki-*ras* oncogene activation in mucous cell hyperplasias of pancreas suffering from chronic inflammation. Cancer Res 1993, 53:953–956.
22. Tada M, Ohashi M, Shiratori Y, et al. Analysis of K-ras gene mutation in hyperplastic duct cells of the pancreas without pancreatic disease. Gastroenterology 1996, 110:227–231.
23. Moskaluk CA, Hruban RH, Kern SE. p16 and K-ras gene mutations in the intraductal precursors of human pancreatic adenocarcinoma. Cancer Res 1997, 57:2140–2143.
24. Lüttges J, Schlehe B, Menke MA, et al. The K-ras mutation pattern in pancreatic ductal adenocarcinoma usually is identical to that in associated normal, hyperplastic, and metaplastic ductal epithelium. Cancer 1999, 85(8):1703–1710.
25. Hruban RH, van Mansfeld ADM, Offerhaus GJ, et al. K-*ras* oncogene activation in adenocarcinoma of the human pancreas. A study of 82 carcinomas using a combination of mutant-enriched polymerase chain reaction analysis and allele-specific oligonucleotide hybridization. Am J Pathol 1993, 143(2):545–554.
26. Hruban RH, Goggins M, Parsons JL, et al. Progression model for pancreatic cancer. Clin Cancer Res 2000, 6:2969–2972.
27. Caldas C, Hahn SA, da Costa LT, et al. Frequent somatic mutations and homozygous deletions of the p16 (MTS1) gene in pancreatic adenocarcinoma. Nat Genet 1994, 8:27–32.
28. Schutte M, Hruban RH, Geradts J, et al. Abrogation of the Rb/p16 tumor-suppressive pathway in virtually all pancreatic carcinomas. Cancer Res 1997, 57:3126–3130.
29. Wilentz RE, Geradts J, Maynard R, et al. Inactivation of the p16 (INK4A) tumor-suppressor gene in pancreatic duct lesions: loss of intranuclear expression. Cancer Res 1998, 58:4740–4744.
30. Fukushima N, Sato N, Ueki T, et al. Aberrant methylation of preproenkephalin and p16 genes in pancreatic intraepithelial neoplasia and pancreatic ductal adenocarcinoma. Am J Pathol 2002, 160(5):1573–1581.
31. Yamano M, Fujii H, Takagaki T, et al. Genetic progression and divergence in pancreatic carcinoma. Am J Pathol 2000, 156(6):2123–2133.
32. Heinmöller E, Dietmaier W, Zirngibl H, et al. Molecular analysis of microdissected tumors and preneoplastic intraductal lesions in pancreatic carcinoma. Am J Pathol 2000, 157(1):83–92.
33. Hustinx SR, Leoni LM, Yeo CJ, et al. Concordant loss of MTAP and p16/CDKN2A expression in pancreatic intraepithelial neoplasia: evidence of homozygous deletion in a noninvasive precursor lesion. Mod Pathol 2005, 18(7):959–963.
34. Lüttges J, Galehdari H, Brocker V, et al. Allelic loss is often the first hit in the biallelic inactivation of the p53 and DPC4 genes during pancreatic carcinogenesis. Am J Pathol 2001, 158(5):1677–1683.
35. Boschman CR, Stryker S, Reddy JK, et al. Expression of p53 protein in precursor lesions and adenocarcinoma of human pancreas. Am J Pathol 1994, 145:1291–1295.
36. DiGiuseppe JA, Hruban RH, Goodman SN, et al. Overexpression of p53 protein in adenocarcinoma of the pancreas. Am J Clin Pathol 1994, 101:684–688.
37. McCarthy DM, Brat DJ, Wilentz RE, et al. Pancreatic intraepithelial neoplasia and infiltrating adenocarcinoma: analysis of progression and recurrence by *DPC4* immunohistochemical labeling. Hum Pathol 2001, 32:638–642.
38. Wilentz RE, Iacobuzio-Donahue CA, Argani P, et al. Loss of expression of Dpc4 in pancreatic intraepithelial neoplasia: evidence that DPC4 inactivation occurs late in neoplastic progression. Cancer Res 2000, 60:2002–2006.
39. van Heek NT, Meeker AK, Kern SE, et al. Telomere shortening is nearly universal in pancreatic intraepithelial neoplasia. Am J Pathol 2002, 161(5):1541–1547.

40. Hruban RH, Adsay NV, Albores-Saavedra J, et al. Pathology of genetically engineered mouse models of pancreatic exocrine cancer: consensus report and recommendations. Cancer Res 2006, 66(1):95–106.
41. Hingorani SR, Petricoin EF, Maitra A, et al. Preinvasive and invasive ductal pancreatic cancer and its early detection in the mouse. Cancer Cell 2003, 4(6):437–450.
42. Hingorani SR, Wang L, Multani AS, et al. Trp53R172H and KrasG12D cooperate to promote chromosomal instability and widely metastatic pancreatic ductal adenocarcinoma in mice. Cancer Cell 2005, 7(5):469–483.
43. Aguirre AJ, Bardeesy N, Sinha M, et al. Activated Kras and Ink4a/Arf deficiency cooperate to produce metastatic pancreatic ductal adenocarcinoma. Genes Dev 2003, 17(24):3112–3126.
44. Bardeesy N, Morgan J, Sinha M, et al. Obligate roles for p16(Ink4a) and p19(Arf)-p53 in the suppression of murine pancreatic neoplasia. Mol Cell Biol 2002, 22(2):635–643.
45. Prasad NB, Biankin AV, Fukushima N, et al. Gene expression profiles in pancreatic intraepithelial neoplasia reflect the effects of Hedgehog signaling on pancreatic ductal epithelial cells. Cancer Res 2005, 65(5):1619–1626.
46. Heidenblut AM, Lüttges J, Buchholz M, et al. aRNA-longSAGE: a new approach to generate SAGE libraries from microdissected cells. Nucleic Acids Res 2004, 32(16):e131.
47. Buchholz M, Braun M, Heidenblut A, et al. Transcriptome analysis of microdissected pancreatic intraepithelial neoplastic lesions. Oncogene 2005.
48. Adsay NV, Merati K, Andea A, et al. The dichotomy in the preinvasive neoplasia to invasive carcinoma sequence in the pancreas: differential expression of MUC1 and MUC2 supports the existence of two separate pathways of carcinogenesis. Mod Pathol 2002, 15(10):1087–1095.
49. Kim GE, Bae HI, Park HU, et al. Aberrant expression of MUC5AC and MUC6 gastric mucins and sialyl Tn antigen in intraepithelial neoplasms of the pancreas. Gastroenterology 2002, 123(4):1052–1060.
50. Swartz MJ, Batra SK, Varshney GC, et al. MUC4 expression increases progressively in pancreatic intraepithelial neoplasia. Am J Clin Pathol 2002, 117(5):791–796.
51. Maitra A, Ashfaq R, Gunn CR, et al. Cyclooxygenase 2 expression in pancreatic adenocarcinoma and pancreatic intraepithelial neoplasia: an immunohistochemical analysis with automated cellular imaging. Am J Clin Pathol 2002, 118(2):194–201.
52. Duxbury MS, Matros E, Clancy T, et al. CEACAM6 is a novel biomarker in pancreatic adenocarcinoma and PanIN lesions. Ann Surg 2005, 241(3):491–496.
53. Maitra A, Adsay NV, Argani P, et al. Multicomponent analysis of the pancreatic adenocarcinoma progression model using a pancreatic intraepithelial neoplasia tissue microarray. Mod Pathol 2003, 16(9):902–912.
54. Brat DJ, Lillemoe KD, Yeo CJ, et al. Progression of pancreatic intraductal neoplasias to infiltrating adenocarcinoma of the pancreas. Am J Surg Pathol 1998, 22(2):163–169.
55. Brockie E, Anand A, Albores-Saavedra J. Progression of atypical ductal hyperplasia/carcinoma in situ of the pancreas to invasive adenocarcinoma. Ann Diagn Pathol 1998, 2(5):286–292.
56. Brentnall TA, Bronner MP, Byrd DR, et al. Early diagnosis and treatment of pancreatic dysplasia in patients with a family history of pancreatic cancer. Ann Intern Med 1999, 131(4):247–255.
57. Canto MI, Goggins M, Yeo CJ, et al. Screening for pancreatic neoplasia in high-risk individuals: An EUS-based approach. Clin Gastroenterol Hepatol 2004, 2(7):606–621.
58. Canto MI, Goggins M, Hruban RH, et al. Screening for early pancreatic neoplasia in high-risk individuals: a prospective controlled study. Clin Gastroenterol Hepatol 2006, 4(6):766–781.
59. Spinelli KS, Fromwiller TE, Daniel RA, et al. Cystic pancreatic neoplasms: observe or operate. Ann Surg 2004, 239(5):651–657.
60. Tada M, Kawabe T, Arizumi M, et al. Pancreatic cancer in patients with pancreatic cystic lesions: a prospective study in 197 patients. Clin Gastroenterol Hepatol 2006.
61. Allen PJ, D'Angelica M, Gonen M, et al. A selective approach to the resection of cystic lesions of the pancreas: results from 539 consecutive patients. Ann Surg 2006, 244(4):572–582.
62. O'Shaughnessy JA, Kelloff GJ, Gordon GB, et al. Treatment and prevention of intraepithelial neoplasia: an important target for accelerated new agent development. Clin Cancer Res 2002, 8(2):314–346.

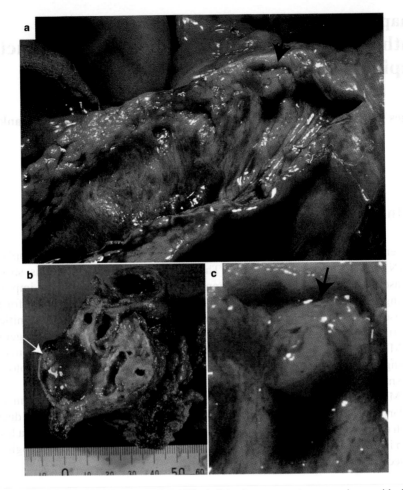

Fig. 4.1 Gross pathologic features of IPMN. **A.** Distal pancreatectomy specimen with dilated main pancreatic duct opened longitudinally showing main duct IPMN throughout the distal lining of the duct and a prominent polypoid area indicated by arrow. Close-up view shown in (**C**). **B.** Whipple pancreatico-duodenectomy specimen showing gross features of IPMN. Note dilated ductal system, and papillae of IPMN indicated by arrow and adjacent reflection produced by secreted mucous. (Image (**B**) kindly provided by A/Prof. R Eckstein, Royal North Shore Hospital, Sydney, Australia.)

An invasive component may be suspected by the presences of sclerotic or mucoid (colloid-like) areas (7). However, it should also be noted that the pancreas surrounding IPMNs is often pale and firm due to associated chronic obstructive pancreatitis.

3   Histologic Features of IPMN

The well-differentiated tumors are usually characterized by tall, well-formed papillae with fibrovascular cores lined by a layer of columnar, mucin-secreting epithelium, although areas of flat epithelium or denuded foci may also be present. The low power architecture of higher grade tumors is more complex with branching papillae, pseudopapillary structures, and cribriform regions (Fig. 4.2) (3, 7–9).

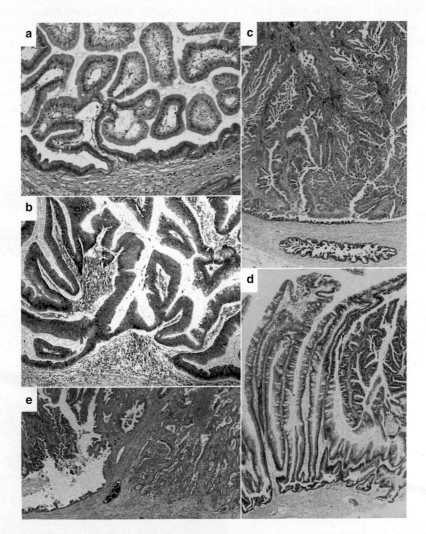

Fig. 4.2 Low power photomicrographs showing (**A**) IPMN adenoma, (**B**) IPMN borderline, (**C**) IPMC, (**D**) mixed IPMN adenoma to the left and IPMN borderline to the right, (**E**) IPMC to the left with associated invasive carcinoma to the right. (Reproduced in part from ref 30 with permission.)

In the WHO classification IPMNs are divided into benign (IPMN adenoma), borderline (IPMN borderline) and malignant noninvasive (intraductal papillary-mucinous carcinoma, IPMC) or invasive (IPMC + invasion) categories according to the greatest degree of dysplasia present (*3*). IPMN adenomas are lined by epithelium composed of regular tall columnar cells demonstrating only slight or minimal atypia. IPMN borderline show moderate dysplasia with some nuclear crowding, nuclear enlargement and hyperchromatism plus an increased nucleocytoplasmic ratio and pseudostratification. Mitotic figures may be identified. In IPMC there is severe dysplasia with more loss of polarity, higher nucleocytoplasmic ratios, reduction in cytoplasmic mucin, cellular pleomorphism and more frequent mitotic figures (*3*, *9*). An invasive component is present in 20–40% of IPMN and may be in the form of mucinous noncystic carcinoma (40%) or conventional tubular ductal adenocarcinoma (60%) (Fig. 4.3) (*7*, *10*).

The grade of dysplasia commonly varies from area to area within IPMN (see Fig. 4.2D), hence it is important to sample these tumors thoroughly. For this reason, a recent consensus publication has recommended that all IPMN should be wholly

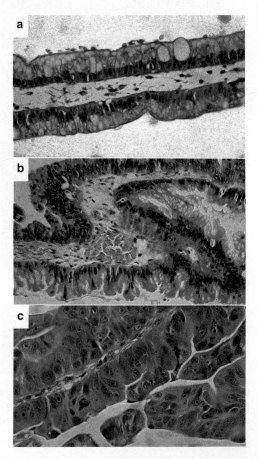

Fig. 4.3 High-power photomicrographs showing (**A**) IPMN adenoma, note goblet cells, (**B**) IPMN borderline, and (**C**) IPMN carcinoma, with visible atypical mitotic figure. (Reproduced in part from ref 30 with permission.)

embedded and examined microscopically to avoid missing areas of high-grade dysplasia or invasion (*1*).

Recently, Adsay and colleagues proposed the subclassification of IPMN into intestinal, pancreatobiliary, null, and mixed types on morphologic and immunohistochemical features (*7, 11*). The histologic subtypes varied in the grade of dysplasia present, the prevalence and type of associated invasive carcinoma (more commonly mucinous noncystic carcinoma with intestinal-type IPMN and tubular ductal adenocarcinoma with pancreatobiliary-type IPMN), and in the expression of CDX2, MUC2, and MUC1. There was a tendency for the pancreatobiliary-type IPMN to have a more aggressive clinical course while the null type was rarely associated with invasion (*11*). Similar subtypes were subsequently incorporated into a consensus subclassification of IPMN with Adsay's null-type being renamed as the gastric-type (Table 4.1, Fig. 4.4) (*12*). Interestingly, areas of lower-grade null/gastric-type epithelium are often associated with larger, higher-grade areas of other subtypes and it has been suggested that the null/gastric type epithelium may represent a common precursor to the other types (*11*).

Intraductal oncocytic papillary neoplasm is a closely related tumor that has recently been incorporated into the proposed consensus subclassification of IPMN

Table 4.1 Nomenclature and criteria for classification of four types of intraductal papillary-mucinous neoplasms of the pancreas

Type	Criteria	Atypia	MUC1	MUC2	MUC5AC
Gastric	Thick finger-like papillae, eosinophilic > basophilic cytoplasm, basally located nuclei. This type may have abundant flat areas.	Mild/ Low-grade	–	–	+
Intestinal	Villous papillae, basophilic > eosinophilic cytoplasm, enlarged oval and hyperchromatic nuclei with pseudostratification. This type may show low papillae consisting of cells with amphophilic cytoplasm.	Moderate or severe/ High-grade	–	+	+
Pancreatobiliary	Thin branching complex papillae, moderate eosinophilic cytoplasm, enlarged hyperchromatic nuclei.	Severe/ High-grade	+	–	+
Oncocytic	Thick branching complex papillae with intracellular and intraepithelial lumina, abundant eosinophilic (oncocytic) cytoplasm, large round nuclei with prominent nucleoli.	Severe/ High-grade	+	–	+

Reproduced from Furukawa et al., ref *12*, with permission.

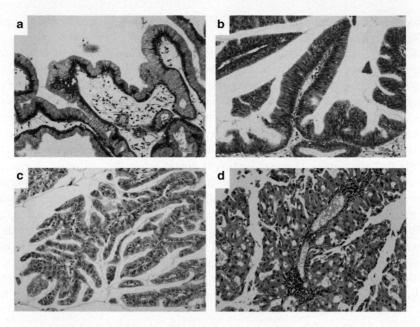

Fig. 4.4 Photomicrographs showing morphological appearance of (**A**) gastric-type IPMN, (**B**) intestinal-type IPMN, (**C**) pancreatobiliary-type IPMN, and (**D**) oncocytic-type IPMN. (Images courtesy of Dr. T. Furukawa, Tohoku University School of Medicine, Sendai, Japan, from ref. 12, with permission.)

as the oncocytic subtype (*12*). This tumor has a similar gross appearance to conventional IPMN and is histologically characterized by stratified oncocytic epithelial cells with eosinophilic finely granular cytoplasm. Small intraepithelial mucin-containing "lumina" are often prominent (*3, 13*).

4 Differential Diagnosis

Intraductal papillary mucinous neoplasm was often misdiagnosed as a mucinous cystic neoplasm (MCN) prior to the widespread recognition of IPMN in the late 1980s and early 1990s (*14*). IPMN often presents as a mucin-filled cystic mass like MCN and microscopically both lesions are lined by variably dysplastic, mucin secreting columnar epithelium. However, in MCN the papillae are generally less well developed and a characteristic cellular "ovarian" stroma is typically present (*3, 9*). Moreover, MCN usually occurs in women with a younger median age, are generally located in the tail or body of the pancreas, and rarely communicate with the pancreatic ductal system (*4, 15*).

Differentiating between IPMNs and some pancreatic intraepithelial neoplasia (PanIN) can also be problematic given that both lesions consist of intraductal neoplastic proliferations of mucin-producing columnar cells with a variable degree of papilla formation (1). Although PanIN typically arise in the small ducts, they may occasionally involve larger ducts. Conversely, although IPMNs generally arise in the larger ducts, they can involve smaller ducts. Indeed, both lesions may coexist in the one pancreas, possibly accounting for the development of pancreatic ductal carcinoma several years after "curative" resection for noninvasive IPMN and the presence of ductal adenocarcinoma distant from an IPMN (5, 7, 16, 17). A consensus conference in 2003 proposed revised definitions for these lesions with PanIN being characterized as a microscopic lesion usually involving ducts less than 5 mm in diameter, while IPMN is typically a grossly visible lesion greater than 10 mm in diameter arising from the main pancreatic duct or branch ducts (1). These new guidelines have resulted in more consistent classification and nomenclature of these lesions, although some distinctions, particularly with regard to grading, remain problematic (18).

5   Cytologic Diagnosis

The cytologic diagnosis of intraductal mucinous neoplasm has received increasing attention in the literature, particularly with more widespread use of endoscopic-guided fine-needle aspiration cytology (EUS-guided FNAC) in the preoperative investigation of cystic pancreatic lesions (19–26). However, there is considerable overlap in cytologic features between IPMN and other pancreatic lesions, especially MCN and mucinous ductal adenocarcinoma (19, 20, 24), and hence FNAC should always be correlated with the clinical presentation and imaging appearances. Reported values for the sensitivity of EUS-guided FNAC for the diagnosis of IPMN vary from 38 to 100%. Likewise, there is considerable variation in reported specificity, in one series it was 98%, although in another there were five false-positive diagnoses out of 18 cases (19, 20, 22, 26). These variations probably reflect a number of factors including the skill of the endoscopic aspirator and adequacy of the sample, the experience of the cytopathologist, whether the cytopathologist attends the FNA procedure, the use of adjunct techniques such as liquid-based collection methods, and the rigor with which the clinicopathologic correlation is performed (20, 22, 24). The most consistent cytologic finding in IPMN is abundant thick colloid-like mucin, whereas the presence of papilliform fragments and intracellular mucin appear to be the most specific features (19, 20).

Studies of the preoperative grading of IPMN utilizing cytology have demonstrated features that correlate with moderate dysplasia (tight epithelial clusters) or carcinoma in situ (abundant background inflammation and parachromatin clearing). The presence of necrosis has been found to be strongly suggestive of invasion (25). The sensitivity of EUS-guided FNAC for the prediction of malignancy in IPMN is ~60%, whereas the specificity is 100% (19, 21). However, the sensitivity of FNAC is significantly limited by the focal nature of malignancy in many IPMN with the attendant risk of sampling error leading to underestimation of tumour grade (19, 23).

Brushing and biopsy specimens obtained during endoscopic retrograde pancreatography have also been utilized for the diagnosis and grading of IPMN with similar results to EUS-guided FNAC (23). Ultimately, the accuracy of cytologic diagnosis and its value as a tool in the preoperative assessment of IPMN is dependent on close correlation with the clinical and imaging information.

6 Frozen Section Diagnosis

Frozen section examination has been advocated principally for assessment of the pancreatic transection margin during resection of intraductal papillary mucinous neoplasms. Recent studies have reported that routine frozen section examination during pancreatico-duodenectomy or distal pancreatectomy resulted in the detection of IPMN at the resection margin, followed by additional resection, in 23–30% of patients (27, 28). Discrepancy between frozen section and subsequent definitive paraffin section examination was low and there was no recurrence of noninvasive IPMN (27–29). However, given that a small proportion of IPMN are multifocal within the pancreatic duct system, inevitably some patients will still have undetected tumor in the pancreatic remnant even when the surgical resection margin is clear (4–6, 27).

7 Molecular Pathology of IPMN

A better understanding of the molecular pathology of IPMN will assist in defining the natural history of these lesions, most importantly the risk of invasive malignancy, and facilitate the development of novel diagnostic and therapeutic strategies. IPMN demonstrate molecular genetic aberrations of some oncogenes and tumor suppressor genes common to premalignant lesions and cancers of other organs, including activating K-ras mutations, p53 mutation, cyclin D1 overexpression and loss of p16[INK4A] expression (30). Molecular aberrations common to IPMN, PanIN and invasive ductal adenocarcinoma include activating K-ras mutation (31), p53 protein accumulation (8, 31, 32), cyclin D1 overexpression, loss of p16[INK4A] expression (32), HER-2/neu overexpression and aberrant expression of oncofetal antigens such as CEA, CA19-9, and DUPAN-2 (33) have been identified in IPMN and invasive carcinoma. Chromosomal aberrations associated with IPMN and invasive carcinoma of the pancreas also share a similar profile (34, 35). Heterogeneity of allelic loss within IPMN lesions suggests progression within IPMN (34, 35), and as a consequence present further difficulties in developing diagnostic strategies. IPMNs do not commonly demonstrate microsatellite instability (36). Comparison of proliferative indices in IPMN with normal ductal cells and invasive cancer, using immunohistochemistry for Ki-67 and proliferating cell nuclear antigen (PCNA), demonstrates a progressive increase from IPMN adenoma to IPMN borderline, to

IPMC, through to invasive carcinoma (8). Similarly, aberrations in cell cycle regulatory genes increase in frequency with increasing dysplasia in IPMN and appear to be similar to those in PanIN lesions with an equivalent degree of dysplasia (32). High telomerase activity is detectable in IPMC (37) and PC, as is COX-2 expression (38). Furthermore, PanIN lesions found in association with IPMN also demonstrate similar molecular aberrations (17). There are two notable differences in ductal adenocarcinomas that arise from IPMN compared to those that do not. First, approximately 40% of carcinomas arising from IPMN are of the mucinous noncystic (colloid) type with 60% being of the tubular type in contrast to carcinomas arising without IPMN where over 95% are of the tubular type (7, 9, 10). Second, <10% of carcinomas arising from IPMN demonstrate loss of DPC4/Smad4 (39) expression compared to 55% of non-IPMN related carcinomas (40, 41). However, expression of DPC4/Smad4 may be related to the type of IPMN and carcinoma that develops from the IPMN, with tubular-type carcinomas accounting for the vast majority of loss of DPC4/Smad4 expression seen in invasive carcinoma associated with IPMN (32).

Potentially the greatest insights into the underlying molecular events that contribute to the development of IPMN come from recent studies that have classified IPMN into the four distinct morphological groups described earlier, based on epithelial phenotype (gastric, intestinal, pancreatobiliary and oncocytic; see Table 4.1) (12). Although oncocytic-type IPMN are a distinct group, the other three suggest that epithelial transdifferentiation, which occurs in precursor lesions of other gastrointestinal tract cancer, notably the esophagus (Barrett's esophagus) and stomach (intestinal metaplasia), may occur in the development of IPMN. Recent studies have shown that molecular mechanisms important in vertebrate pancreas development are also important in the evolution of PanIN. During embryogenesis, hedgehog signaling regulates endodermal cell fate with an absence of hedgehog expression differentiating the nascent pancreas from the primitive gut (42). Activation of hedgehog signalling is a feature of PanIN (43) with misexpression of hedgehog ligand in murine pancreas leading to the evolution of PanIN (44). Although a potential role for hedgehog signalling in IPMN is yet to be reported, the morphologic appearances of IPMN show features of gastrointestinal epithelium, suggesting that transdifferentiation may occur. Expression of the transcription factors CDX1 and/or 2 in hedgehog expressing endoderm appears to promote intestinal epithelial differentiation (45), whereas the lack of CDX and the presence of Sox2 and/or GATA5 promotes gastric epithelial differentiation (46). Intestinal-type IPMN demonstrate CDX2 and MUC2 expression, which is transcriptionally regulated by CDX (46) further supporting transdifferentiation of pancreatic ductal epithelium in the evolution of IPMN. Gastric-type IPMN do not express CDX2 or MUC2, and the pancreatobiliary-type IPMN express neither, but express MUC1, whereas the other two do not. Finally, PanIN lesions appear to share some similar molecular aberrations with pancreatobiliary-type IPMN in that PanIN express MUC1 and MUC5AC (47), but not CDX or MUC2 (43).

There is some evidence to suggest that gastric-type IPMN are associated with only mild/low-grade atypia, intestinal-type IPMN with moderate to severe atypia, and that pancreatobiliary and oncocytic-type IPMN with severe atypia (*11*, *12*). This putative association, together with the occurrence of mixed IPMN, reported genetic heterogeneity of IPMN (*34*), and the observation that the majority of invasive carcinoma arise in association with higher-grade IPMN, suggests that there may be progression of IPMN from IPMN adenoma, through IPMN borderline to IPMC and subsequent invasive carcinoma. Gastric-type IPMN usually demonstrate mild atypia and may represent a common precursor that progresses through IPMN borderline and IPMC to invasive carcinoma. Current research efforts investigating molecular genetic aberrations will lead to a better understanding of the molecular evolution of IPMN, allowing more reliable definition of their natural history as well as the development of novel strategies for the early detection of IPMN, and the determination of the risk of progression to invasive carcinoma for an individual IPMN.

References

1. Hruban RH, Takaori K, Klimstra DS, et al. An illustrated consensus on the classification of pancreatic intraepithelial neoplasia and intraductal papillary mucinous neoplasms. Am J Surg Pathol 2004, 28:977–987.
2. Furukawa T, Takahashi T, Kobari M, et al. The mucus-hypersecreting tumor of the pancreas. development and extension visualised by three-dimensional computerised mapping. Cancer 1992, 70:1505–1513.
3. Longnecker DS, Hruban RH, Adler G, et al. Intraductal papillary-mucinous neoplasms of the pancreas. In: (Hamilton SR, Aaltonen LA, eds.) WHO classification of tumours. pathology and genetics. Tumours of the digestive system. Lyon, IARC Press, 2000:237–240.
4. Milchgrub S, Campuzano M, Casillas J, et al. Intraductal carcinoma of the pancreas. Cancer 1992, 69:651–656.
5. Sho M, Nakajima Y, Kanehiro H, et al. Pattern of recurrence after resection for intraductal papillary mucinous tumors of the pancreas. World J Surg 1998, 22:874–878.
6. Kitagawa Y, Unger TA, Taylor S, et al. Mucus is a predictor of better prognosis and survival in patients with intraductal papillary mucinous tumor of the pancreas. J Gastrointest Surg 2003, 7:12–18; discussion 18–19.
7. Adsay NV, Conlon KC, Zee SY, et al. Intraductal papillary-mucinous neoplasms of the pancreas: an analysis of in situ and invasive carcinomas in 28 patients. Cancer 2002, 94:62–77.
8. Kench JG, Eckstein RP, Smith RC. Intraductal papillary-mucinous neoplasm of the pancreas: a report of five cases with immunohistochemical findings. Pathology 1997, 29:7–11.
9. Solcia E, Capella C, Kloppel G. Tumors of the exocrine pancreas In: Rosai J, Sobin L series editors. Atlas of tumor pathology. Fascicle 20, 3rd series. Tumors of the pancreas. Washington, AFIP 1997, 53–64.
10. Sohn TA, Yeo CJ, Cameron JL, et al. Intraductal papillary mucinous neoplasms of the pancreas: an updated experience. Ann Surg 2004, 239:788–797; discussion 797–799.
11. Adsay NV, Merati K, Iacobuzio-Donahue C, et al. Pathologically and biologically distinct types of epithelium in intraductal papillary mucinous neoplasms: delineation of an "intestinal" pathway of carcinogenesis in the pancreas. Am J Surg Pathol 2004, 28:839–848.
12. Furukawa T, Kloppel G, Adsay NV, et al. Classification of types of intraductal papillary-mucinous neoplasm of the pancreas: a consensus study. Virchows Arch 2005, 447:794–799.
13. Adsay NV, Adair CF, Heffess CS, et al. Intraductal oncocytic papillary neoplasms of the pancreas. Am J Surg Pathol 1996, 20:980–994.
14. Warshaw AL. Mucinous cystic tumors and mucinous ductal ectasia of the pancreas. Gastrointest Endosc 1991, 37:199–201.

15. Warshaw AL, Compton CC, Lewandrowski K, et al. Cystic tumors of the pancreas. New clinical, radiologic, and pathologic observations in 67 patients. Ann Surg 1990, 212:432–443; discussion 444–445.
16. Holme JB, Jacobsen NO, Rokkjaer M, et al. Total pancreatectomy in six patients with intraductal papillary mucinous tumour of the pancreas: the treatment of choice. HPB 2001, 3:257–262.
17. Biankin AV, Kench JG, Biankin SA, et al. Pancreatic intraepithelial neoplasia in association with intraductal papillary mucinous neoplasms of the pancreas: implications for disease progression and recurrence. Am J Surg Pathol 2004, 28:1184–1192.
18. Longnecker DS, Adsay NV, Fernandez-del Castillo C, et al. Histopathological diagnosis of pancreatic intraepithelial neoplasia and intraductal papillary-mucinous neoplasms: interobserver agreement. Pancreas 2005, 31:344–349.
19. Layfield LJ, Cramer H. Fine-needle aspiration cytology of intraductal papillary-mucinous tumors: a retrospective analysis. Diagn Cytopathol 2005, 32:16–20.
20. Frossard JL, Amouyal P, Amouyal G, et al. Performance of endosonography-guided fine needle aspiration and biopsy in the diagnosis of pancreatic cystic lesions. Am J Gastroenterol 2003, 98:1516–1524.
21. Brandwein SL, Farrell JJ, Centeno BA, et al. Detection and tumor staging of malignancy in cystic, intraductal, and solid tumors of the pancreas by EUS. Gastrointest Endosc 2001, 53:722–727.
22. Stelow EB, Stanley MW, Bardales RH, et al. Intraductal papillary-mucinous neoplasm of the pancreas. The findings and limitations of cytologic samples obtained by endoscopic ultrasound-guided fine-needle aspiration. Am J Clin Pathol 2003, 120:398–404.
23. Maire F, Couvelard A, Hammel P, et al. Intraductal papillary mucinous tumors of the pancreas: the preoperative value of cytologic and histopathologic diagnosis. Gastrointest Endosc 2003, 58:701–706.
24. Stelow EB, Bardales RH, Stanley MW. Pitfalls in endoscopic ultrasound-guided fine-needle aspiration and how to avoid them. Adv Anat Pathol 2005, 12:62–73.
25. Michaels PJ, Brachtel EF, Bounds BC, et al. Intraductal papillary mucinous neoplasm of the pancreas: cytologic features predict histologic grade. Cancer 2006, 108:163–173.
26. Emerson RE, Randolph ML, Cramer HM. Endoscopic ultrasound-guided fine-needle aspiration cytology diagnosis of intraductal papillary mucinous neoplasm of the pancreas is highly predictive of pancreatic neoplasia. Diagn Cytopathol 2006, 34:457–462.
27. Couvelard A, Sauvanet A, Kianmanesh R, et al. Frozen sectioning of the pancreatic cut surface during resection of intraductal papillary mucinous neoplasms of the pancreas is useful and reliable: a prospective evaluation. Ann Surg 2005, 242:774–778, discussion 778–780.
28. Gigot JF, Deprez P, Sempoux C, et al. Surgical management of intraductal papillary mucinous tumors of the pancreas: the role of routine frozen section of the surgical margin, intraoperative endoscopic staged biopsies of the Wirsung duct, and pancreaticogastric anastomosis. Arch Surg 2001, 136:1256–1262.
29. Paye F, Sauvanet A, Terris B, et al. Intraductal papillary mucinous tumors of the pancreas: pancreatic resections guided by preoperative morphological assessment and intraoperative frozen section examination. Surgery 2000, 127:536–544.
30. Biankin AV, Kench JG, Biankin SA, et al. Molecular pathogenesis of precursor lesions of pancreatic ductal adenocarcinoma. Pathology 2003, 35:14–24.
31. Satoh K, Shimosegawa T, Moriizumi S, et al. K-ras mutation and p53 protein accumulation in intraductal mucin-hypersecreting neoplasms of the pancreas. Pancreas 1996, 12:362–368.
32. Biankin AV, Biankin SA, Kench JG, et al. Aberrant p16INK4A and *DPC4*/Smad4 expression in intraductal papillary mucinus tumours of the pancreas is associated with invasive ductal adenocarcinoma. Gut 2002, 50:861–868.
33. Terada T, Ohta T, Nakanuma Y. Expression of oncogene products, anti-oncogene products and oncofetal antigens in intraductal papillary-mucinous neoplasm of the pancreas. Histopathology 1996, 29:355–361.

34. Fujii H, Inagaki M, Kasai S, et al. Genetic progression and heterogeneity in intraductal papillary-mucinous neoplasms of the pancreas. Am J Pathol 1997, 151:1447–1454.
35. Soldini D, Gugger M, Burckhardt E, et al. Progressive genomic alterations in intraductal papillary mucinous tumours of the pancreas and morphologically similar lesions of the pancreatic ducts. J Pathol 2003, 199:453–461.
36. Luttges J, Beyser K, Pust S, et al. Pancreatic mucinous noncystic (colloid) carcinomas and intraductal papillary mucinous carcinomas are usually microsatellite stable. Mod Pathol 2003, 16:537–542.
37. Inoue H, Tsuchida A, Kawasaki Y, et al. Preoperative diagnosis of intraductal papillary-mucinous tumors of the pancreas with attention to telomerase activity. Cancer 2001, 91:35–41.
38. Niijima M, Yamaguchi T, Ishihara T, et al. Immunohistochemical analysis and in situ hybridization of cyclooxygenase-2 expression in intraductal papillary-mucinous tumors of the pancreas. Cancer 2002, 94:1565–1573.
39. Iacobuzio-Donahue CA, Klimstra DS, Adsay NV, et al. Dpc-4 protein is expressed in virtually all human intraductal papillary mucinous neoplasms of the pancreas: comparison with conventional ductal adenocarcinomas. Am J Pathol 2000, 157:755–761.
40. Hruban RH, Offerhaus GJ, Kern SE, et al. Tumor-suppressor genes in pancreatic cancer. J Hepato-Biliary-Panc Surg 1998, 5:383–391.
41. Biankin AV, Kench JG, Morey AL, et al. Overexpression of p21WAF1/CIP1 is an early event in the development of pancreatic intraepithelial neoplasia. Cancer Res 2001, 61:8830–8837.
42. Hebrok M, Kim SK, St Jacques B, et al. Regulation of pancreas development by hedgehog signaling. Development 2000, 127:4905–4913.
43. Prasad NB, Biankin AV, Fukushima N, et al. Gene expression profiles in pancreatic intraepithelial neoplasia reflect the effects of Hedgehog signaling on pancreatic ductal epithelial cells. Cancer Res 2005, 65:1619–1626.
44. Thayer SP, Di Magliano MP, Heiser PW, et al. Hedgehog is an early and late mediator of pancreatic cancer tumorigenesis. Nature 2003, 425:851–856.
45. Silberg DG, Sullivan J, Kang E, et al. Cdx2 ectopic expression induces gastric intestinal metaplasia in transgenic mice. Gastroenterology 2002, 122:689–696.
46. Tsukamoto T, Inada K, Tanaka H, et al. Down-regulation of a gastric transcription factor, Sox2, and ectopic expression of intestinal homeobox genes, Cdx1 and Cdx2: inverse correlation during progression from gastric/intestinal-mixed to complete intestinal metaplasia. J Cancer Res Clin Oncol 2003, 130:135–145.
47. Kim GE, Bae HI, Park HU, et al. Aberrant expression of MUC5AC and MUC6 gastric mucins and sialyl Tn antigen in intraepithelial neoplasms of the pancreas. Gastroenterology 2002, 123:1052–1060.

Chapter 5
Familial Pancreatic Cancer

Kieran A. Brune and Alison P. Klein

1 Introduction

In 2008, 37,680 individuals in the United States will be diagnosed with pancreatic cancer (*1*) and approximately 5–10% of these cases will have a familial basis (*2*). Because of the location of the pancreas deep in the abdominal cavity, detection of this disease in its early stages is difficult such that over 80% of pancreatic cancers have metastasized prior to diagnosis. For this reason, it is estimated that in 2008, 34,290 individuals in the United States will die from the disease this year, making the death rate from pancreatic cancer similar to its incidence. Therefore, it is important to identify individuals who are at high risk, such as those with a family history, as these patients may benefit from early detection screening, which may reduce the mortality of this disease. Furthermore, understanding the genetic basis of both inherited and noninherited pancreatic cancer will provide great insight into the etiology of this cancer.

Little is known about the etiology of pancreatic cancer, but the two best established risk factors for the development of this cancer include cigarette smoking and a family history of pancreatic cancer. The following chapter provides a brief overview of the general epidemiology of pancreatic cancer and then focuses on the role of familial risk in the development of this disease.

2 Epidemiology and Biology

Pancreatic cancer is the fourth leading cause of cancer death in the United States and represents 2% of cancer diagnoses worldwide but leads to 5% of all cancer deaths (*1*). The overall age-adjusted incidence rate for the United States was 11.3/100,000 in 2000–2003 (*3*). The incidence of pancreatic cancer is higher in developed nations versus developing nations, but a portion of this difference may be attributable to the difficulty in diagnosing this disease, and therefore under reporting of disease incidence in nations that lack diagnostic equipment (*4*). However, differences in the prevalence of known and suspected risk factors such as cigarette smoking, diabetes, obesity, and dietary factors, may also play a role.

A.M. Lowy et al. (eds.), *Pancreatic Cancer.*
doi: 10.1007/978-0-387-69252-4, © Springer Science+Business Media, LLC 2008

The 5-year survival rate for pancreatic cancer is less than 5%, the poorest of any major cancer sites (1). Pancreatic cancer is primarily a cancer of older individuals. In the United States, the median age at diagnosis is 72, and 69% of the patients over the age of 65 at diagnosis (3). Pancreatic cancer is slightly more common in men than women; however, as the smoking prevalance between men and women equalizes, the difference in incidence decreases. Incidence is also greater in the African-American population (14.9/100,000) than in Caucasian Americans (11.2/100,000). Native American and Hispanic-American individuals have lower rates at around 10.8 per 100,000 and 10.3 per 100,000, respectively. Asian Americans have the lowest incident rate at 9 per 100,000 (3).

3   Risk Factors

In addition to the inherited risk factors that will be discussed in detail in the next section, there are known and suggested environmental risk factors for pancreatic cancer.

The most consistent and well-established environmental risk factor is cigarette smoking. Cigarette smoking has been estimated to account for 25–35% of this disease (5) and the risk of pancreatic cancer in current smokers is about two- to threefold higher than that of nonsmokers (5–7). There also appears to be a dose–response relationship with increasing amount smoked or increasing the duration of the smoking habit (5, 8, 9). Quitting smoking reduces this risk such that among former smokers the risk of dying from pancreatic cancer decreases with the increasing numbers of years since quitting (10).

Type II diabetes (11), pancreatitis (12), and obesity (13), as well as certain occupational exposures have also been suggested to increase the risk pancreatic cancer. Although approximately 80% of persons who have been diagnosed with pancreatic cancer have impaired glucose metabolism, impaired glucose tolerance, or diabetes mellitus, it is unclear what proportion of this impairment in glucose tolerance/metabolism is the causative reason of the cancer and what proportion is a consequence of a growing lesion in the pancreas. Among patients with newly diagnosed diabetes, 0.85% went on to be diagnosed with pancreatic cancer within 3 years of their diabetes diagnoses (14), supporting diabetes as an early symptom of pancreatic cancer. By contrast, type II diabetes of at least 5 years duration has been shown to increase the risk of pancreatic cancer twofold (11). A large US prospective cohort study of 467,922 men and 588,321 women, reported type II diabetes was significantly associated with pancreatic cancer in men (RR = 1.48, 95% CI: 1.27, 1.73) and women (RR = 1.44, 95% CI: 1.21, 1.72) (15).

Chronic pancreatitis, a progressive inflammatory disorder of the pancreas, has also been associated with an increased risk of pancreatic cancer (16). Chronic pancreatitis can be caused by alcohol use and genes as well as other factors. Lowenfels et al. found that the cumulative incidence of pancreatic cancer in individuals with alcohol induced pancreatitis was 1.8% and 4.0% 10 and 20 years after a diagnosis of chronic pancreatitis (*16*). In addition, Lowenfels found that the cumulative life-time cumulative incidence (to the age of 70) of developing pancreatic cancer in patients with hereditary chronic pancreatitis was 40% (*12*). Cigarette smoking seems to further increase this risk (*17*).

The risk of pancreatic cancer has been shown to increase as body mass index increases. Examination of data the Nurses' Health Study and the Health Professionals follow-up study demonstrated a relative risk of pancreatic cancer is 1.72 (95% CI 1.19–2.48) in individuals with a BMI >30 kg/m^2 compared to individuals with a BMI <23 kg/m^2. Similar effect was observed when meta-analysis of data from several European cohort studies was performed (*18*).

4 Case Reports and Registries

One of the greatest risk factors for pancreatic cancer is having a family history of this cancer. It is estimated that up to 10% of pancreatic cancers have a familial basis (*2*).

In 1973, MacDermott and Kramer described a family in which four of six sib-lings developed pancreatic cancer (*19*). This first report was followed by reports of other families (*20, 21*) with a clustering of pancreatic cancer. One of the largest clusterings was reported by Evans and colleagues in which nine cases of pancreatic cancer were identified among 50 individuals in four generations (*22*).

Registries of families with multiple cases of pancreatic cancer were created to gain a better understanding of the familial clustering of pancreatic cancer. One of the largest of these registries is the National Familial Pancreas Tumor Registry (NFPTR). The NFPTR was created at Johns Hopkins in 1994 and as of March 5, 2008 2042 families (Table 5.1) from around the world, including the United States, Europe, and Asia, have enrolled in the NFPTR. The NFPTR helped to define "Familial Pancreatic Cancer" as a kindred in which a pair of first-degree relatives (parents, siblings, children) are affected (*23*). Of the over 2,739 families enrolled in the NFPTR, 961 of these families meet this definition of familial pancreatic cancer. Within these familial kindreds, the number of affected family members range from

Table 5.1 Kindreds enrolled in the national familial pancreas tumor registry as of 3/5/2008

Familial kindreds	961
Nonfamilial kindreds	1,778
Total	2,739

Breakdown of Number of Affected members in Familial Kindreds	
5 or More pancreatic cancers	33
4 Pancreatic cancers	73
3 Pancreatic cancers	237
2 Pancreatic cancers	618

two to seven. For the remaining 1,778 families, at least one family member has been diagnosed with pancreatic cancer but there is not a pair of affected first degree relatives (these kindred are referred to as nonfamilial or sporadic pancreatic cancer kindreds).

In 2000, the Pancreatic Cancer Genetic Epidemiology Consortium (PACGENE) was created to combine the resources of several pancreatic cancer research centers in an effort to identify pancreatic cancer susceptibility genes using linkage methods (24). Because of the rarity of families with multiple cases of pancreatic cancer on whom DNA samples are available on affected pedigree members (25), collaboration of multiple pancreatic cancer family registries is critical to the success of this study.

5   Case-Control Studies

Numerous case-control studies have demonstrated that a family history of pancreatic cancer is associated with an increased risk of pancreatic cancer (Table 5.2). For example, Falk et al. performed a case-control study in Louisiana from 1979 to 1983. They found an increased risk of pancreatic cancer among individuals who reported a close relative with pancreatic cancer, reporting an odds ratio (OR) of 5.25, (95% CI: 2.08–13.21) (8). Ghadirian et al. performed a population based case-control study involving 179 cases and 179 controls matched for age, sex, and language. They found 7.8% of the pancreatic cancer patients reported a positive family history of the disease as compared with only 0.6% among controls, which translated to a 13-fold difference between cases and controls. It is important to note that the authors also concluded that this difference in risk was most likely not due to environmental factors alone but that hereditary factors must play an important role in the etiology of pancreatic cancer (26). Similarly, Fernandez et al. found there was a significant association between family history of pancreatic cancer and the risk of this cancer (OR = 2.8; 95% CI 1.3–6.3) (27) when he studied a group of cases and controls from Northern Italy.

Moreover, in a study of 484 cases and 2,099 controls, ascertained through population based registries in three regions of the United States (Atlanta, Detroit, and

Table 5.2   Case-control studies of pancreatic cancer risk associated with family history

	Study population	Results	Reference
Falk et al.	363 Cases and 1,234 controls	OR = 5.3 (2.1–13.2)	8
Ghadirian et al.	179 Cases and 179 controls	OR = 13-fold ($p < 0.001$)[a]	71
Fernandez et al.	362 Cases and 1,408 controls	OR = 2.8 (1.3–6.3)[b]	72
Silverman et al.	484 Cases and 2,099 controls	OR = 3.2 (1.8–5.6)	6
Schenk et al.	247 Cases and 420 controls	RR = 2.5 (1.3–4.7)[c]	7

[a]Age, sex, and language (French) matched.
[b]Adjusted for tobacco, dietary factors, and history of diabetes and pancreatitis, crude OR 3.0.
[c]Adjusted for age, sex, ethnicity, ever smoking, proband ever smoking, diabetes, age of proband.

New Jersey), it was found that individuals with a first degree relative of pancreatic
cancer had an OR of 3.2 (95% CI 1.8–5.6), and the risk was higher (OR = 3.6; 95%
CI 1.5–8.7) among those with an affected sibling compared to those with an
affected parent (OR = 2.6; 95% CI 1.2–5.4). A higher risk due to family history was
apparent in individuals who smoked for >20 years (OR = 5.3; 95% CI 2.1–13.4)
compared to individuals who did not smoke or smoked for <20 years (OR = 2.2;
95% CI 1.0–7.9) (6). Schenk et al. studied a group of 247 cases and 420 population-based controls and found that a family history of pancreatic cancer approximately doubled the risk of developing pancreatic cancer (RR = 2.49; 95% CI
1.32–4.69) (7).

6   Prospective Studies

Prospective studies allow for assesment of family history prior to the development of
cancer and thus are not biased by differential recall of family history in individuals
with and without pancreatic cancer. Table 5.3 summarzes cohort studies of pancreatic
cancer. Coughlin et al. followed a cohort of 483,109 men and 619,199 as part of the
American Cancer Society's Cancer Prevention Study II to evaluate the risk factors for
pancreatic cancer. After adjusting for age, the relative risk of pancreatic cancer in
individuals who reported a positive family history of pancreatic cancer at baseline
was 1.5 (95% CI 1.1–2.1) (10). This risk estimate was not changed when further
adjusted for history of gallstones, body mass index, smoking history, alcohol consumption, history of diabetes, and several dietary factors.

A study of over 10.2 million people using the Swedish registry reported a 1.73-
fold increased risk of developing pancreatic cancer (28). Similar results were
observed in the Icelandic population. In a study of 678,500 individuals there was a
reported relative risk of 2.33 (90% CI 1.83–2.96) of developing pancreatic cancer
among individuals with a first-degree relative with pancreatic cancer compared to
these without. Risk was elevated, although not significantly, among individuals
with a second-, third-, or fourth-degree relative with pancreatic cancer (29).

Table 5.3 Cohort studies of pancreatic cancer risk associated with family history

Study location	Demographics	Result	Reference
United States	3,751 cases among 1,102,308 individuals	RR = 1.5 (1.1–2.1)[a]	10
Sweden	21,000 cases among 10.2 million individuals	RR = 1.73	28
Iceland	930 cases among 687,500 individuals	RR2 = 2.33 (90% CI 1t.83–2.96)	29

[a]Adjusted for dietary factors, BMI, gallstone history, cholecystectomy history, diabetes, age, race, years of education.

Klein et al. studied 5,179 individuals from 838 kindreds enrolled in the NFPTR. The study period ran from the time of entry into the NFPTR until the end of 2002 and included over 14,000 person-years of follow-up. The number of incident pancreatic cancers that developed in these kindreds was compared to the number expected based on the Surveillance, Epidemiology, and End Results (SEER) database. The standardized incidence ratio (SIR) for pancreatic cancer was significantly higher in familial pancreatic cancer (FPC) kindreds (9.0; 95% CI 4.5–16.1) but not in sporadic pancreatic cancer kindreds (1.8; 95% CI 0.22–6.4). The risk in FPC kindreds was elevated in individuals with three (32.0-fold increased risk; 95% CI 10.2–74.7), two (6.4-fold increased risk; 95% CI 1.8–6.4), or one (4.6-fold increased risk; 95% CI 0.5–16.4) first-degree relative(s) with pancreatic cancer, but was not elevated in 369 spouses or genetically unrelated individuals (30). Consistent with previous studies, the risk was further increased in smokers as compared to nonsmokers (30).

These large prospective studies stress the importance of family history in pancreatic cancer and highlight that genetic factors do play a role in the development of some pancreatic cancers.

7   Precursor Lesions in Familial PC

Precursor lesions to familial pancreatic cancer have not been well characterized; however, two recent studies have begun to examine early changes in the pancreas among individuals with a family history of pancreatic cancer, providing some insight into the biology of familial pancreatic cancer. Brune et al. studied resection specimens from 8 high-risk individuals from familial pancreatic cancer kindreds enrolled in the Cancer of the Pancreas Screening Study (CAPS) who were found to have early pancreatic neoplasia after screening with endoscopic ultrasound (EUS) and CT scan (37, 38). In all eight pancreata, PanINs ranging in grade from PanIN 1 to PanIN 3, were identified, with the majority being PanIN 1 and PanIN 2. Overall, PanINs were significantly more common in the eight cases (mean of 10.7% of the duct profiles) than in the age-matched controls (mean 1.9%). Additionally, IPMNs were identified in four of the eight cases, including two pancreata each having two distinct IPMNs. Lobular parenchymal atrophy was associated with the IPMNs and the PanINs, including the low-grade PanIN-1 lesions. This study concluded that some individuals with a strong family history of pancreatic cancer develop multifocal, noninvasive epithelial precursor lesions of the pancreas, which can include obstructive lobular atrophy, which is likely the source of the chronic pancreatitis-like changes observed by imaging studies in these individuals (39).

Meckler et al. noted similar changes in the pancreata resected from 11 individuals from a kindred with an extensive history of pancreatic cancer and pancreatic insufficiency. In particular, they noted fibrocystic lobulocentric pancreatic atrophy that was patchy to diffuse in distribution. Again they noted PanINs that ranged in severity from PanIN 2 to PanIN 3 (40).

Table 5.4 Known genetic syndromes associated with an increased risk of pancreatic cancer

Syndrome	Gene (location)	Increased risk of pancreatic cancer	Estimated cumulative incidence of pancreatic cancer by age 70	References
No history	—	RR = 1	0.5%	
Hereditary breast and ovarian cancer	BRCA2 (13q12–q13)	3.5–10x	5%	41–44
FAMMM1	p16 (9p21)	9–38x	5–19%	45, 47
Peutz-Jeghers syndrome	STK11/LKB1 (19p13)	75–132x	30–60%	52, 73
HNPCC2	hMLH1; hMSH2	?	?	53
Hereditary pancreatitis	PRSS1 (7q35)	50–80x	25–40%	12, 17, 74, 75

FAMMM, familial atypical multiple mole and melanoma; 2HNPCC, hereditary nonpolyposis colorectal cancer.

8 Known Genetic Syndromes

An increased risk of pancreatic cancer has been demonstrated for several known genetic syndromes, for which causative genes have been identified. These syndromes include familial breast cancer, familial atypical multiple mole and melanoma, Peutz-Jeghers syndrome (PJS), hereditary nonpolyposis colorectal cancer syndrome (HNPCC), and hereditary chronic pancreatitis. Of these syndromes, familial breast cancer due to BRCA2, accounts for the largest portion of the familial clustering of pancreatic cancer. Each of these syndromes is described in more detail in the following paragraphs (Table 5.4).

9 Hereditary Breast Cancer

BRCA2 is a tumor suppressor gene located on chromosome 13q. Germline mutations in the BRCA2 gene have been implicated in 7% of apparently sporadic pancreatic cancers (41) and 12–17% of familial pancreatic cancers (42–44). Murphy et al. reported that five of 29 pancreatic cancer patients from families with at least three pancreatic cancer cases harbored deleterious mutations in the BRCA2 gene (43). Similarly, Hahn et al. found germline BRCA2 gene mutations in three of 26 (12%) European pancreatic cancer patients from families with two or more pancreatic cancer cases (42). Remarkably, in both studies, many of the kindreds that harbored deleterious mutations did not present as typical hereditary breast cancer families highlighting the fact that germline BRCA2 mutations can not be ruled out as a cause of familial pancreatic cancer even among patients with no family history of breast or ovarian cancer.

(*60*). Since the findings are limited to one familial pancreatic cancer kindred further studies need to be done to evaluate the importance of palladin in other familial pancreatic cancer kindreds. Other studies have been unable to replicate linkage to the 4q region for pancreatic cancer. Earl et al. examined this region in a set of European Familial Pancreatic cancer kindreds and did not replicate linkage to this region (*61*). Similarly, Klein et al.'s study of 42 kindreds enrolled in the PACGENE Consortium could not confirm linkage to the 4q region (*62*). However, because it is likely that pancreatic cancer is a genetically heterogeneous disease both studies could not rule out the possibility that a subset of families may be linked to the 4q region (*61, 62*).

15 Segregation Analysis

These known genetic syndromes account for <20% of the familial clustering of pancreatic cancer, suggesting the possibility of another gene or genes important in the development of familial pancreatic cancer. Indeed, segregation analysis of 287 families recruited from The Johns Hopkins Medical Institutions showed major evidence of a gene that influenced the development of pancreatic cancer in some families. From this study it was estimated that 7/1,000 individuals were estimated to carry this high-risk gene, which confers a lifetime (age 85) risk of pancreatic cancer of 32% (*63*).

16 Risk Assessment and Genetic Counseling

Clinical genetic testing is available for several of the known genetic syndromes including *BRCA2*, FAMMM, PJS, HNPCC, and hereditary pancreatitis, and individuals from familial pancreatic cancer kindreds can be tested to determine if they have inherited mutations in one of these genes. Individuals found to carry a mutation that increases the risk of developing pancreatic cancer may benefit from close surveillance. However, since the majority of familial aggregation of pancreatic cancer is not due to mutations in these known genes, predictive testing will not be useful for most families. A study by Axilbund et al. examined the benefits of genetic counseling in the absence of predictive testing among individuals at high-risk of developing pancreatic cancer due to their family history. More than 93% of the participants believed that genetic counseling was helpful despite the fact that no gene had yet been identified (*64*).

In conjuction with genetic counseling risk prediction models, such as PancPRO, a Mendelian risk prediction tool for pancreatic cancer can provide accurate assesment of pancreatic cancer risk. PancPRO software is open source and available free of charge via the Bayes Mendel (*66*) or CancerGene (*67*).

17 Screening

Having established that there is strong evidence supporting the concept of familial pancreatic cancer, the next questions become what individuals are most at risk of developing pancreatic cancer and how do we screen these at risk individuals. Individuals harboring a germline mutation in one of the genes associated with the described syndromes are at an increased risk and may benefit from future surveillance of their pancreas. In addition, the prospective study done by Klein et al. established that individuals with two or more affected first-degree relatives are at a significantly increased risk of developing this cancer (*30*) and therefore may benefit from surveillance as well.

Canto et al. have shown that detection of early neoplasms of the pancreas is possible using a combination of EUS and CT scan. Canto et al. screened 116 patients in two phases of a screening study called Cancer of the Pancreas Screening Study 1 and 2 (CAPS 1 and 2). They found the diagnostic yield for detecting significant pancreatic neoplasm was 5.3% for CAPS 1 (2 of 38 screened) and 10% (8 of 78 screened) in CAPS 2. Indeed they were able to detect one adenocarcinoma of the pancreas at such an early stage that the patient is alive and cancer free 6 years post-surgery. Other lesions detected with EUS included several IPMNs and PanINs ranging in grade from IA to III (*37, 38*).

In a similar study, Brentnall et al. have also shown that a combination of EUS and endoscopic retrograde cholangiopancreatography (ERCP) is an effective way to screen individuals at an increased risk of developing pancreatic cancer. Brentnall et al. found evidence of chronic pancreatitis like changes in high-risk patients screened as part of this study and suggested that these changes were associated with pancreatic dysplasia or PanIN. In 2002, 12 patients at their center had been sent for a complete pancreatectomy based upon findings on screening EUS/ERCP. All surgically resected specimens were found to have diffuse dysplasia and PanINs but no IPMNs or invasive cancer (*58, 68*).

It is hoped that in the future, a simple blood marker for early pancreatic cancer could be identified and used to screen at risk individuals. However, until this marker is identified and its sensitivity and specificity is shown to be high, the best options to screen at-risk individuals seem to be a combination of EUS and ERCP at a center with expertise in these procedures.

18 Future Directions

Although significant advances have been made in understanding familial pancreatic cancer, there is still room for much progress. For example, it is clear that we have not identified all of the genes responsible for familial pancreatic cancer, as the syndromes identified thus far only account for <20% of the observed familial clustering in this cancer. One of the limitations to identifying other genes is the lack of DNA from affected individuals in the same family, hindering complex genetic studies such as linkage and lists. In addition, collaborative registries such as PACGENE could greatly facilitate the speed with which new genes are identified. Furthermore, rapid advances in genotyping and sequencing technology will greatly increase our ability to identify the genetic changes involved in cancer susceptibility and progression (69).

Another challenge of pancreatic cancer is early detection. It is imperative that this cancer be caught at an early stage, preferably at the precursor stage, to offer the best chance of surgical resection and therefore long-term survival for patients. In addition to early detection screens relying on visualization of early changes (EUS, CT, etc.), early detection efforts would be greatly facilitated by the identification of novel early detection markers. For example, Koopmann et al. found that measuring serum levels of MIC-1 was better at differentiating pancreatic cancer patients from normal controls than CA19–9 (70). However, additional studies are needed before MIC-1 or other markers can be used clinically. Identification of individuals at high-risk of developing pancreatic cancer using risk modeling (65) along with genetic counseling (64) and when indicated genetic testing followed by appropriate early detection screening provides the best hope for reducing the burden of this disease.

References

1. Jemal A, Siegel R, Ward E, et al. Cancer statistics, CA A Cancer Journal for Clinicians, 2008, 58:71–96.
2. Lynch HT, Smyrk T, Kern SE, et al. Familial pancreatic cancer: a review. Semin Oncol 1996, 23:251–275.
3. Surveillance, EaERSPwscg. SEER*Stat Database: Incidence SEER 9 Regs, Nov 2002 Sub (1973–2000). (released April 2003, based on the November 2002 submission). 2003. National Cancer Institute, DCCPS, Surveillance Research Program, Cancer Statistics Branch.
4. Ferley J, Bray P, Pisani P, et al. GLOBOCAN2000: cancer incidence, mortality and prevalence worldwide, version 1.0. Lyon, IARC Press, 2001.
5. Fuchs CS, Colditz GA, Stampfer MJ, et al. A prospective study of cigarette smoking and the risk of pancreatic cancer. Arch Intern Med 1996, 156:2255–2260.
6. Silverman DT. Risk factors for pancreatic cancer: a case-control study based on direct interviews. Teratog Carcinog Mutagen 2001, 21:7–25.
7. Schenk M, Schwartz AG, O'Neal E, et al. Familial risk of pancreatic cancer. J Natl Cancer Inst 2001, 93:640–644.
8. Falk RT, Pickle LW, Fontham ET, et al. Life-style risk factors for pancreatic cancer in Louisiana: a case-control study. Am J Epidemiol 1988, 128:324–336.
9. Howe GR, Jain M, Burch JD, et al. Cigarette smoking and cancer of the pancreas: evidence from a population-based case-control study in Toronto, Canada. Int J Cancer 1991, 47:323–328.
10. Coughlin SS, Calle EE, Patel AV, et al. Predictors of pancreatic cancer mortality among a large cohort of United States adults. Cancer Causes Control 2000, 11:915–923.
11. Everhart J, Wright D. Diabetes mellitus as a risk factor for pancreatic cancer. A meta-analysis. JAMA 1995, 273:1605–1609.
12. Lowenfels AB, Maisonneuve P, DiMagno EP, et al. Hereditary pancreatitis and the risk of pancreatic cancer. International Hereditary Pancreatitis Study Group. J Natl Cancer Inst 1997, 89:442–446.
13. Michaud DS, Giovannucci E, Willett WC, et al. Physical activity, obesity, height, and the risk of pancreatic cancer. JAMA 2001, 286:921–929.

14. Chari ST, Leibson CL, Rabe KG, et al. Probability of pancreatic cancer following diabetes: a population-based study. Gastroenterology 2005, 129:504–511.
15. Coughlin SS, Calle EE, Teras LR, et al. Diabetes mellitus as a predictor of cancer mortality in a large cohort of US adults. Am J Epidemiol 2004, 159:1160–1167.
16. Lowenfels AB, Maisonneuve P, Cavallini G, et al. Pancreatitis and the risk of pancreatic cancer. International Pancreatitis Study Group. N Engl J Med 1993, 328:1433–1437.
17. Lowenfels AB, Maisonneuve P, Whitcomb DC, et al. Cigarette smoking as a risk factor for pancreatic cancer in patients with hereditary pancreatitis. JAMA 2001, 286:169–170.
18. Berrington de GA, Sweetland S, Spencer E. A meta-analysis of obesity and the risk of pancreatic cancer. Br J Cancer 2003, 89:519–523.
19. MacDermott RP, Kramer P. Adenocarcinoma of the pancreas in four siblings. Gastroenterology 1973, 65:137–139.
20. Danes BS, Lynch HT. A familial aggregation of pancreatic cancer. An in vitro study. JAMA 1982, 247:2798–27802.
21. Lynch HT, Fitzsimmons M, Smyrk TC. Familial pancreatic cancer: Clinicopathological study of 18 nuclear families. Am J Gastroenterol 1990, 85:54–60.
22. Evans JP, Burke W, Chen R, et al. Familial pancreatic adenocarcinoma: association with diabetes and early molecular diagnosis. J Med Genet 1995, 32:330–335.
23. Hruban RH, Petersen GM, Ha PK, et al. Genetics of pancreatic cancer. From genes to families. Surg Oncol Clin North Am 1998, 7:1–23.
24. Petersen GM, de AM, Goggins M, et al. Pancreatic cancer genetic epidemiology consortium. Cancer Epidemiol Biomarkers Prev 2006, 15:704–710.
25. Klein AP. Overview of linkage analysis: application to pancreatic cancer. Methods Mol Med 2005, 103:329–341.
26. Ghadirian P, Boyle P, Simard A, et al. Reported family aggregation of pancreatic cancer within a population based case-control study in the Francophone community in Montreal, Canada. Int J Pancreatol 1991, 10:183–196.
27. Fernandez E, LaVecchia C, D'Avanzo B, et al. Family history and the risk of liver, gallbladder, and pancreatic cancer. Cancer Epidemiol Biomarkers Prev 1994, 3:209 –212.
28. Hemminki K, Li X: Familial and second primary pancreatic cancers: a nationwide epidemiologic study from Sweden. Int J Cancer 2003, 103:525–530.
29. Amundadottir LT, Thorvaldsson S, Gudbjartsson DF, et al. Cancer as a complex phenotype: pattern of cancer distribution within and beyond the nuclear family. PLoS Med 2004, 1:e65 .
30. Klein AP, Brune KA, Petersen GM, et al. Prospective risk of pancreatic cancer in familial pancreatic cancer kindreds. Cancer Res 2004, 64:2634–2638.
31. Canto M, Goggins M, Hruban R, et al. Screening for early pancreatic neoplasia in high-risk individuals: a prospective controlled study. Clin Gast Hepatol 2006, 4(6):766–781.
32. Canto MI, Goggins M, Yeo CJ, et al. Screening for pancreatic neoplasia in high-risk individuals: an EUS-based approach. Clin Gastroenterol Hepatol 2004, 2:606–621.
33. Brune K, Abe T, Canto M, et al. Multifocal neoplastic precursor lesions associated with lobular atrophy of the pancreas in patients having a strong family history of pancreatic cancer. Am J Surg Pathol 2006, 30:1067–1076.
34. Meckler KA, Brentnall TA, Haggitt RC, et al. Familial fibrocystic pancreatic atrophy with endocrine cell hyperplasia and pancreatic carcinoma. Am J Surg Pathol 2001, 25:1047–1053.
35. Goggins M, Schutte M, Lu J, et al. Germline BRCA2 gene mutations in patients with apparently sporadic pancreatic carcinomas. Cancer Res 1996, 56:5360–5364.
36. Hahn SA, Greenhalf B, Ellis I, et al. BRCA2 germline mutations in familial pancreatic carcinoma. J Natl Cancer Inst 2003, 95:214–221.
37. Murphy KM, Brune KA, Griffin C, et al. Evaluation of candidate genes MAP2K4, MADH4, ACVR1B, and BRCA2 in familial pancreatic cancer: deleterious BRCA2 mutations in 17%. Cancer Res 2002, 62:3789–3793.
38. Lal G, Liu G, Schmocker B, et al. Inherited predisposition to pancreatic adenocarcinoma: role of family history and germ-line p16, BRCA1, and BRCA2 mutations. Cancer Res 2000, 60:409–416.

39. Goldstein AM, Fraser MC, Struewing JP, et al. Increased risk of pancreatic cancer in melanoma-prone kindreds with p16INK4 mutations. N Engl J Med 1995, 333:970–974.
40. Borg A, Sandberg T, Nilsson K, et al. High frequency of multiple melanomas and breast and pancreas carcinomas in CDKN2A mutation-positive melanoma families. J Natl Cancer Inst 2000, 92:1260–1266.
41. Vasen HF, Gruis NA, Frants RR, et al. Risk of developing pancreatic cancer in families with familial atypical multiple mole melanoma associated with a specific 19 deletion of p16 (p16-Leiden). Int J Cancer 2000, 87:809–811.
42. Kamb A, Shattuck-Eidens D, Eeles R, et al. Analysis of the p16 gene (CDKN2) as a candidate for the chromosome 9p melanoma susceptibility locus. Nat Genet 1994, 8:23–26.
43. Schutte M, Hruban RH, Geradts J, et al. Abrogation of the Rb/p16 tumor-suppressive pathway in virtually all pancreatic carcinomas. Cancer Res 1997, 57:3126–3130.
44. Caldas C, Hahn SA, da Costa LT, et al. Frequent somatic mutations and homozygous deletions of the p16 (MTS1) gene in pancreatic adenocarcinoma. Nat Genet 1994, 8:27–32.
45. Su GH, Hruban RH, Bansal RK, et al. Germline and somatic mutations of the STK11/LKB1 Peutz-Jeghers gene in pancreatic and biliary cancers. Am J Pathol 1999, 154:1835–1840.
46. Giardiello FM, Brensinger JD, Tersmette AC, et al. Very high risk of cancer in familial Peutz-Jeghers syndrome. Gastroenterology 2000, 119:1447–1453.
47. Lynch HT, Voorhees GJ, Lanspa SJ, et al. Pancreatic carcinoma and hereditary nonpolyposis colorectal cancer: a family study. Br J Cancer 1985, 52:271–273.
48. Wilentz RE, Goggins M, Redston M, et al. Genetic, immunohistochemical, and clinical features of medullary carcinoma of the pancreas: a newly described and characterized entity. Am J Pathol 2000, 156:1641–1651.
49. van der Heijden MS, Yeo CJ, Hruban RH, et al. Fanconi anemia gene mutations in young-onset pancreatic cancer. Cancer Res 2003, 63:2585–2588.
50. van der Heijden MS, Brody JR, Dezentje DA, et al. In vivo therapeutic responses contingent on Fanconi anemia/BRCA2 status of the tumor. Clin Cancer Res 2005, 11:7508–7515.
51. Rogers CD, van der Heijden MS, Brune K, et al. The genetics of FANCC and FANCG in familial pancreatic cancer. Cancer Biol Ther 2004, 3:167–169.
52. Brentnall TA, Bronner MP, Byrd DR, et al. Early diagnosis and treatment of pancreatic dysplasia in patients with a family history of pancreatic cancer. Ann Intern Med 1999, 131:247–255.
53. Eberle MA, Pfutzer R, Pogue-Geile KL, et al. A new susceptibility locus for autosomal dominant pancreatic cancer maps to chromosome 4q32-34. Am J Hum Genet 2002, 70:1044–1048.
54. Pogue-Geile KL, Chen R, Bronner MP, et al. Palladin mutation causes familial pancreatic cancer and suggests a new cancer mechanism. PLoS Med 2006, 3:e516.
55. Earl J, Yan L, Vitone LJ, et al. Evaluation of the 4q32-34 locus in European familial pancreatic cancer. Cancer Epidemiol Biomarkers Prev 2006, 15:1948–1955.
56. Klein AP, de Andrade M., Hruban RH, et al. Linkage analysis of chromosome 4 in families with familial pancreatic cancer. Cancer Biol Ther 2007, 3:167–169.
57. Klein AP, Beaty TH, Bailey-Wilson JE, et al. Evidence for a major gene influencing risk of pancreatic cancer. Genet Epidemiol 2002, 23:133–149.
58. Axilbund JE, Brune KA, Canto MI, et al. Patient perspective on the value of genetic counseling for familial pancreas cancer. Hered Cancer Clin Pract 2005, 3:115–122.
59. Wang W, Chen S, Brune KA, et al. Development and validation of a risk assessment tool for individuals with a family history of pancreatic cancer: PancPRO. J Clin Oncol 2007, 25(11):1417–1422.
60. Chen S, Wang W, Broman KW, et al. Bayes Mendel: and R environment for Mendelian risk prediction. Stat Appl Genet Mol Biol 2004, 3.
61. Euhus D: Risk modeling in breast cancer. Breast J 2004, 10 Suppl 1:S10–S12.
62. Kimmey MB, Bronner MP, Byrd DR, et al. Screening and surveillance for hereditary pancreatic cancer. Gastrointest Endosc 2002, 56:S82–S86.
63. Sjoblom T, Jones S, Wood LD, et al. The consensus coding sequences of human breast and colorectal cancers. Science 2006, 314:268–274.

64. Koopmann J, Buckhaults P, Brown DA, et al. Serum macrophage inhibitory cytokine 1 as a marker of pancreatic and other periampullary cancers. Clin Cancer Res 2004, 10:2386–2392.
65. Ghadirian P, Boyle P, Simard A, et al. Reported family aggregation of pancreatic cancer within a population-based case-control study in the Francophone community in Montreal, Canada. Int J Pancreatol 1991, 10:183–196.
66. Fernandez E, La Vecchia C, d'Avanzo B, et al. Family history and the risk of liver, gallbladder, and pancreatic cancer. Cancer Epidemiol Biomarkers Prev 1994, 3:209–212.
67. Giardiello FM, Welsh SB, Hamilton SR, et al. Increased risk of cancer in the Peutz-Jeghers syndrome. N Engl J Med 1987, 316:1511–1514.
68. Whitcomb DC, Gorry MC, Preston RA, et al. Hereditary pancreatitis is caused by a mutation in the cationic trypsinogen gene [see comments]. Nat Genet 1996, 14:141–145.
69. Whitcomb D, Preston R, Aston CE, et al. A gene for hereditary pancreatitis maps to chromosome 7q35. Gastroenterology 1996, 110:1975–1980.

Chapter 6
Hereditary Pancreatitis and Pancreatic Cancer

Julia B. Greer, Narcis O. Zarnescu, and David C. Whitcomb

1   Hereditary Pancreatitis: Background

Hereditary pancreatitis (HP) is a rare disorder characterized by recurrent attacks of acute pancreatitis, chronic pancreatitis, and a high incidence of adenocarcinoma of the pancreas. *Hereditary pancreatitis* **specifically refers to otherwise unexplained pancreatitis in an individual from a family in which the pancreatitis phenotype appears to be inherited through a disease-causing gene mutation that is expressed in an autosomal dominant pattern** (*1*). *Familial pancreatitis* **refers to pancreatitis from *any* cause that occurs in a family with an incidence greater than expected by chance alone, given the size of the family and incidence of pancreatitis within a defined population** (*1*). HP typically presents in childhood with an attack of acute pancreatitis. Recurrent acute pancreatitis advances to become chronic pancreatitis in about 50% of patients (*2, 3*). Chronic pancreatitis is a progressive inflammatory process that destroys pancreatic function and results in the malabsorption of nutrients (exocrine failure) and diabetes mellitus (endocrine failure). Additional complications of chronic pancreatitis that are seen in many, but not all, patients include severe and persistent pain, strictures of the common bile duct, pancreatic pseudocysts, and pancreatic duct stones that may require interventional or surgical treatment. Of those patients who develop a chronic course, about 40% develop pancreatic cancer (PC) (*4, 5*).

The early age of onset and distinct phenotypical features of HP allowed Whitcomb et al. to use genetic linkage analysis to identify the disease locus on chromosome 7q35 (*6*). Shortly thereafter, the disease-causing mutation was identified as R122H (originally numbered as R117H), in the third exon of the cationic trypsinogen gene (protease serine 1, *PRSS1*) (*7*). Since the discovery of the R122H mutation in 1996, about 20 other mutations have been categorized in *PRSS1*, including N29I (*2*), and A16V (*8*). There are few phenotypic differences in disease manifestation between these *PRSS1* mutations, although some individuals with the most common mutation, R122H, present with pancreatitis earlier and are more likely to require surgical intervention than those with less frequently observed mutations (*9, 10*). However, carrying the R122H mutation does not always translate into more aggressive disease or a greater number of complications of chronic

A.M. Lowy et al. (eds.), *Pancreatic Cancer.*
doi: 10.1007/978-0-387-69252-4, © Springer Science+Business Media, LLC 2008

Table 6.1 Hereditary pancreatitis: diagnostic criteria

1. Recurrent acute or chronic pancreatitis with R122H or N29I mutation of cationic trypsinogen gene (PRSS1)
2. Recurrent acute or chronic pancreatitis with a family history of ≥ 2 affected patients, irrespective of generation
3. No known etiological factors (such as alcohol) in at least one of the patients.
4. In cases of siblings only, the onset of the disease in at least one of the patients is below age 40.

Diagnosis of hereditary pancreatitis is established when either criterion 1 or the combination of criterion 2, 3, and 4 are fulfilled.

pancreatitis. Additionally, trypsinogen mutations do not account for all mutations causing HP because some families with HP do not have identifiable *PRSS1* mutations (Table 6.1) (*11*).

The *PRSS1* gene codes for cationic trypsinogen, the proenzyme (i.e., zymogen) that becomes trypsin upon activation through cleavage of an N-terminal octapeptide, trypsinogen activation peptide (TAP). Trypsin is a serine protease that attacks internal arginine or lysine amino acid residues. It is also the master enzyme of pancreatic digestive enzymes. Trypsin activates other pancreatic zymogens, a process that typically occurs in the duodenum, where the zymogen activation cascade is initiated by the cleavage of TAP from trypsinogen by enterokinase. Trypsinogen is also activated when TAP is cleaved by trypsin (autoactivation). In addition, trypsin inactivates trypsin by cleaving the molecule at R122 (autolysis). Trypsinogen contains two calcium-binding pockets, and binding of calcium determines whether trypsin will activate trypsinogen or inactivate trypsinogen and trypsin. Thus, the calcium concentration serves as the "on/off" switch for trypsin activity. High calcium levels facilitate activation and prevent inactivation and low calcium levels limit the degree of activation and permit autolysis to occur. The arginine to histidine amino acid substitution at residue 122 results in a gain-of-function mutation because it changes the autolysis site to an amino acid that is not recognized by trypsin, preventing trypsin's inactivation in low calcium solutions (*12*). Gain-of-function mutations often result in an autosomal dominant inheritance pattern as seen in HP. Only one of the two trypsinogen alleles must code for a superfunctional trypsin in order to produce inappropriate enzyme activity, induce injury, and cause acute pancreatitis. The recurrent injury leads to chronic inflammation, progressive glandular autodigestion, and chronic pancreatitis (*13*).

Individuals from HP kindreds with a causative *PRSS1* mutation commonly present in childhood or early adulthood with acute pancreatitis that is clinically indistinguishable from acute pancreatitis of other etiology. Classic symptoms of acute pancreatitis include epigastric abdominal pain radiating to the back, nausea and vomiting, and pancreatic serum amylase and lipase levels that are elevated to at least three times the upper limit of normal (*14*). A number of individuals with detected *PRSS1* mutations have subclinical disease and may progress to chronic pancreatitis or pancreatic adenocarcinoma with few typical warning signs. However, some families appear to have more severe attacks, with nearly 90% of those affected reporting more than five hospitalizations and serious complications occurring, such as splenic vein thrombosis (*2*, *15*). Chronic pancreatitis in HP is indistinguishable in pathology from chronic pancreatitis of other causes (*16*), and is suggested by the combination of recurrent acute pancreatitis attacks, laboratory findings of endocrine and exocrine insufficiency, malabsorption of fat-soluble vitamins A, D, E, and K, steatorrhea, and weight loss. A more definitive diagnosis of chronic pancreatitis can be made by identifying pancreatic calcifications and morphologic changes on abdominal imaging studies such as computed tomography (CT), magnetic resonance imaging (MRI), endoscopic ultrasound (EUS), or pancreatic ductal changes on ERCP, and/or (*3*) typical histology on an adequate surgical pancreatic specimen (*17*, *18*). Comprehensive diagnostic criteria of chronic pancreatitis have been proposed by the Marseilles classification (*19*), the Japanese Society of Gastroenterology, and the Japan Pancreas Society (JPS) (*20*, *21*).

2 Hereditary Pancreatitis Leads to Pancreatic Cancer

While HP incurs numerous complications as a result of fibrosis and chronic inflammation, the most serious complication of HP is pancreatic adenocarcinoma, which has been estimated to have a 53-fold increase in risk of development after age 50 (*22*). An increased risk of PC in individuals with HP was initially observed in case studies from the 1970s, when Kattwinkel et al. reported eight of 54 family members in three large kindreds with HP dying of suspected PC (*23*), and Malik et al. observed that one of his nine HP patients developed PC.

In 1997, Lowenfels et al. attempted to formally define the relationship between HP and cancer in a large, international study that included families from 10 countries on three separate continents (*24*). A total of 246 (125 male and 121 female) patients with HP were followed for 8,531 person-years. The mean age of pancreatitis symptom onset was 13.9 ± 12.2 years. Against a background expected number of predicted cancers of 0.15, eight cases of PC were observed, resulting in a standardized incidence ratio (SIR) of 53 (95% CI 23, 105). Although eight of the reported 20 deaths were due to PC, the frequency of other tumors was not increased: SIR = 0.7 (95% CI 0.3, 1.6). In these HP families, the estimated overall accumulated risk of PC by age 70 was 40%. A paternal pattern of mutation inheritance was associated with an even higher accumulated PC risk of 75% by age 70, implying that genetic imprinting—differential expression of maternally or paternally inherited copies of a gene—may influence the effects of mutation.

The largest study to date of HP was the EUROPAC study, which reported the incidence of PC in 418 HP-affected individuals in 112 families from 14 countries (*25*). Fifty-eight (52%) of families carried the R122H mutation, 24 (21%) carried N29I, 5 (4%) carried A16V, two had rare mutations, and 21 (19%) had no *PRSS1* mutation detected by the researchers' analysis methods. Interestingly, the median age for first symptoms for R122H was 10 years of age, but was 14 years for N29I, and 14.5 for mutation-negative patients ($p = 0.032$). The cumulative risk by age 50 years was 37.2% for exocrine failure, 47.6% for endocrine failure, and 17.5% for pancreatic resection due to pain. Cumulative risk of PC from time of symptom onset for the 233 subjects with complete information was 1.5% at 20 years, 2.5% at 30 years, 8.5% at 40 years, 14.6% at 50 years, 25.3% at 60 years, and 44.0% at 70 years, giving an SIR of 67. There was no difference in cancer risk based on the type of mutation (e.g., R122H, N29I, or no identified mutation). Additional studies have demonstrated that the risk of PC is not related to the particular *PRSS1* mutation type (*26*).

2.1   All Types of Chronic Pancreatitis Are Associated with Pancreatic Cancer

The question may arise whether pancreatitis of hereditary origin is uniquely associated with PC, or whether it is observed in all forms of chronic pancreatitis. HP is actually a rare form of pancreatitis. Chronic pancreatitis is most commonly associated with excessive alcohol intake (70% of cases) and is defined as idiopathic in about 10–20% of cases (*27*). Recent research has theorized, however, that unrecognized genetic aberrations, such as *PRSS1* mutations and the mutation that causes cystic fibrosis (*28, 29*), are often underlying supposedly idiopathic cases of pancreatitis (*10, 30*) and a genetic predisposition to alcoholic pancreatitis is suspected based on population studies, although this has not yet been proved (*27*). Small case-control studies from the 1970s and 1980s noted insignificant increases in PC cases in individuals treated for chronic pancreatitis (*31, 32*) and additional studies in the early 1990s documented minimally increased PC risk in chronic pancreatitis patients (*33–35*).

In 1993, Lowenfels et al. published a landmark paper reporting the results of the International Pancreatitis Study Group's multicenter historical cohort study of 2,015 subjects with chronic pancreatitis recruited from clinical centers in six countries (*4*). With a mean follow-up of 7.4 ± 6.2 years, a total of 56 pancreatic cancers were identified, giving an SIR of 14.4 for subjects with a minimum of 5 years of follow-up against the number of sex- and age-adjusted cancer cases predicted from country-specific incidence data. The cumulative risk in this study of PC in chronic pancreatitis subjects for 10 and 20 years was 1.8% and 4.0%, respectively.

Furthermore, the risk of PC has been shown to be greatly increased in syndromes in which chronic pancreatitis is a central feature. For example, tropical pancreatitis is a form of idiopathic pancreatitis occurring in young nonalcoholic individuals in tropical Asia and Africa (*36*). The disease manifests early with recurrent attacks of abdominal pain, diabetes mellitus, and intraductal pancreatic calculi (*37*). A mutation in the serine protease inhibitor, Kazal type 1 (*SPINK1*) gene (also known as pancreatic secretory trypsin inhibitor, *PSTI*) has recently been shown to be strongly associated with tropical pancreatitis in a subset of patients, suggesting that a major underlying predisposing factor is genetic (*38–40*).

The link between tropical pancreatitis and PC is strong. Augustine and Ramesh identified 22 pancreatic cancers among 266 patients with tropical pancreatitis over an 8-year period (8.3%) (*41*). Risk among this cohort was highest after age 40, and resected pancreatic specimens from individuals with tropical pancreatitis displayed features of dysplasia as well as neoplasia. In 1994, Chari et al. reported following 185 patients with tropical pancreatitis over a 4.5-year period, and noted that of 24 subjects who had died during that period, six (25%) had died due to PC (*42*). The average age of onset of PC in this cohort was 45 ± 7 years, and they determined the risk of PC in those with tropical pancreatitis compared to those without it was 100 times higher.

Cystic fibrosis (CF) is another condition similar to hereditary pancreatitis in its characteristic genetic basis and childhood onset. CF is an autosomal recessive illness caused by mutations in the cystic fibrosis transmembrane receptor (*CFTR*) gene that codes for an anion channel critical for proper function of pancreatic duct and other anion-secreting cells, such as those of the respiratory system and sweat glands (*13*). Moderate to severe dysfunction of *CFTR*-mediated secretory capability markedly limits pancreatic capacity to efficiently flush digestive enzymes out of the pancreas, especially following the activation of trypsin, when the risk of autodigestion and pancreatitis is high. Severe *CFTR* mutations lead to recurrent acute or chronic pancreatitis (*43*). When CF was first described in 1938, the average lifespan for an affected individual was only 6 months, and just decades ago CF patients rarely survived into their twenties (*44*). However, the currently successful treatment of CF-related nutrition, diabetes, pulmonary disease, and pancreatic insufficiency now allows individuals to live well into their thirties and forties (*45*). Ironically, due to improved disease management, the increased duration of long-term pancreatic inflammation from CF may raise these patients' risk of developing PC.

A number of groups have examined PC risk in adult CF patients. In 1993, Sheldon et al. described their study of 412 subjects with CF and found two cases of PC (*46*). With an expected 0.008 cases, this gave an odds ratio of 61 ($p = 0.001$). An increased risk of digestive cancers, but not cancer in general, was then confirmed in 1995 by Neglia et al. among 28,511 CF patients in Canada and the United States (risk ratio 6.5) and Europe (risk ratio 6.4) (*47*). Although they identified only two pancreatic tumors, that these subjects were in their thirties when PC developed is extremely rare, resulting in an odds ratio of PC of 31.5 when compared with controls.

Thus, evidence shows that long-standing chronic pancreatitis is associated with an increased risk of developing PC. PC develops in the setting of chronic pancreatitis of any etiology and the duration of exposure to inflammation appears to be the predominant factor involved in the transition from a benign to a malignant condition (*48*).

2.2 Does the PRSS1 Mutation Actually Cause Cancer?

The carcinogenic process in the pancreas is posited to be genetically induced via a recognizable pattern of mutation accumulation. The pattern has been organized into the pancreatic intraepithelial neoplasm (PanIN) system, a standardized method of classifying pathologically abnormal pancreatic ductal epithelium linked to genetic alterations (49). Numerous studies confirm that this pattern of accumulating mutations parallels progressive dysplasia and usually begins with mutations in K-ras2, Id-1/Id-2, p53, and cyclin D1 (36, 50–52). Abnormalities that typically occur later in the progression of PanIN include P16/CDKN2A, DPC4/MADH4, and BRCA1/2 mutations (53–56). This pattern occurs similarly in sporadic pancreatic adenocarcinoma as well as in PC arising in the context of chronic inflammation, and suggests that the high risk of PC in patients with chronic pancreatitis is due to mutation accumulation rather than a unique process.

In the evolution of tumor formation, positive selection is placed on tumor cells which are able to alter rate-limiting regulatory pathways (51). As a corollary, a mutation of one gene abrogates the need for alteration of another gene in the same pathway, and the coexistence of mutations in disparate genes in a solitary tumor implies their involvement in distinct tumor-suppressive pathways. The PRSS1 gene is not an oncogene or a tumor suppressor gene, but rather codes for a digestive enzyme. If the PRSS1 mutation were an oncogene in which somatic mutation was important in the development of carcinogenesis, it would be found in sporadic PC as well as in hereditary syndromes associated with increased PC risk. As evidence, Hengstler et al. analyzed genomic DNA for the presence of the R122H mutation in the trypsinogen gene (PRSS1) in PC tissue samples from 34 patients and corresponding normal tissue from 28 of the same individuals (57). No PRSS1 mutations were found. These data suggest that underlying trypsinogen gene mutations are uncommon in sporadic PC, and that trypsinogen R122H mutations are not likely to be an important step in pancreatic carcinogenesis.

2.3 PRSS1: Inflammation and Cancer

Epidemiologic and molecular studies in vitro and in vivo similarly support the hypothesis that inflammation plays a critical role in both the initiation and progression of pancreatic tumors (58). During acute pancreatitis, the release of proinflammatory mediators may expand a local disturbance into a systemic inflammatory response (59). Chronic pancreatitis develops at least a decade after recurrent acute attacks, and a key feature is demonstrated by the persistent, dysregulated and heightened inflammatory process (43).

Nearly 200 years ago, French surgeon Jean Nicholas Marjolin hypothesized that there was a causative link between chronic inflammation and cancer when he observed the development of squamous cell carcinoma at the site of a chronically inflamed open wound (60). In 1863, Rudolf Virchow noted the presence of leukocytes in neoplastic tissue, which he felt reflected the origin of cancer at sites of chronic inflammation (61). In recent years, various inflammatory diseases and viruses have been shown to contribute to the development of a variety of cancers, including many cancers of the GI tract (Table 6.2). For example, hepatitis B and C have been shown to incite hepatic carcinoma, esophageal cancer is linked to chronic

Table 6.2 Association between inflammation and cancer risk

Malignancy	Inflammatory stimulus or condition
Bladder	Schistosomiasis
Bronchial	Silica, asbestos, cigarette smoking
Cervical	Human papillomavirus (HPV)
Colorectal	Inflammatory bowel disease
Esophageal	Barrett's esophagus
Gastric	H. pylori-induced gastritis
Hepatocellular	Hepatitis virus (B and C)
Kaposi's sarcoma	Human herpesvirus type B
Mesothelioma	Asbestos
Ovarian	Pelvic inflammatory disease/talc/asbestos
Pancreas	Chronic pancreatitis/hereditary pancreatitis

esophagitis, and gastric cancer develops after chronic gastritis due to *Helicobacter pylori* infection (*13, 62, 63*). Additionally, patients with inflammatory bowel disease involving the colon demonstrate an increased risk of developing colon cancer and anti-inflammatory medications may decrease the risk of developing colon and other cancers (*64, 65*). Furthermore, in at least one large study, aspirin was observed to significantly decrease the risk of developing PC (*66*).

How does chronic inflammation accelerate the oncogenic process, and why does it take decades before cancer develops in a certain percentage of patients with chronic inflammatory diseases? An initial observation is noted in chronic inflammatory diseases in which the process driving oncogenesis is likely a "landscaper" defect rather than a germline genetic "gatekeeper" or "caretaker" defect (*67*). Landscaper defects reflect factors that cause an abnormal microenvironment due to inflammation, and those same factors in the microenvironment increase the risk of neoplastic transformation (*13*). In fact, many response agents associated with chronic inflammation appear to increase genomic damage and cellular proliferation, which favor malignant transformation of pancreatic cells (*68*). Various cytokines, reactive oxygen species, and mediators of the inflammatory pathway increase cell cycling, cause loss of tumor suppressor function and stimulate oncogene expression, all of which may lead to pancreatic malignancy.

Results of a number of studies suggest that PC begins with the establishment of chronic inflammation (*48, 69, 70*). The release of cytokines, production of reactive oxygen species and the up-regulation of proinflammatory transcription factors are all associated with PC and can induce genetic damage, cell proliferation, and inhibition of apoptosis in the pancreas. In PC, inflammatory mediators such as nuclear factor-kappa B (NF-κB), cyclo-oxygenase-2 (Cox-2), and tumor necrosis factor alpha (TNFα), are known to facilitate tumor cell growth and metastasis (*68*). In addition, NF-κB and interleukin-8 (IL-8) are important mediators of the inflammatory process in chronic pancreatitis and both have been implicated in the development of a variety of other malignancies (*68, 71*). A chronic inflammatory environment causes the activation of stellate cells and the combination of an inflammatory infiltrate and proliferating mesenchymal cells leads to the development of pancreatic fibrosis. Inflammation can also induce stroma formation that, via the secretion of epidermal growth factor and the production of proinvasive factors, can facilitate the growth of transformed cells. Cox-2 is a key modulatory molecule involved in inflammation and cancer, and recent evidence shows that in PanIN lesions, Cox-2 expression increases in parallel with the escalating severity of PanIN change (72).

A recent evaluation of inflammatory factors common to chronic pancreatitis and PC used laser capture microdissection, gene array, and immunohistochemistry to compare tissue from normal pancreas, chronic pancreatitis and PC (70). Data showed that while certain inflammatory components were specific either to chronic pancreatitis or pancreatic tumor tissue, increased staining of both the p50 NF-κB subunit and IKKα kinase (a protein that permits activation of NF-κB) was noted both in chronic pancreatitis and pancreatic neoplasia. These results demonstrate that similar inflammatory components and downstream effectors are present in chronic pancreatitis as well as in PC.

2.4   Interactions in Hereditary Pancreatitis

In relation to chronic HP, some kindred appear to demonstrate higher rates of cancer occurrence than others—a finding that suggests that risk factors aside from inflammation are important in oncogenesis. The coinheritance of oncogenic germline mutations and environmental factors must be carefully evaluated in HP kindred since their modulation may represent risk-reducing, preventative strategies against PC in predisposed individuals.

2.4.1   Gene–Gene Interactions

There is growing evidence from familial and epidemiologic studies that nonspecific oncogenes, tumor suppressor genes, or pancreas-specific genes may predispose individuals to PC. In a population-based case-control study of PC involving 484 cases and 2,099 controls, Silverman et al. recently reported that 21% of cases compared with 13% of controls had a first-degree relative with at least one type of cancer (73). At 18- to 57-fold, the risk and incidence of PC is exceptionally high among at-risk first-degree relatives in PC kindreds. Observations from the Pittsburgh-Midwest Multicenter Pancreatic Study Group (74) suggest that other germline mutations may play a role in patients with HP, because PC appeared to be clustered in a subset of families and a number of cancer cases demonstrated vertical transmission. If the high PC risk in HP was due to inflammation alone, one would anticipate widespread and randomly distributed PC throughout the HP families, which was not observed.

The co-inheritance of high-risk genetic factors with cationic trypsinogen mutations or other chronic pancreatitis susceptibility genes will also alter the general risk of PC among patients with HP (*75, 76*). A number of well-defined syndromes demonstrate PC as a major feature. Hereditary nonpolyposis colorectal cancer (HNPCC) is an autosomal dominant disorder caused by mutations in mismatch repair genes, particularly *MLH1, MLH2* and *MSH6*. Germline mutations in *BRCA2* have been shown to segregate in at least 5–10% of sporadic PC cases (*77*) and have been estimated to be associated with a relative risk of 3.51 (*78*). Germline mutations in *p16* predispose to melanoma and PC and genetic mutations in *STK11/LKB1* are associated with PC in the Peutz-Jeghers syndrome. In addition, Park et al. found that cancer at an early age, and PC in particular, were independent predictive factors for germline mutations in a Korean subset of patients (*79*). How these mutations interact with *PRSS1* mutations, and whether they accelerate pancreatic carcinogenesis in chronic pancreatitis patients, however, is an area of research that remains to be examined.

2.4.2 Gene–Environment Interactions

In a number of studies, the single most important environmental factor associated with PC has been demonstrated to be cigarette smoking. Cigarette smoking increases the risk of PC approximately twofold, and evidence suggests that cigarette smoking and a positive family history of PC are synergistic. Schenk et al. examined the relative risk in smokers and in families with a positive history of PC and found that each factor approximately doubled the risk of developing pancreatic adenocarcinoma (*80*). The relative risk for a positive family history of PC was 2.49 and for individuals with a history of smoking was 2.04. However, among individuals who smoked and who had a family member diagnosed with PC prior to age 60, the risk jumped to 8.23.

Cigarette smoking apparently compounds the inflammatory effects of HP. Studies have shown that among very high-risk individuals with HP, cigarette smoking doubles PC risk and reduces the age of cancer onset by about 20 years (*81*). Smoke not only influences pancreatic secretions from its nicotine constituent, but it induces inflammatory reactions and exerts carcinogenic effects with numerous other components (*82*). Additionally, smoke has been shown to enhance ethanol-induced pancreatic injury and to accelerate the development and progression of chronic pancreatitis, regardless of underlying etiology. A retrospective study of 934 patients with chronic alcoholic pancreatitis found that tobacco smoking was associated with an earlier diagnosis of chronic alcoholic pancreatitis (on average 4.7 years earlier) and was also associated with the appearance of calcifications and diabetes, independent of level of alcohol consumption (*83*).

Recently, Wittel et al. evaluated chronic pancreatic inflammation induced by environmental tobacco smoke inhalation in rats, comparing the long-term effects of cigarette smoke on the development of chronic pancreatitis and pancreatic adenocarcinoma (*84*). The study found that 58% of animals that were exposed to cigarette smoke for 70 minutes twice a day for 12 weeks displayed a chronic pancreatic inflammatory process with scarring and fibrosis of pancreatic acinar structures.

Many animals with these fibrotic alterations demonstrated an induction of pancreatic procollagen 1 gene expression and an infiltration of immune cells accompanied by the expression of inflammatory mediators MIP-1α, IL-1β, and TGF-β. MIP-1α has been shown to promote PC cell migration as well as the invasion of type IV collagen (85). Thus, exposure to cigarette smoke, in the setting of a pre-existing inflammatory environment, would theoretically be particularly carcinogenic, and the duration of exposure to coexisting inflammation may influence the transition to neoplastic development.

2.5   Risk Reduction Strategies

HP patients exhibit a 53-fold increased risk of PC with a cumulative risk of 40% by age 70; thus, screening of HP kindred is essential. Although inherited genetic factors cannot be altered, environmental and behavioral factors are modifiable. The greatest risk factor for chronic pancreatitis is heavy consumption of alcohol (83), and cigarette smoking is known to be a risk factor both for PC (48, 81, 86, 87) and chronic pancreatitis (88, 89). A recent cohort study of Italian men concluded that alcohol and cigarette smoking are independent risk factors for chronic pancreatitis and that the combined effect of both factors increased the risk of pancreatitis synergistically, thereby increasing PC risk (90). Thus, high-risk patients, such as those from HP kindreds, are advised to limit their alcohol intake and refrain from smoking cigarettes.

Future cancer risk reduction and prevention strategies are likely to include chemoprevention (91) and/or vaccination (92). Small case reports of surgery for the treatment of chronic pancreatitis, such as enteric-drained pancreas transplantation, have been shown to successfully treat pancreatic exocrine and endocrine failure, but these studies are still in their infancy (93). Additionally, HP causes diffuse, rather than focal, pancreatic tissue damage and the only way to remove all of the tissue at risk of malignant transformation is to perform a total pancreatectomy (94). As the interactive relationship between inflammation and carcinogenesis involved in PC becomes better defined, therapies that target the inflammatory process may help to prevent cancer development as well as cancer invasion and metastasis (85).

2.6   Screening and Surveillance Recommendations

Due to the retroperitoneal location of the pancreas, its great reserve of exocrine cells, and the nonspecific symptoms of pancreatic malignancy, patients usually present at an advanced stage when treatment options are limited and cure is unlikely. Screening of high-risk patients provides one of the only methods currently available for detecting this cancer at an early stage. However, the pancreas is difficult to evaluate by current imaging modalities in the context of chronic pancreatitis and it is the preinvasive, rather than the established, lesion that physicians prefer to identify. In April 2001, a large group of physicians and scientists convened at the Third International

Symposium on Inherited Diseases of the Pancreas in Milan, Italy, and their committee provided recommendations for physicians caring for patients with HP (95, 96). It was the unanimous opinion to screen patients suspected for HP at ≥40 years of age. Optimally, screening should be done at medical centers that are expert in caring for HP patients using state-of-the-art technology. In addition, screening should be considered yearly within the context of multicenter protocols assessing the efficacy of EUS, multiphasic helical CT, or MRI/MRCP in conjunction with standardized collection and storage of blood, serum, and pancreatic juice for future analysis.

The experts recognized the limitation of EUS to identify suspicious lesions in the context of chronic pancreatitis; therefore, no recommendation of the modality of screening was reached. Several investigators argued for the use of ERCP because it facilitates detection and sampling of ductal pancreatic dysplasia/malignancy while allowing for optimal collection of pancreatic juice. Others felt that the same objectives could be accomplished with lower morbidity and mortality through EUS with needle biopsy of suspicious lesions and aspiration of duodenal contents following secretin stimulation. Thus, although a definite need for screening and counseling HP patients is recognized, the mode and timing of screening remains debatable.

This diagnostic dilemma has been addressed by a group from the University of Pittsburgh through analysis of fluid and cells obtained from pancreatic brushing, fine needle aspirations and juice collection employing endoscopic approaches (e.g., ERCP and EUS). Developed by Sydney Finkelstein (Redpath Integrated Pathology, Pittsburgh, PA), this technique takes advantage of the fact that PC is characterized by chromosomal instability, rather than microsatellite instability. The technique involves selection of abnormal-appearing groups of cells from a cytology smear, and additional cells from a cheek swab, blood sample, or other normal sites. DNA is extracted and PCR is used to amplify specific microsatellite regions flanking the major tumor suppressor genes to identify loss of heterozygosity (LOH) in suspicious appearing cells. Detection of LOH in a group of cells suggests clonal expansion linked to loss of a tumor suppressor gene, implying that there is a mutation in the tumor suppressor gene on the opposite arm. This process is far less expensive and technically robust than screening for mutations in various tumor suppressor genes. Furthermore, it is possible to test for LOH in more than a dozen tumor suppressor genes from a single sample. K-ras2 exon 12 and 13 mutations, which are present in >95% of pancreatic cancers, are also detected. In clinical practice, this approach appears to be the most sensitive and specific of all currently used techniques (97–99). Furthermore, it is possible to detect precancerous lesions (e.g., with LOH in one or two sites), allowing patients to be categorized into high-risk groups for more aggressive evaluation or intervention.

3 Conclusions

HP, which is caused by specific *PRSS1* gain-of-function mutations, is one of the strongest known risk factors for PC. The natural progression of HP from recurrent acute pancreatitis attacks to pancreatic adenocarcinoma involves a significant duration of chronic pancreatitis as a necessary intermediary step. The autosomal dominant inheritance pattern, high phenotypic penetrance of HP, and ability to confirm the diagnosis through genetic testing, make HP kindred an ideal group for prevention and screening protocols (96).

References

1. Whitcomb DC. Hereditary diseases of the pancreas. In: Yamada T, Albers DH, Laine L, et al. (eds.) Textbook of gastroenterology. Philadelphia, Lippincott Williams & Wilkins, 2003, 2147–2165.
2. Gorry MC, Gabbaizedeh D, Furey W, et al. Mutations in the cationic trypsinogen gene are associated with recurrent acute and chronic pancreatitis. Gastroenterology 1997, 113(4):1063–1068.
3. Whitcomb DC. Hereditary pancreatitis: new insights into acute and chronic pancreatitis. Gut 1999, 45:317–322.
4. Lowenfels AB, Maisonneuve P, Cavallini G, et al. Pancreatitis and the risk of pancreatic cancer. International Pancreatitis Study Group. N Engl J Med 1993;328(20):1433–1437.
5. Lowenfels AB, Maisonneuve P, Lankisch PG. Chronic pancreatitis and other risk factors for pancreatic cancer. Gastroenterol Clin North Am 1999, 28(3):673–685.
6. Whitcomb DC, Preston RA, Aston CE, et al. A gene for hereditary pancreatitis maps to chromosome 7q35. Gastroenterology 1996, 110(6):1975–1980.
7. Whitcomb DC, Gorry MC, Preston RA, et al. Hereditary pancreatitis is caused by a mutation in the cationic trypsinogen gene. Nat Genet 1996, 14(2):141–145.
8. Witt H, Luck W, Becker M. A signal peptide cleavage site mutation in the cationic trypsinogen gene is strongly associated with chronic pancreatitis. Gastroenterology 1999, 117:7–10.
9. Howes N, Greenhalf W, Stocken DD, et al. Cationic trypsinogen mutations and pancreatitis. Clin Lab Med 2005, 25(1):39–59.
10. Charnley RM. Hereditary pancreatitis. World J Gastroenterol 2003, 9(1):1–4.
11. Otsuki M. Chronic pancreatitis. The problems of diagnostic criteria. Pancreatology 2004, 4(1):28–41.
12. Whitcomb DC, Lowe ME. Pancreatitis: acute and chronic. In: Walker WA, Goulet O, Kleinman RE, et al. (eds.) Pediatric gastrointestinal disease: pathophysiology, diagnosis, management. Hamilton, ON: BC Decker, 2004, 1584–1597.
13. Whitcomb DC. Inflammation and cancer V. Chronic pancreatitis and pancreatic cancer. Am J Physiol Gastrointest Liver Physiol 2004, 287(2):G315–19.
14. Whitcomb DC. Clinical practice. Acute pancreatitis. N Engl J Med 2006, 354(20): 2142–2150.
15. McElroy R, Christiansen PA. Hereditary pancreatitis in a kinship associated with portal vein thrombosis. Am J Med 1972, 52(2):228–241.
16. Shrikhande SV, Martignoni ME, Shrikhande M, et al. Comparison of histological features and inflammatory cell reaction in alcoholic, idiopathic and tropical chronic pancreatitis. Br J Surg 2003, 90(12):1565–1572.
17. Etemad B, Whitcomb DC. Chronic pancreatitis: diagnosis, classification, and new genetic developments. Gastroenterology 2001, 120:682–707.
18. Axon AT, Classen M, Cotton PB, et al. Pancreatography in chronic pancreatitis: international definitions. Gut 1984, 25(10):1107–1112.
19. Sarles H. [Classification and definition of pancreatitis. Marseilles-Rome 1988]. Gastroenterologie Clinique et Biologique 1989, 13(11):857–859.
20. Homma T, Harada H, Koizumi M. Diagnostic criteria for chronic pancreatitis by the Japan Pancreas Society. Pancreas 1997, 15(1):14–15.

21. The Criteria Committee for Chronic Pancreatitis of the Japan Pancreas Society. Clinical diagnostic criteria of chronic pancreatitis. (in Japanese). Suizo (Journal of the Japan Pancreas Society) 2001, 16:560–561.

22. Lowenfels AB, Maisonneuve P, Cavallini G, et al. Pancreatitis and the risk of pancreatic cancer. International Pancreatitis Study Group. [see comment] N Engl J Med 2003, 328(20):1433–1437.

23. Kattwinkel J, Lapey A, Di SAP, et al. Hereditary pancreatitis: three new kindreds and a critical review of the literature. Pediatrics 1973, 51(1):55–69.

24. Lowenfels A, Maisonneuve P, DiMagno E, et al. Hereditary pancreatitis and the risk of pancreatic cancer. J Natl Cancer Inst 1997, 89(6):442–446.

25. Howes N, Wong T, Greenhalf W, et al. Pancreatic cancer risk in hereditary pancreatitis in Europe. Digestion 2000, 61:300.

26. Lee SK. [Hereditary pancreatitis]. Korean Journal of Gastroenterology/Taehan Sohwagi Hakhoe Chi 2005, 46(5):358–367.

27. Pitchumoni CS. Chronic pancreatitis: a historical and clinical sketch of the pancreas and pancreatitis. Gastroenterologist 1998, 6(1):24–33.

28. Sharer N, Schwarz M, Malone G, et al. Mutations of the cystic fibrosis gene in patients with chronic pancreatitis. N Engl J Med 1998, 339(10):645–652.

29. Cohn JA, Friedman KJ, Noone PG, Knowles MR, Silverman LM, Jowell PS. Relation between mutations of the cystic fibrosis gene and idiopathic pancreatitis. N Engl J Med 1998, 339(10):653–658.

30. Creighton J, Lyall R, Wilson DI, et al. Mutations of the cationic trypsinogen gene in patients with chronic pancreatitis [letter]. Lancet 1999, 354(9172):42–43.

31. Mack TM, Yu MC, Hanisch R, et al. Pancreas cancer and smoking, beverage consumption and past medical history. J Natl Cancer Inst 1986;76:49–60.

32. Gold EB, Gordis L, Diener MD, et al. Diet and other risk factors for cancer of the pancreas. Cancer 1985, 55:460–467.

33. Farrow DC, Davis S. Risk of pancreatic cancer in relation to medical history and use of tobacco, alcohol and coffee. Intl J Cancer 1990, 45:816–820.

34. Jain M, Howe GR, St. Louis P, et al. Coffee and alcohol as determinants of risk of pancreatic cancer: a case-control study from Toronto. Intl J Cancer1991, 47:384–389.

35. Kalapothaki V, Tzonou A, Hsieh CC, et al. Tobacco, ethanol, coffee, pancreatitis, diabetes mellitus, and cholelithiasis as risk factors for pancreatic carcinoma. Cancer Causes Control 1993, 4:1433–1437.

36. Whitcomb DC, Pogue-Geile K. Pancreatitis as a risk for pancreatic cancer. Gastroenterol Clin North Am 2002, 31(2):663–678.

37. Pitchumoni CS, Mohan V. Pancreatitis: juvenile tropical pancreatitis. In: Walker WA, Goulet O, Kleinman RE, et al. (eds.) Pediatric gastrointestinal disease: pathophysiology, diagnosis, management. Hamilton, ON, BC Decker, 2004, 1598–1605.

38. Pfützer RH, Barmada MM, Brunskil APJ, et al. SPINK1/PSTI polymorphisms act as disease modifiers in familial and idiopathic chronic pancreatitis. Gastroenterology 2000, 119:615–623.

39. Rossi L, Pfützer RL, Parvin S, et al. SPINK1/PSTI mutations are associated with tropical pancreatitis in Bangladesh: a preliminary report. Pancreatology 2001, 1(3):242–245.

40. Whitcomb DC. Genetic predispositions to acute and chronic pancreatitis. Med Clin North Am 2000, 84(2):531–547.

41. Augustine P, Ramesh H. Is tropical pancreatitis premalignant? Am J Gastroenterol 1992, 87(8):1005–1008.

42. Chari ST, Mohan V, Pitchumoni CS, et al. Risk of pancreatic carcinoma in tropical calcifying pancreatitis: an epidemiologic study. Pancreas 1994, 9:62–66.

43. Whitcomb DC. Chronic pancreatitis and pancreatic cancer. Am J Physiol Gastrointest Liver Physiol 2004, 287:G315–G319.

44. Davis PB. Cystic fibrosis since 1938. Am J Respir Crit Care Med 2006, 173(5): 475–482.

45. Aronson BS, Marquis M. Care of the adult patient with cystic fibrosis. MEDSURG Nursing 2004, 13(3):143–154.
46. Sheldon CD, Hodson ME, Carpenter LM, et al. A cohort study of cystic fibrosis and malignancy. Br J Cancer 1993, 68(5):1025–1028.
47. Neglia JP, FitzSimmons SC, Maisonneuve P, et al. The risk of cancer among patients with cystic fibrosis. Cystic Fibrosis and Cancer Study Group. N Engl J Med 1995, 332(8):494–499.
48. Maisonneuve P, Lowenfels AB. Chronic pancreatitis and pancreatic cancer. Dig Dis 2002, 20(1):32–37.
49. Hruban RH, Adsay NV, Albores-Saavedra J, et al. Pancreatic intraepithelial neoplasia: a new nomenclature and classification system for pancreatic duct lesions. Am J Surg Pathol 2001, 25(5):579–586.
50. Hruban RH, Wilentz RE, Kern SE. Genetic progression in the pancreatic ducts. Am J Pathol 2000, 156(6):1821–1825.
51. Rozenblum E, Schutte M, Goggins M, et al. Tumor suppressive pathways in pancreatic carcinoma. Cancer Res 1997, (57):1731–1734.
52. Kern SE. Molecular genetic alteration in ductal pancreatic adenocarcinomas. In: Whitcomb DC, Cohn JA, UlrichII CD (eds.) Inherited diseases of the pancreas. Philadelphia, WB Saunders, 2000, 691–696.
53. Wilentz RE, Iacobuzio-Donahue CA, Argani P, et al. Loss of expression of Dpc4 in pancreatic intraepithelial neoplasia: evidence that DPC4 inactivation occurs late in neoplastic progression. Cancer Res 2000, 60:2002–2006.
54. Wong T, Howes N, Threadgold J, et al. Molecular diagnosis of early pancreatic ductal adenocarcinoma in high-risk patients. Pancreatology 2001, 1(5):480–503.
55. Shi X, Friess H, Kleef J, et al. Pancreatic cancer: factors regulating tumor development, maintenance and metastasis. Pancreatology 2001, 1(5):511–518.
56. Caldas C, Hahn SA, Da Costa L, et al. Frequent somatic mutations and homozygous deletion of the p16 (MTS1) gene in pancreatic adenocarcinoma. Nat Genet 1994, 8:27–32.
57. Hengstler JG, Bauer A, Wolf HK, et al. Mutation analysis of the cationic trypsinogen gene in patients with pancreatic cancer. Anticancer Res 2000, 20(5A):2967–2974.
58. Garcea G, Dennison AR, Steward WP, et al. Role of inflammation in pancreatic carcinogenesis and the implications for future therapy. Pancreatology 2005, 5(6):514–529.
59. Adler G. Has the biology and treatment of pancreatic diseases evolved? Best Practice Res Clin Gastroenterol 2004, 18:83–90.
60. Marjolin J. Dictionnaire de Medecine, vol. 21 Pratique, 1828.
61. Balkwill F, Mantovani A. Inflammation and cancer: back to Virchow? Lancet 2001, 357(9255):539–545.
62. Eslick GD, Lim LL, Byles JE, et al. Association of *Helicobacter pylori* infection with gastric carcinoma: a meta-analysis. Am J Gastroenterol 1999, 94(9):2373–2379.
63. Blaser MJ, Perez-Perez GI, Kleanthous H, et al. Infection with Helicobacter pylori strains possessing cagA is associated with an increased risk of developing adenocarcinoma of the stomach. Cancer Res 1995, 55(10):2111–2115.
64. Harris RE, Beebe-Donk J, Doss H, et al. Aspirin, ibuprofen, and other non-steroidal anti-inflammatory drugs in cancer prevention: a critical review of non-selective COX-2 blockade (review). [see comment] Oncol Rept 2005, 13(4):559–583.
65. Smith ER, Daly MB, Xu XX. A mechanism for cox-2 inhibitor anti-inflammatory activity in chemoprevention of epithelial cancers. Cancer Epidemiol Biomark Prev 2004, 13(1):144–145.
66. Hitt E. Aspirin may lower risk of pancreatic cancer. Lancet Oncol 2002, 3(9).
67. Kinzler KW, Vogelstein B. Landscaping the cancer terrain. Science 1998, 280(5366):1036–1037.
68. Farrow B, Evers BM. Inflammation and the development of pancreatic cancer. Surg Oncol 2002, 10(4):153–169.

69. Hedin KE. Chemokines: new, key players in the pathobiology of pancreatic cancer. Intl J Gastrointest Cancer 2002, 31(1–3):23–29.
70. Farrow B, Sugiyama Y, Chen A, et al. Inflammatory mechanisms contributing to pancreatic cancer development. Ann Surg 2004, 239(6):763–769.
71. Rayet B, Gelinas C. Aberrant rel/nfkb genes and activity in human cancer. Oncogene 1999, 18(49):6938–6947.
72. Albazaz R, Verbeke CS, Rahman SH, et al. Cyclooxygenase-2 expression associated with severity of PanIN lesions: a possible link between chronic pancreatitis and pancreatic cancer. Pancreatology 2005, 5(4–5):361–369.
73. Silverman DT, Dunn JA, Hoover RN, et al. Cigarette smoking and pancreas cancer: a case-control study based on direct interviews. J Natl Cancer Inst 1994, 86(20):1510–1516.
74. Applebaum-Shapiro SE, Finch R, Pfützer RH, et al. Hereditary pancreatitis in North America: The Pittsburgh-Midwest Multi-Center Pancreatic Study Group Study. Pancreatology 2001, 1(5):439–443.
75. Hruban RH, Petersen GM, Goggins M, et al. Familial pancreatic cancer. Annals of Oncology 1999, 4:69–73.
76. Whitcomb DC, Ulrich II CD. Hereditary pancreatitis: new insights, new directions. Bailliere's Clin Gastroenterol 1999, 13(2):253–263.
77. Goggins M, Schutte M, Lu J, et al. Germline BRCA2 gene mutations in patients with apparently sporadic pancreatic carcinomas. Cancer Res 1996, 56(23):5360–5364.
78. Anonymous. Cancer risks in BRCA2 mutation carriers. The Breast Cancer Linkage Consortium. J Natl Cancer Inst 1999, 91(15):1310–1316.
79. Park JG, Park YJ, Wijnen JT, et al. Gene-environment interaction in hereditary nonpolyposis colorectal cancer with implications for diagnosis and genetic testing. Intl J Cancer 1999, 82(4):516–519.
80. Schenk M, Schwartz AG, O'Neal E, et al. Famlial risk of pancreatic cancer. J Natl Cancer Inst 2001, 93:640–644.
81. Lowenfels AB, Maisonneuve P, Whitcomb DC, et al. Cigarette smoking as a risk factor for pancreatic cancer in patients with hereditary pancreatitis. JAMA 2001, 286(2):169–170.
82. Malfertheiner P, Schutte K. Smoking—a trigger for chronic inflammation and cancer development in the pancreas. [comment] Am J Gastroenterol 2006, 101(1):160–162.
83. Maisonneuve P, Lowenfels AB, Mullhaupt B, et al. Cigarette smoking accelerates progression of alcoholic chronic pancreatitis. Gut 2005, 54(4):510–514.
84. Wittel UA, Pandey KK, Andrianifahanana M, et al. Chronic pancreatic inflammation induced by environmental tobacco smoke inhalation in rats. [see comment] Am J Gastroenterol 2006, 101(1):148–159.
85. Kimsey TF, Campbell AS, Albo D, et al. Co-localization of macrophage inflammatory protein-3alpha (Mip-3alpha) and its receptor, CCR6, promotes pancreatic cancer cell invasion. [erratum appears in Cancer J 2005, 11(4):354 Note: Wilson, M [added]]. Cancer J 2004, 10(6):374–380.
86. Boyle P, Maisonneuve P, Bueno de Mesquita B, et al. Cigarette smoking and pancreas cancer: a case control study of the search programme of the IARC. Intl J Cancer 1996, 67(1):63–71.
87. Warshaw AL, Fernandez-del Castillo C. Pancreatic carcinoma. N Engl J Med 1992, 326(7):455–465.
88. Bourliere M, Barthet M, Berthezene P, et al. Is tobacco a risk factor for chronic pancreatitis and alcoholic cirrhosis? Gut 1991, 32(11):1392–1395.
89. Lowenfels AB, Zwemer FL, Jhangiani S, et al. Pancreatitis in a native American Indian population. Pancreas 1987, 2(6):694–697.
90. Talamini G, Bassi C, Falconi M, et al. Alcohol and smoking as risk factors in chronic pancreatitis and pancreatic cancer. Dig Dis Sci 1999, 44(7):1301–1311.
91. Hruban RH, Canto MI, Yeo CJ. Prevention of pancreatic cancer and strategies for management of familial pancreatic cancer. Dig Dis 2001, 19(1):76–84.
92. Finn OJ. Cancer vaccines: between the idea and the reality. Nat Rev Immunol 2003, 3(8):630–641.

93. Connolly EM, Osborne H, Hickey DP. A novel treatment for chronic pancreatitis. Irish J Med Sci 2003, 172(4):202–203.
94. Kekis PB, Friess H, Kleeff J, et al. Timing and extent of surgical intervention in patients from hereditary pancreatic cancer kindreds. Pancreatology 2001, 1(5):525–530.
95. Whitcomb DC, Ulrich DC, Learch MM, et al. Conference Report: Third International Symposium on Inherited Diseases of the Pancreas. Pancreatology 2001, 1(5):423–431.
96. Ulrich II CD. Pancreatic cancer in hereditary pancreatitis—Consensus guidelines for prevention, screening, and treatment. Pancreatology 2001, 1(5):416–422.
97. Khalid A, Pal R, Sasatomi E, et al. Use of microsatellite marker loss of heterozygosity in accurate diagnosis of pancreaticobiliary malignancy from brush cytology samples. Gut 2004, 53(12):1860–1865.
98. Khalid A, McGrath KM, Zahid M, et al. The role of pancreatic cyst fluid molecular analysis in predicting cyst pathology.[see comment]. Clin Gastroenterol Hepatol 2005, 3(10):967–973.
99. Khalid A, Finkelstein S, McGrath K. Molecular diagnosis of solid and cystic lesions of the pancreas. Clin Lab Med 2005, 25(1):101–116.

Section II
Pancreatic Cancer Biology

Chapter 7
Pancreatic Progenitor Cells in Injury and Regeneration

Solomon Afelik and Jan Jensen

1 Introduction

The pancreas is presently receiving attention for different reasons. Pancreatic cancer is among the most lethal cancers, and treatment options are limited. Treatment modalities for acute or chronic pancreatitis are similarly narrow. Furthermore, as the organ is the home turf for the endocrine islets of Langerhans, it is also a keen subject for researchers investigating issues related to the etiology, and possible cures, of type I and II diabetes. It is now known that both the exocrine and endocrine pancreas share a common progenitor. This progenitor may be the culprit in pancreatic cancer development, and at the same time represent the cell type providing most hope to successfully developing an islet cell replacement therapy for diabetes. No wonder then, "pancreatic progenitor existence" as a subject is receiving attention. This chapter provides a review of current issues on the nature and function of both embryonic, and adult pancreatic progenitor cells, finding that research in pancreatic cancer, embryonic development, and adult regeneration starts to build a picture of adult cell plasticity that one day might be harnessed for therapeutic use.

2 Do Adult Pancreatic Stem Cells Exist?

The adult pancreas consists of endocrine and exocrine compartments, which are involved in the regulation of blood glucose levels and intestinal food digestion, respectively. The endocrine pancreas is made up of different hormone producing cells organized into islets of Langerhans, which are closely associated with blood vessels. The exocrine pancreas consists of digestive zymogen-producing acinar cells connected to a network of duct cells that serve as conduits through which the contents of the acini are channeled into the gastrointestinal tract. Although structurally and functionally distinct, both exocrine and endocrine cells of the mature pancreas differentiate from a common pool of pancreatic progenitors that are specified in the posterior foregut endoderm during early embryogenesis. Much is known from mouse pancreatic development, and it is generally

A.M. Lowy et al. (eds.) *Pancreatic Cancer*.
doi: 10.1007/978-0-387-69252-4, © Springer Science+Business Media, LLC 2008

recognized that common gene regulatory networks exist between mouse and human, although differences must exist in the growth and development between these species given the difference in overall size and gestational duration. In the mouse, it is known that the common pancreatic progenitor is determined by the expression of *Pdx1/Ipf1* and *Ptf1a* genes (*1, 2*). Several other gene regulatory factors are also expressed in this progenitor cell type, many of which are shared among endodermal regions (*3–5*). A series of intercellular signals between the prepancreatic endoderm and a number of neighboring embryonic tissues are involved in the specification of the pancreatic endoderm. Importantly, under the influence of mesenchymal signals, the early pancreatic progenitor cells undergo a phase of proliferation, characterized by active Notch signaling, prior to differentiation. Notch signaling is often involved in maintaining progenitor populations both during embryogenesis, as well as during adult stem cell maintenance in adult, such as in the neurogenic zones of the brain, the intestinal crypt of Lieberkühn, and the dermal stem cells of the skin as a few examples. The segregation of endocrine and exocrine precursors from the common progenitor pool (*6, 7*) is also under the influence of Notch signaling and this mechanism is perhaps the best-described aspect of Notch function in the pancreas (*8, 9*). In the course of embryogenesis and fetal development, the early pancreatic progenitor cells undergo differentiation, resulting in a mature pancreas with fully differentiated pancreatic cells, whereas the early progenitor cells seem to disappear, i.e., cells coexpressing Pdx1, Ptf1a, and active Notch signaling can not be detected in the adult homeostatic organ. Consequently, although embryonic pancreatic progenitor cells are well defined, their presence in the mature pancreas is a subject of controversy. While adult stem cells residing in defined progenitor niches have been well characterized in the skin (basal cells), intestinal epithelium (crypt cells), bone marrow (the marrow can be viewed as the "niche" of the blood), and brain (subventricular zone), there is no concrete evidence of such a spatial niche in the adult pancreas. Alternatively, in multiple differentiated tissues, maintenance and regeneration may be accomplished by resident "adult stem cells," which do not reside in a spatially defined niche. These are described as undifferentiated cells that have an unlimited ability for self-renewal and give rise to progenitor cells that differentiate into multiple lineages (*10–12*). Definition and proof of such cells is not straightforward, and often based on a method known as "BrdU labeling retention" (*13, 14*).

For a group of cells to be unequivocally established as adult stem cells of the pancreas, it is expected that such cells would have a less differentiated phenotype, capable of self-renewal and generate cells that can replenish multiple cell lineages of the pancreas. In an ideal situation, a visualization of the spatial location of such cells relative to differentiated cells with the aid of appropriate molecular markers can be done. To date no cells have been identified in the mature pancreas that fit these criteria; lineage tracing data to track such a defined population has not been possible given lack of a defined marker to initiate the labeling required. A BrdU retention study was described by Duviellie et al. indicating the presence of slow-cycling label-retaining cells located within and around pancreatic islets.

These cells, which were hormone negative and stained positive for Pdx1, were shown to be capable of undergoing β-cell differentiation when cultured in vitro and as such thought of as stem cells for β cells (15). Besides the lack of evidence for the in vivo differentiation potential of these cells, care should be exerted, however, as it has been shown that BrdU is capable of cell-cycle arresting cells while incorporating DNA at early S-phase (16). Also, BrdU is a known differentiation-suppression agent, which is capable of inhibiting differentiation, with no effect on viability (17). Thus, there are two general caveats in the label-retaining assay, strongly suggesting that the use of this assay should be paired with complementary approaches. Notwithstanding, there is no shortage of cells claimed likely to be of a "progenitor" or "stem cell" type in the adult organ, despite the general lack of concrete evidence for such properties. A brief account of such cells is provided in the following.

3 Putative Pancreatic Progenitor-Like Cell Types

3.1 Nestin-Positive Cells

One type of putative pancreatic stem cells are the Nestin-positive cells isolated from rat and human islets. When cultured in vitro, these cells were found to express liver and both exocrine and endocrine-specific genes (18). Nestin-positive cells with a high proliferative rate have also detected within neogenic ducts following subtotal pancreatectomy. These observations, have led to the suggestion that islet and duct-derived Nestin-positive cells may constitute pancreatic stem cell sources for pancreatic regeneration. For these to satisfy the criteria as pancreatic stem cells there is need to verify if, in the in vivo context, they do generate the different cell types seen in vitro and whether or not these cells are functional. To address this, Treutelaar et al. performed an in vivo Cre/loxP based lineage tracing study using a Nestin promoter–driven Cre-recombinase. Within the embryonic pancreas, Cre recombinase activity was detected in Nestin-positive cells within the pancreatic mesenchyme, whereas in adult mice the progeny of the Nestin-positive cells were traced to vascular endothelial cells of the islets. Furthermore, duct explants from these grown in culture could be differentiated into cell clusters containing insulin and Nestin-positive cells, but the insulin-positive cells did not show any lineage relationship to Nestin-positive cells (19). The use of Nestin as a marker of putative pancreatic stem cell is a subject of controversy, as Nestin appears to be expressed in a heterogeneous population of cells within the pancreas. Expression analysis, including the use of lineage tracing both in vitro and in vivo indicates that Nestin is expressed in mesenchymal and exocrine precursor cells of the embryonic pancreas (20–22), whereas in the adult pancreas, Nestin-positive precursor cells contribute to diverse cell lineages, including acinar, ducts, fibroblasts, and vascular cells, but not endocrine cells (20).

3.2   c-Met–Expressing Progenitor Cells

Suzuki et al. have suggested that a group of cells residing in the acinar and ductal compartment of the adult pancreas, positive for the hepatocyte growth factor receptor c-Met, could be pancreatic stem cells. Although these cells form colonies in vitro and appear capable of differentiating into multiple pancreatic lineages, the functionality of these cells, as they exist in vivo, is yet to be proved. Moreover, these cells also give rise to cells that express markers of liver and intestinal cells (*23*). Normal pancreatic progenitors in the rat use c-Met during normal growth (*24*). Also, regenerating adult pancreas reactivates c-Met expression (*25*) and c-Met is up-regulated in pancreatic cancer (*26, 27*), supporting these studies. Also, in the liver, c-Met has been found to be a marker of adult liver stem cells (oval cells), which have been demonstrated to have self-renewal capacity and multilineage potential (*28, 29*).

3.3   Centroacinar Cells

A number of studies in various regeneration models suggest the centroacinar cells may have stem cell–like properties. The centroacinar cell represents the terminal end bud of the ductal system, and shares markers with the intercalated ductal cells. Thus, the nature of the centroacinar cell is elusive; it appears best defined by a strictly spatial criterion. Nonetheless, this spatial localization is unique, and the cell may experience a distinctive cellular signaling environment, contacting both the acinar cells, as well as the intercalated ductal tree. Streptozotocin mediated β-cell damage has been shown to induce β cell neogenesis from centroacinar and intercalated duct cells (*30*). Pancreatic progenitor characteristics have also been detected in centroacinar cells during pancreatic regeneration following surgical wrapping (*31*). Hayashi et al. proposed, upon studying endocrine cell neogenesis following 90% pancreatectomy in the rat, the existence of presence of endocrine stem cells within intercalated duct cells and centroacinar cells (*23, 32*). Given the general absence of lineage tracing of centroacinar cells, and the absence of defined markers characterizing this cell type, formal proof of the unique involvement of the centroacinar cell in regeneration is yet to be obtained. It appears equally likely that under circumstances of regeneration and growth, the microenvironment may uniquely affect cells having the spatial localization of the centroacinar cell/or intercalated duct.

4   Adult Pancreatic Cell Plasticity: Recreation of an Embryonic Progenitor Niche?

While conclusive evidence for the existence of pancreatic stem cells in the homeostatic adult pancreas is still lacking at present, a number of experimental data suggest that the events of neogenesis seen during multiple types of regeneration emanate from fully differentiated adult pancreatic cells. These studies indicate that upon injury fully differentiated acinar and/or ductal cells dedifferentiate into "progenitor-like" cells that give rise to different pancreatic cell lineages. Some lineage tracing studies has provided evidence of these claims. Thus differentiated cells of the mature pancreas apparently possess plasticity and can transdifferentiate into other pancreatic cell types under certain conditions. This is important, as it changes the question of the existence of the "adult stem cell" to not *where* it may reside, but to one of *when* it exists. In light of the well-established progenitor-maintenance environment in the embryo, paraphrasing the preceding question may become: "Under what conditions does the adult organ display similar modes of signaling, remodeling, and growth, whereby it may mimic the environment found in the embryo?" For experimental use, it then becomes important to better define the embryonic progenitor cells, and look to the adult organ for any possible reactivation of such signals. For that reason, the remainder of the present chapter focuses on a comparative manner on cellular plasticity and how important intercellular signaling pathways involved in both embryonic development and pancreatic cancer also play a role during adult organ regeneration from injury.

5   Plasticity of Adult Pancreatic Cells

As stated, the differentiated cells of the adult pancreas derive from a common progenitor earlier on in development. Interestingly, a number of studies have provided evidence to suggest that the terminally differentiated cells of the adult pancreas posses an inherent plasticity whereby a fully differentiated cell can dedifferentiate to assume a progenitor like state and subsequently differentiate into other cell lineages. This plastic nature of differentiated cells of the adult pancreas seems to play a vital role in regeneration of damaged pancreatic tissue; as such adult pancreatic cells may serve as functional stem cells.

5.1   *Ductal Cell Transdifferentiation*

Studies of pancreatic regeneration following 90% pancreatectomy in adult rats suggest that in this model regeneration is achieved via replication of pre-existing endocrine and exocrine cells as well as proliferation and transdifferentiation of duct cells to multiple pancreatic lineages (*33, 34*). Following partial pancreatectomy (Ppx), differentiated duct cells undergo extensive proliferation, and transiently become less differentiated, as shown by the loss of typical duct markers trefoil factor 2 and 3 and mucin 5AC while regaining expression of Pdx1 (*34*). The ability of duct cells to give rise to β cells has also been reported in studies of in vitro culture of enriched human ductal cells (*35, 36*). Obesity generally causes an adaptive increase β cell mass (*37*) and examination of human obese pancreatic tissue samples suggests the presence of hormone-positive neogenic regions that suggestively bud from duct cells (33, 38, 39). Also, pancreatic islet neogenesis from duct cells has been reported in various mouse regeneration models such as transgenic mice overexpressing interferon gamma (IFN-γ) (40) or transforming growth factor α (TGF-α) (41) as well as in mice given extendin-4 (42) or betacellulin (43). In these studies, overexpression of TGFα was achieved by expression under the metal-lothionein promoter (MT-TGFα), which is induced by Zn-administration, whereas IFN-γ expression was driven by the rat insulin promoter (RIP-IFN-γ) (40, 44, 45). Although multiple reports claimed de novo islet formation from pancreatic ductal cells, more recently, lineage-tracing has challenged this view as no conversion of non-islet cells were found occur either over an extended period (1 year) or following partial pancreatectomy (46).

5.2　Acinar Cell Transdifferentiation

There is also evidence for transdifferentiation of pancreatic acinar cells to ductal and suggestively endocrine pancreatic lineages. Pancreatic acinoductal metapla-sia is associated with various pathologic conditions of the pancreas, such as pan-creatitis and pancreatic cancer (47). Also, transgenic mice overexpressing c-myc in pancreatic acinar cells develop mixed acinar/ductal pancreatic adenocarcino-mas (48), suggesting that pancreatic acinar cells could be the origin of adenocar-cinomas (49). A number of experimental models of pancreatic regeneration also display acinoductal metaplasia. In vitro culture of enriched human acinar cells led to a loss of acinar phenotype while gaining expression of ductal markers like cytokeratin 19 (CK19) and mucin (50). Studies in the RIP-IFNγ transgenic mouse model suggest that islet neogenesis in this model proceeds through an acinar-derived acinoductal cell type, characterized by the coexpression of the duct marker carbonic anhydrase II and the exocrine marker amylase (40, 51). Similarly, upon metaplastic development, acinar cells in the MT-TGFα transgenic mouse model appear to adopt a ductal phenotype (52, 53). The spontaneous conversion of acinar cells to ductal cells in response to EGFR signaling represents an addi-tional support for acinoductal metaplasia (54). Tokoro et al. have reported the presence of acinoductal cells in the regenerating foci in the regenerating pancreas of 90% pancreatectomized rat, indicating that acinar cells, and not only ducts, may contribute to the regenerative process in Ppx. Following pancreatectomy, a transient presence of cells arising from acinar cells and becoming positive for both amylase and CK19 was observed (55). Similar observations have been reported following pancreatic duct ligation (56).

Another model of pancreatic regeneration is that of supramaximal cerulein administration (Fig. 7.1). Cerulein mimics cholecystokinin as a secretagogue for exocrine secretion, and continuous cerulein administration led to necrotizing pancreatitis in mice within 8–12 hours from the start of administration (57). Cerulein stimulates the secretion of large amount of pancreatic enzymes and pancreatic fluid by acinar cells resulting in a mild edematous pancreatitis

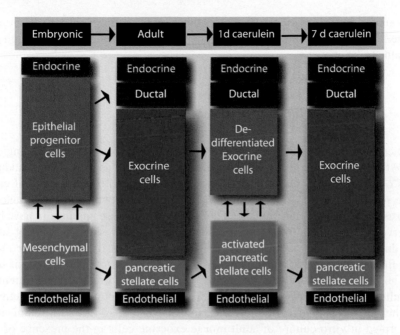

Fig. 7.1 Exocrine cell plasticity during cerulein-induced regeneration. Embryonic pancreatic progenitor cells give rise to mature exocrine, endocrine and ductal cells. Upon exocrine insult, as elicited through supramaximal cerulein administration, surviving exocrine cells initiate a dedifferentiation and redifferentiation program, whereby strong similarity to embryonic progenitors is observed. Restoration of a fully functional exocrine mass is accomplished by 7 days. These changes are prefigured by intraorgan expansion and activation of resident pancreatic stellate cells. Manipulation of stellate cell activation using Gleevec (imatinib mesylate) in turn regulates the epithelial regenerative program (JN Jensen et al., unpublished). This argues for cell–cell interactions possibly mimicking the signaling observed between pancreatic embryonic mesenchyme and epithelium in normal development.

accompanied by high serum amylase level, interstitial edema, leukocyte infiltration, and the vacuolation of acinar cells (*58, 59*). The general effect of cerulein is cathepsin B-mediated intrapancreatic trypsin activation (*60*). The resulting autodigestion leads to a general loss of the acinar cell population (*61*). We have shown that following cerulein-induced pancreatitis in the mouse, organ restoration occurs mainly through a process of exocrine pancreas de- and re-differentiation whereby multiple markers of embryonic progenitors are reactivated. These included the increased expression of β-catenin and E-cadherin, Pdx1, and components of the Notch pathway. Lineage tracing using conditional Ela-CreERT mice confirmed the dynamics of the exocrine populations going from the fully differentiated, to a dedifferentiated, and then redifferentiated state (Jensen et al., unpublished). No transdifferentiation was observed to nonexocrine fates, nor did it appear that nonexocrine cells contributed to any large extent to the exocrine restoration. Given the integrity of both islets, and ducts, in the cerulein model, this may not be surprising. However, the general resemblance to embryonic progenitor cells may indicate competence to nonexocrine fates, although this remains to be shown.

5.3   Acinar-to-Endocrine Conversion

Studies using many of the experimental systems described in the preceding conclude that acinar-to-endocrine transformation may occur as well. The acinoductal cells observed following rat duct ligation are thought to be the source of endocrine neogenesis in this model, since β-cell expansion occurs in the absence of mitosis (62). Indeed, transitional cell coexpressing amylase and insulin have been observed in this model (63). The presence of cells coexpressing markers of acinar and ducts cells or acinar and endocrine cells in the RIP-IFNγ transgenic model (51) further suggest that acinar cells are the origin of endocrine neogenesis here. The ability of AR42J cells, a rat amphicrine tumor cell line to transdifferentiate in culture into insulin producing cells using a given combination of factors is another situation of exocrine-to-endocrine conversion (64, 65). Minami et al. performed in vitro culture of adult mouse exocrine cells in the presence of epidermal growth factor (EGF) and nicotinamide and observed an increase in insulin producing cells from 0.1% to about 5% of the original cell preparation. Using the Cre/loxP based lineage system they demonstrate that the newly made insulin cells, which responded to glucose stimulation, were truly derived from amylase and elastase expressing cells (66). Also, recent evidence from the group of F. Levine indicate that nonendocrine pancreatic epithelial cells (NEPECs) purified from human pancreatic islets are capable of differentiating into endocrine cells upon transplantation together with fetal pancreatic cells under the kidney capsule of immunodeficient mice (67) . Fetal pancreatic cells appear to induce survival and endocrine differentiation potential of NEPEC in this assay as less endocrine differentiation is observed in their absence. It is likely that NEPECs were derived from mature cells through a dedifferentiation process, although this still remains to be shown. Nonetheless, this study provides compelling evidence of the endocrine differentiation potential of NEPECs or a population of cells within them, further characterization of the organization and differentiation potential as well as the inductive signal(s) that appear provided by the embryonic cells should provide further insight about the nature of these cells and their competence for endocrine development.

Finally, perhaps the most dramatic evidence of pancreatic plasticity is that seen in cases of transdifferentiation of pancreas to liver. Copper deficient diet has been shown to lead to the transdifferentiaton of pancreatic acinar cells into hepatocytes (67, 68). This change may be orchestrated by C/EBPβ (69—72), and is likely mediated by changes in DNA methylation, as another model of pancreatic regeneration; the ethionine-supplemented/methionine–deficient diet shows a similar effect.

5.4 Pancreatic Progenitor Cell Characteristics in Relation to the Transformed Phenotype

Pancreatic cancer displays multiple characteristics reminiscent of normal embryonic progenitor cells. This is not unique; it appears as in most cancers some elements of progenitor cell programs are reactivated (73). This phenomenon has been brought to bear by the growing knowledge in both pancreas development and pancreatic cancer, where it has become apparent that in the pancreatic cancer state a number of signaling mechanisms operate that are known to play pivotal roles in embryonic pancreas development—and regeneration as well. It is not the point of this chapter to extensively discuss the molecular pathways of pancreatic development and pancreatic cancer. However, details of these studies allow bridging between the embryonic and transformed organ in a natural manner via the regenerative state. Some of the pathways shared by the developing pancreas and pancreatic cancer are the transforming growth factor-β, Notch, Wnt, EGF, VEGF, and Hedgehog (Hh) signaling pathway. Some of these, Notch, EGF, and Hh pathways provide concrete insight into the nature of normal pancreatic progenitors, and the cellular plasticity of the adult organ, as well as cancer.

6 The Notch Pathway

Notch signaling is conserved across species and known for its pivotal role in cell fate specification. The specification of the endocrine lineage in the common pancreatic progenitor pool is mediated by Notch signaling through the process of lateral inhibition whereby ligand-expressing Ngn3+ cells induce activation of the Notch receptor in neighboring cells. This results in the activation of the bHLH genes of the Hairy and Enhancer of Split (HES) family, which act as transcriptional repressors of prodifferentiation factors such as Ngn3. As such, loss of function of various Notch pathway genes (Hes1, Dll1, Rbp-jκ) leads to up-regulation of Ngn3, and a consequent increase in endocrine formation (8, 74). Notwithstanding the role of Notch in differentiation, the constitutive activation of Notch signaling in the developing pancreas results in repression of differentiation and the maintenance of cells in the progenitor state (75–78). Active Notch signaling represses acinar cell differentiation by inhibiting the transcriptional activity of the exocrine transcription factor complex, Ptf1 (79). Importantly, in transgenic mice overexpressing FGF10 in the developing pancreatic epithelium, Notch signaling is continuously activated, which suggests a role of FGF10 and Notch pathway interaction, plausibly mediated through FGF10-induced Jagged activation of Notch (76, 78). Both FGF10 and Notch are capable of inhibiting endocrine and exocrine differentiation leading to pancreatic progenitor cell expansion. A required role for the jagged-type ligand remains to be shown, but data from Zebrafish development point toward such a role in the fish (80). It is fair to conclude that during pancreas development Notch signaling is required for cell fate determination and the maintenance of progenitor cell state, which ensures an increase in pancreatic progenitor cells mass prior to differentiation. Not surprising, Notch signaling is associated with pancreatic cancer. Increased expression of Notch receptors and ligands as well as the Notch target gene Hes1 occurs in human pancreatic ductal adenocarcinomas (*81*). Also, in the mouse transgenic model of TGFα-induced pancreatic cancer, acinar-to-ductal metaplasia mediated by a loss of acinar cell structure and expansion of a population of Pdx1-positive progenitor-like cells also active in Notch signaling. Ectopic activation of the Notch pathway in normal pancreatic epithelial explants (*81*), or the expression of constitutively active Notch (NICD) (*75, 77*) result in epithelial metaplasia, quite similar to what is observed during pancreatic cancer progression. The role of Notch signaling in pancreatic neoplasia was further demonstrated by the ability of Notch signaling inhibitors to abolish the induction of pancreatic neoplasia in normal pancreatic epithelium cultured in vitro with soluble TGFα (*81*). The activation of Notch signaling during pancreatic cancer progression, therefore, appear to recapitulate aspects of embryonic pancreas development, in which Notch signaling plays an important role in preventing premature differentiation allowing pancreatic progenitor cell expansion. Notch signaling is reactivated during regeneration of the adult pancreas, when the exocrine compartment recovers from cerulein-induced pancreatitis. Adult Notch signaling is likely to be important for attenuation of the terminal gene expression pattern, and the adoption of a proliferative progenitor cell–like state, from which forward differentiation may occur.

7   Epidermal Growth Factor Receptor Pathway

The EGF-pathway appears similarly linked to pancreatic development, regeneration and cancer. This family consists of several ligands, many of which appear to play a role in the pancreas (EGF, TGFα, heparin binding–epidermal growth factor [HB-EGF], and Betacellulin). EGF potently stimulates ductal cell proliferation and EGF and its homologue TGFα are both expressed in pancreatic ducts and acinar cells, in which EGF receptors are found on acinar cells and the apical surface of duct cells arguing for an autocrine pathway (*82–84*). Several studies have indicated the importance of epidermal growth factor receptor-mediated signaling in embryonic pancreas development. The EGF family member, HB-EGF is abundantly expressed in endocrine cells of the fetal pancreas and primitive duct-like cells, and its expression seem to be regulated by Pdx1 (*85*). EGF receptor (EGF-R) null mice display impaired pancreatic epithelial branching and morphogenesis and a significant reduction in β cells (*86*). Furthermore, in vitro culture of embryonic pancreatic epithelium in the presence of EGF results in increased epithelial proliferation with compromised differentiation, whereas the absence of EGF results in premature differentiation into predominantly insulin-positive cells (*87*). Furthermore, induction of EGF signaling in fully differentiated acinar cells in vitro, results in acinar to ductal metaplasia mediated by a dedifferentiated stage (*88*). These effects are quite similar to that of increased Notch signaling in pancreatic progenitor cells and the fully differentiated pancreas. Human pancreatic adenocarcinomas are characterized by an elevated expression of multiple receptors (EGFR, ErbB2, ErbB3) and ligands of the EGF pathway (EGF and TGFα) (89, 90). The elevated level of EGF signaling in cases of pancreatic cancer and pancreatitis is thought to be sustained by an autocrine loop of EGF signalling (83, 91). MT-TGFα mice develop epithelial tubular structures, fibrosis, and eventually ductal pancreatic (44, 45, 92). The mouse TGFα model of pancreatic cancer is a good demonstration of the role of EGF signaling in pancreatic cancer development. In these mice TGFα induces acinar to ductal metaplasia, which result in pancreatic intraepithelial neoplasia (PanIN), which constitute malignant epithelial precursors (53, 93–95). As discussed, one mode of TGFα-induced PanIN is by activation of notch signaling.

The human pancreatic carcinoma cell line PANC-1, like the majority of human pancreatic adenocarcinomas, possesses an activating mutation of K-ras. However, a number of studies have failed to reveal a constitutively active ERK pathway in pancreatic cancer cells with activating K-ras mutation (96–101). Instead, the Ras-MAPK cascade is activated in PANC-1 cells by EGF, which was required for fetal calf serum–induced proliferation of these cells (96). Neurotensin and EGF have been shown to synergistically induce rapid ERK activation and anchorage independent growth in human pancreatic carcinoma cells (102). Indeed, proliferation of PANC-1 cells is suppressed by an anti-TGFα monoclonal antibody (61).

In the model of pancreatic regeneration induced by ectopic interferon-γ, several components of the EGF pathway are up-regulated, including EGF, TGFα, and the EGF receptor in acinar cells, again showing evidence of conversion into duct-like structures (103). A subsequent study indicated the expression of the EGF receptors ErbB2, 3, and 4 as well as the ligand heregulin in the regenerating pancreas of these mice (104). Here, significant expression of ErbB receptors and ligand were detectable in primitive ducts of the fetal pancreas, declining postnatally. EGF has also been used to maintain a dedifferentiated population of exocrine cells in culture (105). Interestingly, if EGF was added to cultured acinar fractions in the presence of LIF (which activates the JAK-STAT pathway), re-expression of Ngn3 and Hnf6—both genes normally only expressed during developmental stages—was observed (3, 5). This indicates that simultaneous activation of specific pathways may lead to restoration of a more embryonic-like progenitor state. Interestingly, these conditions allowed for generation of pancreatic β cells, which strongly support that the differentiation plasticity of the adult exocrine cells include that of the terminally differentiated endocrine type.

Given the importance of the EGF and Notch pathways in growth and neoplasia of the pancreas, it would be expected that these would be excellent markers of stem/progenitor-like cells in the adult homeostatic organ. However, this appears not to be the case, and the described studies therefore reinforce the view that progenitor cell-like characteristics are reactivated in more terminally differentiated cells, rather than providing an explanation of pancreatic regeneration through rapid expansion of a rare intraorgan stem cell.

8 Hedgehog Signaling Pathway

Hedgehog signaling plays an important role in multiple stages of pancreas development. The presumptive pancreatic endoderm shows a characteristic lack of hedgehog signaling components like the hedgehog ligands sonic hedgehog (Shh) and indian hedgehog (Ihh), which are otherwise pan-endodermally expressed (*106–108*). Several studies suggest that the activity and expression pattern of Hh in the developing endoderm serves to demarcate the boundaries of the developing pancreas (*109–114*). It is quite well established that Shh signaling in the nonpancreatic endoderm acts to control radial mesenchymal patterning, and such a role has been confirmed in the pancreas as well, where overexpression of Shh (*115*) leads to gut-type mesenchymal development in the pancreas. Although the early mouse pancreas is devoid of Hh signaling, in the course of development, starting from e13.5, Hh ligands Ihh, and inhibitors patched1 (Ptch1) and human hedgehog inhibitory protein (Hhip) become detectable in the pancreatic epithelium (*110, 111*), suggesting that a tight modulation of Hh signaling continues within the pancreatic epithelium in the course of pancreas development. This later role of Hh signaling is still not understood. The hedgehog pathway may indirectly play a role in modulating the proliferative capacity of the pancreatic epithelium, as ectopic expression of Hh in mouse pancreatic epithelium through targeted deletion of Hedgehog inhibitors results in a reduction in Fgf10 expression (*111*). Fgf10 is required for the proliferation of the pancreatic epithelium prior to the secondary transition (78). Even later, hedgehog signaling has been observed within the islets and duct cells of the mature pancreas, as indicated by the expression of ligands and receptor of hedgehog signaling, namely Ihh, desert hedgehog (Dhh), Hhip, and Ptch1. In vitro cell culture studies, where insulinoma-type (INS1) cells were grown in the presence of exogenous shh or hh inhibitor cyclonamine implied that hh signaling positively regulate insulin production. Notwithstanding the involvement of Hh signaling activity in the adult pancreas, deregulated hh signaling in the adult pancreas is clearly associated with pancreatic cancer. Both human pancreatic cancer tissues and pancreatic cancer cell lines show a strong up-regulation of hh signaling (*116, 117*). This is evidenced by the high level expression of the ligands Shh and Ihh, the receptors Ptch1 and Smo, and the Hh target Gli1. Another hallmark of pancreatic cancer is the reduced levels of the Hh inhibitor Hhip. Indeed, the Hhip promoter has been shown to be hypermethylated in pancreatic cancer and pancreatic cancer cell lines, and exogenous Hhip has been shown to reduce pancreatic cell growth (*118*). Further evidence of a role of Hh signaling in pancreatic cancer progression and maintenance is derived from studies with ectopic expression of shh under the Pdx1 promoter. Not only do these mice develop intraepithelial lesions characteristic of human pancreatic cancer, but the mutations also showed mutations in K-ras and elevated expression in the EGF receptor ErbB-2 (*117*). Thus, hedgehog signaling appears to be involved in the progression of pancreatic cancer in a way that is linked to EGF signaling and K-ras mutation.

The role of the hedgehog pathway in pancreatic regeneration is not as well understood as that of the Notch and EGF pathways. However, the hedgehog pathway appears to be crucial for the re-differentiation events needed to restore the organ following cerulein-mediated pancreatitis in the mouse (S. Leach, personal communication). This is highly interesting as it discriminates among molecular events needed for the coordinated regenerative response, which previously was not known.

9 Conclusions

Although the inherent plastic nature of the mature pancreas is the basis of pancreatic diseases such as chronic pancreatitis and pancreatic cancer, it also serves as a potential source of cells for therapeutic purposes. The recent success in restoring normoglycemia in diabetes patients by islet transplantation presents a promise for a cure of diabetes but is not widely applicable due to inadequate supply of donor tissue. Therefore, identification of a pancreatic progenitor/stem cell niche in the adult pancreas holds enormous promise for the treatment of diabetes. Thus far the lack of solid evidence for adult pancreatic stem cells has increased the focus for other cell replacement sources ranging from embryonic stem cells to nonpancreatic organs such as the liver. Although these approaches hold promise, it is becoming evident from the plastic nature of the adult pancreas that the organ itself may represent a feasible source for the generation of pancreatic β cells. The fact that normal β cells are normally derived from a common endocrine/exocrine embryonic progenitor cell type makes the prospect of adult dedifferentiated cell conversion quite enticing. Furthermore, such a therapy holds the prospect of allowing a diabetic patient to supply "self" tissue for therapeutic use, which is clinically beneficial as auto- versus allo-transplantation reduces the issue of immunomodulatory intervention post-transplantation to one of tolerance induction, rather than allo-type rejection. Another advantage is that this would represent an ethically acceptable method compared with the prospective use of an embryonic stem cell–based therapy. Notwithstanding, given the current increase in knowledge of cellular dynamics and pathway involvement of the regenerating pancreas, it might be expected that novel intervention and preventative strategies for pancreatic diseases such as acute pancreatitis and pancreatic cancer—both presently difficult if not impossible to treat— will eventually find their way to the clinic.

Acknowledgments This work was supported by the American Diabetes Association (JJ) and the NIH-(R01 DK070636, JJ). SA is a recipient of a Barbara Davis Center Blum-Kovler fellowship.

References

1. Afelik S, Chen Y, Pieler T. Combined ectopic expression of Pdx1 and Ptf1a/p48 results in the stable conversion of posterior endoderm into endocrine and exocrine pancreatic tissue. Genes Dev 2006, 20(11):1441–1446.

 2. Kawaguchi Y, Cooper B, Gannon M, et al. The role of the transcriptional regulator Ptf1a in converting intestinal to pancreatic progenitors. Nat Genet 2002, 32(1):128–134.
 3. Jensen J. Gene regulatory factors in pancreatic development. Dev Dyn 2004, 229(1):176–200.
 4. Lantz KA, Kaestner KH. Winged-helix transcription factors and pancreatic development. Clin Sci (Lond) 2005, 108(3):195–204.
 5. Servitja JM, Ferrer J. 2004, Transcriptional networks controlling pancreatic development and beta cell function. Diabetologia 47(4):597–613.
 6. Gu G, Dubauskaite J, Melton DA. 2002, Direct evidence for the pancreatic lineage: NGN3+ cells are islet progenitors and are distinct from duct progenitors. Development 129(10):2447–2457.
 7. Herrera PL, Huarte J, Zufferey R, 1994, Ablation of islet endocrine cells by targeted expression of hormone-promoter-driven toxigenes. Proc Natl Acad Sci U S A 91(26):12999–13003.
 8. Apelqvist A, Li H, Sommer L, 1999, Notch signalling controls pancreatic cell differentiation. Nature 400(6747):877–881.
 9. Jensen J, Heller RS, Funder-Nielsen T, 2000, Independent development of pancreatic alpha- and beta-cells from neurogenin3-expressing precursors: a role for the notch pathway in repression of premature differentiation. Diabetes 49(2):163–176.
10. Shih CC, DiGiusto D, Mamelak A, 2002, Hematopoietic potential of neural stem cells: plasticity versus heterogeneity. Leuk Lymphoma 43(12):2263–2268.
11. Torella D, Ellison GM, Mendez-Ferrer S, 2006, Resident human cardiac stem cells: role in cardiac cellular homeostasis and potential for myocardial regeneration. Nat Clin Pract Cardiovasc Med 3(Suppl 1):S8–13.
12. Vescovi A, Gritti A, Cossu G, 2002, Neural stem cells: plasticity and their transdifferentiation potential. Cells Tissues Organs 171(1):64–76.
13. Bergstrom M, Lu L, Fasth KJ, 1998, In vitro and animal validation of bromine-76-bromodeoxyuridine as a proliferation marker. J Nucl Med 39(7):1273–1279.
14. Gardelle O, Roelcke U, Vontobel P, 2001, [76Br]Bromodeoxyuridine PET in tumor-bearing animals. Nucl Med Biol 28(1):51–57.
15. Duvillie B, Attali M, Aiello V, 2003, Label-retaining cells in the rat pancreas: location and differentiation potential in vitro. Diabetes 52(8):2035–2042.
16. Brown EH, Schildkraut CL. 1979, Perturbation of growth and differentiation of Friend murine erythroleukemia cells by 5-bromodeoxyuridine incorporation in early S phase. J Cell Physiol 99(2):261–278.
17. Tapscott SJ, Lassar AB, Davis RL, 1989, 5-bromo-2Î-deoxyuridine blocks myogenesis by extinguishing expression of MyoD1. Science 245(4917):532–536.
18. Zulewski H, Abraham EJ, Gerlach MJ, 2001, Multipotential nestin-positive stem cells isolated from adult pancreatic islets differentiate ex vivo into pancreatic endocrine, exocrine, and hepatic phenotypes. Diabetes 50(3):521–533.
19. Treutelaar MK, Skidmore JM, Dias-Leme CL, 2003, Nestin-lineage cells contribute to the microvasculature but not endocrine cells of the islet. Diabetes 52(10):2503–2512.
20. Delacour A, Nepote V, Trumpp A, 2004, Nestin expression in pancreatic exocrine cell lineages. Mech Dev 121(1):3–14.
21. Esni F, Stoffers DA, Takeuchi T, 2004, Origin of exocrine pancreatic cells from nestin-positive precursors in developing mouse pancreas. Mech Dev 121(1):15–25.
22. Selander L, Edlund H. 2002, Nestin is expressed in mesenchymal and not epithelial cells of the developing mouse pancreas. Mech Dev 113(2):189–192.
23. Suzuki T, Kadoya Y, Sato Y, 2003, The expression of pancreatic endocrine markers in centroacinar cells of the normal and regenerating rat pancreas: their possible transformation to endocrine cells. Arch Histol Cytol 66(4):347–358.
24. Calvo EL, Boucher C, Pelletier G, 1996, Ontogeny of hepatocyte growth factor and c-met/hgf receptor in rat pancreas. Biochem Biophys Res Commun 229(1):257–263.
25. Otte JM, Kiehne K, Schmitz F, 2000, C-met protooncogene expression and its regulation by cytokines in the regenerating pancreas and in pancreatic cancer cells. Scand J Gastroenterol 35(1):90–95.

26. Furukawa T, Duguid WP, Kobari M, 1995, Hepatocyte growth factor and Met receptor expression in human pancreatic carcinogenesis. Am J Pathol 147(4):889–895.
27. Kiehne K, Herzig KH, Folsch UR. 1997, c-met expression in pancreatic cancer and effects of hepatocyte growth factor on pancreatic cancer cell growth. Pancreas 15(1):35–40.
28. Suzuki A, Zheng YW, 2002, Clonal identification and characterization of self-renewing pluripotent stem cells in the developing liver. J Cell Biol 156(1):173–184.
29. Zheng YW, Taniguchi H. 2003, Diversity of hepatic stem cells in the fetal and adult liver. Semin Liver Dis 23(4):337–348.
30. Nagasao J, Yoshioka K, Amasaki H, 2003, Centroacinar and intercalated duct cells as potential precursors of pancreatic endocrine cells in rats treated with streptozotocin. Ann Anat 185(3):211–216.
31. Hosotani R, Ida J, Kogire M, 2004, Expression of pancreatic duodenal hoemobox-1 in pancreatic islet neogenesis after surgical wrapping in rats. Surgery 135(3):297–306.
32. Hayashi KY, Tamaki H, Handa K, 2003, Differentiation and proliferation of endocrine cells in the regenerating rat pancreas after 90% pancreatectomy. Arch Histol Cytol 66(2):163–174.
33. Bonner-Weir S, Toschi E, Inada A, 2004, The pancreatic ductal epithelium serves as a potential pool of progenitor cells. Pediatr Diabetes 5(Suppl 2):16–22.
34. Sharma A, Zangen DH, Reitz P, 1999, The homeodomain protein IDX-1 increases after an early burst of proliferation during pancreatic regeneration. Diabetes 48(3):507–513.
35. Bonner-Weir S, Taneja M, Weir GC, 2000, In vitro cultivation of human islets from expanded ductal tissue. Proc Natl Acad Sci U S A 97(14):7999–8004.
36. Gao R, Ustinov J, Korsgren O, et al. Maturation of in vitro-generated human islets after transplantation in nude mice. Mol Cell Endocrinol 2006, online.
37. Kloppel G, Lohr M, Habich K, 1985, Islet pathology and the pathogenesis of type 1 and type 2 diabetes mellitus revisited. Surv Synth Pathol Res 4(2):110–125.
38. Butler AE, Janson J, Bonner-Weir S, 2003, Beta-cell deficit and increased beta-cell apoptosis in humans with type 2 diabetes. Diabetes 52(1):102–110.
39. Yoon KH, Ko SH, Cho JH, 2003, Selective beta-cell loss and alpha-cell expansion in patients with type 2 diabetes mellitus in Korea. J Clin Endocrinol Metab 88(5):2300–2308.
40. Gu D, Sarvetnick N. 1993, Epithelial cell proliferation and islet neogenesis in IFN-g transgenic mice. Development 118(1):33–46.
41. Wang TC, Bonner-Weir S, Oates PS, 1993, Pancreatic gastrin stimulates islet differentiation of transforming growth factor alpha-induced ductular precursor cells. J Clin Invest 92(3):1349–1356.
42. Stoffers DA, Kieffer TJ, Hussain MA, 2000, Insulinotropic glucagon-like peptide 1 agonists stimulate expression of homeodomain protein IDX-1 and increase islet size in mouse pancreas. Diabetes 49(5):741–748.
43. Yamamoto K, Miyagawa J, Waguri M, 2000, Recombinant human betacellulin promotes the neogenesis of beta-cells and ameliorates glucose intolerance in mice with diabetes induced by selective alloxan perfusion. Diabetes 49(12):2021–2027.
44. Jhappan C, Stahle C, Harkins RN, 1990, TGF alpha overexpression in transgenic mice induces liver neoplasia and abnormal development of the mammary gland and pancreas. Cell 61(6):1137–1146.
45. Sandgren EP, Luetteke NC, Palmiter RD, 1990, Overexpression of TGF alpha in transgenic mice: induction of epithelial hyperplasia, pancreatic metaplasia, and carcinoma of the breast. Cell 61(6):1121–1135.
46. Dor Y, Brown J, Martinez OI, 2004, Adult pancreatic beta-cells are formed by self-duplication rather than stem-cell differentiation. Nature 429(6987):41–46.
47. Bockman DE. 1997, Morphology of the exocrine pancreas related to pancreatitis. Microsc Res Tech 37(5–6):509–519.
48. Sandgren EP, Quaife CJ, Paulovich AG, 1991, Pancreatic tumor pathogenesis reflects the causative genetic lesion. Proc Natl Acad Sci U S A 88(1):93–97.

49. Bockman DE. 1981, Cells of origin of pancreatic cancer: experimental animal tumors related to human pancreas. Cancer 47(6 Suppl):1528–1534.
50. Hall PA, Lemoine NR. 1992, Rapid acinar to ductal transdifferentiation in cultured human exocrine pancreas. J Pathol 166(2):97–103.
51. Gu D, Sarvetnick N. 1994, A transgenic model for studying islet development. Recent Prog Horm Res 49:161–165.
52. Bockman DE, Merlino G. 1992, Cytological changes in the pancreas of transgenic mice over-expressing transforming growth factor alpha. Gastroenterology 103(6):1883–1892.
53. Wagner M, Luhrs H, Kloppel G, 1998, Malignant transformation of duct-like cells originating from acini in transforming growth factor transgenic mice. Gastroenterology 115(5):1254–1262.
54. Means AL, Meszoely IM, Suzuki K, 2005, Pancreatic epithelial plasticity mediated by acinar cell transdifferentiation and generation of nestin-positive intermediates. Development 132(16):3767–3776.
55. Tokoro T, Tezel E, Nagasaka T, 2003, Differentiation of acinar cells into acinoductular cells in regenerating rat pancreas. Pancreatology 3(6):487–496.
56. Wang RN, Kloppel G, Bouwens L. 1995, Duct- to islet-cell differentiation and islet growth in the pancreas of duct-ligated adult rats. Diabetologia 38(12):1405–1411.
57. Neuschwander-Tetri BA, Ferrell LD, Sukhabote RJ, 1992, Glutathione monoethyl ester ameliorates caerulein-induced pancreatitis in the mouse. J Clin Invest 89(1):109–116.
58. Frossard JL, Bhagat L, Lee HS, 2002, Both thermal and non-thermal stress protect against caerulein induced pancreatitis and prevent trypsinogen activation in the pancreas. Gut 50(1):78–83.
59. Wagner AC, Mazzucchelli L, Miller M, 2000, CEP-1347 inhibits caerulein-induced rat pancreatic JNK activation and ameliorates caerulein pancreatitis. Am J Physiol Gastrointest Liver Physiol 278(1):G165–G172.
60. Halangk W, Lerch MM, Brandt-Nedelev B, 2000, Role of cathepsin B in intracellular trypsinogen activation and the onset of acute pancreatitis. J Clin Invest 106(6):773–781.
61. Watanabe O, Baccino FM, Steer ML, 1984, Supramaximal caerulein stimulation and ultrastructure of rat pancreatic acinar cell: early morphological changes during development of experimental pancreatitis. Am J Physiol 246(4 Pt 1):G457–G467.
62. Rooman I, Heremans Y, Heimberg H, Bouwens L. 2000, Modulation of rat pancreatic acinoductal transdifferentiation and expression of PDX-1 in vitro. Diabetologia 43(7):907–914.
63. Bertelli E, Bendayan M. 1997, Intermediate endocrine-acinar pancreatic cells in duct ligation conditions. Am J Physiol 273(5 Pt 1):C1641–C1649.
64. Mashima H, Shibata H, Mine T, 1996, Formation of insulin-producing cells from pancreatic acinar AR42J cells by hepatocyte growth factor. Endocrinology 137(9):3969–3976.
65. Mashima H, Ohnishi H, Wakabayashi K, 1996, Betacellulin and activin A coordinately convert amylase-secreting pancreatic AR42J cells into insulin-secreting cells. J Clin Invest 97(7):1647–1654.
66. Minami K, Okuno M, Miyawaki K, 2005, Lineage tracing and characterization of insulin-secreting cells generated from adult pancreatic acinar cells. Proc Natl Acad Sci U S A 102(42):15116–15121.
67. Hao E, Tyrberg B, Itkin-Ansari P, Lakey JR, Geron I, Monsov EZ, Barcova M, Mercola M, Levine F, 2006, Beta-cell differentiation form non-neuroendocrine epithelial cells of the adult human pancreas. Nat Med 12(3):273–274.
68. Rao MS, Dwivedi RS, Yeldandi AV, 1989, Role of periductal and ductular epithelial cells of the adult rat pancreas in pancreatic hepatocyte lineage. A change in the differentiation commitment. Am J Pathol 134(5):1069–1086.
69. Scarpelli DG, Rao MS. 1981, Differentiation of regenerating pancreatic cells into hepatocyte-like cells. Proc Natl Acad Sci U S A 78(4):2577–2581.
70. Kurash JK, Shen CN, Tosh D. 2004, Induction and regulation of acute phase proteins in transdifferentiated hepatocytes. Exp Cell Res 292(2):342–358.
71. Shen CN, Slack JM, Tosh D. 2000, Molecular basis of transdifferentiation of pancreas to liver. Nat Cell Biol 2(12):879–887.

72. Shen CN, Seckl JR, Slack JM, 2003, Glucocorticoids suppress beta-cell development and induce hepatic metaplasia in embryonic pancreas. Biochem J 375(Pt 1):41–50.
73. Tosh D, Shen CN, Slack JM. 2002, Conversion of pancreatic cells to hepatocytes. Biochem Soc Trans 30(2):51–55.
74. Heiser PW, Hebrok M. 2004, Development and cancer: lessons learned in the pancreas. Cell Cycle 3(3):270–272.
75. Jensen J, Pedersen EE, Galante P, 2000, Control of endodermal endocrine development by Hes-1. Nat Genet 24(1):36–44.
76. Hald J, Hjorth JP, German MS, 2003, Activated Notch1 prevents differentiation of pancreatic acinar cells and attenuate endocrine development. Dev Biol 260(2):426–437.
77. Hart A, Papadopoulou S, Edlund H. 2003, Fgf10 maintains notch activation, stimulates proliferation, and blocks differentiation of pancreatic epithelial cells. Dev Dyn 228(2):185–193.
78. Murtaugh LC, Stanger BZ, Kwan KM, 2003, Notch signaling controls multiple steps of pancreatic differentiation. Proc Natl Acad Sci U S A 100(25):14920–14925.
79. Norgaard GA, Jensen JN, Jensen J. 2003, FGF10 signaling maintains the pancreatic progenitor cell state revealing a novel role of Notch in organ development. Dev Biol 264(2):323–338.
80. Esni F, Ghosh B, Biankin AV, 2004, Notch inhibits Ptf1 function and acinar cell differentiation in developing mouse and zebrafish pancreas. Development 131(17):4213–4224.
81. Zecchin E, Filippi A, Biemar F, et al. Distinct delta and jagged genes control sequential segregation of pancreatic cell types from precursor pools in zebrafish. Dev Biol 2006, online.
82. Miyamoto Y, Maitra A, Ghosh B, 2003, Notch mediates TGF alpha-induced changes in epithelial differentiation during pancreatic tumorigenesis. Cancer Cell 3(6):565–576.
83. Hormi K, Onolfo JP, Gres L, 1995, Developmental expression of transforming growth factor-alpha in the upper digestive tract and pancreas of the rat. Regul Pept 55(1):67–77.
84. Korc M, Chandrasekar B, Yamanaka Y, 1992, Overexpression of the epidermal growth factor receptor in human pancreatic cancer is associated with concomitant increases in the levels of epidermal growth factor and transforming growth factor alpha. J Clin Invest 90(4):1352–1360.
85. Verme TB, Hootman SR. 1990, Regulation of pancreatic duct epithelial growth in vitro. Am J Physiol 258(6 Pt 1):G833–G840.
86. Kaneto H, Miyagawa J, Kajimoto Y, 1997, Expression of heparin-binding epidermal growth factor-like growth factor during pancreas development. A potential role of PDX-1 in transcriptional activation. J Biol Chem 272(46):29137–29143.
87. Miettinen PJ, Huotari M, Koivisto T, 2000, Impaired migration and delayed differentiation of pancreatic islet cells in mice lacking EGF-receptors. Development 127(12):2617–2627.
88. Cras-Meneur C, Elghazi L, Czernichow P, 2001, Epidermal growth factor increases undifferentiated pancreatic embryonic cells in vitro: a balance between proliferation and differentiation. Diabetes 50(7):1571–1579.
89. Means AL, Meszoely IM, Suzuki K, 2005, Pancreatic epithelial plasticity mediated by acinar cell transdifferentiation and generation of nestin-positive intermediates. Development 132(16):3767–3776.
90. Barton CM, Hall PA, Hughes CM, 1991, Transforming growth factor alpha and epidermal growth factor in human pancreatic cancer. J Pathol 163(2):111–116.
91. Friess H, Berberat P, Schilling M, 1996, Pancreatic cancer: the potential clinical relevance of alterations in growth factors and their receptors. J Mol Med 74(1):35–42.
92. Lemoine NR, Hughes CM, Barton CM, 1992, The epidermal growth factor receptor in human pancreatic cancer. J Pathol 166(1):7–12.
93. Greten FR, Wagner M, Weber CK, 2001, TGF alpha transgenic mice. A model of pancreatic cancer development. Pancreatology 1(4):363–368.
94. Hruban RH, Wilentz RE, Goggins M, 1999, Pathology of incipient pancreatic cancer. Ann Oncol 10(Suppl 4):9–11.
95. Song SY, Gannon M, Washington MK, 1999, Expansion of Pdx1-expressing pancreatic epithelium and islet neogenesis in transgenic mice overexpressing transforming growth factor alpha. Gastroenterology 117(6):1416–1426.

96. Wagner M, Greten FR, Weber CK, 2001, A murine tumor progression model for pancreatic cancer recapitulating the genetic alterations of the human disease. Genes Dev 15(3):286–293.

97. Giehl K, Skripczynski B, Mansard A, et al.2000, Growth factor-dependent activation of the Ras-Raf-MEK-MAPK pathway in the human pancreatic carcinoma cell line PANC-1 carrying activated K-ras: implications for cell proliferation and cell migration. Oncogene 19(25):2930–2942.

98. Guha S, Lunn JA, Santiskulvong C, 2003, Neurotensin stimulates protein kinase C-dependent mitogenic signaling in human pancreatic carcinoma cell line PANC-1. Cancer Res 63(10):2379–2387.

99. Ryder NM, Guha S, Hines OJ, 2001, G protein-coupled receptor signaling in human ductal pancreatic cancer cells: neurotensin responsiveness and mitogenic stimulation. J Cell Physiol 186(1):53–64.

100. Seufferlein T, Lint J, Van Liptay S, 1999, Transforming growth factor alpha activates Ha-Ras in human pancreatic cancer cells with Ki-ras mutations. Gastroenterology 116(6):1441–1452.

101. Yip-Schneider MT, Lin A, Barnard D, 1999, Lack of elevated MAP kinase (Erk) activity in pancreatic carcinomas despite oncogenic K-ras expression. Int J Oncol 15(2):271–279.

102. Yip-Schneider MT, Lin A, Marshall MS. 2001, Pancreatic tumor cells with mutant K-ras suppress ERK activity by MEK-dependent induction of MAP kinase phosphatase-2. Biochem Biophys Res Commun 280(4):992–997.

103. Kisfalvi K, Guha S, Rozengurt E. 2005, Neurotensin and EGF induce synergistic stimulation of DNA synthesis by increasing the duration of ERK signaling in ductal pancreatic cancer cells. J Cell Physiol 202(3):880–890.

104. Arnush M, Gu D, Baugh C, 1996, Growth factors in the regenerating pancreas of gamma-interferon transgenic mice. Lab Invest 74(6):985–990.

105. Kritzik MR, Krahl T, Good A, 2000, Expression of ErbB receptors during pancreatic islet development and regrowth. J Endocrinol 165(1):67–77.

106. Baeyens L, Bonne S, German MS, 2006, Ngn3 expression during postnatal in vitro beta cell neogenesis induced by the JAK/STAT pathway. Cell Death Differ 13(11):1892–1899.

107. Bitgood MJ, McMahon AP. 1995, Hedgehog and Bmp genes are coexpressed at many diverse sites of cell-cell interaction in the mouse embryo. Dev Biol 172(1):126–138.

108. Echelard Y, Epstein DJ, Jacques B, St. 1993, Sonic hedgehog, a member of a family of putative signaling molecules, is implicated in the regulation of CNS polarity. Cell 75(7):1417–1430.

109. Ramalho-Santos M, Melton DA, McMahon AP. 2000, Hedgehog signals regulate multiple aspects of gastrointestinal development. Development 127(12):2763–2772.

110. Hebrok M, Kim SK, Melton DA. 1998, Notochord repression of endodermal Sonic hedgehog permits pancreas development. Genes Dev 12(11):1705–1713.

111. Hebrok M, Kim SK, Jacques B, St. 2000, Regulation of pancreas development by hedgehog signaling. Development 127(22):4905–4913.

112. Kawahira H, Ma NH, Tzanakakis ES, 2003, Combined activities of hedgehog signaling inhibitors regulate pancreas development. Development 130(20):4871–4879.

113. Kawahira H, Scheel DW, Smith SB, 2005, Hedgehog signaling regulates expansion of pancreatic epithelial cells. Dev Biol 280(1):111–121.

114. Kim SK, Hebrok M, Melton DA. 1997, Notochord to endoderm signaling is required for pancreas development. Development 124(21):4243–4252.

115. Kim SK, Hebrok M, Li E, 2000, Activin receptor patterning of foregut organogenesis. Genes Dev 14(15):1866–1871.

116. Apelqvist A, Ahlgren U, Edlund H. 1997, Sonic hedgehog directs specialised mesoderm differentiation in the intestine and pancreas. Curr Biol 7(10):801–804.

116. Berman DM, Karhadkar SS, Maitra A, 2003, Widespread requirement for Hedgehog ligand stimulation in growth of digestive tract tumours. Nature 425(6960):846–851.

117. Thayer SP, Magliano MP, di Heiser PW, 2003, Hedgehog is an early and late mediator of pancreatic cancer tumorigenesis. Nature 425(6960):851–856.

118. Kayed H, Kleeff J, Esposito I, 2005, Localization of the human hedgehog-interacting protein (Hip) in the normal and diseased pancreas. Mol Carcinog 42(4):183–192.

Chapter 8
Development of the Endocrine and Exocrine Pancreas

L. Charles Murtaugh, Jared Cassiano, and Jean-Paul De La O

1 Introduction

Is the field of pancreas developmental biology relevant to human disease? An affirmative answer is certainly given by proponents of "regenerative medicine," which aims to treat disease through stem cell transplantation, tissue engineering and similar interventions. Type I diabetes, in which insulin-producing β cells are lost to autoimmunity, is regarded as a test case for cell-based therapies, and a major goal of research into pancreas development is to translate an understanding of β-cell development into an approach to generating such cells de novo (1). Pancreas developmental biologists are increasingly aware that their insights might also apply to pancreatic cancer research, particularly as regards the cellular and molecular origins of the disease. The cell type from which pancreatic cancer arises remains unknown, but may be discovered through the use of experimental paradigms and reagents appropriated from embryology (2). In addition, tumorigenesis in the pancreas appears to be accompanied by reactivation of signaling systems normally active in the developing organ, such as the Notch pathway (ref. 3, and see following discussion). We therefore hope that understanding what goes right in pancreas development will shed light on what goes wrong in neoplasia.

This chapter briefly surveys the current understanding of pancreas development. We recommend several excellent reviews, recent and classic, for a more comprehensive view (4–7). Our focus is on embryonic pancreas development: How do specific regions of the developing gut assume a pancreatic identity, what controls growth and morphogenesis of the organ, and how do cells differentiate into specific mature cell types? In rodents, generation of new endocrine and exocrine cells—barring injury or disease—occurs predominantly prenatally, and further growth of the pancreas appears to rely on division of differentiated cells, rather than recruitment of dedicated stem cells (8, 9, and see the chapter by Jensen et al. in this volume). Toward the end of this chapter, however, we briefly review the pathologic phenomenon of metaplasia, when differentiated cells of the adult appear to relax their normal discipline and resume embryonic-like behavior.

A.M. Lowy et al. (eds.) *Pancreatic Cancer*.
doi: 10.1007/978-0-387-69252-4, © Springer Science+Business Media, LLC 2008

2 Early Specification of the Pancreas

Figure 8.1 summarizes pancreatic organogenesis in the mouse, the organism of choice for most of the field (although we discuss important contributions from other organisms, most notably zebrafish *[Danio rerio]* and frog *[Xenopus laevis]*). Figure 8.2 shows representative photomicrographs of developing mouse pancreata. For obvious reasons, prenatal development of the human pancreas is less well studied, but its overall anatomical pattern appears similar to that of the mouse (*10, 11*).

Figure 8.1 also depicts the spatiotemporal expression patterns of several regulatory factors that prefigure anatomical changes in the pancreas, the roles of which will be discussed in the next sections. Some of these genes, such as the homeodomain transcription factor *Pdx1*, are expressed in the earliest precursors of the pancreas, and can serve as markers for establishment of the "pancreatic state" (*12, 13*). Other markers are expressed in specific lineages of the pancreas: the basic helix-loop-helix (bHLH) transcription factor *Ngn3* (Mouse Genomic Informatics [MGI] gene symbol *Neurog3*), for example, is expressed in cells largely or entirely fated to give rise to islets (*13, 14*). Relationships between marker expression and lineage have been found using the Cre-loxP system (*15*), one of many genetic tools that ensure a continued foremost place for the mouse in pancreas developmental biology.

Expression of *Pdx1* initiates in the posterior foregut at roughly 8.5 days postfertilization (E8.5) in the mouse, prior to any morphologic changes within the prepancreatic endoderm (see Figs. 8.1A and 8.2A) (*12*). This timing closely correlates with that of pancreatic specification, defined by classic in vitro culture experiments (*16*).

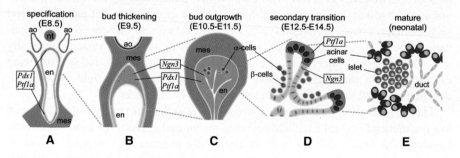

Fig. 8.1 Mammalian pancreas development. Schematized "cross-sections" through the developing pancreas at various stages (timepoints listed for mouse embryogenesis). **A.** Expression of *Pdx1* and *Ptf1a* marks the early pancreatic progenitors at ~E8.5 *(purple)*, both dorsal and ventral. **B.** The pancreatic epithelia subsequently thicken as the first *Ngn3⁺* pro-endocrine cells appear *(dark blue)*, and the mesenchyme *(orange)* moves medially to surround the future dorsal bud (the ventral pancreas is omitted for clarity). **C.** Subsequent outgrowth produces a dense, convoluted epithelial bud, comprised primarily of progenitor cells with a small number of early α cells *(green)*. **D.** During the secondary transition, *Pdx1* expression is downregulated in the core epithelium *(light purple)*, which begins to produce abundant β cells *(light blue)* and other islet cells. (The mesenchyme is omitted for clarity, but continues to surround the epithelium.) At the same time, *Ptf1a* expression becomes restricted to peripheral regions, which undergoes acinar differentiation *(red)*. **E.** By birth, all of the mature cell types have developed, and islets assume their characteristic arrangement of cell types. Abbreviations: *ao*, aorta, *en*, endoderm, *mes*, mesenchyme, *nt*, notochord

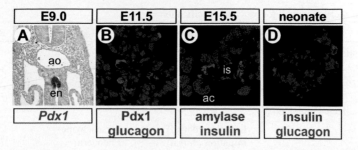

Fig. 8.2 Snapshots of mouse pancreas development. **A.** Pdx1 expression (blue, transverse section of an Xgal-stained *Pdx1*[LacZ] mouse) (*37*) in the E9.0 dorsal bud, shortly after the mesenchyme has separated the pancreas from the overlying aorta. (Photomicrograph provided by Dr. Ondine Cleaver, University of Texas Southwestern Medical Center.) **B.** Emergence of early α cells *(green)* among Pdx1+ progenitor cells *(red)* at E11.5. **C.** At E15.5, primitive islet cells (including β cells, *green*) cluster in the core of the developing pancreas, surrounded by amylase+ acinar cells *(red)*. **D.** Islets achieve mature organization by birth, with a large number of β cells *(red)* surrounded by a smaller number of α cells *(green)*. Abbreviations: *ac*, acinar cells, *ao*, aorta, *en*, endoderm, *is*, islet cells

Approximately a day later, thickenings of the dorsal and ventral surfaces of the gut tube endoderm provide the first visible sign of pancreas development (see Fig. 8.1B). These thickenings will ultimately give rise to the tail and head of the pancreas, respectively. Over the next several days (E9.5-E11.5), the pancreatic primordia expand into the surrounding mesenchyme as compact, convoluted epithelial buds (see Figs. 8.1C and 8.2B) (*17*), whereas the ventral pancreas emerges close to the future liver and gallbladder, the dorsal is well separated and thus easily dissected and cultured. Classic studies showed that the dorsal pancreatic epithelium at this stage will undergo growth and acinar differentiation in vitro, but only when co-cultured with adjacent mesenchyme (*18*). Interestingly, other sources of embryonic mesenchyme can substitute for that of the pancreas, suggesting that its role is *permissive* in nature, supporting the execution of an intrinsic developmental program.

When and how is this program established, i.e., when does the prepancreatic endoderm receive the *instructive* signals that confer its future identity? Table 8.1 lists genes that act early in development to induce and stabilize pancreatic identity, in most cases ascertained by the effects of knockout mutations on expression of *Pdx1*. Although space does not permit an exhaustive treatment of this list, several themes emerge. First, the genetic requirements for dorsal and ventral pancreas are not identical. Second, some genes are required for the initiation of *Pdx1* expression, whereas others are required for its maintenance and the continued execution of the pancreatic program. Third, most of these genes encode transcription factors, and close study of the mutant phenotypes suggest that they act within the pancreas itself.

Most of those genes that are required outside the pancreas—e.g., *Flk1* (*19*) and *Isl1* (*20*)—mediate permissive signaling to the dorsal pancreas. The dorsal pancreas sequentially contacts three independent tissues that each appear to provide permissive signals (*6*): notochord (*21*), aorta (*22*), and mesenchyme (*20*). (The ventral pancreas, by contrast, develops in continuous contact with splanchnic mesenchyme,

Table 8.1 Genes required for pancreas specification

Gene	Step affected in knockout	Site of action	Reference
Both dorsal and ventral lobes affected			
Sox17	Initiation	Endoderm	*123*
Hnf6/Fgf10 (double mutant)	Initiation	Endoderm	*56*
Tcf2/Hnf1	Initiation/stabilization	Endoderm	*124*
One lobe affected preferentially			
Raldh2	Initiation (dorsal)	Mesenchyme	*28, 29*
Hlxb9	Initiation (dorsal)	Endoderm	*125, 126*
Isl1	Stabilization (dorsal)	Mesenchyme	*20*
Flk1	Stabilization (dorsal)	Vasculature	*19*
N-cadherin	Stabilization (dorsal)	Mesenchyme	*127*
Ptf1a	Initiation (ventral)	Endoderm	*30*
Hex	Initiation (ventral)	Endoderm (nonpancreatic)	*128*
Other (see text)			
Hes1	Initiation	Endoderm	*31, 32*

Listed are genes required for either initiation or stabilization of pancreatic fates (in the latter class of mutants, *Pdx1* expression initiates but disappears prior to bud emergence), separated according to whether they are required in both dorsal and ventral buds, or preferentially in one or the other. Also indicated is the tissue in which the genes are most likely required, those acting outside the endoderm are thought to directly or indirectly mediate signaling to the endoderm.

which produces unknown instructive cues for its specification (*23*)). Instructive patterning of the dorsal pancreas precedes these permissive interactions, and is mediated in part by retinoic acid (RA) signaling. Initial studies in zebrafish showed that blocking RA synthesis or response prevents endocrine and exocrine development (*24, 25*). Ectopic RA signaling, conversely, can expand the pancreatic domain, a hallmark of an instructive cue (*24, 26*). Zebrafish studies also indicate that RA is required during gastrulation (*24*), well before *Pdx1* is expressed. Loss of function studies in frog (*27*) and mouse (*28, 29*) confirm that RA is required for pancreas specification, although in these species it is selectively required dorsally but not ventrally.

In a rapidly growing embryo such as the mouse, defects in survival or proliferation may mimic defects in specification. The strongest possible evidence for misspecification is to find affected cells adopting alternate fates, and studies of *Ptf1a* (*30*) and *Hes1* (*31, 32*) knockouts are among the few that irrefutably demonstrate this. *Ptf1a* encodes a bHLH transcription factor that was identified as a positive regulator of exocrine-specific genes (*33*). Mice and humans lacking functional *Ptf1a/PTF1A* have a dramatic reduction in pancreas size and islet cell number, and completely fail to develop acini (*34, 35*). Further study showed that *Ptf1a* expression initiates far in advance of acinar gene expression, approximately coincident with *Pdx1*, and lineage tracing showed that *Ptf1a*-expressing cells contribute exclusively to pancreas (*30*). When *Ptf1a* is mutated, however, these same cells instead form intestinal tissue (*30*). *Ptf1a* is thus required to specify pancreas in cells otherwise fated to generate intestine.

As mentioned, *Ptf1a* was originally characterized for its role in acinar development, yet proved to have additional functions. A similar story can be told about the *Hes1* transcription factor, a downstream target of the Notch signaling pathway that was originally characterized as a negative regulator of endocrine development (*36*, and see the following). Further examination of *Hes1* knockout mice found that they also developed *ectopic* pancreas tissue, deriving from cells of the bile ducts (*31*), posterior stomach and duodenum (*32*). These tissues all express *Pdx1* during their normal development, albeit with a delay relative to the pancreas (*37*), and in the absence of *Hes1* they also ectopically express *Ptf1a* (*32*). *Hes1* (and by extension the Notch pathway, although this remains to be proven) thus acts to limit pancreas specification to a subset of *Pdx1*-expressing tissues, apparently by repressing *Ptf1a* expression outside the prospective pancreas.

3 Growth and Differentiation: Intercellular Signals

As described, the dorsal and ventral pancreata initially grow out of the gut tube as dense, convoluted epithelial buds, surrounded by mesenchymal cells (*17*). As shown in Fig. 8.2B, a small number of endocrine cells—primarily glucagon-producing α cells—differentiate during this period (E9.5-E11.5), but the majority of cells remain undifferentiated *Pdx1*-positive progenitors (*38*). The functional significance of the early endocrine cells in rodents is unclear: They do not express markers typical of their mature counterparts (*38–40*), they differentiate in the background of mutations that abolish or inhibit mature islet development (*37*, *41–43*), and they do not develop in the early human pancreas (*11*). A similar population of early islet cells, with apparently unique developmental programs, also appears in zebrafish (*44*) and Xenopus (*45*).

Most mature endocrine cells are born during the so-called "secondary transition," a developmental period when insulin and acinar enzyme levels, barely detectable in the emergent pancreatic buds, undergo exponential increases (*4*). In mice, this begins at approximately E13.5, as the epithelium expands and branches into the surrounding mesenchyme. During this process, large numbers of progenitor cells in the central regions of the pancreas turn on *Ngn3*, delaminate from the epithelium, and assume endocrine fates (see Figs. 8.1D–E and 8.2C). As shown in Fig. 8.2D, these cells subsequently aggregate to establish proto-islet arrangements by birth (*11*, *46*). β cells comprise the majority (≥75%) of endocrine cells in rodents, and tend to segregate to the islet core; the b-cell proportion is smaller in humans (≥50%), and the distribution of cells within the islets is consequently more heterogeneous (*47*). The remaining islet cell types, which also differentiate in utero albeit with slightly different kinetics from the β cells (*11*, *46*), each expresses a distinctive peptide hormone such as glucagon (α cells), somatostatin (δ cells), or pancreatic polypeptide (PP cells). Recent work has identified a fifth islet cell type, the ghrelin-producing ε cells (*48*, *49*). Although the proportions vary between species, α cells are usually the next most abundant cell type after β cells, with the other cell types comprising relatively small minorities.

Just as β cells begin to appear, acinar differentiation initiates in more peripheral regions of the epithelium (see Fig. 8.2C); unlike islet cells, which do not divide in utero, newly-formed acinar cells are highly proliferative, and rapidly expand to comprise the majority of pancreatic cells by birth (4, 7). Cells expressing ductal markers also begin to appear at these stages, although it should be noted that many ductal antigens are also expressed in progenitor cells (11, 50), and relatively little is known about the molecular mechanisms of duct development.

The secondary transition occurs as the pancreatic epithelium expands into the surrounding mesenchyme (Figs. 8.1C–D), which provides critical pro-growth/pro-acinar signals to the budding stage (E10.5-E11.5) pancreas (16, 18). The mesen-chyme also appears to suppress endocrine development within the epithelium, suggesting that islet differentiation represents a "default" fate in the pancreas (51–54). Such studies must be interpreted with the caveat that in vitro culture cannot perfectly mimic the environment in which the pancreas normally develops, and minor differences in technique may skew results between investigators. Although the pancreatic mesenchyme is likely to produce multiple signals, only one has been validated by in vivo experiments: the fibroblast growth factor (FGF) family mem-ber encoded by the *Fgf10* gene (55).

Expression of *Fgf10* initiates in the mesenchyme shortly after that of *Pdx1* in the endoderm (56), and persists through E11.5 (55). *Fgf10* is listed in Table 8.1 among the genes required for pancreas specification, but this requirement is uncovered only in the absence of *Hnf6*: Embryos lacking both *Hnf6* and *Fgf10* lack early pan-creatic buds (56), while those lacking *Fgf10* alone exhibit normal specification and bud outgrowth (55). Subsequent development of *Fgf10* knockout pancreata is dra-matically impaired, however, producing a hypoplastic organ that lacks mature islet cells. Interestingly, the decreased growth of *Fgf10* mutant pancreata is prefigured by a premature depletion of *Pdx1*-expressing progenitor cells, as their proliferation fails to keep pace with their differentiation (55). When *Fgf10* expression is artifi-cially maintained, conversely, progenitors not only proliferate but fail to differenti-ate altogether (57, 58).

Fgf10 appears to inhibit differentiation by indirectly activating another signaling pathway, mediated by the Notch receptor family (59). Mouse knockout studies showed that several members of this pathway, including the upstream *Delta1* ligand (60) and the downstream transcription factor *Hes1* (36), act to prevent premature endocrine differentiation. Subsequent work in mice and zebrafish established that Notch also inhibits acinar (61–63) and duct development (64), and therefore exerts a general suppressive effect on pancreatic progenitor differentiation. Interestingly, the Notch pathway is up-regulated in human pancreatic cancer (65), as well as mouse models of the disease (66, 67), where it may act to prevent tumor cells from differentiating and ceasing their malignant growth.

It is unclear how the Notch pathway is activated in tumors, but one possibility is that it responds to Fgf10-like signals, as it does during organogenesis. In the embry-onic pancreas, Fgf10 and other signals from the mesenchyme activate Notch in the epithelium, and this activation is required to inhibit differentiation (54, 57, 58, 68). Although there is no consensus on how Fgf10 or other signals promote Notch

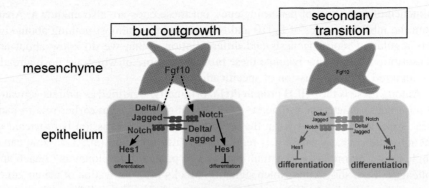

Fig. 8.3 Regulation of differentiation by Fgf10 and Notch signaling. During bud outgrowth *(left)*, high levels of Fgf10 from the mesenchyme indirectly up-regulate the Notch pathway within the epithelium, repressing differentiation via *Hes1*. This may occur via up-regulation of Notch ligands (Delta and Jagged family members) throughout the epithelium *(58)*, although other mechanisms are also possible *(57, 68)*. As *Fgf10* expression declines prior to the secondary transition *(right)*, Notch activity is downregulated and differentiation regulators (e.g., *Ngn3*) are up-regulated

activation, these results together suggest that the mesenchyme represses epithelial differentiation via secreted signals, including Fgf10, that indirectly upregulate Notch signaling (Fig. 8.3).

This simple model makes an imperfect fit to a complex reality. For example, pancreata overexpressing Fgf10 are larger than normal *(57, 58)*, whereas those expressing constitutive Notch are smaller *(62, 63)*, indicating that Fgf10 does more than just activate Notch. Perhaps more importantly, the superficial resemblance between *Fgf10* knockout pancreata and those lacking Notch signaling (in vivo) or mesenchyme (in vitro) obscures an important qualitative difference: While both classes of pancreas are smaller than normal, the former are made up of acini and few or no islets, whereas the latter comprise islets with little or no acinar tissue. Additional cues are thus likely to derive from the mesenchyme, acting to promote growth and differentiation. Among the candidates for such signals, for which further experimental support is required, are members of the laminin *(69, 70)*, TGFβ *(52, 71–74)*, and Wnt *(75–80)* families.

4   Growth and Differentiation: Transcriptional Regulation

Although the secondary transition is marked by the simultaneous onset of acinar and β-cell differentiation, we know frustratingly little about the timing mechanisms involved. We also know little about how cells decide between endocrine or exocrine fates, although studies of Notch- or mesenchyme-deprived pancreata certainly imply that the early epithelium is comprised of multipotent progenitors. The pancreatic epithelium appears to be partitioned into islet- and acinar-forming domains at the onset of the secondary transition (see Figs. 8.1D and 8.2C), suggesting the influence of some sort of patterning cues, but these cues are also unknown. Apart from the inhibitory roles of Fgf10 and Notch, we know almost nothing about signals regulating morphogenesis and differentiation. What we do know about are transcription factors that regulate these processes, some of which we have already encountered in our discussion of specification.

Among these is the bHLH protein Ptf1a, originally identified as a direct activator of numerous acinar gene promoters (*33*). Although it plays an earlier role in pancreas specification, discussed in the preceding, its later expression is restricted to the acinar lineage, in which it is required for differentiation (*30, 34*). How can a single transcription factor play multiple roles in pancreas development? Leach and colleagues have shown that Notch signaling blocks Ptf1a activation of acinar genes prior to the secondary transition (*61, 81*); one possibility is that Ptf1a activates acinar genes in the absence of Notch activity, and early specification genes when Notch is active. The relationship between Notch signaling and Ptf1a function is likely to be complex, and further progress may require identifying those Ptf1a target genes that are involved in specification.

Duct development is still largely a mystery, in part because of the difficulty in distinguishing between uncommitted progenitor cells and differentiated ducts (*4, 11*). Lineage-tracing studies indicate that at least a subset of the duct-like structures present in the embryonic pancreas are actually islet precursors, whereas others are more likely to be "true" ducts (*13, 14*); we cannot yet distinguish these structures a priori. Interestingly, *Hnf6* knockout pancreata exhibit a selective impairment of large duct morphogenesis (*50*) (among other abnormalities) (*82, 83*), suggesting that underlying developmental mechanisms differ between large, branching ducts and their terminal, intercalated counterparts. The ductal phenotype in these mice may be caused by aberrant ciliogenesis (*50, 84*), and further studies of *Hnf6* and ciliogenesis genes should advance our understanding of this embarrassingly little-understood cell type.

By far the best-understood aspect of pancreas development is endocrine specification, which begins with expression of the transcription factor *Ngn3*. *Ngn3* is absolutely required for development of all islet cells (*85*), and ectopic *Ngn3* expression induces α-cell differentiation in the pancreas as well as elsewhere in the developing gut (*60, 86, 87*). *Ngn3* expression—and thus its potent pro-endocrine function—is kept in check by the Notch pathway prior to the secondary transition (*60, 88*). The only endocrine cells that normally differentiate at these stages are α cells, but *Ngn3* is transiently expressed in the precursors of all the other islet cell types (*13, 14*), and presumably acts to initiate their development later in organogenesis. It also seems safe to assume—pending experimental support—that *Ngn3* expression remains under the leash of the Notch pathway during these later stages, when β cell and other endocrine subtypes are produced. *Ngn3* alone, however, cannot account for the specificity of endocrine development, as it appears to confer only α-cell identity. Additional factors, discussed below, must cooperate with *Ngn3* to specify the appropriate temporal pattern of endocrine cell genesis.

Table 8.2 lists transcription factors required for endocrine development. Like *Ngn3*, several of these genes appear to function in a "core program" of endocrine

Table 8.2 Genes required for endocrine development

Gene	Islet cell types affected in knockout	Reference
Core endocrine program		
Prox1	All (reduced)	*42*
Hnf6	All (reduced)	*82*
Ngn3	All (absent)	*85*
Isl1	All (absent)	*20*
NeuroD	All (reduced).	*89*
Islet subtype development		
Nkx6.1/Nkx6.2 (double-mutant)	β Cells (absent), α-cells (reduced)	*94*
Nkx2.2	β Cells (absent)	*90*
Nkx6.1	β Cells (absent)	*43*
Hlxb9	β Cells (reduced)	*125, 126*
Pax6	α, β, and δ Cells (reduced)	*129–131*
	ε Cells (increased)	
	β Cells (strongly reduced)	
Pax4	δ Cells (absent)	*91, 93*
	α Cells (increased)	
Arx	α Cells (absent), β cells (increased), δ cells (increased)	*92*

Listed are genes required for various aspects of endocrine development, indicating the specific islet cell types that are increased in numbers, reduced or absent in the respective knockout mice. We have divided the genes into those likely to act in all endocrine cells, either upstream or downstream of *Ngn3* (arranged in order accordingly), as well as those apparently required only in a subset of islet cell types.

differentiation. Some of the core regulators, such as *NeuroD* (*89*) and *Isl1* (*20*), appear to act downstream of *Ngn3*, whereas others, such as *Prox1* (*42*) and *Hnf6* (*82*), may act upstream or in parallel. Other transcription factors are selectively required for development of specific islet cell types, such as *Nkx2.2* (*90*) and *Pax4* (*91*). The severity of the phenotypes in mice lacking these genes varies widely, and it is rarely obvious whether they reflect defects in specification or survival.

Double-mutant studies to address cross-talk between the subtype-specification factors have begun to yield interesting and unexpected results. For instance, the genes *Pax4* and *Arx* are required for β- and a-cell development, respectively, and each appears to inhibit expression of the other (*91, 92*). When both genes are disrupted, however, endocrine cells appear to preferentially adopt a somatostatin-producing δ-cell fate (*93*). Double-mutant studies of *Nkx6*-family transcription factors underscore the complexity of endocrine specification: Both genes are expressed beginning prior to the secondary transition, and whereas *Nkx6.2* knockouts have normal pancreata, those lacking *Nkx6.1* fail to generate β cells (*43, 94*). *Nkx6.1/Nkx6.2* double mutants, however, are deficient in both β and a cells (*94*). Other redundancies and interactions no doubt remain to be identified.

4.1 Pdx1: Master Regulator of Pancreas Development?

We have until now neglected (except as a "marker gene") the most famous and important transcriptional regulator of pancreas development: *Pdx1*. The Pdx1 protein was originally identified as β-cell–specific binding activity on the *Insulin* promoter (*95*), from whence it derived its original name, *Insulin promoter factor-1* (*Ipf1*). Once cloned, the gene proved to be homologous to a *Xenopus* homeobox gene, *Xlhbox8*, and expressed (like *Xlhbox8*) in both the pancreas and duodenum (*12*, *96*). (Hence its most-common and offical name, *Pancreatic and duodenal homeobox-1*).

Pdx1 is expressed throughout the early embryonic pancreas, and initial studies found that *Pdx1* knockout mice die shortly after birth due to pancreatic agenesis (*97*). Closer examination revealed that budding initiates normally in *Pdx1* mutants, as does differentiation of early endocrine cells (*37, 41*). Further growth and branching, however, fail to occur, as does the secondary transition of islet and acinar differentiation. Subsequent work showed that *Pdx1* plays distinct, critical roles at multiple stages of pancreas development.

To address the potential role of *Pdx1* after bud formation (i.e., at stages beyond which the null mutant does not develop), Holland et al. (*98*) generated compound transgenic/gene-targeted mice in which *Pdx1* expression could be turned off by doxycycline administration. Treating pregnant females with doxycycline permitted these authors to inactivate *Pdx1* at specific developmental stages, and they went on to show that *Pdx1* was required during all stages of exocrine pancreas development (*98, 99*). At stages prior to the secondary transition, shut-down of *Pdx1* leads to a complete arrest in outgrowth and branching; as the pancreas enters the secondary transition, *Pdx1* shut-down has relatively little effect on growth and branching, but prevents acinar differentiation (*99*).

In the adult, *Pdx1* expression is largely restricted to β cells, where the protein was originally hypothesized to transactivate the *Insulin* promoter. To test this, Ahlgren et al. (*100*) used the Cre-loxP system to bypass the early developmental arrest of *Pdx1* nulls, and instead delete the gene specifically from β cells. The result was loss of insulin production and diabetes, showing that although *Pdx1* acts early to promote pancreas growth and differentiation, it also acts later to maintain β-cell function. (An identical phenotype was obtained by doxycycline administration to adult mice carrying the regulatable *Pdx1* allele described in the preceding.) (*98*) Together, these studies suggest that *Pdx1* is necessary for nearly every aspect of pancreas development and function. Can *Pdx1* be used as a tool to generate exogenous pancreatic tissue, and in particular β cells?

In fact, several studies have found that misexpression of *Pdx1* outside the pancreas fails to induce ectopic pancreatic tissue (*87, 101, 102*). Pdx1 normally functions as a transcriptional activator, but its ability to activate target genes depends on interactions with various cofactor proteins (*103–106*). Ectopically expressed *Pdx1*, in the absence of these cofactors, might not activate its full range of target genes. To bypass these issues, Slack and colleagues fused *Pdx1* to the VP16 transcriptional activation domain, producing a form of Pdx1 protein that should activate target genes without needing cofactors (*107*). When this was expressed in transgenic *Xenopus* embryos, under control of the liver-specific *Transthyretin* promoter, part or all of the liver transdifferentiated into endocrine and exocrine pancreas (*107*). This occurred after the liver had begun to differentiate, and thus constitutes a form of metaplasia, i.e., replacement of one differentiated tissue type by another. Importantly, the transdifferentiated cells lose expression of liver genes, and hence of the *Transthyretin*-driven *Pdx1-VP16* transgene itself, yet the pancreatic markers remain expressed. Activation of Pdx1 target genes is thus sufficient to initiate a stable program of pancreas development, both endocrine and exocrine. These authors went on to show identical results in cultured mammalian hepatoma cells (*107, 108*), suggesting that this approach could be useful in generating functional β cells from nonpancreatic sources such as liver cells.

These striking results raise several questions, including exactly what downstream target genes mediate ectopic pancreas induction by Pdx1-VP16, and how wild-type Pdx1 activates these targets during normal development. One possibility is that Pdx1 activates an early pancreas program in collaboration with Ptf1a. As noted, ectopic pancreas formation in *Hes1* null mice occurs only where *Pdx1* is normally expressed, and is accompanied by and dependent on up-regulation of *Ptf1a* in these regions (*32*). A very recent study, also performed in *Xenopus*, shows that coexpression of *Pdx1* and *Ptf1a* (but neither gene alone) converts posterior endoderm into pancreas (*45*).

A major challenge for the future will be to disentangle the many roles of *Pdx1*. Although future efforts to generate new β cells will likely exploit its apparent "master regulator" properties, *Pdx1* may also have pathologic activities relevant to pancreas cancer. Thus, Pdx1 over-expression has been observed in a subset of human pancreatic tumors, apparently correlating with worse outcome (*109*). *Pdx1* is also reactivated in the premalignant lesions seen in several mouse models of the disease (*66, 67, 110*), and Miyatsuka et al. (*111*) recently showed that re-expressing *Pdx1* in differentiated acinar cells causes them to adopt a duct-like phenotype. As discussed in the final section, this so-called acinar-ductal metaplasia occurs in a number of pathologic contexts, and may represent the origin of pancreatic cancer.

5   Cell Fate Maintenance and Metaplasia

Once cells differentiate, what keeps them that way? In most cases, the differentiated state is maintained by a transcriptional network established during development; *Pdx1* functions in such a network in the adult β-cell, the disruption of which leads to maturity-onset diabetes of the young (MODY) (*112*). In other pathologic circumstances, particularly within the exocrine pancreas, differentiated cells appear to change their fates altogether, a phenomenon termed metaplasia (*113, 114*).

As noted, *Pdx1-VP16* can induce hepatocyte-to-pancreas transdifferentiation (*107*), suggesting that the liver developmental program is close enough to that of the pancreas that it can be "flipped" with a single gene. Further evidence for this close relationship derives from studies of the opposite phenomenon, i.e., pancreas-to-liver transdifferentiation. This was first described in regenerating, carcinogen-treated hamster pancreas (*115*), and an identical phenomenon occurs in adult rats fed a peroxisome proliferator drug (*116*). This can be mimicked in vitro, in an aci-nar cell line as well as mouse embryonic pancreas, by treatment with glucocorti-coid, an effect mediated by induction of the transcription factor C/EBPβ (*117*). Together, these results suggest that acinar or other adult pancreatic cells have a latent capacity for transdifferentiation to a liver fate.

Cell fate maintenance appears to be especially labile in acinar cells, which undergo apparent transdifferentiation in response to numerous stimuli. These include overexpression of *Pdx1*, as described (*111*), as well as a number of injury models (*113*), most of which result in replacement of acini by cells expressing duct/progenitor markers. The acinar-specific transcription factor *Mist1* is required to suppress metaplasia, as *Mist1*-deficient pancreata exhibit a pancreatitis-like phe-notype accompanied by the appearance of cells coexpressing acinar and ductal markers (*118*). The phenomenon of metaplasia is likely to be of wide relevance to pancreatic disease: On the one hand, metaplastic acini have been suggested to give rise to new islet cells under some circumstances (*110, 119*), and to serve as the ori-gin of pancreatic cancer under others (*120, 121*).

Metaplasia and transdifferentiation are not necessarily identical: The former term is agnostic as to the fate of the old cells and the source of the new. For exam-ple, an apparent change in cell phenotype could actually reflect the death of one cell type and its rapid replacement by another. To address this, Means et al. (*122*) recently used genetic lineage tracing to mark pre-existing acinar cells, and trace their fate during TGFα-induced metaplasia in vitro. TGFα, an EGF receptor ligand, induces acinar-ductal metaplasia in vivo and in vitro, in a Notch-dependent manner (*65, 110*). Marking acinar cells prior to TGFα treatment revealed that they were the true source of the metaplastic duct-like cells, supporting (but not yet proving) the hypothesis of similar plasticity in vivo (*122*).

Quite different results were obtained by Stanger et al. (*67*), in studying the source of metaplastic ducts induced by loss of the tumor suppressor gene *Pten*. Deleting *Pten* throughout the pancreas caused widespread metaplasia, but deletion specifically from acinar cells had no effect. Further study suggested that what looked like transdifferentiation was actually replacement, as terminal ductal cells expanded to supplant dying acinar cells (*67*). These two studies, of course, used quite different experimental systems, and the precise mode of metaplasia may depend on the nature of the inducing stimulus. What is without question is that careful lineage tracing, such as used by these authors, will be as essential to study-ing metaplasia as it has been to studying organogenesis.

6   Conclusions

Pancreas developmental biology has flourished in the past decade, as the field has embraced new techniques, new model organisms, and (most importantly) new hypotheses. Nonetheless, as emphasized in this chapter, a number of questions remain unanswered. For example, what aspects of cell fate determination are regulated by intercellular signals, from the mesenchyme or within the epithelium itself? When various specification events fail, what happens to the unspecified precursor cells? What (if anything) are the defining characteristics of progenitor cells that distinguish them from mature ducts? How is the "pancreatic state" defined, and how malleable is this definition? Are cells in the adult pancreas fixed with respect to their identity, or is there potential for re-programming under physiologic or experimental conditions? These questions are of clear relevance to diabetes research, a goal of which is to generate new functional β-cells. Insofar as developmental controls go awry during tumorigenesis—e.g., metaplasia of acinar cells into progenitor-like cells, inhibition of differentiation, disruption of inhibitory cell–cell interactions—further progress should also inform pancreatic cancer research, hopefully identifying new avenues for prevention and treatment.

Acknowledgments The authors thank Ondine Cleaver for her unpublished $Pdx1^{LacZ}$ photomicrograph, and Ben Stanger, Sheldon Rowan, Kristen Kwan, and Matthew Firpo for comments on the manuscript. Work in the lab of LCM is supported by the NIH, the Lustgarten Foundation for Pancreatic Cancer Research, and the Searle Scholars Program.

References

1. Madsen OD. 2005, Stem cells and diabetes treatment. APMIS 113(11–12):858–875.
2. Stanger BZ, Dor Y. 2006, Dissecting the cellular origins of pancreatic cancer. Cell Cycle 5(1):43–46.
3. Lomberk G, Fernandez-Zapico ME, Urrutia R. 2005, When developmental signaling pathways go wrong and their impact on pancreatic cancer development. Curr Opin Gastroenterol 21(5):555–560.
4. Pictet R, Rutter WJ. 1972, Development of the embryonic endocrine pancreas. In: Steiner D, Freinkel N (eds.) Handbook of physiology, section 7. Williams & Wilkins, Baltimore, 25–66.
5. Slack JM. 1995, Developmental biology of the pancreas. Development 121(6):1569–1580.
6. Edlund H. 2002, Pancreatic organogenesis--developmental mechanisms and implications for therapy. Nat Rev Genet 3(7):524–532.
7. Jensen J. 2004, Gene regulatory factors in pancreatic development. Dev Dyn 229(1):176–200.
8. Dor Y, Brown J, Martinez OI, et al. 2004, Adult pancreatic beta-cells are formed by self-duplication rather than stem-cell differentiation. Nature 429(6987):41–46.
9. Magami Y, Azuma T, Inokuchi H, et al. 2002, Heterogeneous cell renewal of pancreas in mice: (^{3}H)-thymidine autoradiographic investigation. Pancreas 24(2):153–160.
10. O'Rahilly R. 1978, The timing and sequence of events in the development of the human digestive system and associated structures during the embryonic period proper. Anat Embryol (Berl) 153(2):123–136.
11. Piper K, Brickwood S, Turnpenny LW, et al. 2004, Beta cell differentiation during early human pancreas development. J Endocrinol 181(1):11–23.
12. Ohlsson H, Karlsson K, Edlund T. 1993, IPF1, a homeodomain-containing transactivator of the insulin gene. EMBO J 12(11):4251–4259.
13. Gu G, Dubauskaite J, Melton DA. 2002, Direct evidence for the pancreatic lineage: NGN3+ cells are islet progenitors and are distinct from duct progenitors. Development 129(10):2447–2457.

14. Schonhoff SE, Giel-Moloney M, Leiter AB. 2004, Neurogenin 3-expressing progenitor cells in the gastrointestinal tract differentiate into both endocrine and non-endocrine cell types. Dev Biol 270(2):443–454.
15. Branda CS, Dymecki SM. 2004, Talking about a revolution: the impact of site-specific recombinases on genetic analyses in mice. Dev Cell 6(1):7–28.
16. Wessells NK, Cohen JH. 1967, Early pancreatic organogenesis: morphogenesis, tissue interactions and mass effects. Dev Biol 15:237–270.
17. Pictet RL, Clark WR, Williams RH, et al. 1972, An ultrastructural analysis of the developing embryonic pancreas. Dev Biol 29(4):436–467.
18. Golosow N, Grobstein C. 1962, Epitheliomesenchymal interaction in pancreatic morphogenesis. Dev Biol 4:242–255.
19. Yoshitomi H, Zaret KS. 2004, Endothelial cell interactions initiate dorsal pancreas development by selectively inducing the transcription factor Ptf1a. Development 131(4):807–817.
20. Ahlgren U, Pfaff SL, Jessell TM, et al. 1997, Independent requirement for ISL1 in formation of pancreatic mesenchyme and islet cells. Nature 385(6613):257–260.
21. Kim SK, Hebrok M, Melton DA. 1997, Notochord to endoderm signaling is required for pancreas development. Development 124(21):4243–4252.
22. Lammert E, Cleaver O, Melton D. 2001, Induction of pancreatic differentiation by signals from blood vessels. Science 294(5542):564–567.
23. Kumar M, Jordan N, Melton D, et al. 2003, Signals from lateral plate mesoderm instruct endoderm toward a pancreatic fate. Dev Biol 259(1):109–122.
24. Stafford D, Prince VE. 2002, Retinoic acid signaling is required for a critical early step in zebrafish pancreatic development. Curr Biol 12(14):1215–1220.
25. Nadauld LD, Sandoval IT, Chidester S, et al. 2004, Adenomatous polyposis coli control of retinoic acid biosynthesis is critical for zebrafish intestinal development and differentiation. J Biol Chem 279(49):51581–51589.
26. Stafford D, White RJ, Kinkel MD, et al. 2006, Retinoids signal directly to zebrafish endoderm to specify insulin-expressing beta-cells. Development 133(5):949–956.
27. Chen Y, Pan FC, Brandes N, et al. 2004, Retinoic acid signaling is essential for pancreas development and promotes endocrine at the expense of exocrine cell differentiation in Xenopus. Dev Biol 271(1):144–160.
28. Martin M, Gallego-Llamas J, Ribes V, et al. 2005, Dorsal pancreas agenesis in retinoic acid-deficient Raldh2 mutant mice. Dev Biol 284(2):399–411.
29. Molotkov A, Molotkova N, Duester G. 2005, Retinoic acid generated by Raldh2 in mesoderm is required for mouse dorsal endodermal pancreas development. Dev Dyn 232(4):950–957.
30. Kawaguchi Y, Cooper B, Gannon M, et al. 2002, The role of the transcriptional regulator Ptf1a in converting intestinal to pancreatic progenitors. Nat Genet 32(1):128–134.
31. Sumazaki R, Shiojiri N, Isoyama S, et al. 2004, Conversion of biliary system to pancreatic tissue in Hes1-deficient mice. Nat Genet 36(1):83–87.
32. Fukuda A, Kawaguchi Y, Furuyama K, et al. 2006, Ectopic pancreas formation in Hes1-knockout mice reveals plasticity of endodermal progenitors of the gut, bile duct, and pancreas. J Clin Invest 116(6):1484–1493.
33. Krapp A, Knofler M, Frutiger S, et al. 1996, The p48 DNA-binding subunit of transcription factor PTF1 is a new exocrine pancreas-specific basic helix-loop-helix protein. EMBO J 15(16):4317–4329.
34. Krapp A, Knofler M, Ledermann B, et al. 1998, The bHLH protein PTF1-p48 is essential for the formation of the exocrine and the correct spatial organization of the endocrine pancreas. Genes Dev 12(23):3752–3763.
35. Sellick GS, Barker KT, Stolte-Dijkstra I, et al. 2004, Mutations in PTF1A cause pancreatic and cerebellar agenesis. Nat Genet 36(12):1301–1305.
36. Jensen J, Pedersen EE, Galante P, et al. 2000, Control of endodermal endocrine development by Hes-1. Nat Genet 24(1):36–44.
37. Offield MF, Jetton TL, Labosky PA, et al. 1996, PDX-1 is required for pancreatic outgrowth and differentiation of the rostral duodenum. Development 122(3):983–995.

38. Oster A, Jensen J, Serup P, et al. 1998, Rat endocrine pancreatic development in relation to two homeobox gene products (Pdx-1 and Nkx 6.1). J Histochem Cytochem 46(6):707–715.
39. Pang K, Mukonoweshuro C, Wong GG. 1994, Beta cells arise from glucose transporter type 2 (Glut2)-expressing epithelial cells of the developing rat pancreas. Proc Natl Acad Sci U S A 91(20):9559–9563.
40. Wilson ME, Kalamaras JA, German MS. 2002, Expression pattern of IAPP and prohormone convertase 1/3 reveals a distinctive set of endocrine cells in the embryonic pancreas. Mech Dev 115(1–2):171–176.
41. Ahlgren U, Jonsson J, Edlund H. 1996, The morphogenesis of the pancreatic mesenchyme is uncoupled from that of the pancreatic epithelium in IPF1/PDX1-deficient mice. Development 122(5):1409–1416.
42. Wang J, Kilic G, Aydin M, et al. 2005, Prox1 activity controls pancreas morphogenesis and participates in the production of "secondary transition" pancreatic endocrine cells. Dev Biol 286(1):182–194.
43. Sander M, Sussel L, Conners J, et al. 2000, Homeobox gene Nkx6.1 lies downstream of Nkx2.2 in the major pathway of beta-cell formation in the pancreas. Development 127(24):5533–5540.
44. Field HA, Dong PD, Beis D, et al. 2003, Formation of the digestive system in zebrafish. II. Pancreas morphogenesis. Dev Biol 261(1):197–208.
45. Afelik S, Chen Y, Pieler T. 2006, Combined ectopic expression of Pdx1 and Ptf1a/p48 results in the stable conversion of posterior endoderm into endocrine and exocrine pancreatic tissue. Genes Dev 20(11):1441–1446.
46. Herrera PL, Huarte J, Sanvito F, et al. 1991, Embryogenesis of the murine endocrine pancreas, early expression of pancreatic polypeptide gene. Development 113(4):1257–1265.
47. Cabrera O, Berman DM, Kenyon NS, et al. 2006, The unique cytoarchitecture of human pancreatic islets has implications for islet cell function. Proc Natl Acad Sci U S A 103(7):2334–2339.
48. Wierup N, Svensson H, Mulder H, et al. 2002, The ghrelin cell: a novel developmentally regulated islet cell in the human pancreas. Regul Pept 107(1–3):63–69.
49. Prado CL, Pugh-Bernard AE, Elghazi L, et al. 2004, Ghrelin cells replace insulin-producing beta cells in two mouse models of pancreas development. Proc Natl Acad Sci U S A 101(9):2924–2929.
50. Pierreux CE, Poll AV, Kemp CR, et al. 2006, The transcription factor hepatocyte nuclear factor-6 controls the development of pancreatic ducts in the mouse. Gastroenterology 130(2):532–541.
51. Gittes GK, Galante PE, Hanahan D, et al. 1996, Lineage-specific morphogenesis in the developing pancreas: role of mesenchymal factors. Development 122(2):439–447.
52. Miralles F, Czernichow P, Scharfmann R. 1998, Follistatin regulates the relative proportions of endocrine versus exocrine tissue during pancreatic development. Development 125(6):1017–1024.
53. Li Z, Manna P, Kobayashi H, et al. 2004, Multifaceted pancreatic mesenchymal control of epithelial lineage selection. Dev Biol 269(1):252–263.
54. Duvillie B, Attali M, Bounacer A, et al. 2006, The mesenchyme controls the timing of pancreatic beta-cell differentiation. Diabetes 55(3):582–589.
55. Bhushan A, Itoh N, Kato S, et al. 2001, Fgf10 is essential for maintaining the proliferative capacity of epithelial progenitor cells during early pancreatic organogenesis. Development 128(24):5109–5117.
56. Jacquemin P, Yoshitomi H, Kashima Y, et al. 2006, An endothelial-mesenchymal relay pathway regulates early phases of pancreas development. Dev Biol 290(1):189–199.
57. Hart A, Papadopoulou S, Edlund H. 2003, Fgf10 maintains notch activation, stimulates proliferation, and blocks differentiation of pancreatic epithelial cells. Dev Dyn 228(2):185–193.
58. Norgaard GA, Jensen JN, Jensen J. 2003, FGF10 signaling maintains the pancreatic progenitor cell state revealing a novel role of Notch in organ development. Dev Biol 264(2):323–338.

59. Lai EC. 2004, Notch signaling: control of cell communication and cell fate. Development 131(5):965–973.
60. Apelqvist A, Li H, Sommer L, et al. 1999, Notch signalling controls pancreatic cell differentiation. Nature 400(6747):877–881.
61. Esni F, Ghosh B, Biankin AV, et al. 2004, Notch inhibits Ptf1 function and acinar cell differentiation in developing mouse and zebrafish pancreas. Development 131(17):4213–4224.
62. Hald J, Hjorth JP, German MS, et al. 2003, Activated Notch1 prevents differentiation of pancreatic acinar cells and attenuate endocrine development. Dev Biol 260(2):426–437.
63. Murtaugh LC, Stanger BZ, Kwan KM, et al. 2003, Notch signaling controls multiple steps of pancreatic differentiation. Proc Natl Acad Sci U S A 100(25):14920–14925.
64. Fujikura J, Hosoda K, Iwakura H, et al. 2006, Notch/Rbp-j signaling prevents premature endocrine and ductal cell differentiation in the pancreas. Cell Metab 3(1):59–65.
65. Miyamoto Y, Maitra A, Ghosh B, et al. 2003, Notch mediates TGF alpha-induced changes in epithelial differentiation during pancreatic tumorigenesis. Cancer Cell 3(6):565–576.
66. Hingorani SR, Petricoin EF, Maitra A, et al. 2003, Preinvasive and invasive ductal pancreatic cancer and its early detection in the mouse. Cancer Cell 4(6):437–450.
67. Stanger BZ, Stiles B, Lauwers GY, et al. 2005, Pten constrains centroacinar cell expansion and malignant transformation in the pancreas. Cancer Cell 8(3):185–195.
68. Miralles F, Lamotte L, Couton D, et al. 2006, Interplay between FGF10 and Notch signalling is required for the self-renewal of pancreatic progenitors. Int J Dev Biol 50(1):17–26.
69. Crisera CA, Kadison AS, Breslow GD, et al. 2000, Expression and role of laminin-1 in mouse pancreatic organogenesis. Diabetes 49(6):936–944.
70. Jiang FX, Cram DS, DeAizpurua HJ, et al. 1999, Laminin-1 promotes differentiation of fetal mouse pancreatic beta-cells. Diabetes 48(4):722–730.
71. Jiang FX, Stanley EG, Gonez LJ, et al. 2002, Bone morphogenetic proteins promote development of fetal pancreas epithelial colonies containing insulin-positive cells. J Cell Sci 115(Pt 4):753–760.
72. Sanvito F, Herrera PL, Huarte J, et al. 1994, TGF-beta 1 influences the relative development of the exocrine and endocrine pancreas in vitro. Development 120(12):3451–3462.
73. Dichmann DS, Miller CP, Jensen J, et al. 2003, Expression and misexpression of members of the FGF and TGFbeta families of growth factors in the developing mouse pancreas. Dev Dyn 226(4):663–674.
74. Smart NG, Apelqvist AA, Gu X, et al. 2006, Conditional expression of Smad7 in pancreatic beta cells disrupts TGF-beta signaling and induces reversible diabetes mellitus. PLoS Biol 4(2):e39.
75. Heller RS, Dichmann DS, Jensen J, et al. 2002, Expression patterns of Wnts, Frizzleds, sFRPs, and misexpression in transgenic mice suggesting a role for Wnts in pancreas and foregut pattern formation. Dev Dyn 225(3):260–270.
76. Dessimoz J, Bonnard C, Huelsken J, et al. 2005, Pancreas-specific deletion of beta-catenin reveals Wnt-dependent and Wnt-independent functions during development. Curr Biol 15(18):1677–1683.
77. Papadopoulou S, Edlund H. 2005, Attenuated Wnt signaling perturbs pancreatic growth but not pancreatic function. Diabetes 54(10):2844–2851.
78. Murtaugh LC, Law AC, Dor Y, et al. 2005, Beta-Catenin is essential for pancreatic acinar but not islet development. Development 132(21):4663–4674.
79. Kim HJ, Schleiffarth JR, Jessurun J, et al. 2005, Wnt5 signaling in vertebrate pancreas development. BMC Biol 3:23.
80. Heiser PW, Lau J, Taketo MM, et al. 2006, Stabilization of {beta}-catenin impacts pancreas growth. Development 133(10):2023–2032.
81. Ghosh B, Leach SD. 2006, Interactions between hairy/enhancer of split-related proteins and the pancreatic transcription factor Ptf1-p48 modulate function of the PTF1 transcriptional complex. Biochem J 393(Pt 3):679–685.
82. Jacquemin P, Durviaux SM, Jensen J, et al. 2000, Transcription factor hepatocyte nuclear factor 6 regulates pancreatic endocrine cell differentiation and controls expression of the proendocrine gene ngn3. Mol Cell Biol 20(12):4445–4454.

83. Jacquemin P, Lemaigre FP, Rousseau GG, 2003, The Onecut transcription factor HNF-6 (OC-1) is required for timely specification of the pancreas and acts upstream of Pdx-1 in the specification cascade. Dev Biol 258(1):105–116.

84. Cano DA, Murcia NS, Pazour GJ, et al. 2004, Orpk mouse model of polycystic kidney disease reveals essential role of primary cilia in pancreatic tissue organization. Development 131(14):3457–3467.

85. Gradwohl G, Dierich A, LeMeur M, et al. 2000, neurogenin3 is required for the development of the four endocrine cell lineages of the pancreas. Proc Natl Acad Sci U S A 97(4):1607–1611.

86. Schwitzgebel VM, Scheel DW, Conners JR, et al. 2000, Expression of neurogenin3 reveals an islet cell precursor population in the pancreas. Development 127(16):3533–3542.

87. Grapin-Botton A, Majithia AR, Melton DA. 2001, Key events of pancreas formation are triggered in gut endoderm by ectopic expression of pancreatic regulatory genes. Genes Dev 15(4):444–454.

88. Lee JC, Smith SB, Watada H, et al. 2001, Regulation of the pancreatic pro-endocrine gene neurogenin3. Diabetes 50(5):928–936.

89. Naya FJ, Huang HP, Qiu Y, et al. 1997, Diabetes, defective pancreatic morphogenesis, and abnormal enteroendocrine differentiation in BETA2/neuroD-deficient mice. Genes Dev 11(18):2323–2334.

90. Sussel L, Kalamaras J, Hartigan-O'Connor DJ, et al. 1998, Mice lacking the homeodomain transcription factor Nkx2.2 have diabetes due to arrested differentiation of pancreatic beta cells. Development 125(12):2213–2221.

91. Sosa-Pineda B, Chowdhury K, Torres M, et al. 1997, The Pax4 gene is essential for differentiation of insulin-producing beta cells in the mammalian pancreas. Nature 386(6623):399–402.

92. Collombat P, Mansouri A, Hecksher-Sorensen J, et al. 2003, Opposing actions of Arx and Pax4 in endocrine pancreas development. Genes Dev 17(20):2591–2603.

93. Collombat P, Hecksher-Sorensen J, Broccoli V, et al. 2005, The simultaneous loss of Arx and Pax4 genes promotes a somatostatin-producing cell fate specification at the expense of the alpha- and beta-cell lineages in the mouse endocrine pancreas. Development 132(13):2969–2680.

94. Henseleit KD, Nelson SB, Kuhlbrodt K, et al. 2005, NKX6 transcription factor activity is required for alpha- and beta-cell development in the pancreas. Development 132(13):3139–3149.

95. Ohlsson H, Thor S, Edlund T. 1991, Novel insulin promoter- and enhancer-binding proteins that discriminate between pancreatic alpha- and beta-cells. Mol Endocrinol 5(7):897–904.

96. Wright CV, Schnegelsberg P, De Robertis EM, 1989, XlHbox 8: a novel Xenopus homeo protein restricted to a narrow band of endoderm. Development 105(4):787–794.

97. Jonsson J, Carlsson L, Edlund T, et al. 1994, Insulin-promoter-factor 1 is required for pancreas development in mice. Nature 371(6498):606–609.

98. Holland AM, Hale MA, Kagami H, et al. 2002, Experimental control of pancreatic development and maintenance. Proc Natl Acad Sci U S A 99(19):12236–12241.

99. Hale MA, Kagami H, Shi L, et al. 2005, The homeodomain protein PDX1 is required at mid-pancreatic development for the formation of the exocrine pancreas. Dev Biol 286(1):225–237.

100. Ahlgren U, Jonsson J, Jonsson L, et al. 1998, Beta-cell-specific inactivation of the mouse Ipf1/Pdx1 gene results in loss of the beta-cell phenotype and maturity onset diabetes. Genes Dev 12(12):1763–1768.

101. Heller RS, Stoffers DA, Hussain MA, et al. 1998, Misexpression of the pancreatic homeodomain protein IDX-1 by the Hoxa-4 promoter associated with agenesis of the cecum. Gastroenterology 115(2):381–387.

102. Ferber S, Halkin A, Cohen H, et al. 2000, Pancreatic and duodenal homeobox gene 1 induces expression of insulin genes in liver and ameliorates streptozotocin-induced hyperglycemia. Nat Med 6(5):568–572.

103. Asahara H, Dutta S, Kao HY, et al. 1999, Pbx-Hox heterodimers recruit coactivator-corepressor complexes in an isoform-specific manner. Mol Cell Biol 19(12):8219–8225.

104. Dutta S, Gannon M, Peers B, et al. 2001, PDX:PBX complexes are required for normal proliferation of pancreatic cells during development. Proc Natl Acad Sci U S A 98(3):1065–1070.

105. Kim SK, Selleri L, Lee JS, et al. 2002, Pbx1 inactivation disrupts pancreas development and in Ipf1-deficient mice promotes diabetes mellitus. Nat Genet 30(4):430–435.

106. Swift GH, Liu Y, Rose SD, et al. 1998, An endocrine-exocrine switch in the activity of the pancreatic homeodomain protein PDX1 through formation of a trimeric complex with PBX1b and MRG1 (MEIS2). Mol Cell Biol 18(9):5109–5120.

107. Horb ME, Shen CN, Tosh D, et al. 2003, Experimental conversion of liver to pancreas. Curr Biol 13(2):105–115.

108. Li WC, Horb ME, Tosh D, et al. 2005, In vitro transdifferentiation of hepatoma cells into functional pancreatic cells. Mech Dev 122(6):835–847.

109. Koizumi M, Doi R, Toyoda E, et al. 2003, Increased PDX-1 expression is associated with outcome in patients with pancreatic cancer. Surgery 134(2):260–266.

110. Song SY, Gannon M, Washington MK, et al. 1999, Expansion of Pdx1-expressing pancreatic epithelium and islet neogenesis in transgenic mice overexpressing transforming growth factor alpha. Gastroenterology 117(6):1416–1426.

111. Miyatsuka T, Kaneto H, Shiraiwa T, et al. 2006, Persistent expression of PDX-1 in the pancreas causes acinar-to-ductal metaplasia through Stat3 activation. Genes Dev 20(11):1435–1440.

112. Hattersley AT. 2003, Maturity-onset diabetes of the young. In: Pickup JC, Williams G, eds. Textbook of diabetes, 3Blackwell Science, Malden, MA, 1–12rd ed.

113. Lardon J, Bouwens L. 2005, Metaplasia in the pancreas. Differentiation 73(6):278–286.

114. Tosh D, Slack JM. 2002, How cells change their phenotype. Nat Rev Mol Cell Biol 3(3):187–194.

115. Scarpelli DG, Rao MS. 1981, Differentiation of regenerating pancreatic cells into hepatocyte-like cells. Proc Natl Acad Sci U S A 78(4):2577–2581.

116. Reddy JK, Rao MS, Qureshi SA, et al. 1984, Induction and origin of hepatocytes in rat pancreas. J Cell Biol 98(6):2082–2090.

117. Shen CN, Slack JM, Tosh D. 2000, Molecular basis of transdifferentiation of pancreas to liver. Nat Cell Biol 2(12):879–887.

118. Pin CL, Rukstalis JM, Johnson C, et al. 2001, The bHLH transcription factor Mist1 is required to maintain exocrine pancreas cell organization and acinar cell identity. J Cell Biol 155(4):519–530.

119. Wang RN, Kloppel G, Bouwens L. 1995, Duct- to islet-cell differentiation and islet growth in the pancreas of duct-ligated adult rats. Diabetologia 38(12):1405–1411.

120. Bockman DE, Black O Jr, Mills LR, et al. 1978, Origin of tubular complexes developing during induction of pancreatic adenocarcinoma by 7,12-dimethylbenz(a)anthracene. Am J Pathol 90(3):645–658.

121. Meszoely IM, Means AL, Scoggins CR, et al. 2001, Developmental aspects of early pancreatic cancer. Cancer J 7(4):242–250.

122. Means AL, Meszoely IM, Suzuki K, et al. 2005, Pancreatic epithelial plasticity mediated by acinar cell transdifferentiation and generation of nestin-positive intermediates. Development 132(16):3767–3776.

123. Kanai-Azuma M, Kanai Y, Gad JM, et al. 2002, Depletion of definitive gut endoderm in Sox17-null mutant mice. Development 129(10):2367–2379.

124. Haumaitre C, Barbacci E, Jenny M, et al. 2005, Lack of TCF2/vHNF1 in mice leads to pancreas agenesis. Proc Natl Acad Sci U S A 102(5):1490–1495.

125. Harrison KA, Thaler J, Pfaff SL, et al. 1999, Pancreas dorsal lobe agenesis and abnormal islets of Langerhans in Hlxb9-deficient mice. Nat Genet 23(1):71–75.

126. Li H, Arber S, Jessell TM, et al. 1999, Selective agenesis of the dorsal pancreas in mice lacking homeobox gene Hlxb9. Nat Genet 23(1):67–70.

127. Esni F, Johansson BR, Radice GL, et al. 2001, Dorsal pancreas agenesis in N-cadherin-deficient mice. Dev Biol 238(1):202–212.
128. Bort R, Martinez-Barbera JP, Beddington RS, et al. 2004, Hex homeobox gene-dependent tissue positioning is required for organogenesis of the ventral pancreas. Development 131(4):797–806.
129. Sander M, Neubuser A, Kalamaras J, et al. 1997, Genetic analysis reveals that PAX6 is required for normal transcription of pancreatic hormone genes and islet development. Genes Dev 11(13):1662–1673.
130. St-Onge L, Sosa-Pineda B, Chowdhury K, et al. 1997, Pax6 is required for differentiation of glucagon-producing alpha-cells in mouse pancreas. Nature 387(6631):406–409.
131. Heller RS, Jenny M, Collombat P, et al. 2005, Genetic determinants of pancreatic epsilon-cell development. Dev Biol 286(1):217–224.

Chapter 9
Models of Pancreatic Cancer: Understanding Disease Progression

Laleh G. Melstrom and Paul J. Grippo

1 Introduction

This book focuses on pancreatic cancer, which is a highly aggressive cancer that kills more than half of all of its victims within 6 months after the initial diagnosis. This dismal prognosis is due to late diagnosis, an incomplete knowledge of the pathways that generate invasive and metastatic disease, and a lack of efficacious therapies. Since patients present at such a late stage, it is extremely difficult to improve our understanding of markers of early detection, causative genetic events, and effective targets for treatment. Thus, investigations must initially concentrate on modeling systems that recapitulate the human disease at both the cellular and tissue levels. It is these systems that shed light onto the etiology of pancreatic cancer and provide the means of experimentation aimed at improving overall patient survival. Hence, the theme of this chapter is on models of pancreatic cancer and how these models help address important issues in this field of research.

One of the most pressing needs in regard to pancreatic cancer research is understanding the transitional step between PanIN development and invasive disease. Herein lies the key between early lesions and lethal cancer—identifying the causative genetic events that can serve as targets for earlier detection, chemoprevention, and therapy. Unfortunately, these types of evaluations in humans are restricted by presentation of this disease at a very late stage (metastasis). To begin unraveling the genetic alterations and epigenetic contributions that promote progression to cancer, a variety of modeling systems are needed. These models can be used in various applications, but for the sake of this chapter, attention is focused on the in vitro, ex vivo, and in vivo models of pancreatic precancer and cancer that highlight various aspects of the invasive phenotype in humans. A brief discussion of many of these models will help guide investigations focused on understanding the progression from precancer to adenocarcinoma and how particular models can suit a specific analysis.

Many of these models help address critical issues regarding the invasive nature of pancreatic cancer while providing the means with which to assess early detection schemes and evaluate novel chemoprevention and anticancer compounds. This chapter is divided into four broad sections: (*1*) pancreatic cancer cells in culture, (*2*) subcutaneous/orthotopic xenografts, (*3*) chemically induced rodents, and (*4*) genetically engineered mice.

A.M. Lowy et al. (eds.) *Pancreatic Cancer.*
doi: 10.1007/978-0-387-69252-4, © Springer Science+Business Media, LLC 2008

2 Pancreatic Cancer Cells in Culture

One of the major challenges in treating patients with pancreatic cancer is that
>80% of these patients present with advanced metastatic disease. It is important to
study the morphologic and genetic changes that lead to invasive and metastatic
tumors. The study of these alterations is difficult to do at the tissue level because
multiple cell types are involved. Therefore, pancreatic cancer cells in vitro offer an
opportunity to study these phenotypic and molecular alterations in cells derived
from various stages of invasion and metastasis, thus allowing for the study of different cell types within or associated to the pancreas.

Currently, there are a large number of stable pancreatic cancer cell lines available. Work has been done to characterize them by cataloging their primary source,
genetic profile, histology, and tumor grade (particularly after transplantation into
nude or SCID mice) (Table 9.1) (*1, 2*). The various sources of pancreatic cancer cell
lines can arise from primary tumors, liver metastasis, ascites, and lymph node

Table 9.1 Origin, genetic alterations, histology, and grade of pancreatic ductal adenocarcinoma
cell lines transplanted into SCID or nude mice

Cell line	Primary source	Genetic mutations	Histology & tumor grade
A818.4	Ascites	K-ras, p53, p16	PDAC, G2
AsPC-1	Ascites	K-ras, p53, p16	PDAC, G2/G3
BI		K-ras, p53, p16, DPC4	
BJ		K-ras, p53, p16, DPC4	
BxPc3	Primary tumor	p53, p16, DPC4	PDAC, G2/G3
Capan-1	Liver metastasis	K-ras, p53, p16, DPC4	PDAC, G1
Capan-2	Primary tumor	K-ras, p16, DPC4	PDAC, G1
CFPAC1	Liver metastasis	K-ras, p53, p16, DPC4	
Colo357	Lymph node mets.	K-ras, DPC4	PDAC, G2
FA6		K-ras, p53, p16, DPC4	
Ger	Primary tumor	K-ras, p53, p16, DPC4	
HPAF-2	Ascites	K-ras, p53, p16	PDAC, G2
IMIM-PC2	Primary tumor	K-ras, p53, p16	
MDAPanc3	Liver metastasis	K-ras, p53, p16	
MiaPaCa-2	Primary tumor	K-ras, p53, p16	PDAC, G3
PaCa3	Primary tumor	p16	
PaCa44		K-ras, p53, p16	
Panc1	Primary tumor	K-ras, p53, p16	PDAC, G3
Panc89	Lymph node mets.	p53, p16	PDAC, G2
PancTu-I	Primary tumor	K-ras, p53, p16	PDAC, G3
PC		K-ras, p53, p16, DPC4	
PSN1	Primary tumor	K-ras, p53, p16, DPC4	
Pt45P1	Primary tumor	K-ras, p53, p16	PDAC, G3
RWP1	Liver metastasis	K-ras, p53, p16	
SK-PC 1	Primary tumor	K-ras, p53, p16, DPC4	
SUIT-2	Liver metastasis	K-ras, p53, p16	
T3M4	Lymph node mets.	p53, p16	

metastasis (*1*). Each of these sources yields a cancer that has both shared and unique molecular profiles evident in genetic mutations.

2.1   Genetic Alterations and Downstream Events

The most common mutations in pancreatic adenocarcinoma include alterations in K-ras, *p16, p53,* and *DPC4/Smad4* (*1, 3–11*). The majority (90%) of pancreatic ductal adenocarcinomas (PDACs) harbor a gain of function mutation of K-ras (*3, 12*). Ras is a GTP-binding protein involved in several growth factor-mediated signal transduction pathways (*12*). Homozygous deletion of the 9p21 region, which harbors CDKN2A/INK4A/p16, is frequently seen in PDAC. CDKN2A/p16 is a cyclin-dependent kinase inhibitor that binds to CDK4 and prevents the interaction between CDK4 and CCND1. CCND1 functions with Rb to induce cell cycle arrest at the G1 phase (*13*). The p53 gene is also frequently mutated in pancreatic ductal adenocarcinoma. P53/TP53 is a DNA binding protein that functions as a transcription factor modulating molecules pertinent to a variety of functions primarily involved in cell cycle arrest and apoptosis (*14*). SMAD4/DPC4 is located in the region 18q21.1 and is lost in approximately 50% of pancreatic ductal adenocarcinomas by either homozygous deletion or mutation (*15*). SMAD4/DPC4 is a signal mediator involved in the transforming growth factor-β signaling pathway that plays an important role in the negative regulation of cell proliferation and the induction of extracellular matrices, angiogenesis, and immune suppression (*12, 16*). In a study of 22 pancreatic cancer cell lines, >90% possessed mutations in the K-ras, p53, and p16 genes, and 36% had genetic alterations in the DPC4/SMAD4 gene (*1*).

2.2   Histology and Molecular Grades

Sipos et al. studied 12 of these pancreatic ductal adenocarcinoma cell lines to categorize them in grade as a function of cell morphology using light microscopy and ultra structural features. The cells were classified into three grades similar to the World Health Organization (WHO) grading system which allows using tumor grade as a prognostic marker. The features that separated grades 1 and 2 (G1 and G2) cell lines were cellular and nuclear polymorphism and loss of polarity of the outer cell layer. G2 and G3 cell lines were distinguished mainly by the decreased number of mucin granules and cell organelles. Based on their grading, most (>80%) of the analyzed cell lines fell into either G2 (50%) or G3 (33.3%) with only 16.7% of the pancreatic cancer cell lines identified as G1. Interestingly, this categorization does not parallel the same distribution seen in pancreatic adenocarcinoma tumors, which is 33% G1, 51% G2, and 16% G3 (*17*). This difference can be accounted for in the inherent difficulty in culturing cell lines from well differentiated tumors. Due to the possible limitations in the number of cell lines evaluated, the authors were not able to correlate the grade of the cell lines to K-ras, p53, p16, or DPC4/smad4 mutation rates. There was, however, a relationship between grade and population doubling time, with G1 cells having a significantly higher doubling time than G3 cell lines.

Sipos et al also studied immunocytochemical features of monolayer cultures and spheroids generated from cultured pancreatic ductal adenocarcinoma cells stained for cytokeratin 7, 8, 18, and 19, vimentin, MUC1, 5, 6, carcinoembryonic antigen (CEA) and pancytokeratin. In vivo, the expression of cytokeratins 7, 8, 18, and 19 is a well-defined characteristic of pancreatic adenocarcinoma (18–21). In contrast, vimentin is a marker of undifferentiated carcinomas and is more frequently absent in differentiated PDAC in vivo (22). Based on their findings, vimentin was present in 10 of the 12 pancreatic adenocarcinoma cell lines studied as well as variable expression of cytokeratins 7, 8, 18, and 19. In addition none of the other markers evaluated (including MUC1, 2, 5, 6, CEA, synaptophysin, and chromogranin A) had a direct relationship with the grade of the cell lines (2). Therefore, these immunohistochemical markers do not seem to be useful for the categorization of pancreatic cancer cell lines with regard to their phenotypic qualities and differentiation status.

The degree of differentiation or grade has been deemed as a surrogate for the aggressiveness of a tumor. A progression model for PDAC has been proposed with the classification of preinvasive ductal lesions called pancreatic intraepithelial neoplasia (PanIN) that are hyperplastic and progress through a series of architectural and cytological changes to become malignant (23). PanINs are subclassified into PanIN-1A, PanIN-1B, PanIN-2, and PanIN-3. However, the global definition of a PanIN is a microscopic papillary or flat, noninvasive, epithelial neoplasm arising in the pancreatic ducts. PanINs are characterized by columnar-to-cubical cells with varying amounts of mucin and degrees of cytologic and architectural atypia (24). PanINs usually involve ducts <5 mm in diameter (24). In addition to PanINs, intraductal papillary mucinous neoplasms (IPMNs) and mucinous cystic neoplasms (MCNs) have also been thought to be noninvasive precursors of invasive ductal adenocarcinoma of the pancreas (24). Since these preinvasive lesions are observed in the pancreatic ducts, these cells have become the target of in vitro isolation and maintenance techniques.

2.3   Therapeutic Evaluations

The last point to make regarding cell culture of pancreatic cancer cells is that not only can they be evaluated for genetic and morphologic changes, but the response to various therapeutics can also be obtained. If a primary tumor is established in culture, response to chemotherapeutics can be determined in an in vitro setting. This is particularly relevant to patient/tumor specific therapeutics. Prior to any testing in animal models or humans, novel pharmacological agents must undergo evaluation for the ability to inhibit cell proliferation, identify mechanisms of action, and determine dose efficacy. Although gemcitabine with or without other agents is the present standard, there are a multitude of novel cytotoxic agents and targeted therapies (e.g., VEGFR, EGFR, TGF-β, HER-2/neu, MEK, proteasome, Ras, TNF-α, and CDK inhibitors) that may function as multitargeted molecular therapies for the individualized care of pancreatic cancer patients (25).

Since PanINs and most pancreatic cancers are observed in the ducts, the general consensus is that PDAC is derived in the ducts. Although not conclusive, the argument is reasonable enough to derive a near-normal ductal cell line with which to use for investigations.

2.4   Human Pancreatic Ductal Epithelial (HPDE) Cells in Culture

The limitations involved in maintaining pancreatic ductal cells in vitro include the relatively small percentage of ductal cells (5–10%) in the human pancreas, their phenotypic instability in culture, their cellular senescence, and a decline in normal enzymatic activity over time (26). The ability to culture normal ductal epithelial cells would allow testing of various carcinogens and a more precise ability to observe genetic changes that occur in the progression from a hyperplastic to malignant phenotype. Initially, small dissected ductal fragments could be obtained in culture for up to 4 months (27). This was further developed using various extracellular matrices, although the limitation was still that the cultures grew slowly and eventually become senescent. Fetal pancreas tissue has also been explanted and is more easily cultured. Fetal pancreas tissue in culture also produced bicarbonate and expressed cytokeratins 18 and 19, consistent with that of adult ductal cells.

The more common culture protocols are to either explant tissue or to enzymatically digest cells. Ductal cells are dissected from explants and then minced and placed into plastic dishes where they can grow as cell monolayers in several different media types including RPMI-1640, CMR1066, DMEM, and DME/F12. Use of collagenase for enzymatic digestion or tissue disruption can be applied to whole or dissected ductal tissue.

Another limitation of culturing ductal epithelial cells is that they have been observed to be phenotypically unstable over time. It has been observed that adult human ductal epithelial cells of the pancreas acquire a fibroblastic morphology or are overgrown by fibroblasts (28). Interestingly, adult acinar cells produce both acinar and ductal antigens and, in vitro, have been reported to transdifferentiate to a ductal phenotype before, eventually becoming senescent (29). With each normal human cell division, telomeres are shortened and this eventually leads to telomere-controlled senescence in HPDE cells (30). The transfer of hTERT cDNA (which encodes the catalytic subunit of human telomerase) can immortalize human cells without changing their phenotype (31–33). However, this has not been well established in HPDE cells (26). At this point, premature senescence is overcome with use of viral oncogenes such as HPV 16 E6/E7 or the SV40 large T antigen (34–36). Several groups have established lines of immortalized HPDE cells with these oncogenes and Lawson et al. describe their method with HPV16 E6/E7 (26). The major limitation for this technique is that the resulting cell lines cannot be used for molecular biological studies with regard to defining genetic changes that occur with cell differentiation and transformation (*37*).

In general, one major limitation of studying pancreatic cancer in vitro is that through isolation, purification, and maintenance of the cells, their interaction with their in vivo milieu has been changed or lost at both the cellular and molecular levels. In an attempt to re-establish these and other interactions, cultured and primary pancreatic cancer cells can be introduced into immunocompromised mice.

3 Subcutaneous/Orthotopic Xenografts

Another mechanism to study the biology of pancreatic cancer employs xenograft transplantation into either athymic or severe combined immunodeficient (SCID) mice. Nude or athymic mice are characterized by aberrant development of the thymus and thus lack T-lymphocytes (*38*). SCID mice are defective in immunoglobulin gene and T-cell receptor gene rearrangements and therefore lack mature B- and T-lymphocytes (*38*). Xenograft transplantation involves the injection or surgical anchoring of either established pancreatic cancer cell lines or tumor pieces from primary pancreatic neoplasms injected either subcutaneously or orthotopically into the pancreas. This allows for the study of pancreatic cancer cells in an in vivo setting in the context of invasion, metastasis, angiogenesis, rate of growth, and response to therapeutics.

3.1 Subcutaneous Model

The subcutaneous injection of pancreatic cancer cell lines or primary tumors into mice is a reasonable model to assess tumor growth either independently or in response to various therapeutics. In this manner, tumor volume can be estimated by measuring the tumor dimensions in a temporal fashion. In addition, tumor mass can be calculated at the end of an experiment following tissue/tumor resection. The healthy nude or SCID mouse can be useful as an in vivo model for assessing the metastatic potential of human pancreatic cancers, selecting and maintaining cell variants of high metastatic potential from heterogeneous human tumors and studying therapeutic agents directed against metastatic cell proliferation in visceral organs (*39*). Another advantage of this approach is the ability to obtain a library of human pancreatic carcinomas in nude mice that includes various degrees of histologic differentiation (*40*). However, although the subcutaneous xenografts generally grow well and may be locally invasive and malignant, they rarely metastasize (*41*). With this shortcoming, the subcutaneous xenografts do not display the signs and symptoms that may arise as a consequence of tumor growth within visceral organs (*42*). In addition, intrasplenic, hepatic, or intravenous xenotransplantation has been used to create metastatic models, but these bypass multiple steps in the metastatic cascade (43). Finally, it has been established that pancreatic cancer cells and malignancies in general interact with the extracellular matrix and local milieu to establish invasion and metastatic potential. Therefore an additional limitation of the subcutaneous xenotransplantation model is that the important interaction between stroma and tumor cells is lost, including the exchange of enzymes and cytokines which modify the extracellular matrix, stimulate cell migration, promote cell proliferation, and increase tumor cell survival (44–47).

3.2 Orthotopic Model

Although technically more challenging, the orthotopic model is thought to be a better method to evaluate local and distant metastases in terms of mimicking the disease in humans. The orthotopic model has undergone modifications and refinements to decrease trauma to the pancreas and prevent intraperitoneal tumor spillage. It is possible to directly inject human pancreatic cancer cells into the pancreas (48–50). Some authors have described techniques for injecting about 1×10^6 cells in a 15-μl aliquot of PBS into the proximal part of the pancreas (51). The cells are injected to visibly infiltrate the pancreatic tissue. The limitation of this technique is the potential for intra-abdominal hemorrhage, disruption of the pancreatic capsule, and concomitant significant intra-peritoneal tumor spillage (40). An alternative approach is to anchor a solid tumor fragment into the pancreas with surgical sutures. One group describes securing a 1-mm³ tumor fragment onto the pancreas with 1 6-0 Dexon II suture (43). Several weeks after this procedure, a solid mass on or replacing the mouse pancreas can be observed with both the retained histological appearance of the original tumor and the expression of tumor-associated antigens (40, 52, 53). Luokopoulos et al. evaluated 10 pancreatic cancer cell lines and 12 primary tumors after orthotopic transplantation into SCID mice (43). The cell line-derived xenografts represented the entire expected range of histologic differentiation and the overall metastatic rate was moderate to high. The primary tumor-derived xenografts retained histologic and biological similarity to their corresponding original tumors. K-ras, p53, p16, and DPC4/SMAD4 aberrations were in 80%, 70%, 50%, and 40% of the cell lines and 100%, 33%, 75%, and 58% of the primary tumor derived xenografts, respectively. The metastatic behavior of the xenografts was significantly associated with the degree of histologic differentiation, number of genes altered, and p53 status. This technique has reliably generated pancreatic tumors with subsequent metastasis to regional lymph nodes, liver and lungs (52–54). Implantation rates can range from 66% to 100% using this technique and there is good correlation between the histology of the primary tumor and the growing mass (40).

One of the limitations of anchoring tumor pieces to the pancreas is that the use of sutures is traumatic and the suture itself can induce an inflammatory response. Hotz et al. conducted a study comparing the intrapancreatic injections of human tumor cells to the atraumatic pancreatic implantation of two fragments from subcutaneous donor tumors (*55*). Primary tumor volume, local infiltration and systemic metastasis were assessed and analyzed 14 weeks after implantation or immediately after death. Their findings were that the rate of implantation was 100% for all four cell lines. There were marked differences with regard to tumor size, metastatic spread, and survival depending on the differentiation status of the cells. Less differentiated cells caused higher dissemination scores and mortality than well-differentiated cells. In the orthotopic tumor cell injection group, there was incomplete tumor take rate with early artificial abdominal tumor spread, likely secondary to microscopic cell loss during the injection.

Regardless of the method of orthotopic transplantation used, there are several biological aspects that can be studied. First, the rate of tumor establishment in the pancreas is anywhere from 50 to 100%. Regarding metastasis, in contrast to subcutaneous implantation where local growth is absent, orthotopic implantation more closely reproduces human tumors with up to 60% of tumors disseminating (*40, 43*). The variability comes with the organs that are the recipients of the metastatic cells. In the study of cell lines injected into the pancreas, there was significant metastasis to the peritoneum (43%), liver (58%), lungs (22%) and lymph nodes (33%) (*43*). In another study, results were similar, only reflecting differences in metastatic potential as a function of grade or degree of differentiation of the cell lines (*55*). One shortcoming in the implantation of tumor fragments was that although there was lymphatic, blood-borne and peritoneal dissemination, there was less perineural and lymph node invasion (*40, 53*).

3.3 *Imaging of Xenograft Models*

The ultimate value in developing these models of pancreatic cancer is to mimic the disease for early detection and therapeutic trials. Novel imaging techniques can be used to follow the growth of lesions and possibly serve as translational models for detecting preclinical disease in humans. Positron emission tomography (PET) has been used to monitor the growth of transplanted tumors without the need of euthanizing the animal (*56*). Other groups have introduced the green fluorescent protein (GFP) coding region into the pancreatic cancer cell line prior to explant (*57*). Another group used a fluorescent, highly metastatic, orthotopic model of human pancreatic cancer, where MIA PaCa-2 cells were engineered to selectively express high levels of a red fluorescent protein (*58, 59*). Imaging of orthotopically implanted primary tumors and metastases in the same animals by both fluorescent protein imaging (FPI) and high-resolution MRI at various time points allowed the comparison of these two techniques (*58*). Their findings were that MRI enables tissue structure to be visualized and that FPI provides high resolution with instant image capture. The advantage with FPI is that the animals do not need to be anesthetized or given a contrast agent. The data from the above study indicate a complimentary role of FPI and MRI in monitoring the growth of primary tumors and metastases in addition to their responsiveness to therapeutic agents in a noninvasive fashion.

Although not ideal, the various xenograft models allow for the study of various pancreatic cancer cell lines and primary tumors in an in vivo setting. In addition, imaging of these models allows for the temporal monitoring of their biology and response to therapeutics. However, the major limitation with these methodologies is that cancer does not develop spontaneously from carcinogens and/or genetic alterations. Thus, carcinogen-induction and genetically modified pancreas cells become the next set of models critical for understanding these pathways in the development and progression of pancreatic cancer.

4 Chemically Induced Rodents

There are a variety of rodents that have been used for the administration of chemical carcinogens in order to generate pancreatic lesions and pancreatic adenocarcinoma, including hamsters, rats, guinea pigs, and mice.

4.1 Nitrosamine-Induced Pancreatic Cancer in Hamsters

The most widely used rodent model of pancreatic cancer is chemically induced in the Syrian golden hamster through the administration of N-nitroso-bis(2-oxopropyl)amine (BOP) or N-nitroso-bis(2-hydroxypropyl)amine (BHP), which was initially characterized about 30 years ago. One of the first characteristics observed with this approach was that the type of nitrosamine and the parameters of administration employed made a difference in regard to the phenotype. Using blood and urine levels of the BOP and BHP metabolite N-nitroso-(2-hydroxypropyl)(2-oxopropyl)amine (HPOP), it was discovered that HPOP was more readily produced from BOP compared to BHP, which might explain the differences in potency and organ sensitivity (60). However, administration of HPOP to hamsters generated a multiplicity of tumors not unique to the pancreas (61). Likewise, administration of N-nitroso-bis(2-acetoxypropyl)amine (BAP) also led to the development of pancreatic neoplasia with the primary metabolite in the urine being BHP (60). Another carcinogen that induces pancreatic cancer is N-nitrosomethyl(2-oxopropyl)amine (MOP), which is a potent methylating agent that was used to generate methylguanine adducts that are commonly observed in liver and pancreatic cancers. MOP simulates additional cancers in the liver, kidney, and vascular compartment (e.g., BOP) and at a high incidence in the nasal cavity (unlike BOP) (62). Prior to the use of the nitroso-bis-amines, 2,2″-dihydroxy-di-n-propylnitrosamine (DHPN) was used to generate human-like pancreatic cancer in hamsters, and this served as the predecessor to the BOP-induced hamster model (63). In addition to the type of nitrosamine, the intervals (64) and route (64, 65) of nitrosamine administration and their subsequent metabolism (61) played a significant role in generating and fine-tuning a rodent model of pancreatic cancer.

Rats have also been used to generate carcinogen-induced precancer and carcinoma of the pancreas, and some of these models have been well used in understanding the process of pancreatic carcinogenesis.

4.2   Azaserine-Induced PC in Rats

Azaserine is a potent mutagen that concentrates heaviest in the pancreas and kidney. When administered to rats, azaserine generates atypical nodules, adenomas, and adenocarcinoma of the pancreas in at least 25% of the treated mice with metastases developing in lymph nodes, liver, and lung. The nodules were classified as basophilic or acidophilic, with the latter having greater growth potential and being more responsive to carcinogenic modulators (66). The predominant histotype of this cancer is acinar, though duct and cystic-like lesions can develop (67). Use of another agent, O-(N-methyl-N-nitroso-beta-alanyl)-L-serine, led to similar early lesions but without the development of adenocarcinoma (68). The use of N delta-(N-methyl-N-nitrosocarbamoyl)-L-ornithine (MNCO) can act similarly to azaserine, and at higher doses, can induce the development of cystic and tubular ductal complexes (67). The azaserine-induced lesions and cancer were enhanced following partial pancreatectomy, potentially through a mechanism related to pancreatic regeneration (69). As with nitrosamines in hamsters, the route, dose, and intervals of azaserine administration altered the incidence of pancreatic cancers, although the spectrum of histologic changes were similar (70). Rat strain also played a role in the incidence of azaserine-induced neoplasia as Wistar and W/ LEW rats were highly susceptible to the effects of azaserine compared to that of F344 rats (71).

4.3   DMBA-Induced PC in Rats

Rats implanted with 7,12-dimethylbenz[alpha]anthracene (DMBA) crystals into the head of the pancreas developed adenocarcinoma with pronounced ductal cell characteristics and metastases similar to that observed in the human disease (72). The presence of ductal markers (cytokeratin 19 and 20) with the concomitant loss of acinar and islet cell markers (chymotrypsin and chromogranin A) (33) and reduced levels of amylase (73) further demonstrate the ductal nature of these cells. The process by which pancreatic parenchyma is transformed into ductal carcinoma has been described as the process of acino-ductal transdifferentiation or acinar-to-ductal metaplasia with occasional plasticity of islet cells producing a similar phenotype (74). Although other carcinogens can generate similar metaplastic structures, including ductal hyperplasia and tubular complexes (like methynitro nitrosoguanidine, or ethylnitro nitrosoguanidine), only DMBA has demonstrated the ability to induce ductal carcinoma in rats (75).

4.4   Methylnitroso-Urea-Induced Pancreatic Cancer in Guinea Pigs

The administration of N-methyl-N-nitrosourea (MNU) to guinea pigs led to the development of pancreatic adenocarcinoma in about a third of the animals that survived more than 6 months. Focal alterations in acinar cells were observed with the occasional ductular transformation, suggestive of acinar cell dedifferentiation or acinar-to-ductal metaplasia and accompanying fibrosis (76, 77). A lower incidence of pancreatic tumors with a broad spectrum of additional tumor sites was reported (78), although clear evidence of proliferating acinar cells dedifferentiating into pseudo-ductular lesions and progressing to adenocarcinoma in guinea pig pancreas was observed (79).

The morphologic changes in cells of the pancreas of hamsters, rats, and guinea pigs implies a great degree of plasticity among acinar and perhaps islet cells and their ability to generate ductal adenocarcinoma (80, 81).

4.5   Carcinogen-Induced PC in Mice

Mouse pancreas tends to be rather resistant to the effects of carcinogens, which has limited the development of carcinogen-induced mouse models of pancreatic cancer. About 20% of surviving mice administered MNU developed undifferentiated acinar cell carcinoma at 2 years of age (82). Mice administered BOP beginning as neonates developed acinar adenomas and infrequent carcinomas, although the predominant phenotype of these mice were liver and lung cancers (83). A newer model has emerged that generates precancerous lesions leading to the development of pancreatic adenocarcinoma with a purported ductal histotype in developing PanINs and adenocarcinoma following DMBA implantation in the head of the mouse pancreas (84).

5   Genetically Engineered Rodents

Animal models that recapitulate disease progression observed in humans, including many with accompanying genetic alterations, provide a unique in vivo system with which to study progressive events in pancreatic cancer and eventually evaluate strategies for early detection, chemoprevention, and innovative therapies. The primary rodent for these types of evaluations has fallen heavily upon the mouse due the availability of technologies that manipulate the mouse genome. Only a few other genetically engineered animals have been successfully engineered in other rodents, mainly rats, and these models are infrequently found in the literature. Two transgenic rats that stand out include targeting TAg via the phosphoenolpyruvate carboxykinase promoter (PEPCK), where rats develop pancreatic islet cell hyperplasia and carcinoma (*85*). Metallothionein promoter-drive (MT) expression of spermidine/spermine N(1)-acetyltransferase (SSAT) generated transgenic rats which develop polyamine-induced acute pancreatitis (*86*).

Genetically engineered mice (GEMs) are in vivo models generated by genomic manipulation and employed to study discrete genetic mutations on selected mammalian cells and tissue. One frequently used approach makes use of a common initiating event (a mutation in the K-ras gene) in order to study its effect on the pancreas and identify which additional molecular events contribute to cellular changes leading to cancer. GEMs are generated by transgenesis or manipulation of mouse embryos with targeting vectors that can integrate, knock-out genes, or knock-in mutations at a specific locus. Multiple genetic alterations can be mimicked in vivo by breeding various GEMs, providing an in vivo setting for evaluation of these genetic combinations. Current GEMs are highlighted in Table 9.2.

5.1   Elastase Targeting

Some of the first transgenic mice ever developed targeted the pancreas. These investigations made use of the elastase (EL) promoter to target expression of oncogenes primarily to pancreatic acinar cells. EL was a proven tool for targeting genes selectively to pancreatic acinar cells. Previous targeting of oncogene expression by elastase has proven effective at inducing exocrine pancreatic neoplasms in transgenic mice, including EL-TAg and EL-H*ras* (*87, 88*). Development of cancer in mouse pancreas was further demonstrated by targeting myc and TGFα to mouse pancreatic acinar cells (EL-myc and EL-TGFα), which demonstrated acinar-to-ductal metaplasia leading to exocrine carcinoma, predominantly of an acinar cell histotype, although some cancers contained heterogeneous populations of mixed cellular components, including focally distinct ductal-like lesions (*89–92*). EL-TAg and EL-H*ras* mice develop acinar hyperplasia and carcinoma while the EL-TGF-α mice develop severe fibrosis, tubular complexes, and aberrant cell morphology (*88–90*).

The work done with the EL-TGFα and EL-TGFα/p53 null mice deserves special consideration since the evaluations regarding subsequent genomic and cellular changes has been very well characterized. Beyond the acinar-to-ductal metaplasia, EL-TGFα mice demonstrated marked activation of Erk 1/2 dependent on MEK 1, overexpression of EGFR and p53, and induction of cyclin D1-Cdk 4. Older EL-TGFα mice eventually develop carcinoma, and tumor development is enhanced in a p53 null background and concomitant with partial or whole loss of INK4a or SMAD4 (*93*). The metaplasia in EL-TGFα/p53+/– mice was characterized along with its genomic signature and increased expression of Pdx1 (*94, 95*), a gene necessary for pancreas development and often expressed in pancreatic cancer. Additionally in these mice, STAT 3 and NF-kB induced Bcl expression (*96*), and notch activation led to an increase in Nestin-positive cells with expansion of the ductal epithelium

Table 9.2 Genetically engineered mouse models of pancreatic precancer and cancer

Genetic modification	Lesions/tissue abnormalities	Molecular/marker evaluation	Cancer development (age at onset) (freq)	Organ metastases (frequency)	Strain background	Ref.
EL-TAg	Acinar dysplasia; Pseudoacinar strcts	Reduced RNA-to-DNA ratio	Acinar cell carcinoma (2–3 mos.) (100%)	Kidney, lung (1–2%) peritoneal	B6/SJL F2 chimeras	87
EL-Hras^{G12V}	Disrupted organogenesis	Reduced amylase mRNA	Acinar cell carcinoma (1.5–14 mos.) (100%)	None reported	B6/SJL F2 chimeras	88
EL-myc	Mixed acinar-ductal lesions; tubular complex; lymphocytic infiltrate	AB-PAS; CK19; amylase +	Acinar cell carcinoma (2–4 mos.); some with positive markers for ductal cells (100%)	Liver (10%) (peritoneal surface)	B6/SJL F2 chimeras	91
EL-TGF-α	Pseudoductular acinar metaplasia; hyperplasia; fibrosis; tubular complex	K-ras mutant – nuclear p53; EGFR; Acinar1; amylase; Duct1 +	Cancer w/proliferating tubular complexes; parenchymal invasion (12+ mos.) (20%)	None detected	B6/SJL F2 chimeras; backcross to B6	89, 92
EL-TGF-α/p53 null	Tubular/cystic transfm; acinar hyperplasia	Chr 11,15 gain; CK19+Chr 14 loss (20–35%)	Diff. acinar carcinoma; AC transitional carcin.	None reported	B6; B6/BALB/c chimeras	94
MT-TGF-α/p16/19 null and/or p53 null	Tubular metaplasia	Pdx1; VEGF +Promoter hypermethyl	Serous cystic adenomas	None reported	CD1/B6/CBA/ 129	107
EL-K-ras^{G12D}	Tubular complex; Metaplasia; dCIS	5-Lox; Cox-2; MMP-7; SHH; notch; nestin +	None detected (22+ mos.)	None detected	FVB (low inc) FVB6 (high)	108
EL-K-ras^{G12D} p16 null (PEDF null)	Tubular complex;Metaplasia; dCIS	VEGF, SMA, desmn+ Reduced TSP-1	PDAC w/increased stroma (12+mos.) (50%)	None detected	FVB6 F2 chimeras	MS
CK19-K-ras^{G12V}	Ductal dysplasia/ hyperplasia; lymphocytic infiltrate	N-cad +	None detected	None detected	B6/SJL chimeras	100

(continued)

Table 9.2 (continued)

Genetic modification	Lesions/tissue abnormalities	Molecular/marker evaluation	Cancer development (age at onset) (freq)	Organ metastases (frequency)	Strain background	Ref.
Mist1-K-ras^{G12D} KI p53 +/− or +/+	Acinar-ductal metaplasia	CK19; Alcian blue +	Acinar cell carcinoma; cystic neoplasia; PDAC	Liver (40%) w/p53+/−; Lung (18%) w/p53+/−	B6/129 F1 chimeras	109
Pdx1-SHH	Intestinal phenotype; Tubular complex	Her-2/neu; Ptc; smo + Mutation in K-ras	None detected (mice only live 3 weeks)	None detected	B6/C3 F1 chimeras	101
Pdx1-Cre (p48-Cre) K-ras^{LSLG12D}	Tubular Complex; MPanINs; desmoplas.	CK19; Alcian blue; Muc5 +	PDAC (6–9 mos.) (7%)	Liver (7%); Adrenal cortex, Diaphragm	FVB/B6 chimeras	102
Pdx1-Cre/K-ras^{LSLG12D} p16/p19flox	Ductal lesions; MPanINs (2+ weeks)	CK19; PAS; EGFR; Her-2/neu +	PDAC (2–3 mos.) (100%)	Duodenum, spleen, bile duct, stom., colon, liver	FVB/B6/ FV B chimeras	103
Pdx1-Cre/ K-ras^{LSLG12D} p53LSLR172H/+	Ductal lesions; MPanINs (10 weeks)	Genomic instability; EGFR; Her-2; SHH +	PDAC (2–5 mos.) (~100%)	Liver, Lung, Adrenal, Diaphragm	129/SVJ/B6 chimeras	104
Pdx1-Cre/pTEN^{flox} and/or p53^{flox}	Irreg islets; epith prolif; ductal metaplasia	Reducd pTEN; Muc5+ Increased Akt/PI3K	PDAC (3 mos.) (15%) PDAC (4–6 mo) (40%)	Duodenom (7%)	FVB/B6 chimeras	105
MT-TGF-α/EL-myc	Dyplastic duct lesion; cystic neoplasms	ND for K-ras, p16, Rb	Mixed acinar/ductal carcinoma (2–7 mos.); PDAC w/much stroma	Liver (33%)	B6/SJL/ FVBchimeric	90, 99
CK5-Cox-2	Polycystic pancreas; ductal dilation; fibrosis	Lymphocytic infiltrate CK19; Her-2/ neu; ras +	IPMN or SCA adenoma	None reported	NMRI	106
EL-tTA/TRE-Cre/ K-ras^{LSLG12V} and/ or p53-/-	Tubular complex; Metaplasia; mPanINs	Pdx1; Hes1; Cox-2; Cyclin D1 +	PDAC w/desmoplasia (40%)	Duodenum, stomach	FVB/B6 chimeras	MS

(*97*). Secondary genomic changes and alterations in the immune response profile were also noted (*98*). These types of findings, especially expansion of pancreatic ductal cells, encouraged future acinar cell targeting. Another model (MT-TGF-α/EL-myc) has recently demonstrated that combined expression of both the myc oncogene and TGF-α produce widespread mixed acinar and ductal lesions and adenocarcinoma (*99*). Similar findings were reported earlier (*90*).

The first attempts at targeting mutant K-ras to pancreatic tissue made use of the acinar-specific EL and the ductal cell targeting regulatory elements of cytokeratin 19. The interesting finding was that pancreatic ductal cells appeared relatively resistant to the transforming effects of the K-ras oncogene, although noticeable ductal dysplasia and hyperplasia, accompanied with lymphocytic infiltration along with other mild architectural abnormalities were observed (*100*). Yet, when targeting acinar cells with mutant K-ras, a variety of lesions developed including metaplastic ductal structures and ductal carcinoma in situ (DCIS) reminiscent of human PanINs (*100*). Only very infrequent (<2%) acinar adenomas were observed in these mice. Neither of these mice developed any overt pancreatic cancers. However, EL-K-ras mice in either the p16 or pigment epithelium-derived factor (PEDF) null background developed progression to ductal adenocarcinoma with varying frequencies at about 1 year of age or older (manuscript submitted).

5.2 Pdx1 Targeting

Regulatory elements from the Pdx1 gene have become the most recent means of targeting mouse pancreas. Pdx1-positive cells, which direct transgene expression to embryonic progenitor cells, were targeted with sonic hedgehog (SHH). These young mice developed severely abnormal pancreases with hybrid lesions having both ductal and intestinal characteristics. Some of these lesions expressed mutant K-ras as well as other aberrantly expressed proteins commonly observed in human PanINs and pancreatic cancer (*101*). As a means of avoiding SHH's effects on developing mouse tissue, this system has been moved into an inducible setting (Pdx1-Cre/TRE-SHH) and SHH expression after birth leads to acinar-to-ductal metaplasia and a pronounced desmoplastic response. Another Pdx1 targeting strategy included expression of Cre recombinase (Pdx1-Cre mice) in mice with flanking Lox elements (floxed) that, upon cre-mediated recombination, generated a mutant K-ras in the endogenous mouse allele (termed Pdx1-Cre/K-ras[LSLG12D]). These mice developed ductal lesions and precancer in the pancreas that occasionally progressed to invasive cancer in older mice (*102*). Targeting with Pdx1 demonstrated that mutant K-ras expression in precursor cells or a subset of mature exocrine cells can lead to lesions resembling human PanINs, which have been termed mouse PanINs or mPanINs, which can progress to adenocarcinoma in vivo. It is notable that the mPanINs from these mice also resemble the lesions observed in the EL-K-ras model despite their distinct targeting mechanisms, bringing the cell of origin issue centerfold. Additionally, these mice were further modified by deletion of the p16/

p19, p16, p19, and p53 loci (using crosses with traditional and conditional (floxed) knockout mice for each) (*103*, *104*). The results of these crosses were a multiplicity of mPanINs at all grades, invasive adenocarcinoma, and ultimately metastasis to other organs. p48/PTF1-Cre targeting of these knock-in/knock-out genes led to a similar pattern of cellular changes including the development of mPanINs and adenocarcinoma. Perhaps the best model from these Pdx1-targeted mutant K-ras and TSG knock-out strategies is the Pdx1-Cre/K-ras^{LSLG12D}/p53^{flox}, which develops genomic instability as part of the human-like progression to PDAC (104).

A recent addition to this group of mouse models employs Pdx1-Cre targeted deletion of pTEN (a negative regulator of Akt and PI$_3$K signaling). These mice develop ductal metaplasia from centroacinar cells leading to precancerous lesions with infrequent progression to ductal adenocarcinoma. Hemizygous loss of p53 enhances this progression as demonstrated by increased levels of PanIN-like lesions and PDAC. Use of pTEN deletion in EL positive cells via EL-Cre targeting generated no overt signs of premalignant lesions or cancer in the pancreas (*105*).

Another mouse model targeted COX-2 to ductal cells using the keratin-5 promoter, and these mice developed cystic lesions, ductal dilation, and accompanying fibrosis leading to SCA- and IPMN-like lesions and adenomas (*106*).

5.3   Future Genetically Engineered Mice

There are several newer models on the horizon which make use of Cre-mediated recombination events generating an endogenous mutation in K-ras and loss of additional alleles targeting Pdx1 positive cells. These models include Pdx1-Cre/K-ras^{LSLG12D}/smad4^{flox} (poster at the 2006 Mouse Models of Cancer Conference) and Pdx1-Cre/K-ras^{LSLG12D}/TGFβ^{flox} mice. Early reports indicate progression of both the ductal adenocarcinoma and metastatic phenotypes beyond that of the single oncogenic K-ras event.

Novel targeting of nestin-positive pancreas cells with a mutant K-ras knock-in approach also appears to reproduce a PanIN-to-PDAC progression. Perhaps the most novel and innovative model to appear on the scene makes use of a system employing both inducible and conditional strategies to target EL positive cells in the pancreas. With this approach (EL-tTA/TRE-Cre/K-ras^{LSLG12V}), an endogenous mutation in K-ras led to the development of mPanINs and, in a smaller subset of older mice, ductal adenocarcinoma. However, when adult mouse cells were targeted, the progression from precancer to cancer was not observed without an additional stimulus (manuscript submitted). This modeling system will allow study of the addictive nature of oncogenic insult on the development of both mPanINs and ductal cancer.

Several ideas can be supported by this body of work. One critical finding is the clear in vivo demonstration of mutant K-ras-induced mPanIN development that can lead to ductal adenocarcinoma at a lower frequency and higher latency compared with mutant K-ras mice with lost TSG activity. These results support the causative nature of these genetic events and support how a single initiating event (mutation in K-ras) can, in combination with several different gene loss mutations, lead to adenocarcinoma. In addition, it is becoming clear that at least a few cell types may be able to establish a PanIN-PDAC paradigm of cancer progression. However, despite these insights, the current explosion in genetically modified mouse models has introduced some controversies regarding the cell of origin, the combination of genetic events, and the establishment of cellular phenotypes that resemble varying types of human pancreatic cancers. As a limitation, GEMs do not reproduce the carcinogen-induced genetic and cellular changes and therefore only represent an artificial system for mocking these events. However, carcinogen-induced GEMs may become an improved means of evaluating both genetic background and carcinogen exposure in the same in vivo system.

References

1. Moore PS, Sipos B, Orlandini S, 2001, Genetic profile of 22 pancreatic carcinoma cell lines Analysis f K-ras, p53, p16 and DPC4/Smad4. Virchows Arch 439:798–802.
2. Sipos B, Moser S, Kalthoff H, 2003, A comprehensive characterization of pancreatic ductal carcinoma cell lines: towards establishment of an in vitro research platform. Virchows Arch 442:444–452.
3. Almoguera C, Shibata D, Forrester K, 1988, Most human carcinomas of the exocrine pancreas contain mutant c-Kras genes. Cell 53;549–54.
4. Caldas C, Hahn SA, Costa L, da 1994, Frequent somatic mutations and homozygous deletions of the p16 (MTS1) gene in pancreatic adenocarcinoma. Nat Genet 8:27–32.
5. Kalthoff H, Schmiegel W, Roeder C, 1993, p53 and K-RAS alteration in pancreatic epithelial cell lesions. Oncogene 8:289–298.
6. Lemoine NR, Jain S, Hughes CM, 1992, Ki-ras oncogene activation in preinvasive pancreatic cancer. Gastroenterology 102:230–236.
7. Redston MS, Caldas C, Seymour AB, 1994, p53 mutations in pancreatic carcinoma and evidence of common involvement of homocopolymer tracts in DNA microdeletions. Cancer Res 54:3025–3033.
8. Ruggeri B, Zhang SY, Caamano J, 1992, Human pancreatic carcinomas and cell lines reveal frequent and multiple alterations in the p53 and Rb-1 tumor-suppressor genes. Oncogene 7:1503–1511.
9. Scarpa A, Capelli P, Mukai K, 1993, Pancreatic adenocarcinoma frequently show p53 gene mutations. Am J Pathol 142:1534–1543.
10. Scarpa A, Capelli P, Villanueva A, 1994, ;Pancreatic cancer in Europe: Ki-ras gene mutation pattern shows geographical differences. Int J Cancer 57:167–171.
11. Smit V, Boot AM, Smits AM, 1988, K-ras codon 12 mutations occur very frequently in pancreatic adenocarcinoma. Nucleic Acids Res 16:7773–7782.
12. Furukawa T, Sunamura M, Horii A, 2006, Molecular mechanisms of pancreatic carcinogenesis. Cancer Sci 97:1–7.
13. Serrano M, Hannon GJ, Beach D, 1993, A new regulatory motif in cell-cycle control causing specific inhibition of cyclin D/CDK4. Nature 366:704–707.
14. Nakamura Y. 2004, Isolation of p53-target genes and their functional analysis. Cancer Sci 95:7–11.
15. Hahn SA, Schutte M, Hogque AT, 1996, DPC4, a candidate tumor suppressor gene at human chromosome 18q21.1. Science 271:350–353.

16. Miyazono K, Suzuki H, Imamura T, 2003, Regulation of TGF-beta signalling and its roles in progression of tumors. Cancer Sci 94:230–234.
17. Luttges J, Schemm S, Vogel I, 2000, The grade of pancreatic ductal carcinoma is an independent prognostic factor and is superior to the immunohistochemical assessment of proliferation. J Pathol 191:154–161.
18. Herzig KH, Altmannsberger M, Folsche UR, 1994, Intermediate filaments in rat pancreatic acinar tumors, human ductal carcinomas, and other gastrointestinal malignancies. Gastroenterology 106:1326–1332.
19. Heyderman E, Larkin SE, O'Donnell PJ, 1990, Epithelial markers in pancreatic adenocarcinoma: immunoperoxidase localisation of DD9, CEA, EMA and CAM 5.2. J Clin Pathol 43:448–452.
20. Rafiee P, Ho SB, Bresalier RS, 1992, Characterization of the cytokeratins of human colonic, pancreatic, and gastric adenocarcinoma cell lines. Pancreas 7:123–131.
21. Santini D, Ceccarelli C, Martinelli GN, 1994, Expression of intermediate filaments in normal and neoplastic exocrine pancreas. Zentralbl Pathol 140:247–258.
22. Hoorens A, Prenzel K, Lemoine NR, 1998, Undifferentiated carcinoma of the pancreas: analysis of intermediate filament profile and Ki-ras mutations provides evidence of a ductal origin. J Pathol 185:53–60.
23. Cubilla AL, Fitzgerald PJ, 1976, Morphological lesions associated with human primary invasive nonendocrine pancreas cancer. Cancer Res 36:2690–2698.
24. Hruban RH, Takaori K, Klimstra DS, 2004, An illustrated consensus on the classification of panreatic intraepithelial neoplasia and intraductal papillary mucinous neoplasms. Am J Surg Pathol 28:977–987.
25. Eckel F, Schneider G, Schmid R, 2006, Pancreatic cancer: a review of recent advances. Epert Opin Ivestig Drugs 15(11):1395–1410.
26. Lawson T, Ouellette M, Kolar C, 2005, Culture and immortalization of pancreatic ductal epithelial cells. methods in molecular medicine pancreatic cancer. Methods Protocols 103:113–122.
27. Jones RT, Hudson EA, Resau JH. 1981, A review of in vitro and in vivo culture techniques for the study of pancreatic carcinogenesis. Cancer 47:1490–1406.
28. Gmyr V, Kerr-Conte J, Vanderwalle B, 2001, Human pancreatic ductal cells: Large scale isolation and expansion. Cell Transplant 10:109–121.
29. Lisle RC, de Logsdon CD. 1990, Pancreatic acinar cells in culture: expression of acinar and ductal antigens in a growth-related manner. Eur J Cell Biol 51:64–75.
30. Ouellette MM, Lee K. 2001, Telomerase: diagnostics, cancer therapeutics and tissue engineering. Dru Discov Today 6:1231–1237.
31. Bodnar AG, Ouellette M, Frolkis M, 1998, Extension of life-span by introduction of telomerase into normal human cells. Science 279:349–352.
32. Morales CP, Holt SE, Ouellet MM, 1999, Absence of cancer-associated changes in human fibroblasts immortalized with telomerase. Nat Genet 21:115–118.
33. Jiang XR, Jimenez G, Change E, 1999, Telomerase expression in human somatic cells does not induce changes associated with a transformed phenotype. Nat Genet 21:111–114.
34. Jesnowski R, Muller P, Schareck W, 1999, Immortalized pancreatic duct cells in vitro and in vivo. Ann N Y Acad Sci 880:50–65.
35. Furukawa T, Duguid WP, Rosenberg L, 1996, Long-term culture and immortalization of epithelial cells from normal adult human pancreatic ducts transfected by the E6E7 gene of human papilloma virus 16. Am J Pathol 148:1763–1770.
36. Jesnowski R, Liebe S, Lohr M. 1998, Increasing the transfection efficacy and subsequent long-term culture of resting human pancreatic duct epithelial cells. Pancreas 17:262–265.
37. Ulrich AB, Schmied BM, Standop J, 2002, Pancreatic cell lines: a review. Pancreas 24:111–120.
38. Grippo PJ, Sandgren EP, 2005, Modeling pancreatic cancer in animals to address specific hypothesis. Methods Mol, Med 103:217–243.

39. Fidler IJ, 1986, Rationale and methods for the use of nude mice to study the biology and therapy of human cancer metastasis. Cancer Metastasis Rev 5(1):29–49.
40. Capella G, Farre L, Villanueva A, 1999, Orthotopic models of human pancreatic cancer. Ann N Y Acad Sci 880:103–109.
41. Fogh J, Orfeo T, Tiso J, 1980, Twenty-three new human tumor lines established in nude mice. Exp Cell Biol 880:229–239.
42. Alisauskus R, Wong GY, Gold DV, 1995, Initial studies of monoclonal antibody PAM4 targeting to xenografted orthotopic pancreatic cancer. Cancer Res 55:5743s–48s.
43. Luokopoulos P, Kanetaka K, Takamura M, 2004, Orthotopic transplantation models of pancreatic adenocarcinoma derived from cell lines and primary tumors and displaying varying metastatic activity. Pancreas 29:193–203.
44. Ellenrieder V, Adler G, Gress TM, 1999, Invasion and metastasis in pancreatic cancer. Ann Oncol 10(Suppl 4):46–50.
45. Keleg S, Buchler P, Ludwig R, 2003, Invasion and metastasis in pancreatic cancer. Mol Cancer 2:14.
46. L AC. Modulation of response to tumor therapies by the extracellular matrix. Future Oncol 2006, 2(3):417–429.
47. Petrulio CA, Kim-Schulze S, Kaufman HL. 2006, The tumour microenvironment and implications for cancer immunotherapy. Expert Opin Biol Ther 6(7):671–684.
48. Tan MH, Chu TM. 1985, Characterization of the tumorigenic and metastatic properties of a human pancreatic tumor cell line (AsPC-1) implanted orthotopically into nude mice. Tumour Biol 6(1):89–98.
49. Marincola FM, Drucker BJ, Siao DY, 1989, The nude mouse as a model or the study of human pancreatic cancer. J Surg Res 47(6):520–529.
50. Mohammad RM, Al-Katib A, Pettit GR, 1998, An orthotopic model of human pancreatic cancer in severe combined immunodeficient mice: potential application for preclinical studies. Clin Cancer Res 4(4):887–894.
51. Alves F, Contag S, Missbach M, 2001, An orthotopic model of ductal adenocarcinoma of the pancreas in severe combined immunodeficient mice representing all steps of the metastatic cascade. Pancreas 23(3):227–235.
52. Fu X, Guadagni F, Hoffman RM. 1992, A metastatic nude-mouse model of human pancreatic cancer constructed orthotopically with histologically intact patient specimens. Proc Natl Acad Sci USA 89:5645–5649.
53. Reyes G, Villanueva A, Garcia C, 1996, Orthotopic xenografts of human pancreatic carcinomas acquire genetic aberrations during dissemination in nude mice. Cancer Res 56(24):5713–5719.
54. Vezeridis MP, Doremus CM, Tibbetts LM, 1989, Invasion and metastasis following orthotopic transplantation of human pancreatic cancer in the nude mouse. J Surg Oncol 40(4):261–265.
55. Hotz HG, Howard AR, Hotz B, 2003, An orthotopic nude mouse model for evaluating pathophysiology and therapy of pancreatic cancer. Pancreas 26(4):89e–98e.
56. Samnick S, Romeike BF, Kubuschok B, 2004, p-[123I]iodo-L-phenylalanine for detection of pancreatic cancer: basic investigations of the uptake characteristics in primary human pancreatic tumour cells and evaluation in in vivo models of human pancreatic adenocarcinoma. Eur J Nucl Med Mol Imaging 31(4):532–541.
57. Bouvet M, Yang M, Nardin S, 2000, Chronologically-specific metastatic targeting f human pancreatic tumors in orthotopic models. Clin Exp Metastasis 18(3):213–218.
58. Bouvet M, Spernyak J, Katz MH, 2005, High correlation of whole-body red fluorescent protein imaging and magnetic resonance imaging on an orthotopic model of pancreatic cancer. Cancer Res 65(21):9829–9833.
59. Bouvet M, Wang J, Nardin SR, 2002, Real-time optical imaging of primary tumor growth and multiple metastatic events in a pancreatic cancer orthoptic model. Cancer Res 62:1534–1540.
60. Gingell R, Wallcave L, Nagel D, 1976, Metabolism of the pancreatic carcinogens N-nitroso-bis(2-oxopropyl)amine and N-nitroso-bis(2-hydroxypropyl)amine in the Syrian hamster. J Natl Cancer Inst 57(5):1175–1178.

61. Gingell R, Brunk G, Nagel D, 1979, Metabolism of three radiolabeled pancreatic carcinogenic nitrosamines in hamsters and rats. Cancer Res 39(11):4579–4583.
62. Pour P, Gingell R, Langenbach R, 1980, Carcinogenicity of N-nitrosomethyl(2-oxopropyl)amine in Syrian hamsters. Cancer Res 40(10):3585–3590.
63. Pour P, Mohr U, Cardesa A, 1975, Pancreatic neoplasms in an animal model: morphological, biological, and comparative studies. Cancer 36(2):379–389.
64. Pour P, Althoff J. 1977, The effect of N-nitrosobis(2-oxopropyl)amine after oral administration to hamsters. Cancer Lett 2(6):323–326.
65. Gingell R, Pour P. 1978, Metabolism of the pancreatic carcinogen N-nitroso-bis(2-oxopropyl)amine after oral and intraperitoneal administration to Syrian golden hamsters. J Natl Cancer Inst 60(4):911–913.
66. Roebuck BD, Baumgartner KJ, Thron CD. 1984, Characterization of two populations of pancreatic atypical acinar cell foci induced by azaserine in the rat. Lab Invest 50(2):141–146.
67. Longnecker DS. 1984, Lesions induced in rodent pancreas by azaserine and other pancreatic carcinogens. Environ Health Perspect 56:245–251.
68. Longnecker DS, Curphey TJ. 1975, Adenocarcinoma of the pancreas in azaserine-treated rats. Cancer Res 35(8):2249–2258.
69. Konishi Y, Denda A, Maruyama H, 1980, Pancreatic tumors induced by a single intraperitoneal injection of azaserine in partial pancreatectomized rats. Cancer Lett 9(1):43–46.
70. Longnecker DS, Roebuck BD, Yager JD, Jr. 1981, Pancreatic carcinoma in azaserine-treated rats: induction, classification and dietary modulation of incidence. Cancer 47(6 Suppl):1562–1572.
71. Roebuck BD, Longnecker DS. 1977, Species and rat strain variation in pancreatic nodule induction by azaserine. J Natl Cancer Inst 59(4):1273–1277.
72. Dissin J, Mills LR, Mains DL, 1975, Experimental induction of pancreatic adenocarcinoma in rats. J Natl Cancer Inst 55(4):857–864.
73. Hilmy AM, Kandeel KM, Selim NM. 1984, Pancreatic amylase as a tumour marker for pancreatic cancer. Arch Geschwulstforsch 54(6):475–482.
74. Bockman DE, Guo J, Buchler P, 2003, Origin and development of the precursor lesions in experimental pancreatic cancer in rats. Lab Invest 83(6):853–859.
75. Rivera JA, Graeme-Cook F, Werner J, 1997, A rat model of pancreatic ductal adenocarcinoma: targeting chemical carcinogens. Surgery 122(1):82–90.
76. Reddy JK, Rao MS. 1975, Pancreatic adenocarcinoma in inbred guinea pigs induced by n-methyl-N-nitrosourea. Cancer Res 35(8):2269–2277.
77. Reddy JK, Svoboda DJ, Rao MS. 1974, Susceptibility of an ibred strain of guinea pigs to the induction of pancreatic adenocarcinoma by N-methyl-N-nitrosourea. J Natl Cancer Inst 52(3):991–993.
78. Rao MS, Reddy JK. 1977, Pathology of tumors developed in guinea pigs given intraperitoneal injections of N-methyl-N-nitrosourea. Neoplasma 24(1):57–62.
79. Rao MS, Reddy JK. 1980, Histogenesis of pseudo-ductular changes induced in the pancreas of guinea pigs treated with N-methyl-N-nitrosourea. Carcinogenesis 1(12):1027–1037.
80. Longnecker D. 1990, Experimental pancreatic cancer: role of species, sex and diet. Bull Cancer 77(1):27–37.
81. Scarpelli DG, Rao MS, Reddy JK. 1984, Studies of pancreatic carcinogenesis in different animal models. Environ Health Perspect 56:217–227.
82. Zimmerman JA, Trombetta LD, Carter TH, 1982, Pancreatic carcinoma induced by N-methyl-NÎÎ-nitrosourea in aged mice. Gerontology 28(2):114–120.
83. Fujii K, Hayakawa T, Kikuchi M. 1994, Tumor induction in mice administered neonatally with bis(2-oxopropyl)nitrosamine. Tohoku J Exp Med 174(4):361–368.
84. Osvaldt AB, Wendt LR, Bersch VP, 2006, Pancreatic intraepithelial neoplasia and ductal adenocarcinoma induced by DMBA in mice. Surgery 140(5):803–809.
85. Haas MJ, Dragan YP, Hikita H, 1999, Transgene expression and repression in transgenic rats bearing the phosphoenolpyruvate carboxykinase-simian virus 40 T antigen or the phosphoenolpyruvate carboxykinase-transforming growth factor-alpha constructs. Am J Pathol 155(1):183–192.

86. Alhonen L, Parkkinen JJ, Keinanen T, 2000, Activation of polyamine catabolism in transgenic rats induces acute pancreatitis. Proc Natl Acad Sci U S A 97(15):8290–8295.
87. Ornitz DM, Hammer RE, Messing A, 1987, Pancreatic neoplasia induced by SV40 T-antigen expression in acinar cells of transgenic mice. Science 238(4824):188–193.
88. Quaife CJ, Pinkert CA, Ornitz DM, 1987, Pancreatic neoplasia induced by ras expression in acinar cells of transgenic mice. Cell 48(6):1023–1034.
89. Sandgren EP, Luetteke NC, Palmiter RD, 1990, Overexpression of TGF alpha in transgenic mice: induction of epithelial hyperplasia, pancreatic metaplasia, and carcinoma of the breast. Cell 61(6):1121–1135.
90. Sandgren EP, Luetteke NC, Qiu TH, 1993, Transforming growth factor alpha dramatically enhances oncogene-induced carcinogenesis in transgenic mouse pancreas and liver. Mol Cell Biol 13(1):320–330.
91. Sandgren EP, Quaife CJ, Paulovich AG, 1991, Pancreatic tumor pathogenesis reflects the causative genetic lesion. Proc Natl Acad Sci U S A 88(1):93–97.
92. Wagner M, Luhrs H, Kloppel G, 1998, Malignant transformation of duct-like cells originating from acini in transforming growth factor transgenic mice. Gastroenterology 115(5):1254–1262.
93. Greten FR, Wagner M, Weber CK, 2001, TGF alpha transgenic mice. A model of pancreatic cancer development. Pancreatology 1(4):363–368.
94. Schreiner B, Baur DM, Fingerle AA, 2003, Pattern of secondary genomic changes in pancreatic tumors of Tgf alpha/Trp53+/– transgenic mice. Genes Chromosomes Cancer 38(3):240–248.
95. Song SY, Gannon M, Washington MK, 1999, Expansion of Pdx1-expressing pancreatic epithelium and islet neogenesis in transgenic mice overexpressing transforming growth factor alpha. Gastroenterology 117(6):1416–1426.
96. Greten FR, Weber CK, Greten TF, 2002, Stat3 and NF-kappaB activation prevents apoptosis in pancreatic carcinogenesis. Gastroenterology 123(6):2052–2063.
97. Miyamoto Y, Maitra A, Ghosh B, 2003, Notch mediates TGF alpha-induced changes in epithelial differentiation during pancreatic tumorigenesis. Cancer Cell 3(6):565–576.
98. Garbe AI, Vermeer B, Gamrekelashvili J, 2006, Genetically induced pancreatic adenocarcinoma is highly immunogenic and causes spontaneous tumor-specific immune responses. Cancer Res 66(1):508–516.
99. Liao DJ, Wang Y, Wu J, 2006, Characterization of pancreatic lesions from MT-tgfalpha, Ela-myc and MT-tgfalpha/Ela-myc single and double transgenic mice. J Carcinog 5:19.
100. Brembeck FH, Schreiber FS, Deramaudt TB, 2003, The mutant K-ras oncogene causes pancreatic periductal lymphocytic infiltration and gastric mucous neck cell hyperplasia in transgenic mice. Cancer Res 63(9):2005–2009.
101. Thayer SP, di Magliano MP, Heiser PW, 2003, Hedgehog is an early and late mediator of pancreatic cancer tumorigenesis. Nature 425(6960):851–856.
102. Hingorani SR, Petricoin EF, Maitra A, 2003, Preinvasive and invasive ductal pancreatic cancer and its early detection in the mouse. Cancer Cell 4(6):437–450.
103. Aguirre AJ, Bardeesy N, Sinha M, 2003, Activated Kras and Ink4a/Arf deficiency cooperate to produce metastatic pancreatic ductal adenocarcinoma. Genes Dev 17(24):3112–3126.
104. Hingorani SR, Wang L, Multani AS, 2005, Trp53R172H and KrasG12D cooperate to promote chromosomal instability and widely metastatic pancreatic ductal adenocarcinoma in mice. Cancer Cell 7(5):469–483.
105. Stanger BZ, Stiles B, Lauwers GY, 2005, Pten constrains centroacinar cell expansion and malignant transformation in the pancreas. Cancer Cell 8(3):185–195.
106. Muller-Decker K, Furstenberger G, Annan N, 2006, Preinvasive duct-derived neoplasms in pancreas of keratin 5-promoter cyclooxygenase-2 transgenic mice. Gastroenterology 130(7):2165–2178.
107. Bardeesy N, Morgan J, Sinha M, 2002, Obligate roles for p16(Ink4a) and p19(Arf)-p53 in the suppression of murine pancreatic neoplasia. Mol Cell Biol 22(2):635–643.

108. Grippo PJ, Nowlin PS, Demeure MJ, 2003, Preinvasive pancreatic neoplasia of ductal phenotype induced by acinar cell targeting of mutant Kras in transgenic mice. Cancer Res 63(9):2016–2019.
109. Tuveson DA, Zhu L, Gopinathan A, 2006, Mist1-KrasG12D knock-in mice develop mixed differentiation metastatic exocrine pancreatic carcinoma and hepatocellular carcinoma. Cancer Res 66(1):242–247.

Chapter 10
From Inception to Invasion: Modeling Pathways to Pancreatic Cancer

Sunil R. Hingorani

1 Introduction

Despite a relatively modest incidence, pancreatic ductal adenocarcinoma (PDA) is the fourth leading cause of cancer-related deaths in the Western hemisphere (*1*). The reason is straightforward and sobering: with rare exception, pancreas cancer kills every patient it afflicts. The disease is not only uniformly but also rapidly lethal, largely because of delayed detection. Most patients are diagnosed too late in the course of disease progression to permit surgical intervention. Symptoms, when they occur at all, are typically vague and nonlocalizing, and there are currently no biomarkers for early detection. Radiographically evident lesions have already crossed the threshold of curability. Nevertheless, it is difficult to escape the conclusion that the improved survival seen in the first few years after surgery in the fortuitous few results from lead-time bias (*2*); all of these patients also eventually succumb to recurrent and/or metastatic disease. Despite increasingly aggressive surgical procedures and the use of adjuvant chemotherapies and radiation, the result is the same (*3–5*). Anatomy and biology conspire not only to elude early detection but also to hinder scientific inquiry. The pancreas is difficult to access and hazardous to biopsy: the organ does not forgive violation and biopsy can be fraught with the potentially dire consequences of pancreatitis.

These ineluctable truths of pancreas cancer beg the development of animal models that faithfully mimic the disease from its very inception to invasion and metastasis. In fact, driven by the ubiquity and sequelae of diabetes, genetic manipulation of the murine pancreas has a long and rich history that dates to the earliest experiments in transgenesis. Those early years formed the foundation for continuing refinements that have recently achieved notable success. These most recent attempts, specifically employing conditional activation of oncogenic K-ras, to genetically engineer pancreatic ductal adenocarcinoma in the mouse are the prescribed purview of this chapter.

A.M. Lowy et al. (eds.) *Pancreatic Cancer.*
doi: 10.1007/978-0-387-69252-4, © Springer Science+Business Media, LLC 2008

2 Roadmaps and Yardsticks: What Is to Be Modeled?

Insight and analysis of resected human pancreatic tumor specimens have led to the development of histologic and genetic frameworks for the initiation and progression of PDA (6, 7). These schema have guided current efforts to model the disease while also serving as the benchmarks against which any effort must be measured. Preinvasive disease is thought to begin most commonly in the terminal ductules, below the detection threshold of current imaging modalities, and progresses through definable morphologic and genetic changes in the ductal epithelium (Fig. 10.1) (8, 9). These preinvasive lesions, collectively termed pancreatic intraepithelial neoplasias (PanINs), manifest distinct nuclear and architectural changes as they progress from PanIN-1 to PanIN-2 to PanIN-3, or carcinoma in situ (6). Not surprisingly, given their size and peripheral location, PanINs are asymptomatic.

Although by far the most common pathway, the PanIN-to-PDA sequence is not the only route to invasive ductal adenocarcinoma of the pancreas. Distinct adenoma-to-carcinoma sequences exist in which invasive disease arises from cystic neoplasia (10, 11). Although less common and less likely to invade than PanINs, cystic neoplasms can be lethal once they do become invasive. The two major classes of cystic neoplasms, mucinous cystic neoplasms (MCNs) and intraductal papillary mucinous neoplasms (IPMNs), have clearly distinct histological, genetic, clinical and prognostic implications from each other and from PanIN (see Fig. 10.1; Table 10.1) (12, 13). Nevertheless, each pathway can ultimately result in invasive "tubular" (or ductal) adenocarcinomas with similar histologic features.

IPMNs typically arise at the head of the pancreas in the main or branch ducts and are usually asymptomatic, unless they become obstructive and induce pancreatitis. They occur in the eighth decade of life with a slight male preponderance (60%). The lesions characteristically have papillary fronds extending into the lumen with fibrovascular cores. IPMNs most commonly progress to colloid carcinomas, characterized by isolated carcinoma cells floating in pools of extracellular mucin; they can also give rise to more conventional-appearing ductal adenocarcinomas. So as not to obscure the considerable, and likely informative, distinctions between cystic and noncystic routes to ductal carcinomas, I will refer to invasive disease arising from classical PanINs as PDA, and the "tubular," or ductal, adenocarcinomas arising from either IPMNs or MCNs as IDA (invasive ductal adenocarcinoma).

MCNs preferentially form in the body and tail of the gland and likely arise in the terminal ductules, although their precise relationship to the ductal system remains controversial (14–16). As the majority of MCNs do not appear to communicate with the ductal tree, it has been suggested that they represent de novo structures. However, it also possible that a small ductal communication may be missed depending on the method of assessment, or that an original connection is lost as the cysts grow and expand such that they exist apart at the time of diagnosis. MCNs are 20-fold more common in women than men and tend to occur in the fifth decade of life. MCNs are usually asymptomatic until they become very large (≥10 cm), at which point patients often describe vague sensations of abdominal fullness and bloating. One of the defining features of MCNs is their association with a unique "ovarian" stroma,

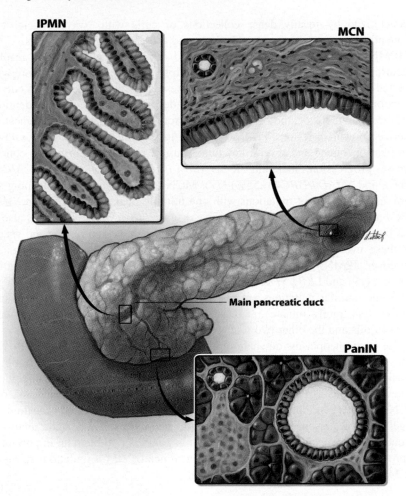

Fig. 10.1 Preinvasive neoplasms of the pancreatic ductal epithelium. The most common precursors to PDA, PanINs, arise in the terminal ductules and typically progress to invasive disease in the head of the pancreas. IPMNs are macroscopic structures that form in the main or branch ducts most commonly in the pancreatic head. MCNs develop in the periphery of the gland, usually in the body and tail, and exhibit a characteristic highly cellular "ovarian stroma." Artwork by D. Ehlert

Table 10.1 Distinct routes to invasive ductal adenocarcinoma of the pancreas

Preinvasive lesion	Anatomic location	Symptoms	Age at diagnosis (y)	Gender ratio (F:M)	Invasive disease	Curable
PanIN	H; Periphery	None	60–70	~1:1	PDA	No
MCN	B/T; Periphery	Vague; abdominal fullness	40–50	>10:1	IDA	Yes
IPMN	H; Central	Rare; pancreatitis	70–80	~1.5:1	Colloid carcinoma; IDA	Yes

H, Head; B, body; T, tail; PDA, pancreatic ductal adenocorcinoma; IDA, invasive ductal adenocarcinoma; IDA, invasive ductal adenocarcinoma

characterized by focally dense collections of cells with "wavy" nuclei which frequently express progesterone (50–75%) and estrogen (~25%) receptors.

IPMNs tend to be multifocal and limited resection therefore often results in "recurrence"—more likely the result of multiple primary lesions in a more widely affected duct. MCNs more commonly progress as isolated lesions and complete resection of the primary lesion is frequently definitive. The genetic epidemiology of these discrete histopathologic routes underscores their distinction. The best characterized precursor lesions, PanINs, show an increasing frequency of mutations in a critical oncogene and several key tumor suppressor genes during the course of disease progression, including K-ras (90%), *TP53* (>75%), *CDKN2A/INK4A* (90%), and *SMAD4/DPC4* (~55%) (*17*). MCNs share a largely overlapping spectrum and frequency of mutations with one notable nuance: mutations in *SMAD4/DPC4* are essentially invariant in invasive disease (*18*). Although IPMNs also possess frequent mutations in these cardinal genes, the reported ranges and specifics for these events are not as congruous as those for the other two routes (*11*). Moreover, IPMNs harbor several unique genetic events including mutations in *PI3KCA* (*19*) and *LKB1/STK1* (~25%) (*20*), the gene associated with Peutz-Jeghers syndrome; similar mutations are not seen in PanIN-PDA or MCN-IDA. Finally, IPMNs very rarely mutate *SMAD4/DPC4* (*21*) perhaps the clearest difference between this and the other two routes to invasive ductal cancers.

The cystic neoplasms do share one important and distinguishing feature, however: they are often curable by resection. This finding is particularly intriguing for invasive MCNs as these neoplasms share virtually identical spectra and incidences of key mutations as PanIN-PDA. Moreover, the invasive disease that arises out of MCNs strongly resembles conventional ductal adenocarcinoma and is distinguished largely by the presence of associated cystic neoplasms. Thus, static analyses of resected tumor specimens do not resolve this paradox, although an important clue is provided by the essentially uniform occurrence of *DPC4* mutations in invasive MCNs (discussed further in the following).

3   Brief History of Modeling in the Mouse Pancreas

The long history of genetic manipulation in the mouse together with the widespread availability of inbred strains and, more recently, embryonic stem cell lines, make the laboratory mouse a particularly attractive vehicle for the study of disease pathogenesis. Interestingly, the murine pancreas, unlike that of the hamster and rat, has been relatively resistant to chemically induced carcinogenesis, a barrier that may have recently been surmounted (*22, 23*). Until recently, it has also resisted attempts to model ductal adenocarcinoma genetically. Among the pioneering experiments to introduce transgenes into the mouse genome were those linking the expression of presumptive oncogenes to pancreas-specific promoters (*24–27*). The transforming effects of *c-myc* (*28*), *SV40 T* and *t* antigens (*29, 30*), and *Hras^{G12V}* (*31*) were probed in this manner and early models of acinar and islet cell neoplasia were developed, some of which continue to be studied today (*32*). More recently, *Elastase* promoter elements have been used to drive expression of *TGFα* (*33–35*) and K-ras^{G12D} (*36*), whereas the ductal-selective *CK-19* promoter has been linked to K-ras^{G12V} (*37*), in model systems that achieved some notable similarities to the human disease. Each of these investigations has yielded critical insights into the functions of specific genes and the apparent requirements for specific cellular contexts and levels of gene expression to recapitulate histopathology. Collectively, they have also laid the foundation for subsequent efforts.

The abilities to target the endogenous locus by homologous recombination in ES cells and to spatially, and even temporally, restrict gene expression have led to a new generation of mouse models of human disease (*38, 39*). Efforts to model pancreas cancer have also benefited from these technologies. Although the considerable differences in biology and physiology (*40*) should necessarily give pause to scientist and physician alike, carefully conceived and constructed animal systems can help illuminate and clarify otherwise obscure questions on mechanisms of human disease. Indeed, informed syntheses of clinical, biological, histologic, and molecular data from cognate human and animal diseases may hold the greatest promise to unravel heretofore intractable questions of human disease.

The studies of human PDA described above have raised a number of pivotal questions, questions that have been or promise to be illuminated by investigations in animal systems:

1. Are PanINs bona fide precursors to invasive PDA?
2. Is there a temporal relationship between the various putative stages of PanIN lesions?
3. Do activating mutations in K-ras initiate disease?
4. Which compartment(s) is competent to initiate disease? In other words, what is the cell-of-origin of PDA?
5. Which, if any, of the identified mutations in the principal tumor suppressor gene pathways play a causal role in disease progression?
6. Do different combinations of mutations define distinct histopathologic forms of the disease?
7. Does the sequence in which the mutations arise help define the ensuing disease?
8. At what point along the continuum of preinvasive disease does invasion pass from the possible to the inevitable? In other words, at what point must we intervene?

4   Pancreas Cancer: *Ras* Reveals the Way

The earliest genetically engineered mouse models involved targeted deletion or "knock-out" of prominent tumor suppressor genes, including those frequently mutated in PDA such as *Trp53* (*41, 42*), *Cdkn2a/Ink4a* (*43*), and *Smad4/Dpc4* (*44–47*). None of these animals revealed any evidence of pancreatic pathology, however.

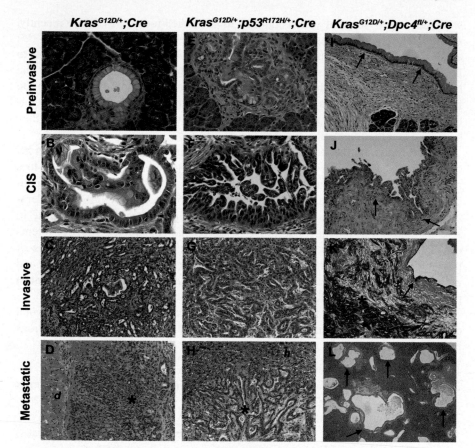

Fig. 10.2 Histologic progression in genetically engineered murine models of pancreatic ductal adenocarcinomas. Early preinvasive, advanced preinvasive (carcinoma in situ), invasive and metastatic neoplasms are shown from K-ras $^{G12D/+}$;Cre (A–D) (47, 49), K-ras$^{G12D/+}$;Trp53$^{R172H/+}$;Cre (E-H) (49) and K-ras$^{G12D/+}$;Dpc4$^{flox/+}$;Cre (I–L) (53) animals. A PanIN-1A lesion (A) denotes a transition from the simple cuboidal epithelium of a normal duct to a columnar phenotype with abundant apical mucin. In a PanIN-3, or carcinoma-in-situ (B), complete loss of polarity, nuclear atypia, and clusters of luminal cells are observed. Progression to invasive disease from these precursors can reveal moderately well-differentiated (C) to poorly differentiated to sarcomatoid or spindle cell morphologies. Metastatic disease (D, *asterisk*), in this case to the diaphragm (*d*), typically retains the morpholigcal features of the primary malignancy. The preinvasive (E, F), invasive (F), and metastatic (H, *asterisk*) disease in K-ras$^{G12D/+}$;Trp53$^{R172H/+}$;Cre animals also follows the classical PanIN-to-PDA progression with a preponderance of well-differentiated histology. The cystic lesions arising in K-ras$^{G12D/+}$;Dpc4$^{flox/+}$;Cre mice reveal all of the diagnostic features of human MCNs including a columnar, mucin-filled epithelial lining without significant papillary projections into the lumen (I, *arrows*). These lesions progress through increasing degrees of dysplasia from low-grade (I), to moderate grade, to high-grade (J; microscopic foci of invasion are also evident, *arrows*). Invasive disease (K, *asterisk*) reveals a glandular histology in clear association with a mucinous cystic neoplasm *(arrow)*. Once again, the metastases arising from invasive MCNs (L, *arrows*), here shown in the liver, retain the cystic morphology of their primary cancers, including recapitulating varying degrees of cellular and nuclear atypia

These studies suggested that an oncogenic mutation may serve as the rate-limiting event and therefore be required to initiate disease. Because embryonic expression of the activated K-ras allele is a lethal event (*48*), studying the potential tumorigenic effects of oncogenic K-ras requires targeted expression to specific tissues postgastrulation. This can be achieved through conditional expression systems using *Cre-Lox* (*49*) or *Flp-Frt* (*50*) technologies. Using these strategies, the physiologic expression of oncogenic K-ras^{G12D} targeted to the *Pdx-1* and *p48*-expressing compartments of the developing murine pancreas resulted in the faithful recapitulation of all three postulated stages of preinvasive lesions, or PanINs (*51*). These lesions progressed over time, accumulating increasing numbers and degrees of cellular and nuclear atypia, ultimately culminating in the development of invasive and metastatic PDA (Fig. 10.2). In addition, a number of signaling pathways were aberrantly activated at even the earliest stages of preinvasive disease, mirroring their behavior in the human disease and implicating oncogenic K-ras in their dysregulation. These pathways further suggest potential targets for chemoprevention and treatment. Finally, a distinctive signature in the low molecular weight serum proteome of animals was preinvasive disease was identified, providing proof-of-principle of the existence of definable markers for the earliest stages of disease.

5 Tumor Suppressor Gene Mutations Shape What K-ras Begins

Similar targeting strategies have been used to systematically evaluate the effects of the other genetic events of postulated importance, both alone and in combination. Unlike tumor suppressor gene mutations commonly encountered in human malignancies, which generally involve genomic deletion and/or epigenetic silencing, mutations in *TP53* found in PDA invariably involve point mutation of one allele at one of several "hot spots" followed by LOH of the locus (*52*). Engineered mutations of one of the most frequently encountered point mutations in human PDA, *Trp53*^{R172H} (corresponding to *TP53*^{R175H}), when concomitantly expressed with K-ras^{G12D}, results in the accelerated evolution of disease with highly glandular histology and widespread metastases (*53*) (Table 10.2). The histological phenotype as well as the sites and frequencies of metastases all closely recapitulate the human disease. Intriguingly, the primary cells isolated from pancreatic tumors and metastatic lesions exhibit high degrees of both simple (numerical) and complex (structural) instability, notable features of human PDA, perhaps reflecting a gain-of-function phenotype associated with point-mutation as opposed to deletion of *Trp53*. Disease progression also invariably involves LOH of the *Trp53* locus, again as is seen in human PDA. Interestingly, rare variants including adenosquamous, sarcomatoid and cystic pathology were also seen again at similar frequencies encountered in human pancreatic cancer. These findings speak to the considerable plasticity exhibited by the target cell in response to a defined set of genetic perturbations and implicate, though by no means prove, a mutated pluripotent progenitor cell as the cell-of-origin. Thus, it appears that the combined physiologic expression of oncogenic

Table 10.2 Phenotypes of genetically engineered mouse models of pancreatic ductal carcinoma

Genotype	Primary disease		Histology	Median survival (mo)	References
	Preinvasive	Invasive			
K-ras$^{G12D/+}$	PanIN	PDA	G, S	15	57, 53
K-ras$^{G12D/+}$;p53$^{R172H/+}$	PanIN	PDA	G	5	53
K-ras$^{G12D/+}$;p16/p19$^{fl/fl}$	*PanIN*	PDA	G, S, A	2	54
K-ras$^{G12D/+}$;p53$^{flox/+}$; p16$^{(+/-)}$	PanIN	PDA	G, S	3.5	56
K-ras$^{G12D/+}$;Dpc4$^{fl/+}$	MCN	IDA	C + G + OS	15	57
K-ras$^{G12D/+}$;Dpc4$^{fl/fl}$	MCN	IDA	C + G + OS	8	57
K-ras$^{G12D/+}$;Dpc4$^{fl/fl}$	IPMN	PDA	C + G	4	58
K-ras$^{G12D/+}$; p16/p19$^{fl/fl}$;Dpc4$^{fl/fl}$	PanIN> IPMN	PDA	G > S	3.5	58
K-ras$^{G12D/+}$;Tgfbr2$^{flox/flox}$	PanIN	PDA	G > S	2	62
K-ras$^{G12D/+}$;CLEG2	PanIN + "lobular"	Undiff. carcinoma	U	1	75

A, anaplastic; C, cystic; G, glandular; OS, ovarian stroma; S, sarcomatoid; U, undifferentiated.

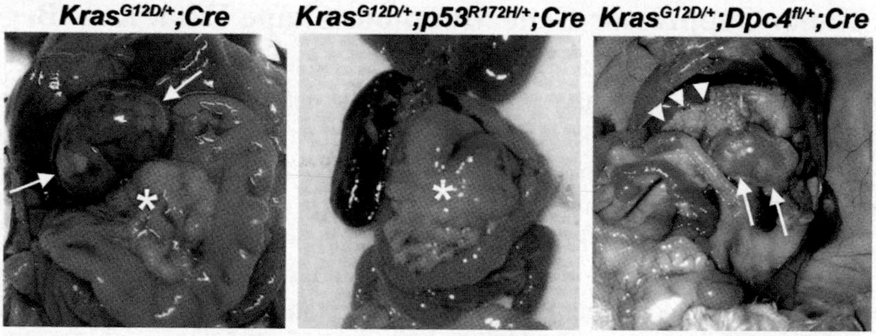

Fig. 10.3 Genotype determines phenotype in mouse models of invasive pancreatic ductal adeno-carcinoma. K-ras$^{G12D/+}$;*Cre* (47, 49) and K-ras$^{G12D/+}$;*Trp53*$^{R172H/+}$;*Cre* (dorsal view) (49) mice typi-cally develop large, firm tumors at the head-of-the-pancreas (asterisks) frequently accompanied by metastatic disease (arrows), here shown to the liver. In contrast, K-ras$^{G12D/+}$;*Dpc4*$^{flox/+}$;*Cre* animals developed multilocular cysts (arrows) in the body and tail of the organ, usually filled with serous fluid. The head of the pancreas was frequently micronodular (*arrowheads*), but lacked a dominant mass or the large cysts noted in more distal portions of the gland

K-ras^{G12D} and *Trp53*^{R172H} faithfully recapitulates the human disease at the molecular, cellular, and organismal levels, including the rare occurrences of alternative histologies. Moreover, the absence of cooperating mutations in the other principal tumor suppressor pathways implicated in pancreatic cancer pathogenesis, led to the postulation that distinct genetic pathways to PDA may exist with unique biological behaviors (Fig. 10.3). The possibility of discrete genetic subtypes of PDA has potentially important implications for disease detection, treatment and chemoprevention strategies (discussed further in the following).

Biallelic deletion of the contiguous *Cdkn2a/Ink4a* (*p16*) and *Cdkn2d/Ink4d* (*p19*) loci also hastens disease progression, resulting in a very aggressive local disease with rare microscopic metastases. Interestingly, these tumors frequently displayed sarcomatoid histology, often as the predominant pattern (*54, 55*). Subsequent studies confirmed this tendency of *p16* mutations, in particular, to steer pathology strongly toward sarcomatoid, or spindle cell, carcinomas (*56*). The uniform sarcomatoid histology seen with *p16*-null animals is pulled toward glandular, and secondarily anaplastic phenotypes with heterozygous mutation of *Trp53*; homozygous mutation of both *p16* and *Trp53* appears to further shift some of the glandular tumors toward an anaplastic phenotype, thought to represent a particularly aggressive form of the disease. Compound heterozygous mutation of *p16* and *p19* similarly results in a modest shift toward glandular phenotypes. Conversely, the strong tendency toward glandular histology seen with mutation of *Trp53* is shifted toward an anaplastic pattern in animals with compound homozygous mutation of *Trp53* and *p16*. In each of the mentioned models, mutation of additional tumor suppressor gene pathways was not observed, suggesting that mutation of the *Ink4a* and *Trp53* pathways represent distinct genetic routes to PDA with definable clinical and histological characteristics. The notion of different genetic routes to PDA was further supported by the identification of distinct clusters of copy number alterations segregating tumors that developed in the context of different TSG mutation combinations (*56*).

From here, studies logically turned to the next most frequently altered signaling pathway in human PDA, the TGFβ cascade. The findings with mutation of *Smad4/Dpc4* in the setting of K-ras^{G12D} were unexpected and startling, although in some respects, clues from human disease progression were perhaps telling.

6   TGFβ Signaling and Cystic Neoplasia: When Matters as Much as Which

As noted, mutations in *SMAD4/DPC4* occur in about half of PanIN-PDA and almost uniformly in MCN-IDA, consistent with a relatively late occurrence in the progression of PanINs while suggesting a potentially earlier event in the progression of MCNs (i.e., mutation of the first allele occurring relatively early allowing sufficient time for mutation of the second allele in virtually all cases). *Smad4* is an essential gene in the mouse, although pancreas-specific deletion does not cause any overt developmental or functional abnormalities (*57, 58*). Consistent with the role of K-ras mutation as the rate-limiting event in pancreatic tumorigenesis, pancreatic pathology only becomes manifest in the setting of concomitant expression of K-ras^{G12D} resulting in the development of cystic neoplasms. Although Bardeesy et al. described the presence of IPMNs (*58*), Hingorani and colleagues found that MCNs developed (*57*). The precise reasons for this difference in observed pathology is unclear, but may have to do with differences in background strains (FVB in the

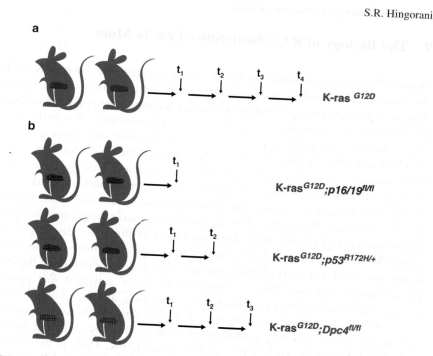

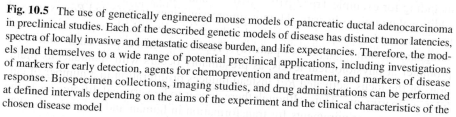

Fig. 10.5 The use of genetically engineered mouse models of pancreatic ductal adenocarcinoma in preclinical studies. Each of the described genetic models of disease has distinct tumor latencies, spectra of locally invasive and metastatic disease burden, and life expectancies. Therefore, the models lend themselves to a wide range of potential preclinical applications, including investigations of markers for early detection, agents for chemoprevention and treatment, and markers of disease response. Biospecimen collections, imaging studies, and drug administrations can be performed at defined intervals depending on the aims of the experiment and the clinical characteristics of the chosen disease model

In the end, the most relevant measure of animal models of human disease, and their greatest potential value, lies in their ability to impact the nature and delivery of clinical care. Specifically, will the mouse models described here prove to be more predictive of the human disease than previous preclinical models? The proof is in the testing. The development of distinct murine models of genetic subtypes of PDA (Fig. 10.5) with apparently unique phenotypes and latencies enables a wide range of investigations into disease detection, treatments, and markers of response. Moreover, if indeed these unique genetic and histopathologic routes to invasive ductal adenocarcinoma of the pancreas have direct equivalents in patients, then each type is also likely to require its own strategies for detection and therapy. As discussed, mice expressing targeted endogenous K-ras^{G12D} develop the full spectrum of PanINs which slowly progress to invasive and metastatic disease (51) (see Fig. 10.5). Thus, this model is ideally suited for studies of early detection of preinvasive disease and of potential chemopreventive agents, for example, which would be particularly appropriate for high-risk cohorts of patients with familial pancreatic cancer

(*90, 91*). Disease and target response would most likely be assessed by pathology at a defined study endpoint. Survival studies, on the other hand, could more readily be performed in models of rapidly advancing disease (*53, 54, 62*) (see Fig. 10.5). Moreover, the different propensities for locally advanced and widely metastatic disease in these models may distinguish the abilities of different agents to target local versus systemic disease burdens.

11   Conclusions and Future Directions

The last several years have seen considerable progress in the faithful modeling of diverse histologic and genetic pathways to invasive ductal cancers of the pancreas. An emerging theme from these models reveals the essential role of oncogenic K-ras in initiating preinvasive disease and the existence of discrete combinations of additional mutations in tumor suppressor genes that influence the differentiation pattern and clinical behavior as disease progresses. Thus, each of the major tumor suppressor pathways critically shapes the course of neoplastic evolution in the pancreas in response to the challenge of an oncogenic K-ras stimulus. Similar approaches can, and undoubtedly will, be used to explore the effects on disease initiation and progression of genetic perturbations of Notch pathway members, Wnt/β-catenin pathway components, matrix metalloproteinases, and so on in the context of K-ras-^{G12D}expression. Recently developed murine models of heritable forms of pancreatitis (*92, 93*) may also be used in conjunction to study the influence of inflammatory injury in promoting K-ras-initiated disease, perhaps illuminating mechanisms behind the increased risk of pancreas cancer in patients with chronic pancreatitis (*94, 95*). Inflammation may induce genetic damage directly, stimulate proliferation of tissue progenitor cells, and/or increase the receptivity of specific cellular compartments to the transforming effects of mutant *Ras*. Finally, combining inducible systems should enable more precise control of the timing of various genetic perturbations, revealing the impact of temporal sequence on shaping the resultant disease. With an expanding array of tools now at hand, the field is poised to make decisive inroads into this formidable disease, transforming fear into hope and bracing humility with confidence.

Acknowledgments Work in my laboratory is supported by CA114028, P30 CA15704, AACR-PanCAN Career Development Award, Canary Foundation, Mead Foundation and Rosenzweig Foundation.

References

1. Jemal A, Siegel R, Ward E, 2007, Cancer statistics, 2007. CA Cancer J Clin 57:43–66.
2. Hingorani SR, Tuveson D. A. 2003, In search of an early warning system for pancreatic cancer. Cancer Biol Ther 2:84–86.

3. Allison DC, Piantadosi S, Hruban RH, 1998, DNA content and other factors associated with ten-year survival after resection of pancreatic carcinoma. J Surg Oncol 67:151–159.

4. Farnell MB, Pearson RK, Sarr MG, 2005, A prospective randomized trial comparing standard pancreatoduodenectomy with pancreatoduodenectomy with extended lymphadenectomy in resectable pancreatic head adenocarcinoma. Surgery 138:618–628; discussion 628–630.

5. Oettle H, Post S, Neuhaus P, 2007, Adjuvant chemotherapy with gemcitabine vs observation in patients undergoing curative-intent resection of pancreatic cancer: a randomized controlled trial. JAMA 297:267–277.

6. Hruban RH, Adsay NV, Albores-Saavedra J, 2001, Pancreatic intraepithelial neoplasia: a new nomenclature and classification system for pancreatic duct lesions. Am J Surg Pathol 25:579–586.

7. Hruban RH, Takaori K, Klimstra DS, 2004, An illustrated consensus on the classification of pancreatic intraepithelial neoplasia and intraductal papillary mucinous neoplasms. Am J Surg Pathol 28:977–987.

8. Cubilla AL, Fitzgerald PJ. 1976, Morphological lesions associated with human primary invasive nonendocrine pancreas cancer. Cancer Res 36:2690–2698.

9. Klimstra DS, Longnecker DS. 1994, K-ras mutations in pancreatic ductal proliferative lesions. Am J Pathol 145:1547–1550.

10. Adsay NV. 2005, Pathological classification of cystic neoplasms of the pancreas. In: Hoff DD, Von Evans DB, Hruban RH (eds.) Pancreatic cancer. Sudbury, Jones and Bartlett, MA, 716–756.

11. Hruban RH. 2006Tumors of the pancreas. In: Hruban RH, Klimstra DS, Pitman MB (eds.) Atlas of tumor pathology, 4Armed Forces Institute of Pathology, Washington, DC, th series ed.

12. Tanaka M, Chari S, Adsay V, 2006, International consensus guidelines for management of intraductal papillary mucinous neoplasms and mucinous cystic neoplasms of the pancreas. Pancreatology 6:17–32.

13. Maitra A, Fukushima N, Takaori K, 2005, Precursors to invasive pancreatic cancer. Adv Anat Pathol 12:81–91.

14. Sugiyama M, Atomi Y. 2003, Recent topics in mucinous cystic tumor and intraductal papillary mucinous tumor of the pancreas. J Hepatobiliary Pancreat Surg 10:123–124.

15. Goh BK, Tan YM, Cheow PC, 2005, Cystic neoplasms of the pancreas with mucin-production. Eur J Surg Oncol 31:282–287.

16. Goh BK, Tan YM, Chung YF, 2006, A review of mucinous cystic neoplasms of the pancreas defined by ovarian-type stroma: clinicopathological features of 344 patients. World J Surg 30:2236–2245.

17. Hruban RH, Goggins M, Parsons J, 2000, Progression model for pancreatic cancer. Clin Cancer Res 6:2969–2972.

18. Iacobuzio-Donahue CA, Wilentz RE, Argani P, 2000, Dpc4 protein in mucinous cystic neoplasms of the pancreas: frequent loss of expression in invasive carcinomas suggests a role in genetic progression. Am J Surg Pathol 24:1544–1548.

19. Schonleben F, Qiu W, Ciau NT, 2006, PIK3CA mutations in intraductal papillary mucinous neoplasm/carcinoma of the pancreas. Clin Cancer Res 12:3851–3855.

20. Sato N, Rosty C, Jansen M, 2001, STK11/LKB1 Peutz-Jeghers gene inactivation in intraductal papillary-mucinous neoplasms of the pancreas. Am J Pathol 159:2017–2022.

21. Iacobuzio-Donahue CA, Klimstra DS, Adsay NV, 2000, Dpc-4 protein is expressed in virtually all human intraductal papillary mucinous neoplasms of the pancreas: comparison with conventional ductal adenocarcinomas. Am J Pathol 157:755–761.

22. Osvaldt AB, Wendt LR, Bersch VP, 2006, Pancreatic intraepithelial neoplasia and ductal adenocarcinoma induced by DMBA in mice. Surgery 140:803–809.

23. Kimura K, Satoh K, Kanno A, 2007, Activation of Notch signaling in tumorigenesis of experimental pancreatic cancer induced by dimethylbenzanthracene in mice. Cancer Sci 98:155–162.

24. Leach SD. 2004, Mouse models of pancreatic cancer: the fur is finally flying! Cancer Cell 5:7–11.

25. Grippo PJ, Sandgren EP. 2005, Modeling pancreatic cancer in animals to address specific hypotheses. Methods Mol Med 103:217–243.
26. Hingorani SR. 2005, Modeling pancreatic ductal adenocarcinoma in the mouse. In: Gress TM, Neoptolemos JP, Lemoine (eds.) NR, Exocrine pancreas cancer. Felsenstein CCCP Publishing, Hannover, 152–171.
27. Lowy AM. 2003, Transgenic models of pancreatic cancer. Int J Gastrointest Cancer 33:71–78.
28. Sandgren EP, Quaife CJ, Paulovich AG, 1991, Pancreatic tumor pathogenesis reflects the causative genetic lesion. Proc Natl Acad Sci U S A, 88:93–97.
29. Hanahan D. 1985, Heritable formation of pancreatic beta-cell tumours in transgenic mice expressing recombinant insulin/simian virus 40 oncogenes. Nature 315:115–122.
30. Ornitz DM, Hammer RE, Messing A, 1987, Pancreatic neoplasia induced by SV40 T-antigen expression in acinar cells of transgenic mice. Science 238:188–193.
31. Quaife CJ, Pinkert CA, Ornitz DM, 1987, Pancreatic neoplasia induced by ras expression in acinar cells of transgenic mice. Cell 48:1023–1034.
32. Hanahan D, Folkman J. 1996, Patterns and emerging mechanisms of the angiogenic switch during tumorigenesis. Cell 86:353–364.
33. Sandgren EP, Luetteke NC, Palmiter RD, 1990, Overexpression of TGF alpha in transgenic mice: induction of epithelial hyperplasia, pancreatic metaplasia, and carcinoma of the breast. Cell 61:1121–1135.
34. Wagner M, Luhrs H, Kloppel G, 1998, Malignant transformation of duct-like cells originating from acini in transforming growth factor transgenic mice. Gastroenterology 115:1254–1262.
35. Wagner M, Greten FR, Weber CK, 2001, A murine tumor progression model for pancreatic cancer recapitulating the genetic alterations of the human disease. Genes Dev 15:286–293.
36. Grippo PJ, Nowlin PS, Demeure MJ, 2003, Preinvasive pancreatic neoplasia of ductal phenotype induced by acinar cell targeting of mutant Kras in transgenic mice. Cancer Res 63:2016–2019.
37. Brembeck FH, Schreiber FS, Deramaudt TB, 2003, The mutant K-ras oncogene causes pancreatic periductal lymphocytic infiltration and gastric mucous neck cell hyperplasia in transgenic mice. Cancer Res 63:2005–2009.
38. Jonkers J, Berns A. 2002, Conditional mouse models of sporadic cancer. Nat Rev Cancer 2:251–265.
39. Dyke T, Van Jacks T. 2002, Cancer modeling in the modern era: progress and challenges. Cell 108:135–144.
40. Rangarajan A, Weinberg RA. 2003, Opinion: comparative biology of mouse versus human cells: modelling human cancer in mice. Nat Rev Cancer 3:952–959.
41. Donehower LA, Harvey M, Slagle BL, 1992, Mice deficient for p53 are developmentally normal but susceptible to spontaneous tumours. Nature 356:215–221.
42. Jacks T, Remington L, Williams BO, 1994, Tumor spectrum analysis in p53-mutant mice. Curr Biol 4:1–7.
43. Serrano M, Lee H, Chin L, 1996, Role of the INK4a locus in tumor suppression and cell mortality. Cell 85:27–37.
44. Sirard C, Pompa JL, de la Elia A, 1998, The tumor suppressor gene Smad4/Dpc4 is required for gastrulation and later for anterior development of the mouse embryo. Genes Dev 12:107–119.
45. Takaku K, Oshima M, Miyoshi H, 1998, Intestinal tumorigenesis in compound mutant mice of both Dpc4 (Smad4) and Apc genes. Cell 92:645–656.
46. Takaku K, Miyoshi H, Matsunaga A, 1999, Gastric and duodenal polyps in Smad4 (Dpc4) knockout mice. Cancer Res 59:6113–6117.
47. Xu X, Brodie SG, Yang X, 2000, Haploid loss of the tumor suppressor Smad4/Dpc4 initiates gastric polyposis and cancer in mice. Oncogene 19:1868–1874.
48. Tuveson DA, Shaw AT, Willis NA, 2004, Endogenous oncogenic K-ras(G12D) stimulates proliferation and widespread neoplastic and developmental defects. Cancer Cell 5:375–387.
49. Sauer B. 1998, Inducible gene targeting in mice using the Cre/lox system. Methods 14:381–392.

50. Branda CS, Dymecki SM. 2004, Talking about a revolution: The impact of site-specific recombinases on genetic analyses in mice. Dev Cell 6:7–28.
51. Hingorani SR, Petricoin EF, Maitra A, 2003, Preinvasive and invasive ductal pancreatic cancer and its early detection in the mouse. Cancer Cell 4:437–450.
52. Hansel DE, Kern SE, Hruban RH. 2003, Molecular pathogenesis of pancreatic cancer. Annu Rev Genomics Hum Genet 4:237–256.
53. Hingorani SR, Wang L, Multani AS, 2005, Trp53R172H and KrasG12D cooperate to promote chromosomal instability and widely metastatic pancreatic ductal adenocarcinoma in mice. Cancer Cell 7:469–483.
54. Aguirre AJ, Bardeesy N, Sinha M, 2003, Activated Kras and Ink4a/Arf deficiency cooperate to produce metastatic pancreatic ductal adenocarcinoma. Genes Dev 17:3112–3126.
55. Hruban RH, Adsay NV, Albores-Saavedra J, 2006, A. Pathology of genetically engineered mouse models of pancreatic exocrine cancer. consensus report and recommendations. Cancer Res 66:95–106.
56. Bardeesy N, Aguirre AJ, Chu GC, 2006, Both p16(Ink4a) and the p19(Arf)-p53 pathway constrain progression of pancreatic adenocarcinoma in the mouse. Proc Natl Acad Sci U S A 103:5947–5952.
57. Izeradjene K, Combs C, Best M, 2007, Kras(G12D) and Smad4/Dpc4 haploinsufficiency cooperate to induce mucinous cystic neoplasms and invasive adenocarcinoma of the pancreas. Cancer Cell 11:229–243.
58. Bardeesy N, Cheng KH, Berger JH, 2006, Smad4 is dispensable for normal pancreas development yet critical in progression and tumor biology of pancreas cancer. Genes Dev 20:3130–3146.
59. Gorelik L, Flavell RA. 2002, Transforming growth factor-beta in T-cell biology. Nat Rev Immunol 2:46–53.
60. Siegel PM, Massague J. 2003, Cytostatic and apoptotic actions of TGF-beta in homeostasis and cancer. Nat Rev Cancer 3:807–821.
61. Bhowmick NA, Neilson EG, Moses HL. 2004, Stromal fibroblasts in cancer initiation and progression. Nature 432:332–337.
62. Ijichi H, Chytil A, Gorska AE, 2006, Aggressive pancreatic ductal adenocarcinoma in mice caused by pancreas-specific blockade of transforming growth factor-beta signaling in cooperation with active Kras expression. Genes Dev 20:3147–3160.
63. Kelly OG, Melton DA. 2000, Development of the pancreas in Xenopus laevis. Dev Dyn 218:615–627.
64. Kim SK, Hebrok M, Melton DA. 1997, Pancreas development in the chick embryo. Cold Spring Harb Symp Quant Biol 62:377–383.
65. Slack JM. 1995, Developmental biology of the pancreas. Development 121:1569–1580.
66. Niihori T, Aoki Y, Narumi Y, 2006, Germline KRAS and BRAF mutations in cardio-facio-cutaneous syndrome. Nat Genet 38:294–296.
67. Schubbert S, Zenker M, Rowe SL, 2006, Germline KRAS mutations cause Noonan syndrome. Nat Genet 38:331–336.
68. Apelqvist A, Li H, Sommer L, 1999, Notch signalling controls pancreatic cell differentiation. Nature 400:877–881.
69. Jensen J, Pedersen EE, Galante P, 2000, Control of endodermal endocrine development by Hes-1. Nat Genet 24:36–44.
70. Miyamoto Y, Maitra A, Ghosh B, 2003, Notch mediates TGF alpha-induced changes in epithelial differentiation during pancreatic tumorigenesis. Cancer Cell 3:565–576.
71. Hebrok M. 2003, Hedgehog signaling in pancreas development. Mech Dev 120:45–57.
72. Berman DM, Karhadkar SS, Maitra A, 2003, Widespread requirement for Hedgehog ligand stimulation in growth of digestive tract tumours. Nature 425:846–851.
73. Thayer SP, di Magliano MP, Heiser PW, 2003, Hedgehog is an early and late mediator of pancreatic cancer tumorigenesis. Nature 425:851–856.
74. Apelqvist A, Ahlgren U, Edlund H. 1997, Sonic hedgehog directs specialised mesoderm differentiation in the intestine and pancreas. Curr Biol 7:801–804.

75. Pasca di Magliano M, Sekine S, Ermilov A, 2006, Hedgehog/Ras interactions regulate early stages of pancreatic cancer. Genes Dev 20:3161–3173.
76. Land H, Parada LF, Weinberg RA. 1983, Tumorigenic conversion of primary embryo fibroblasts requires at least two cooperating oncogenes. Nature 304:596–602.
77. Ruley HE. 1983, Adenovirus early region 1A enables viral and cellular transforming genes to transform primary cells in culture. Nature 304:602–606.
78. Serrano M, Lin AW, McCurrach ME, 1997, Oncogenic ras provokes premature cell senescence associated with accumulation of p53 and p16INK4a. Cell 88:593–602.
79. Malumbres M, Barbacid M. 2003, RAS oncogenes: the first 30 years. Nat Rev Cancer 3:459–465.
80. Almoguera C, Shibata D, Forrester K, 1988, Most human carcinomas of the exocrine pancreas contain mutant c-K-ras genes. Cell 53:549–554.
81. Guerra C, Mijimolle N, Dhawahir A, 2003, Tumor induction by an endogenous K-ras oncogene is highly dependent on cellular context. Cancer Cell 4:111–120.
82. Hamad NM, Elconin JH, Karnoub AE, 2002, Distinct requirements for Ras oncogenesis in human versus mouse cells. Genes Dev 16:2045–2057.
83. Rangarajan A, Hong SJ, Gifford A, 2004, Species- and cell type-specific requirements for cellular transformation. Cancer Cell 6:171–183.
84. Hingorani SR, Tuveson DA. 2003, Ras redux: rethinking how and where Ras acts. Curr Opin Genet Dev 13:6–13.
85. Burris HA 3rdMoore MJ, Andersen J, 1997, Improvements in survival and clinical benefit with gemcitabine as first-line therapy for patients with advanced pancreas cancer: a randomized trial. J Clin Oncol 15:2403–2413.
86 Ko AH, Tempero MA. 2005, Treatment of metastatic pancreatic cancer. J Natl Compr Canc Netw 3:627–636.
87. Cardenes HR, Chiorean EG, Dewitt J, 2006, Locally advanced pancreatic cancer: current therapeutic approach. Oncologist 11:612–623.
88. Xiong HQ, Carr K, Abbruzzese JL. 2006, Cytotoxic chemotherapy for pancreatic cancer: Advances to date and future directions. Drugs 66:1059–1072.
89. Tang PA, Tsao MS, Moore MJ. 2006, A review of erlotinib and its clinical use. Expert Opin Pharmacother 7:177–193.
90. Canto MI, Goggins M, Hruban RH, 2006, Screening for early pancreatic neoplasia in high-risk individuals: a prospective controlled study. Clin Gastroenterol Hepatol 4:766–781; quiz 665.
91. Rulyak SJ, Brentnall TA. 2001, Inherited pancreatic cancer: surveillance and treatment strategies for affected families. Pancreatology 1:477–485.
92. Archer H, Jura N, Keller J, 2006, A mouse model of hereditary pancreatitis generated by transgenic expression of R122H trypsinogen. Gastroenterology 131:1844–1855.
93. Cano DA, Sekine S, Hebrok M. 2006, Primary cilia deletion in pancreatic epithelial cells results in cyst formation and pancreatitis. Gastroenterology 131:1856–1869
94. Lowenfels AB, Maisonneuve P, Cavallini G, 1993, Pancreatitis and the risk of pancreatic cancer. International Pancreatitis Study Group. N Engl J Med 328:1433–1437.
95. Lowenfels AB, Maisonneuve P, DiMagno EP, 1997, Hereditary pancreatitis and the risk of pancreatic cancer. International Hereditary Pancreatitis Study Group. J Natl Cancer Inst 89:442–446.

Chapter 11
Molecular Signaling Pathways in Pancreatic Cancer

Genevieve M. Boland and Sarah P. Thayer

1 Pancreatic Cancer: Background and Clinical Significance

The pancreas is an extremely intriguing organ that has been the topic of discussion and study since its first description by the Greek anatomist and surgeon Herophilus around 300 BC. It is a retroperitoneal gland involved in various processes of human physiology, including blood glucose homeostasis, and secretion of digestive enzymes. In the context of the field of oncology, cancers of the pancreas can be divided into those of exocrine and those of endocrine lineages. The most common tumor of the pancreas is pancreatic adenocarcinoma, responsible for an estimated 37,680 newly diagnosed cases in 2008 with an associated 34,290 deaths from the disease in the same year (www.cancer.org). These numbers are a staggering example of the poor prognosis associated with this disease.

1.1 Definition of Pancreatic Adenocarcinoma

There are many signaling pathways implicated in the development and evolution of pancreatic adenocarcinoma. The role of these signature signaling pathways in driving specific biological behaviors during pancreatic cancer initiation, progression, and migration remains to be defined and thoroughly clarified. Pancreatic cancer is known for its characteristic histologic, genetic, and biologic phenotypes (1–7). Histologically, pancreatic adenocarcinomas are composed of neoplastic cells that demonstrate glandular or ductal differentiation, which has been known to take on many gastrointestinal characteristics (8–11). Pancreatic cancer is defined not only by its abnormal epithelium but also by its extensive non-neoplastic desmoplastic response. This extensive tumor stroma is composed of myofibroblasts, lymphocytes, extracellular matrix (ECM) proteins such as collagen, as well as trapped non-neoplastic pancreatic tissues such as islets. Pancreatic ductal adenocarcinomas (PDACs), unlike pancreatic intraepithelial neoplasias (PanINs), demonstrate an infiltrative growth pattern. The biology of pancreatic cancer is distinguished by its early dissemination even with small primary tumor loads. It also is known for its

A.M. Lowy et al. (eds.) *Pancreatic Cancer.*
doi: 10.1007/978-0-387-69252-4, © Springer Science+Business Media, LLC 2008

propensity for early perineural and peritoneal metastases (*3, 12–14*). Another well-known biologic behavior is the ability of these cancers to be highly resistant to chemotherapy and radiation (*15–17*). Genetically this tumor is noted to be markedly aneuploid, with extensive ongoing chromosomal instability. The molecular mechanisms that control these behaviors are just beginning to be identified and understood, with the eventual goal of regulating these various cellular behaviors through signaling mediators and/or inhibitors.

1.2   History of Pancreatic Signaling Research

Due to the devastating natural course of pancreatic adenocarcinoma, much energy has been focused on the identification, classification, and biology of this cancer (*1–7*). A series of precursor lesions have been identified that correlate with various stages of cancer development. Pancreatic cancer is believed to arise from histologically well-defined precursor lesions termed pancreatic intraepithelial neoplasias (PanINs). In this progression model, the normal cuboidal ductal epithelium is replaced by progressive histologic lesions: PanIN-1A, PanIN-1B, PanIN2, and PanIN3 (carcinoma in situ) (*18*). The key features noted in the sequential progression of PanIN lesions are enhanced mucin production, graded nuclear atypia, and loss of cellular polarity, with increasing abnormality of ductal structures. Additionally, the rate of cellular proliferation increases with advancing stages of PanINs as well as with increased aggressiveness of tumor behavior (*18–22*). These progressive histologic changes have been correlated with progressive genetic mutations and signaling alterations.

During the earliest stages of PanIN formation (i.e., PanIN-1A and PanIN-1B), inciting oncogenic events are thought to be mediated by activating mutations of K-ras (*23–25*), as well as telomere attrition (*7, 26*) and loss of p21 (*7, 21*). Increased EGF signaling, such as in the context of overexpression of Her-2/neu, has also been correlated with these early neoplastic changes (*27*). By the PanIN-2 stage, an intermediate stage in lesion progression, there is additionally the loss of p16 (*22, 28–30*) and loss of PTEN (*31, 32*). In the setting of PanIN-3 (or carcinoma in situ), epithelial cells now demonstrate increased expression of receptor for various signaling pathways. There is an up-regulation of the EGF receptor as well as c-Met (the HGF receptor), concurrent with changes in TGF-β receptor expression level (*27, 33–42*). The loss of Smad4 (DPC4), an intracellular mediator of TGF-β signaling, also compounds the down-regulation of TGF-β receptors and enhances the TGF-β resistance of these oncogenic cell populations (*39, 43–46*). Cell cycle regulators such as p53 and BRCA2 are often mutated or inactivated in more advanced stages of tumorigenesis (Fig. 11.1) (*47–50*). All these molecular events have been catalogued and recognized as integral in establishing the evolution and progression of pancreatic adenocarcinomas. The identification of common mutation patterns suggests that these factors may play key roles in the formation of this tumor as well as may represent common mechanisms of lesion development (*2, 51, 52*).

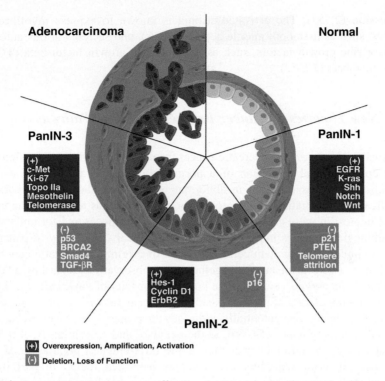

Fig. 11.1 Pancreatic adenocarcinoma: cell-cell and cell-matrix signaling. During the progression of normal ductal epithelium through the stages of PanIN progression and finally to the stage of invasive adenocarcinoma, there are many mutations and alterations in signaling cascades that affect not only the ductal epithelial component, but also the stromal component of the pancreas. This results in the robust desmoplastic reaction characteristic of pancreatic adenocarcinomas. These changes correlate with specific changes in signaling molecules and functional behavior of the epithelial cells themselves. These alterations in local cytoarchitecture contribute to the progressive development of tumors, as previously described. Listed here are known changes associated with these various premalignant and malignant stages in pancreatic cancer formation

1.3 Desmoplasia and the Dynamic Cross-Talk Between the Stroma and the Epithelium

It is well documented that many carcinomas induce a modified stroma during tumor progression. Pancreatic adenocarcinoma is particularly notable for the activation of the stromal compartment into a very robust desmoplastic reaction (8–10). These stromal changes have been ascribed to the induced expression of various growth factors that promote angiogenesis, altered ECM protein expression, increased fibroblast proliferation, and inflammatory cell recruitment. Subsequent studies of this process of tumor–stromal interaction have implicated the stroma as more than a mere reactive process or facilitator of tumorigenesis (52) and many current theories support the stroma as an active inducer of tumor formation and progression (*2*, *53*). The activated stroma is known to express myofibroblast markers, such as α-smooth muscle actin (α-SMA), and secrete various autocrine and paracrine growth factors, such as transforming growth factor-beta (TGF-β) family members (*10*, *52*).

1.4   New Theories of Cancer Progression: New Pathways

Historically, the theory of pancreatic cancer formation through PanIN lesions was based upon a clonal expansion of a normal somatic cell that had undergone sequential mutations resulting in abnormal behavior. In the last 20 years, the identification of somatic stem or progenitor cell niches has resulted in an explosion of interest in these cells, both for regenerative purposes and for understanding pathologic processes in the human, such as cancer. The theory of pancreatic cancer stem cells and/or stem cells as the cell or origin of pancreatic cancer has gained much enthusiasm and ties together many observations regarding a "dedifferentiated" phenotype, as well as the potential capacity of these cells for infinite renewal of a population of phenotypically heterogeneous cells over a long period of time. This theory also potentially addresses the property of cancer precursor or stem cell chemoresistance (*54–56*), as the behavior and susceptibility of this cell population may be different than that of the differentiated population of local cells. This ideology regarding the pancreas has been fueled in part by the observed re-expression or mis-expression of various developmental genes during tumorigenesis, which have been known to play a role in maintaining stem cell niches in adults and/or a progenitor cell population in utero. Some of the pathways now implicated in pancreatic cancer include the Notch, Wnt, and Hedgehog pathways, to name just a few (*51*, *57–71*). Their exact roles in pancreatic morphogenesis, morphostasis, and carcinogenesis remain an area of active investigation and an exciting area of research.

1.4.1   Morphogens and the 3D Theory of Cancer

A multitude of different theories of cancer formation have been posited, many of which have focused on the cells of origin of a particular tumor and the various mutations, alterations, and histologic changes these cells undergo. More recently, the emphasis in the field of cancer research has shifted to a focus on the broader milieu in which tumor formation occurs. Much of this literature has been borrowed from developmental biology, and more recently from the stem cell field, in which the stem cell niche and the morphogenic gradients involved in embryologic development have found new popularity. These models integrate the local cellular environment and intracellular pathways active within a given cell into the larger context of the local environment, tissue architecture, and tissue geography as they influence cellular behavior.

   Morphogens are secreted proteins, described initially in the developing embryo, that are capable of eliciting qualitatively different responses from a target cell depending upon concentration. In this case, the distance and location of the target cell in relationship to the source of the morphogen dictates cellular behavior and subsequent tissue patterning. Interestingly, not only do these morphogens therefore activate or suppress various signaling pathways; their distribution actually precedes and dictates the final tissue pattern. Morphogenesis is the process by which patterned embryonic tissue acquires its final form as a result of directional purposeful movement and targeted differentiation. In contrast, morphostasis is a term coined to describe a process similar to morphogenesis, but one that maintains a previously established tissue template. These concepts have been very nicely reviewed and summarized in an article by Potter (72). This process of morphostasis is applicable to the situation in terminally differentiated adult tissues, where the goal is not to create form but to maintain the established microarchitecture (73, 74). In this way, morphostasis is not controlled by a genetic program active within each cell, but rather is a dynamic process involving a cell's interaction with its environment and the active signaling that occurs between different cell types and tissue compartments. The specific physical conditions important in the maintenance of microarchitecture are the rigidity of the stroma, cytoskeletal tension, interaction of adherens junctions, and maintenance of tissue polarity. Any disruption in these processes can result in a disorder in the local tissue architecture, altering the delicate balance of signals and potentially allowing disordered growth or loss of architecture and therefore, loss of tight cellular control. Of interest, the description of dysregulated morphostasis is quite similar to the well-documented phenomenon of epithelial–mesenchymal transitions (EMT), described at length both in development and in tumor metastasis and invasion (75–77). EMT is a coordinated process occurring in polarized epithelial cells organized in layers in which they become fibroblastoid cells capable of locomotion. During cancer formation and progression, EMT has been associated with tumor invasiveness and metastasis, and has been discussed as a late-stage change in more aggressive or more advanced cancers. Temporally, this process involves the disassembly of cell junctions, cytoskeletal reorganization, loss of epithelial polarity, and remodeling of the cell-matrix adhesions. Implicated in this process of altered morphostasis or EMT are various growth factors and their receptors known to play important roles in cancer, and more specifically, pancreatic cancer development and progression, such as TGF-β, EGF, PDGF, Wnts, MAPK, and various other signaling molecules important in cross-talk between the epithelium and the stroma (75–83). Therefore, the well-known process of EMT may in fact be an alternative description of the process of disrupted morphostasis, with merely a different name ascribed to this process. Regardless of this, it has been overtly clear for a long period of time that one of the most prominent features of cancer is the disruption of normal tissue architecture. Therefore, one of the key initial steps in understanding the development of pancreatic adenocarcinoma is clarifying the native tissue microarchitecture and changes that accompany tumorigenesis (Fig. 11.2).

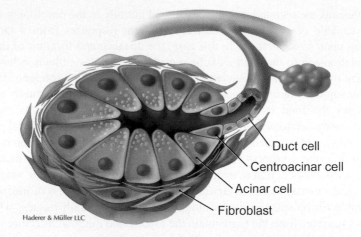

Haderer & Müller LLC

Fig. 11.2 Pancreatic microarchitecture. The pancreas is a glandular organ composed of both endocrine and exocrine components. Of interest to the study of pancreatic adenocarcinoma is the microarchitecture of the distal tubular system. The pancreatic ducts and ductules are lined by epithelial ductal cells. The terminal exocrine structures, the acini, are lined by acinar cells, which are cuboidal cells surrounded by fibroblastic-like cells called pancreatic stellate cells. At the junction of the ductal system and the acini are centroacinar cells, which have been implicated in various processes during tissue injury, regeneration, and oncogenesis

1.5   Implicated Signaling Pathways in Pancreatic Adenocarcinoma

1.5.1   K-ras

The transforming gene from Kirsten rat sarcoma virus (K-ras) (Fig. 11.3) was identified more than 20 years ago. Activating mutations of K-ras constitute one of the most frequently activated oncogenes, with 25% of all human tumors harboring these mutations. In the pancreas, activating mutations in K-ras are regarded as the molecular signature of pancreatic cancer, since nearly 100% of tumors have this feature (*84*), making K-ras one of the most thoroughly studied topics in the field of pancreatic adenocarcinoma research. K-ras is a 21-kDa intracellular, membrane-bound protein, which is a member of the small GTPase superfamily of proteins. K-ras undergoes a multistage post-translational modification with farnesyl, methyl, and palmityl groups in order for it to be membrane-associated, which is vital for its function (*85*). K-ras is known to mediate a multitude of cellular activities, including cellular proliferation, survival, and migration (*86*). Many growth factor receptors utilize K-ras to transduce their downstream signals, and it is a converging point of many disparate signaling pathways. Ras proteins are used to transmit signals from the extracellular to the intracellular environment.

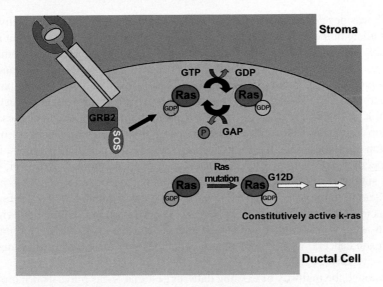

Fig. 11.3 Activation of K-ras protein. K-ras is activated by the binding of various growth factors to membrane-bound receptors and the recruitment of GRB2 and SOS concurrent with the transition of Ras-GDP to the Ras-GTP activated protein form. Under normal conditions, RAS GTPases (GAP proteins) promote GTP hydrolysis and reversal of the Ras activation step. During oncogenic transformation of Ras, the protein is mutated such that it is rendered constitutively activated, incapable of deactivation by the activity of the GAP proteins

Receptor activation of K-ras occurs via the recruitment of the adaptor protein (GRB2), which subsequently recruits guanine exchange factors (SOS1 and CDC25) to the cell membrane. This enables the membrane to interact with K-ras, resulting in the exchange of GDP to GTP, which forms the activated form of K-ras (K-ras-GTP). Normally this pathway is negatively regulated by GAPs (GTPase activating proteins) that convert GTP to RAS-GDP (see Fig. 11.3). Mutations in several K-ras codons (e.g., 12, 13, and 61) have been identified that render K-ras constitutively active and resistant to GAP inactivation. Other mutations have been identified but their biologic significance remains unknown (*23, 87, 88*). However, the most common mutation is a single amino acid substitution in codon 12, which has also been implicated in various malignancies, including pancreatic and lung adenocarcinoma, mucinous adenoma, and colorectal carcinoma (*2, 89*).

In humans K-ras mutations are early events in pancreatic adenocarcinoma formation, identified in PanIN-1A lesions (*90*). However, the mutations in K-ras are identified with increasing frequency with disease progression and are present in nearly 100% of pancreatic adenocarcinomas (*25*). The current theory states that K-ras functions principally as an *initiator* of pancreatic cancer. Mutation in K-ras in multiple mouse models has demonstrated that these mutations are sufficient to cause the formation of lesions that resemble human PanINs. The mouse strain K-ras^{G12D} was developed to study the role of K-ras using a conditionally activatable K-ras allele in these mice. The alleles are silent in the majority of cells but can be heritably activated by Cre-loxP recombination. The promoter most commonly driving expression Cre expression is Pdx1, which is expressed early in pancreatic development in pancreatic precursor cells. Therefore, all cells within the pancreas will harbor this K-ras mutation. The findings from these studies suggest that activation of K-ras plays a role in pancreatic adenocarcinoma initiation, since these mice develop lesions that closely resemble human PanINs. Of interest, K-ras overexpression does not induce the formation of various other pancreatic tumors, implying specificity of this mutation for pancreatic adenocarcinomas. However, only a small subset of mice went on to develop invasive adenocarcinoma. This implies that K-ras is an initiator, but also that it may need other mutations in order for these lesions to progress to pancreatic cancer. K-ras activation in combination with loss of p16 resulted in a higher percentage and shorter latency to the development of pancreatic cancers, with lesions that also demonstrate increased invasiveness and aggressiveness (24, 91).

Although the majority of existing data suggest that K-ras plays its principal role as an initiator, mutations in K-ras may also play an important role in maintenance of the tumor phenotype and for tumor progression (92). Inhibition of K-ras signaling in various tumor cell lines abrogates malignant transformation, suggesting an ongoing need for K-ras signals during cancer progression. One study using immortalized human pancreatic ductal-derived cells was able to demonstrate that activation of K-ras resulted in a loss of density-dependent growth, increasing anchorage independence, and the ability to invade through basement membrane proteins. These studies also showed that these effects were abrogated in the context of MAPK and PI3K inhibition (93). Thus present evidence supports K-ras as a cornerstone of initiating events in pancreatic cancer; however, its in vivo importance as a maintenance factor remains to be determined.

Despite the depth of research into the role of K-ras in cancer formation, the precise mechanism by which oncogenic K-ras contributes to initiation and maintenance of the tumors remains to be determined. K-ras not only has numerous growth factor activators, but it also affects multiple signaling pathways. Oncogenic K-ras propagates its signal through at least three primary Ras binding effectors: (1) the phosphoinositide-3-kinase (PI3K) pathway, which is thought to promote cell survival; (2) the RAF-MAPK pathways, which comprise a family of Raf serine/threonine kinases that activate mitogen-activated protein kinases (MAPKs) and play a key role in cellular proliferation; and (3) the Ral guanine nucleotide exchange factor pathway (RalGEFs), which activates the RalA and RalB Ras-related small GTPases including the Ras-binding family member Ral guanine nucleotide dissociation stimulator (RalGDS) (93–95). The impact of these pathways on K-ras signaling has been studied using various chemical inhibitors of these downstream cascades, particularly MAPK and PI3K pathway inhibitors. Since mutations in K-ras have been identified in various cancers, there has been much interest in RAS inhibitors with an ongoing debate as to the importance of each downstream signaling pathway in specifically mediating K-ras signaling.

1.6   Ras Effectors

1.6.1   RAF-MAP Kinase

One of the most thoroughly characterized Ras effector pathways is that mediated by the mitogen-activated protein kinases (MAPK), also referred to as the extracellular signal-regulated protein kinases (ERKs). These are a group of intracellular protein serine threonine kinases that are known to play important roles in the downstream mediation of various signaling pathways. The MAP kinase pathway consists of three protein kinases. RAF, aka MAPKK kinase or MEKK, phosphorylates and activates a MAPK-kinase (or MEK), which in turn phosphorylates and activates MAPK/ERK. ERK will then activate downstream transcriptional factors to induce transcription of key genes for proliferation (Fig. 11.4) (*96*). Since these enzymes are integral in such a wide variety of processes with many diffuse effects, it is straightforward to observe an effect in vitro via modulation of the MAPK signaling pathway. However, as this family of signaling molecules is a convergence point for many different signaling cascades, it has also been notoriously difficult to utilize that information for therapeutic interventions. In the setting of

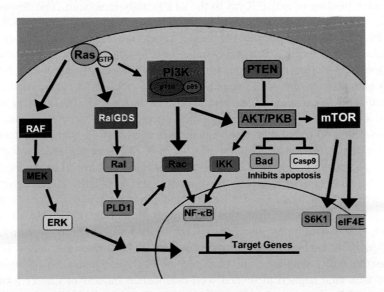

Fig. 11.4 Ras signaling cascades. Signaling via Ras results in the activation of various downstream pathways RAF/MAPK, RalGDS, and PI3K. The downstream RAF/MAPK pathway activates MEK, which then acts to activate either JNK or ERK, resulting in the final output of target gene transcription, particularly affecting cellular proliferation. Alternatively, Ras signaling can be mediated by the RalGDS pathway, with eventually intersecting with the cellular polarity signaling pathways, including Rac. Finally, Ras signaling is often mediated by the PI3K pathway, with resultant activation of the AKT/PKB pathway; this inhibits apoptosis or the Rac and/or IKK pathway, which promotes expression of anti-apoptotic proteins such as NF-κB

pancreatic adenocarcinoma, the RAF-MAP kinase pathway is believed to be critical for the progression and maintenance of tumorigenicity. In vitro studies utilizing dominant negative MEKK demonstrate an inhibition of pancreatic cancer cells' growth with abrogation of MEKK signals (*97*). Inhibition of RAF/MAPK not only results in an inhibition of K-ras–mediated growth, but also facilitates tissue invasion (*93*). In vivo, pharmacologic inhibition of *kinase suppressor of ras-1*, a transducer of the Ras-Raf signaling pathway, is able to inhibit K-ras-mediated pancreatic cancer formation in murine xenografts (*98, 99*).

1.6.2   PI3 Kinase-AKT-PTEN

Phosphatidylinositol-3-kinases (PI3K) constitute a large and complex family of lipid kinases. They are implicated in several different cellular functions, including proliferation, differentiation, chemotaxis, survival, cellular trafficking, and glucose homeostasis (*100*). There are three classes of these proteins with multiple subunits and isoforms. Class IA PI3Ks are heterodimeric proteins composed of a p110 catalytic subunit and a p85 regulatory subunit. These proteins are activated through interaction with the phosphotyrosine residues of various receptor tyrosine kinases or through binding of active K-ras to the p110 catalytic subunit. The downstream signals are mediated through the action of the survival signaling kinase AKT/PKB. AKT/PKB plays a significant role in the regulation of apoptosis through pro-apoptotic proteins such as Bad and caspase 9 (*101*). There are three known sites of mutations that elevate the lipid kinase activity of PIK3CA (a catalytic subunit of PI3K) and activate the AKT signaling pathway (*102*), and many studies have reported high frequencies of somatic mutations in the PIK3CA gene in various human solid tumors (*103*). Studies looking specifically at pancreatic cancer cell lines have demonstrated that PI3K signaling is necessary for growth and survival of tumor cells (*104*), and as a major effector of K-ras signaling, PI3K is well situated to play a role in pancreatic adenocarcinoma. Mice have been engineered in which the endogenous PI3K gene has a mutant p110α subunit, which is enzymatically active but incapable of binding to and interacting with K-ras. Therefore, activation of K-ras signals cannot be transmitted through the PI3K network. In this context, mouse embryonic fibroblasts were treated with various growth factors, including EGF and FGF2, demonstrating an inability of these cells to now respond to growth factor signaling with blockade of PI3K activation. In addition, this system was then applied to several well-established models of cancer formation demonstrating an overt inhibition of oncogenesis with blockade of downstream PI3K signals. These findings suggest that the interaction of K-ras with the PI3K subunit p110α is required for the development and progression of malignancies, likely mediated by various extracellular signaling proteins (*105, 106*). An alternative target of the PI3K pathway is Rac, a G protein that can be activated by phosphatidyl 3,4,5-triphosphate (PIP3) (*107*). Rac is important in regulating anti-apoptotic gene expression through NF-κB, and cytoskeletal rearrangements

(*108*). Ras-controlled membrane remodeling through Rac is dependent on PI3K activity (*109*). Thus, as we begin to know more about affectors and effectors on the PI3K pathway in pancreatic cancer, it appears that PI3K is an important mediator of Ras-induced cell transformation. As the models in which many of these studies are done are murine, the caveat is the unknown relevance these systems may have to the actual situation of humans in vivo (*106*).

1.6.3   AKT/Protein Kinase B (PKB) and PTEN

AKT, also known as protein kinase B (PKB), is a serine-threonine protein kinase known to be a key downstream mediator of the aforementioned PI3K pathway (*110*), and inhibition of AKT via chemical suppression or transgene expression has a clear impact on tumorigenesis, with resultant alterations in cell growth and survival (*110, 111*). AKT is capable of suppression of apoptosis in a transcription-independent manner through direct phosphorylation and inactivation of the apoptotic machinery (*112*). The AKT gene exists in multiple alternatively spliced variants. Of interest to pancreatic cancer research is the fact that this gene is amplified and/or constitutively activated in up to 60% of pancreatic cancers (*111, 113*). Recently the interaction of the AKT inhibitor PTEN has also been examined in the context of pancreatic adenocarcinoma (*51*).

PTEN is an interesting protein, identified as a tumor suppressor and found mutated in multiple different cancers at high frequency (*110*). Functionally, it is a protein tyrosine phosphatase, but unlike most of these phosphatases, this protein preferentially *de*phosphorylates phosphoinositide substrates. It is therefore a negative regulator of various proteins and functions as a tumor suppressor by inhibiting the AKT/PKB signaling pathway (*114*). It has been observed that PTEN point mutations are rare in pancreatic cancer; however, functional inactivation occurs with high frequency. This inactivation occurs through multiple different mechanisms including promoter methylation, inhibition of protein synthesis, and/or mRNA expression (*115, 116*). In order to elucidate the potential role of PTEN in pancreatic cancers, a mouse model with pancreas-specific deletion of the PTEN gene has been created. In these mice with PTEN deletions (and therefore implied activation of AKT signaling) there are progressive pancreatic abnormalities throughout development and maturation, with the development of diffuse ductal mucinous metaplasia as well as the evolution of PanIN lesions with occasional malignant transformation. As PTEN is an inhibitor of PI3K signaling through AKT/PKB, the studies suggest that there may be an association between PI3K signaling and pancreatic cancer (*51*). That said, PTEN has other functions that are independent of its activity as a PI3K antagonist (e.g., p53 modulation) (*117*), and it is unclear to what extent, if any, these factors influence the formation of pancreatic lesions.

Other downstream effectors of AKT, such as mammalian target of rapamycin (mTOR), have recently been under investigation as mediators of tumorigenesis.

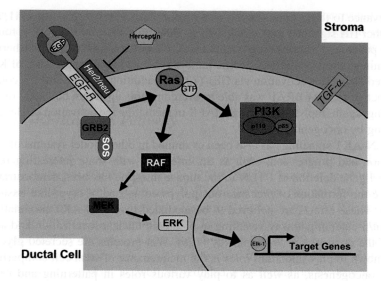

Fig. 11.5 EGF and EGF-related signaling. The epidermal growth factor (EGF) family of receptor tyrosine kinases is composed of various receptors, including the Her2Neu orphan receptor and the EGF-related ligands EGF, TGF-α, amphiregulin, HB-ECF, β-cellulin, neu-differentiation factor, and heregulin, which exist as membrane-bound proteins prior to activation and initiation of signaling. The EGF receptor proteins contain an extracellular ligand-binding region, a transmembrane segment, and a cytoplasmic tyrosine kinase domain. These proteins function as dimers, either heterodimeric or homodimeric complexes, that are capable of activating various downstream pathways including the RAF/MAPK and PI3K pathways. EGF-R dimerization results in the recruitment of various Src homology 2 (SH2)–containing effector proteins to the membrane-bound receptor complex. Upstream of the Ras pathway, the EGF receptor signal activates the GRB2/SOS complex, resulting in Ras activation (as seen previously), with subsequent activation of the PI3K and MAPK pathways

there is also a positive feedback loop in which activation of K-ras actually stimulates the production of EGF receptors, allowing increased responsiveness of the cells to the incoming signals. Pancreatic ductal adenocarcinoma cells (PDACs) express high levels of EGFR, HER-2, HER-3, and, to a more limited extent, HER-4 (*134, 135*). PDACs also express high levels of the EGF family of ligands (see the following) (*136*). EGFs and EGFRs are able to activate autocrine signaling cascades involving PI3K. This activation of EGF signaling is observed in even the earliest PanIN lesions, suggesting that these signals may be active in initiating pancreatic cancer. However, more important than the temporal expression of these proteins in pancreatic lesions is the finding that pancreatic adenocarcinomas undergo growth inhibition in the context of suppression of EGF signaling by blocking antibodies or by dominant negative expression constructs (*2*), thereby demonstrating functional consequences of EGF signal modulation in tumorigenesis. Pancreatic cancers that overexpress ERBB3 (HER3) are known to be sensitive to inhibition by Erlotinib (Tarceva) (*137*). Presently there are clinical trials looking at the efficacy of this drug in humans with pancreatic cancer based upon the favorable in vitro studies. EGFR-related peptide (ERRP), a recently isolated pan-erbB inhibitor that targets multiple members of the EGFR family, seems to attenuate EGFR activation (*138*). ERRP applied to pancreatic adenocarcinoma studies causes marked inhibition of pancreatic cancer cell growth. These changes are accompanied by increased apoptosis and a concomitant attenuation of Notch-1 and NF-κB expression and down-regulation of NF-κB downstream genes, such as *matrix metalloproteinase-9* and *vascular endothelial growth factor*. These changes result in an inhibition of pancreatic cancer cell invasion, as assayed by transit through Matrigel (*139*). Activation of the EGFR pathway is also likely to contribute to the maintenance of tumors by promoting neovascularization through stimulation of vascular endothelial growth factor (VEGF) expression through the JAK/STAT pathway (*140*).

1.10.1 Her-2/neu/ErbB2

Her-2/neu, also known as ErbB2, is a 185 kDa glycoprotein receptor, structurally homologous to the epidermal growth factor (EGF) receptor. There are multiple different transcriptional variants, although the distinctions between these proteins remain to be fully characterized. Of note, Her-2/neu is called an "orphan" receptor due to the fact that, although it bears structural similarity to EGF receptor (EGF-R), it is not capable of binding to EGF ligands. Instead, it is capable of dimerization with EGF-R to form a heterodimer. This interaction stabilizes EGF-R ligand binding and enhances kinase-mediated activation of various downstream signaling pathways, such as the MAPK and PI3K pathways. Amplification and/or overexpression of Her-2/neu have been associated with various cancers, including breast, ovarian, and, of relevance to our studies, pancreatic malignancies. There have been conflicting reports in regard to the importance of this pathway in pancreatic cancer. It was recently demonstrated by FISH analysis that in pancreatic adenocarcinoma 25% of tumors have HER2/neu gene amplification (*141*). Herceptin, a monoclonal antibody to Her2/neu, has been shown to suppress tumor growth both in vivo and in vitro in pancreatic cancer cell lines that overexpress HER-2/neu (*142*). There are also data to suggest that Her-2/neu expression correlates with shorter survival times in patients with pancreatic cancer (*89*), although its predictive or prognostic role remains unclear.

1.10.2 EGFR Ligands

Epidermal growth factor (EGF) is a potent mitogen in a variety of cells, with profound effects on the differentiation of specific cells in vivo and in vitro, including cells of both epidermal and mesenchymal lineages. The EGF precursor protein exists as a membrane-bound molecule, which is proteolytically cleaved upon activation to generate a peptide hormone that stimulates cells to divide. Members of the

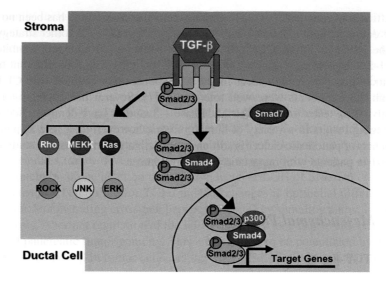

Fig. 11.6 TGF-β signaling. TGF-β proteins bind to a type II receptor dimer, which then recruits a type I receptor dimer to the membrane, resulting in a tetrameric complex of membrane-bound serine/threonine kinase receptors. Receptor-bound Smad 2 is phosphorylated and activated, resulting in an intracellular cascade leading to Smad4 activation and translocation to the nucleus. This initial phosphorylation step can be blocked by the inhibitory Smad, Smad7. Downstream TGF-β signaling is mediated by a combination of Smad2/3 and Smad4 activation. The phosphorylated Smad2/3 and Smad4 complex translocates to the nucleus and activates transcription of various downstream target genes important in cellular proliferation as well as angiogenesis and apoptosis. TGF-β is also capable of activating various non-Smad–dependent pathways as well, including the Rho/ROCK cellular polarity pathway and MAPK pathways

In the setting of pancreatic adenocarcinoma, there is often the expression of three different TGF-β isoforms as well as altered expression of the various TGF-β receptors (*33, 39, 44, 159*). Inactivating mutations of the TGF-β receptors (types I and II) have also been noted in specimens from pancreatic adenocarcinomatous lesions. Similar to observations in other systems, pancreatic cancer cells are often resistant to the growth-inhibitory effects of TGF-β, and this correlates with Smad4 mutations that have been observed in these cancer cells (*43, 153, 153a*). As mentioned, mutations in Smad4 appear to play an integral role in pancreatic carcinogenesis, as demonstrated by the observation that 55% of pancreatic tumors have chromosomal deletions and inactivating mutations in Smad4 (*153a*). Smad4 is a downstream mediator of TGF-β signaling and is implicated in the growth inhibition and anti-angiogenic properties of TGF-β (*164*). TGF-β inhibits the growth of most epithelial types either by blocking the G1-S cell cycle transition or by inducing apoptosis. These cellular responses are partially, but not exclusively, Smad4-dependent (*152, 153*). These alterations in cellular behavior can be enhanced by activated oncogenes, such as K-ras, which cooperates with TGF-β signaling during cellular invasion. In vivo observations have correlated disruption of the TGF-β signaling cascade via Smad7, a TGF-β downstream inhibitor, with premalignant ductal lesions of the pancreas (*139*).

Observations of Smad4 mutations in pancreatic cancer suggest that these mutations occur later in cancer progression, such as at the stage of PanIN3 lesions and adenocarcinomas, as these mutations have not been associated with flat or papillary intraductal neoplasias (*43, 153, 153a*). It is believed that alterations in Smad4 expression may be a molecular prognostic marker for pancreatic cancer. There is increased expression of mutated versions of Smad4 in poorly differentiated versus well-differentiated cancers, and studies of patient outcomes have demonstrated that patients without mutations do better after tumor resection than those with Smad4 mutations (*42, 164a*). Speaking to the importance of modulation of the TGF-β signaling cascade in pancreatic cancer is the observation that mutations in Smad4 are a common genetic alteration identified in pancreatic cancer, while they occur with a low incidence in other cancers (*89*).

1.12.2 Smad4/DPC4

Smad4 is a 64-kDa protein known to be important in gene transcription and growth arrest. During TGF-β–mediated signaling, a downstream cascade results in protein phosphorylation and nuclear translocation of Smad4 in complex with other intracellular proteins (*152, 153, 160*). In the context of pancreatic cancer, the high incidence of loss-of-function mutations in Smad4 and various other disturbances in the TGF-β cascade may result in a loss of tumor suppression and the acquisition of a more proliferative and invasive phenotype. These tumors then become resistant to the antiproliferative effects of TGF-β (*153, 164b*). It remains unclear whether alterations in Smad4 exert their primary effect on the epithelial tissue itself or instead modulate tumor formation through alterations in the tumor-associated stroma. Several studies suggest that the latter might be the case (*164, 165, 166*). Interestingly, re-expression of Smad4 in human colon and pancreatic cancer cells suppresses tumor cell growth in vivo but not in vitro, suggesting that changes in the local tissue environment may contribute to the Smad4-mediated events, which can be seen more readily in the context of the dynamic signaling present in vivo rather than in an in vitro system. Recent studies have examined the role of Smad4 during pancreatic development with, surprisingly, no phenotypic changes in pancreatic tissue development in the absence of Smad4. However, when loss of Smad4 occurs in combination with activation of K-ras, pancreatic neoplasms rapidly form. Isolated expression of K-ras in this system results in PanIN lesions with very slow turnover to malignancy. Yet in K-ras mutant mice with Smad4 deficiencies, tumors rapidly develop (*153a*).

There are several clinical syndromes that have been associated with Smad4 mutations. In juvenile polyposis syndrome (JPS), patients demonstrate an overgrowth of native-type tissue in the intestine, resulting in these multiple polyps. Of note, the loss of normal genetic function in this syndrome occurs predominantly in the interstitial fibroblasts among the colonic polyps. Interestingly, there does not

homodimers or heterodimers depending upon the context, connected via disulfide bonds. PDGF signals through its cognate receptor, PDGFR, which forms a homodimer or heterodimer, which results in receptor autophosphorylation. Studies of PDGF function using knock-out mice have demonstrated cellular effects of these proteins on various cell types. PDGF knock-out mice usually die as embryos or shortly after birth, emphasizing the importance of PDGF in various developmental processes (179). PDGFs and PDGFRs have been implicated in various processes in tumorigenesis, both in the setting of pancreatic cancer as well as other gastrointestinal cancers and other cancer systems. PDGF appears to be involved in growth stimulation of tumor cells, tumor angiogenesis, recruitment of tumor fibroblasts, and the tumor desmoplastic response. Interestingly, PDGF receptors in the tumor stroma have become recent targets of drug therapy as their roles in regulating tumor interstitial fluid pressure, transvascular transport, and tumor drug uptake become more apparent (180, 181). In studies of pancreatic fibroblasts, PDGF has been touted as an effective mitogen, enhancing the migratory capacity of these pancreatic stromal cells (PSCs) and inducing AP-1 binding in these PDGF-activated cells (10). In the context of pancreatic adenocarcinoma, immunohistochemical studies have demonstrated the expression of phosphorylated PDGFR-α or PDGFR-β in both tumor cells and tumor-associated endothelial cells. Comparison of in vivo to in vitro cultures of pancreatic cells demonstrates increased expression of PDGF and PDGFR in in vivo systems. Tumor activity can be functionally inhibited with blockade of PDGF signaling via treatment with the tyrosine kinase inhibitor, STI571 (Gleevec) in combination with gemcitabine, which results in inhibition of tumor growth and metastasis (182).

1.12.5   Matrix Metalloproteinases

Matrix metalloproteinases (MMPs) are a family of enzymatic proteins involved in the breakdown of extracellular matrix (ECM) during normal physiologic processes, such as during embryonic development, reproduction, and tissue remodeling, as well as in cancer metastasis. Most MMPs are secreted as inactive pro-proteins, which are activated through cleavage by extracellular proteinases. These MMPs are capable of degrading various protein types, including collagen subtypes. Many murine models also suggest a role for MMPs in tumor-associated tissue remodeling. In keeping with this theory, levels of MMP activity are found in various tumor types, and in well-established models MMP2 and MMP9 knock-out mice have a reduced susceptibility for lung metastasis. These effects may be mediated by growth factors activated by MMPs, such as IGFs, FGFs, and TGF family members (162). MMPs as targets for cancer therapy have been the focus of several clinical studies with mixed outcomes in regard to the role of MMP inhibitors (MMPIs) on cancer progression. Several Phase III drug trials of MMPIs were discontinued secondary to reports of no clinical efficacy with MMP inhibition in various cancers. However, more recent studies of the role of MMPs in cancer suggest that MMPs may be more active in tumor–stromal interactions and tumor angiogenesis, rather than as effectors on tumor cell behavior directly. This being the case, the role of MMPs in the treatment of cancer may need to be refocused to examine the effect of MMP modulation in earlier stages of cancer or in combination with other therapeutics for a combined effect on tumor cell activity and tumor–stromal interactions (*183*).

1.13 Developmental Regulators

1.13.1 Wnts

Wnt proteins (Fig. 11.8) are a family of secreted glycoproteins responsible for signaling during many stages of embryologic development. Wnts signal through the membrane-bound receptor family, Frizzleds, often in cooperation with the Wnt co-receptors LRP-5 or LRP-6. Downstream Wnt signals mediate a cascade in which β-catenin in the cytoplasm, which is normally serine/threonine phosphorylated and tagged for ubiquitin proteasome degradation, is protected from this

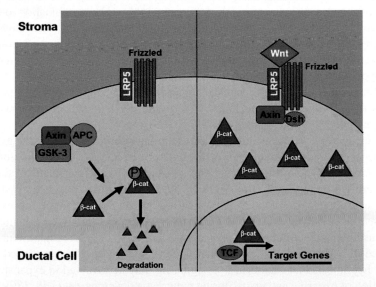

Fig. 11.8 Canonical Wnt signaling. In the absence of Wnt proteins, intracellular complexes composed of Axin, APC, and GSK-3 are formed which are responsible for the serine/threonine phosphorylation of the cytoplasmic pool of β-catenin. This phosphorylating step tags β-catenin for ubiquitin proteasome-mediated degradation, thus keeping intracellular levels of this protein low. In the presence of canonical Wnt signaling, a receptor complex composed of the Wnt receptors Frizzled, as well as the co-receptor LRP5/6, is formed. This leads to a destabilization of this Axin-APC-GSK3 complex and a resultant protection of β-catenin from this phosphorylation step. Cytoplasmic levels of β-catenin increase with translocation of the protein to the nucleus and activation of downstream signaling mediated by the TCF/LEF family of transcriptional activators

degradation and eventually translocates to the nucleus to initiate transcription through the TCF/LEF family of transcriptional activators (*184*). More recently, Wnt signaling has been implicated in the maintenance of various stem cell populations in humans (*185*), which is a logical extension of the presumed mitogenic role Wnt signaling plays during embryogenesis. Wnts have historically enjoyed a high level of interest as developmental regulators as well as oncogenes, with implication of this signaling pathway in various forms of cancer (*186*). During development, Wnts play irreplaceable roles in the formation of various organ systems, directing both organ growth and patterning. In the context of tumorigenesis, Wnts have been studied in depth in various systems. In terms of the gastrointestinal system, the role of Wnt signaling has been clarified quite extensively in the intestine, resulting in a clear model of the Wnt activity in intestinal homeostasis and dysregulation of Wnt signaling in colon cancer formation and tumorigenesis. First, active Wnt signaling has been demonstrated to keep intestinal cells dividing and in a state of continued proliferation. Simultaneously, Wnt activation prevents terminal differentiation of cells as they continue in a proliferative and undifferentiated state. Finally, specific to the intestine, Wnt signaling confers the potential (but not the obligation) to become a secretory cell type (e.g., Paneth cell). In contrast to the Paneth cells, all terminally differentiated cells in the intestine demonstrate no maintenance or persistence of Wnt activation outside of the stem cell compartments or those niches in which oncogenic transformation is occurring (*187*). The combination of these observations clarifies the role of Wnt signaling as a mediator of the intestinal stem cell niche and a key factor in maintenance of an undifferentiated pool of progenitor cells, with release from Wnt control as cells progress toward a differentiated phenotype. Parallel observations have resulted in a large volume of literature describing similar roles for canonical (or β-catenin–mediated) Wnt signaling in various other progenitor populations in the adult system and during oncogenic transformation of various tissue types (*127*, *185*).

In the pancreas, Wnt signaling has been implicated in formation of the exocrine pancreas as well as in maintenance of the endocrine pancreas. Expression of Wnts has been noted in both the epithelial and mesenchymal compartments of the pancreas during organogenesis (*61*). Work by Wells et al. (*188*) has recently demonstrated a critical role for β-catenin signaling in the formation of the exocrine pancreas, as β-catenin knock-out mice (using the Pdx1 promoter) demonstrate hypoplastic pancreata with a significantly decreased exocrine compartment in the presence of a normal islet cell compartment. These observations have led to the current hypothesis that canonical Wnt signaling may be involved in expansion of a population of exocrine precursors during pancreatic development (*188*, *189*), which is congruent with the purported role of Wnt signaling in various other organ systems. Interestingly, deletion of β-catenin in adult acinar cells has no effect on cellular function, suggesting a more isolated role for β-catenin signaling during development and initial differentiation, and a suggestion of potential reactivation in a subset of cells in the setting of chronic injury and/or oncogenesis. This is remarkably similar to the aforementioned role of canonical Wnt signaling in the intestine and other cancer models.

Recent work has demonstrated proliferative effects of Wnts on pancreatic β cells both in vitro and in vivo, with associated functional alterations in β cell activity including alterations in blood glucose homeostasis. This suggests a modulatory role of Wnt signaling in the endocrine pancreas (*190*). In the setting of pancreatic adenocarcinoma, the downstream effector of canonical Wnt signaling, β-catenin, is found localized to the nucleus in various high-grade PanINs and malignant lesions, suggesting re-activation of this signaling system in pancreatic cancer. Nuclear localization of β-catenin correlates with activation of downstream mediators of Wnt signaling, including the LEF/TCF family of transcription factors (*191*). Tumor specimens have also been examined for expression of Wnts and various Frizzled receptors, with observational reports of increased Wnt1 and Fz2 levels, as well as decreased serine/threonine tagged β-catenin (i.e., that subset of β-catenin targeted for degradation) in 65% of tumor specimens, again suggesting canonical Wnt activation during tumor formation (*192*). In a mouse model of Wnt activation, the APC min mouse (with inactivation of a suppressor of Wnt signaling), there is a predisposition of the mice to colon polyps, but also to abnormal acinar foci that demonstrate high levels of β-catenin. Upon further study in this system, the combined activation of Wnt signaling combined with inactivation or loss of p53 results in a progression of these abnormal pancreatic foci to adenocarcinoma, suggesting a role for Wnt signaling and cross-talk with other important oncogenic mediators during tumorigenesis. In studies examining the role of Smad4 in pancreatic adenocarcinoma, TGF-β/Wnt interaction has been suggested by the finding of increased β-catenin levels in abnormal pancreatic lesions in Smad4 mutant mice (*57*).

The previous studies of β-catenin–mediated Wnt signaling are intriguing and suggestive of an important role of canonical Wnt signaling in pancreatic oncogenesis. However, Wnt signaling is slightly more complex than previously described, with various other non-canonical (i.e., not β-catenin–mediated) pathways capable of activation by Wnt ligand binding. One alternative intracellular signaling pathway, termed the non-canonical pathway, is mediated by intracellular calcium signaling and has been associated with various other co-receptors and intracellular mediators. Confusing the field of Wnt research is the fact that Wnt proteins are promiscuous in their ligand/receptor interactions, leading to a lack of specificity in ligand/receptor pairings. This makes it difficult to correlate a given Wnt or Frizzled with activation of a given downstream signaling cascade, as the role of co-receptors and intracellular mediators is crucial in guiding the activation of the canonical versus non-canonical Wnt pathway. However, there is a subset of non-canonical Wnts (e.g., Wnt 5a, Wnt 11) more prone to activation of the non-canonical pathways, mediated by calcium signaling and/or the planar cell polarity pathways, including MAPK signaling, rather than by the traditional β-catenin–mediated cascade (*193–195*). Interestingly, these non-canonical Wnts have also been implicated in pancreatic development and carcinogenesis. During development of the pancreas, Wnt 5a is believed to direct islet formation and positioning (*196*). More recently Wnt 5a overexpression as well as Wnt 5a inhibition has been examined in the context of pancreatic tumorigenesis. In these studies, Wnt 5a expression enhances cellular migration, proliferation, and invasiveness in several in vitro assays. In order to correlate these in vitro findings with in vivo changes, expression of Wnt 5a was examined in tumor specimens and noted to be elevated in PanINs and invasive pancreatic adenocarcinomas, suggesting a role for non-canonical Wnt signaling in these events (*69*). In these studies of Wnt 5a, CUTL1, a homeodomain family member and transcription factor, was also examined and found to act upstream of Wnt 5a (*197*). Interestingly, CUTL1 is known to play important roles in gene expression, morphogenesis, cellular differentiation, and cell cycle progression. CUTL1 is also known to interact with TGF-β and mediate some of the pro-invasive effects of TGF-β later in tumorigenesis (*198, 199*). These findings then may be suggestive of a site of potential for cross-talk between TGF-β and Wnts, a convergence point of two distinct and very powerful signaling pathways, consistent with work in various other systems suggesting interaction and modulation of intracellular signaling by these two divergent pathways.

1.13.2   Notch

Notch proteins (Fig. 11.9) are a family of type I transmembrane proteins that function as receptors for membrane-bound ligands. All Notch proteins demonstrate many structural similarities, including an extracellular domain with multiple EGF repeats, as well as an intracellular domain with divergent domain types. Notch proteins are known to play a role in a variety of developmental processes and to control cell fate decisions by mediating interactions of physically adjacent cells. There are four known Notch genes in humans and two families of Notch ligands, Delta and Jagged (*200*). During development, Notch prevents cellular differentiation and maintains a population of undifferentiated precursor cells (*201*). A similar role has been proposed for Notch signaling in the setting of oncogenesis and maintenance of somatic stem cell pools in the adult. As is the case for Wnt signaling, the role of Notch signaling in cancer formation and progression has been characterized in great detail in various organ systems, for which the model of colon cancer is most relevant to our purposes. In this system the most notable feature of Notch pathway activation is lateral inhibition (*187*). Via lateral inhibition, a single cell is programmed to differentiate while its neighbors remain undifferentiated. This process of lateral inhibition mediated by Notch is also known to play an important role in pancreas development during embryogenesis (*202*), although Notch is also implicated in signaling via other distinct mechanisms during development of the pancreas as well (*203*).

Using the intestine as a model system with well-characterized and defined roles of the various signaling cascades, the Notch, Delta, and Hes proteins in the intestine are primarily expressed in stem cell niches. As has been described, Wnt signaling is well established as a stem cell factor maintaining a pool of progenitor cells in the undifferentiated and highly proliferative state. In the intestinal crypts, the proliferating cells rely on a sequential combination of Wnt and Notch signaling pathways to maintain their proliferative activity. Interestingly, neither pathway in isolation is sufficient to maintain this proliferation. Temporally, Wnt signaling activates Notch signaling, whereas Notch

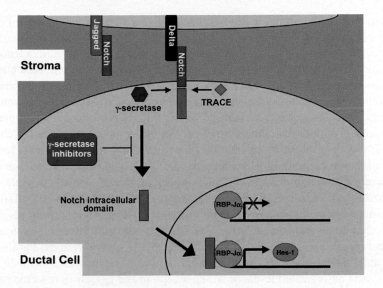

Fig. 11.9 Notch signaling. Notch is a membrane spanning protein in which the extracellular domain interacts with a ligand bound to a neighboring cell. After ligand-ligand interaction, an ADAM family metalloproteases, tumor necrosis factor-α converting enzyme (TACE), cleaves the Notch protein, releasing the extracellular portion of the protein and allowing the cytoplasmic portion to be endocytosed. The intracellular portion of the Notch protein is then modified and eventually translocates to the nucleus, where it activates gene transcription in a complex with various transcriptional co-repressors/co-activators, such as CSL, to activate the expression of Notch-related genes, such as Hes-1

seems to be permissive of the proliferative effect of Wnts. Wnt activation appears to drive the expression of Notch pathway components, whereas Notch activation mediates lateral inhibition within the population with active Wnt signaling (*191*).

In models studying embryologic pancreatic development, suppression of Notch signaling results in a depletion of exocrine precursors and selective differentiation of endocrine cells. This observation is interestingly similar to the role of Notch in intestinal maintenance and oncogenesis, in which Notch mediates lateral inhibition as well as controls the secretory (goblet and enteroendocrine) phenotype. In the intestine, Notch is expressed by cells of the secretory lineage and inhibits neighboring cell differentiation into a similar phenotype. Notch signaling during development has also been demonstrated to play a role in maintenance of a progenitor population of cells. Many theories have surfaced regarding the role of Notch signaling and Notch reactivation in the adult pancreas. In general, evidence of Notch activation is absent in most normal adult pancreatic tissue. Typically, expression of the Notch target gene Hes-1 is limited to centroacinar cells and a small subset of ductal cells. However, during dysplastic transformation, increasing amounts of Hes-1 are observed in PanINs and pancreatic adenocarcinomas. This has led to the speculation that Notch activation may play a role in reactivation of progenitor cells, dedifferentiation of terminally differentiated cells, or some as yet undefined role in cancer progression and development (*51*).

As activation of Notch signaling has been implicated in pancreatic adenocarcinoma formation, there has been much interest in the potential role of Notch signaling in controlling the behavior of pancreatic progenitor cells, maintaining pancreatic stem cell niches, or as an identifier of a progenitor population of cells. Examination of the Notch pathway has also focused on the influence of this signaling pathway in the process of oncogenic transformation. Various components of the Notch pathways are observed to be up-regulated in invasive pancreatic neoplasms. However, many of these observations of up-regulation of Notch and Notch-related genes in bulk tumor material or cancer specimens are suggestive of pathway activation, but are actually quite non-specific findings. Hes-1 is a basic helix-loop-helix transcription factor and is a known downstream mediator of Notch signaling. In pancreatic adenocarcinoma specimens, nuclear Hes-1 expression, indicative of Notch activation, is highest in basal epithelial cells of metaplastic ductal lesions, PanINs, and infiltrating ductal adenocarcinomas. Studies using immunohistochemistry also demonstrate up-regulated levels of Notch receptors and ligands in resected pancreatic adenocarcinoma specimens as well as in PanINs, and although suggestive of pathway activation these studies too lack functional implications.

More functionally relevant studies in vitro suggest that EGF-mediated Notch overexpression in pancreatic explants induces dedifferentiation (*58*). In pancreatic adenocarcinoma, elevated levels of Notch proteins, as well as increased expression of the Notch mediator Hes-1, have been observed in various premalignant and malignant lesions (*66*). In human tissue samples increased expression of Notch mRNA and protein has been correlated with pancreatic cancer as compared with normal pancreatic tissue, and overexpression of Notch pathway components also results in increased levels of VEGF, suggesting cross-talk of this signaling pathway with other oncogenic signaling cascades (*201*). The Notch signaling cascade has been linked to many other important signaling pathways in pancreatic cancer formation. Recently, concurrent inhibition of the EGF and Notch signaling pathways has been demonstrated to result in decreased tumor cell proliferation and increased cellular apoptosis (*204–206*). Some of these effects of Notch inhibition occurred with resultant decrease in the activity of NF-kB and up-regulation of p21 and p27 (*204*). The combined implications of these various studies all suggest a role for Notch signaling in pancreatic oncogenesis, perhaps similar to the role played by Notch in intestinal carcinogenesis.

1.13.3   Hedgehog

Hedgehogs (Fig. 11.10) are a family of secreted proteins known to play key inductive roles during patterning of the ventral neural tube, the anterior-posterior limb axis, ventral somites, and foregut patterning during embryogenesis. The protein is made as a precursor that is autocatalytically cleaved and attached to the cell surface, thereby preventing it from freely diffusing. Defects in this signaling cascade have

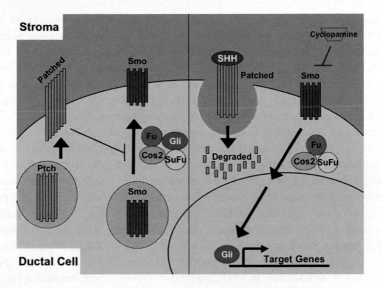

Fig. 11.10 Hedgehog signaling. Hedgehog proteins are capable of autocrine and paracrine signaling. The cell receiving the Hedgehog signals expresses the membrane-bound proteins Patched and Smoothened. In the absence of Hedgehog signaling, the Patched receptor suppresses the activity of a transmembrane receptor, Smoothened. Ptch interferes with the translocation of Smo to the membrane. In the presence of Hedgehog signaling and binding to the Patched protein, the Smoothened receptor is de-repressed, translocates to the cell membrane, leading to activation of this protein with resultant translocation of Gli protein to the nucleus and activation of gene transcription

been associated with holoprosencephaly (HPE), a disorder in which the developing brain does not appropriately separate into right and left hemispheres. It is also implicated in the VACTERL syndrome, characterized by vertebral defects, anal atresia, tracheoesophageal fistula, esophageal atresia, radial and renal dysplasia, cardiac anomalies, and limb abnormalities. These global effects on development speak to the importance of these signaling proteins as morphogens and patterning templates during embryonic organ formation. In addition to its role during development, the Hedgehog family of proteins has also been implicated in various models of oncogenesis. In pancreatic adenocarcinoma, Sonic Hedgehog (Shh) has been implicated in the initiation and maintenance of the process of carcinogenesis.

Shh plays a key role in normal pancreatic development. It appears that down-regulation of Shh is necessary for the induction of pancreatic-specific genes such as PDX1 (see the following). It also has been known to play a key regulatory role in rapidly proliferating epithelia. The role of Shh in the adult is perhaps best understood in the gastrointestinal system. In this system, Shh demarcates villi from crypts and is concentrated in the intervillous regions of the epithelium. The receptors for Shh (Patched 1 and 2) and the effectors of Shh signaling (Gli 1, 2, and 3) are restricted to the underlying mesenchyme. Conversely, Shh and Ihh expression are restricted to the epithelium. In the intestine, Shh and Ihh are produced only in sites where proliferation persists. Therefore, this occurs in intervillous pockets at the base of the crypts where the intestinal stem cell compartment exists. There is the suggestion that the Shh proteins diffuse outward from these sites and exert their effects at a distance. The theory proposes that they function to maintain proper spacing between the crypts, although they likely play a broader role in the proliferative and regenerative capacity of these cellular compartments as well (*187*).

In pancreatic cancer Shh is misexpressed in a majority of PDACs and is identified early in the PanIN progression. Shh is thought to be activated in the context of inflammation and/or repair in response to toxic or caustic stimuli, since it is not normally expressed in the pancreas. Its in role early on may be in regeneration and protection by promoting a GI metaplasia of the pancreatic epithelium. In pancreatic cancer, however, Shh is believe to be important in tumor initiation. Misexpression of Shh in the pancreatic endoderm results in tubular formations that resemble human PanINs; however, activation of Shh signaling alone is not sufficient to induce cancer in a mouse model (*59, 60*). Shh is believed to play an equally important later role in PDAC, where it appears to be important for proliferation and survival at least in a subset of pancreatic cancer cell lines (*59*). It appears that Shh must cooperate with other mutations, such as K-ras, in order to promote and maintain pancreatic tumorigenesis (*68*).

The mechanism by which Shh contributes to pancreatic tumorigenesis is now better understood. Shh expression results in enhanced proliferation of pancreatic ductal epithelial cells (PDECs) through MAPK and PI3K signaling pathways. Shh also has a protective effect of PDECs from apoptosis through a PI3K-dependent mechanism. In PDECs transfected with various combinations of expression constructs, cells expressing both K-ras and Shh undergo significantly increased levels of proliferation. Unexpectedly, this proliferative capability is not inhibited in the presence of inhibitors of the PI3K pathway. In addition, these cells are also refractory to Shh inhibition once the combined activation of K-ras and Shh has begun. Again, this suggests that K-ras and Shh may cooperate in initiation of tumorigenesis, but that these neoplasias may subsequently become pathway independent—and perhaps then chemoresistant. Reassuringly, simultaneous blockade of both cascades in these studies does suppress the oncogenic activity of these cells, perhaps revealing some level of cooperation and redundancy between the two signaling networks (*59, 60, 68*). Shh thus may contribute to pancreatic carcinogenesis by promoting proliferation, inhibition of apoptosis and enhancing chemoresistance.

1.13.4   PDX1

PDX1, also called insulin promoter factor 1 (IPF-1), is an islet-related protein known to activate transcription of the insulin and somatostatin genes. It is an important regulator of islet hormone expression (*207, 208*), as well as a key modulator of pancreatic development (*209*). There is an association between mutations in this gene and various disorders of the pancreas, including diabetes mellitus (DM) (*210*).

During embryologic development, PDX1 is required for the initiating steps of pancreas formation, and the expression of PDX1 correlates with a population of cells capable of giving rise to all of the pancreatic cellular lineages (*211*). In the adult pancreas, PDX1 expression is normally limited to islet cells (*208*). However, PDX1 expression has also been observed in metaplastic ducts in TGF-α–induced models of pancreatic metaplasia as well as PTEN gene knock-out mice (*51*). Interestingly, PDX1 has also been observed to be weakly positive in PanIN lesions in K-ras mutant mice (*212*). Finally, PDX1 is also expressed in many human pancreatic cancers (*1*), and this expression correlates with poor patient outcome (*213*). Therefore, the expression of PDX1 in various malignant and premalignant lesions suggests either activation of an immature cell type, marked by PDX1 expression, or expansion of a cell type with re-acquired PDX1 expression, either of which may be important in pancreatic carcinogenesis (*51*).

2 Maintenance and Progression Factors

2.1 Cell Cycle Regulators

2.1.1 p16 (INK-4A) and p19 (ARF)

The tumor suppressor gene p16 is also known by several different names—INK-4A, CDKN2, and MTS1 (Fig. 11.11). It has been observed that approximately 95% of pancreatic cancers have a loss of function of the p16 gene (*48, 214, 215*). The mechanism for this inactivation can occur by mutation, deletion, or promoter hypermethylation (*91, 215–220*). Conversely, mutations in p16 are very rare in the setting of chronic pancreatitis and, therefore, the absence of p16 in a subset of patients with pancreatitis may indicate a subpopulation at high risk for development of pancreatic adenocarcinoma (*221*). It is thought that mutations in p16 may play a role in the aggressiveness of pancreatic adenocarcinoma. It has been noted that tumors are larger and survival shorter in patients with a p16 mutation (*218, 220*). Mutations in p16 have also been found in the settings of gliomas, melanomas, leukemias, and esophageal squamous carcinomas (*222*). The locus that encodes the p16 protein is 9p21; however, this locus encodes two distinct proteins, INK4A/p16 and ARF/p19 in mice and ARF/p14 in humans, which can be classified into two separate cell cycle regulators (see Fig. 11.11A). Although INK4A and ARF are generated from the same locus, they do not share any amino acid homology. This is a result of a unique first exon (exon 1-β—ARF; exon 1-α—INK4a) being spliced onto common exons 2 and 3. Furthermore, unique translational reading frames result in proteins that share no homology.

INK4A[p16] regulates G1-S cell cycle transition through regulation of RB inhibitors of cyclin-dependent kinases (e.g., CDK4 kinase). INK4Ap16 proteins prevent the phosphorylation of RB, preventing the release of E2F from RB and resulting in

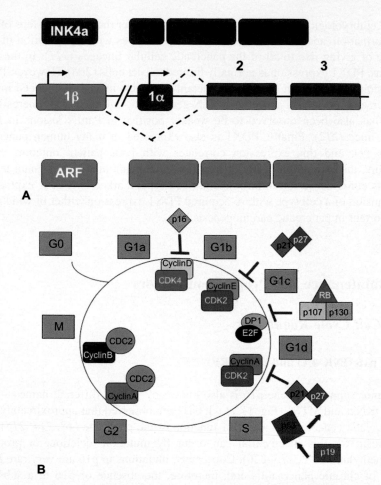

Fig. 11.11 A. INK/ARF locus. The INK4a/ARF locus encode for two distinct proteins. Each protein has a unique first exon INK4A, uses exon 1-α and ARF uses exon 1-β these are spliced on to common downstream exons. Different internal translational reading frames encode unique proteins with limited homology. **B.** Cell cycle. The cell cycle is composed of distinct phases *(in yellow)* including: (1) the G phase, divided into G0 (quiescent/senescent phase), G1a, G1b, G1c, and G1d; (2) the S phase; (3) the G2 phase; and (4) the M phase. The G0 phase is the quiescent or senescent phase of the cell cycle and is often found in terminally differentiated cells. The G1 phase extends from the previous mitosis and cytokinesis until the beginning of DNA synthesis. The S phase commences with DNA synthesis and ends when the amount of DNA has doubled, resulting in sister chromatids. The G2 phase occurs after the S phase until the next mitosis begins, and is a time dedicated to protein synthesis and microtubule formation. Finally, the M phase occurs; this encompasses the processes of mitosis and cytokinesis (cytoplasmic division). Various cyclin-dependent kinases and cyclins participate in this process, and there is a strict regulation system of various proteins that are responsible for halting cell cycle progression at sequential cell cycle checkpoints

cell cycle arrest in G1. In the absence of INK4Ap16, cyclinD1 in association with cyclin-dependent kinase 4/6 (CDK4/6) phosphorylates RB. Hyperphosphorylated RB (pRB) releases E2F, which then transcribes genes necessary for entry into

S phase (see Fig. 11.11). INK4a appears to be dispensable for normal development and homeostasis, as loss-of-function mutations are not lethal (*2*, *223–225*). Interestingly, germline mutations in p16 are associated with the familial atypical mole-malignant melanoma (FAMMM). Bearers of this mutation have a 12-fold increased risk of pancreatic cancer. However, pancreatic cancer is seen in some but not all FAMMM kindreds, suggesting that other mutations or modulating factors contribute to pancreatic cancer formation (*216, 226*).

The alternate protein ARF has been identified to cause G1 arrest by several p53-dependent mechanisms. First, ARF acts as a stabilization factor for p53 by sequestering MDM1, a protein active in p53 degradation. Second, ARF proteins interact with the E2F-1, -2, and -3 transcription activators to inhibit their transcriptional activity and induce their degradation via the 26S proteasome pathway in a p53-dependent manner. The impact of ARF on the E2F proteins provides a mechanism for p53-independent ARF activity on cell cycle progression and tumor susceptibility (*2, 89, 227*). However, the finding that p53 (see below) is frequently mutated in tumors noted to have homozygous deletions of the INK4A locus suggests that ARF may have other p53-independent roles in pancreatic tumorigenesis.

Overall, the current theory regarding the role of p16/p19 in pancreatic adenocarcinoma purports that these mutations are likely important in tumor maintenance and progression rather than tumor initiation, since there is such a low incidence of tumor formation in the setting of germline mutations and the sporadic mutations and subsequent malignancies seem to occur after the initiation of oncogenesis and after the activation of K-ras (*221*). Therefore, these mutations are often identified in PanIN2 or PanIN3 lesions as well as pancreatic adenocarcinomas, rather than in the earlier precursor lesions (*217*). It has been observed that tumors with K-ras activation are often the same subset of tumors in which associated mutations are also found in the p16/p19 genes. In the previously discussed mouse model of K-ras constitutive activation (*91*), these mutations were associated with PanINs but rarely with malignant lesions, whereas mutations in INK4A/ARF were not associated with malignancies. However, in the context of mutations in both K-ras and INK4A/ARF, there was a very rapid evolution of high grade pancreatic neoplasias and subsequent death of the animals (*91*). This again supports the theory of K-ras as an initiator of neoplasia and INK4A/ARF as a maintenance or progression factor as well as a promoter of a less differentiated and more malignant phenotype (*227a, 215, 224, 225, 228*).

2.1.2 p21/WAF1

The potent cyclin-dependent kinase inhibitor p21 has also been called WAF1 and CIP1. p21 acts as a regulator of cell cycle progression at G1 by binding to and inhibiting the activity of cyclin-CDK2 or –CDK4 complexes (*229, 230*). The expression of this protein is tightly controlled by the activity of the tumor suppressor p53, as p21 mediates the p53-dependent cell cycle G1 phase arrest in response to stressful stimuli (*231, 232*). p21 Itself interacts with proliferating cell nuclear antigen (PCNA) to play a regulatory role in S phase DNA replication and repair (*234–235*). p21 Is also activated by caspases and plays a role in apoptosis following caspase activation (*236, 237*). Since its activity is associated with induction of apoptosis, it follows that its inactivation is associated with increased proliferation and decreased apoptosis, which is in keeping with observations in various experimental systems (*232*). In pancreatic cancer, inactivation of the p21 signaling pathway is often noted to coordinate temporally with the onset of K-ras mutations (*233, 234*). The MAPK pathway has been implicated in this p21 activation (*2*). There has also been observed up-regulation of p21 in the context of Notch signaling as well as Shh signaling (*68, 112*).

2.1.3 p53

Mutations in the tumor suppressor p53 are the most common somatic alteration found consistently in various human cancers. Hence, it is a very potent and yet very nonspecific proliferative and/or survival factor. P53 is a cell cycle regulator that is capable or causing G1 or G2 cell cycle arrest. It is well established that p53 plays a role in modulating the cellular response to cytotoxic stress, DNA damage, and/or hypoxia via either cell cycle arrest or apoptosis through an ARF-independent mechanism (*235*). In the pancreatic cancer progression model, p53 mutations occur later at the PanIN-3 stage. In PanIN3 lesions of the pancreas, loss of p53 has been associated with abnormal mitoses and severe nuclear abnormalities (*30*). In pancreatic cancer, p53 mutation can be found in 50–75% of tumors (*236*). These mutations appear to correlate with later lesions demonstrating more severe levels of dysplasia and invasiveness (*2, 89*). These observations imply that genomic instability may be an integral component of tumor progression at these more advanced stages, and this may be mediated in part by inactivation of p53 (see the following) (*237*). Many studies have demonstrated a synchronous interaction between progressive telomere dysfunction and p53 loss or inactivation in the progression of carcinogenesis (*238*). In various systems examining pancreatic adenocarcinoma, loss of p53 function is associated with inappropriate cell growth, increased cellular survival, and genetic instability (*7, 237*). Therefore, p53 is considered a maintenance or progression factor in pancreatic adenocarcinoma, rather than an inductive agent. In addition, this associated chromosomal instability and subsequent gene amplifications and/or deletions are manifestations of the heterogeneity of these tumors.

2.2 Genetic Instability: Progression Factor

2.2.1 Telomere Dysfunction

Telomeres are GC-rich DNA "caps" found on the terminal ends of chromosomes. They consist of highly repetitive DNA that allows transcription of DNA without truncating the end of the message. Telomeres allow faithful replication of DNA and protect against abnormal recombination events and against genomic instability. In general telomeres are sequentially shortened during each replication, and thus in normal somatic cells this phenomenon has been thought to be important for senescence. Telomeres can be extended by telomerases, such as telomerase reverse transcriptase (TERT), in order to maintain telomere length (*239*). In pancreatic cancer telomere dysfunction is thought to contribute to pancreatic cancer progression and maintenance by two mechanisms: (*1*) telomere attrition, and (*2*) telomerase activation.

Shortened telomeres have been found in PanIN1 lesions and are thought to be early markers of neoplasia and important in tumor induction (*26, 240, 241*). It is thought that this telomere shortening and dysfunction may contribute to the formation of free ends that are very susceptible to chromosomal rearrangements and subsequent mutations through breakage-fusion cycles (*242, 243*). Abnormal breakage with chromosomal fusion results in abnormal chromosomes with two centromeres; thus during mitosis they are abnormally segregated. Histologically these are identified as anaphase bridges. The resultant daughter cell not only has abnormal genomic copy numbers, but also has free sticky ends that are highly recombinogenic. This loss of telomeres is of interest in systems in which the cells induced to proliferate are not normally proliferative cells (i.e., in settings of toxin damage or chronic inflammation), since these cells may not contain telomerase, the enzyme necessary for telomere extension and protection. Thus, early in pancreatic carcinogenesis telomere shortening is believed to contribute to pancreatic cancer progression by this genetic instability.

Abnormal activation of telomerase in cancer cells enables them to maintain functional telomeres at the end of chromosomes, preventing them from senescence. Telomerase is consequently a key enzyme in the process of immortalization of cancer cells and is believed to play a pivotal role in carcinogenesis (*244, 245*). In general, telomerase activity is highly overexpressed in malignant cells, compared to normal cells (*246*). With regard to pancreatic cancer, in contrast to the very early alterations seen in telomere size and stability, telomerase activation is a late-stage alteration but one which is present in up to 95% of pancreatic adenocarcinomas (*247*). The mechanism for the misexpression of telomerase is poorly understood. Telomerase is a uniquely appealing target for drug discovery because its expression in normal versus cancer cells suggests it may be a selective target for cancer cells. A variety of approaches to telomerase inhibition are being investigated in human studies.

2.2.2   BRCA2

BRCA2 is a tumor suppressor protein with a well-established correlation with various cancer syndromes, but an incompletely understood mechanism of action (*248*). It is clear that BRCA1 and BRCA2 can activate transcription as well as participate in double-stranded DNA break repair and/or homologous recombination (*248–250*). Thus, mutation in this gene contributes to genetic instability in pancreatic cancer tumorigenesis. Inherited mutations in BRCA2 have been associated with various breast and ovarian cancer syndromes (*49*, *248*, *250*); however, the penetrance for pancreatic cancer appears to be variable. Carriers with this mutation have a 10-fold higher risk for pancreatic cancer as compared to those without the mutation. BRCA mutations are found in 5% of pancreatic cancer patients with no family history and in 17% of those with a family history of pancreatic cancer (*251*). In terms of inherited mutations predisposing to pancreatic adenocarcinoma, BRCA2 is one of the most common mutations found in familial pancreatic cancer syndromes (*252*). In somatic cell acquisition of BRCA2 mutations, it appears to be a later event and to be restricted to the more severely dysplastic lesions, such as PanIN-3 lesions (*253*). Therefore, BRCA2 mutations are thought of as a progression factor likely due to enhanced genetic instability. BRCA-mediated genetic instability may require the inactivation of other tumor suppressor proteins concurrently, such as p53. Experiments in mice have shown that homozygous deletion of BRCA1 can be rescued by mutating p53. Furthermore, in a breast cancer model using serial BRCA, p53 gene mutation suggested that loss of p53 is critical for the development of BRCA associated tumors (*254*).

2.2.3 MicroRNA

MicroRNA are small non-coding RNAs in the size range of approximately 19–25 nucleotides in length. They are spliced into these small segments from larger 70- to 100-nucleotide hairpin RNA molecules by an Rnase called Dicer. These small single-stranded RNA molecules have gained much interest in the last few years, even resulting in the Nobel Prize award to Andrew Fire and Craig Mello for their work in developing this field of research. These small microRNAs bind to their complementary RNA target, resulting in the degradation and suppression of this target mRNA's expression. The interest in these molecules is fueled not merely by their activity in vivo (which is still being clarified), but also by their utility in vitro for the creation of siRNA, small molecules capable of silencing the expression of various RNA products. In the field of cancer research, these molecules have gained much popularity as proto-oncogenes by inhibiting the expression of various tumor suppressors. Several groups have recently utilized these findings to evaluate the microRNA signature of various tissues under different circumstances in order to find a "fingerprint" of the tumor state for identification, risk stratification, and treatment planning, as well as to gain a more basic understanding of the process of tumorigenesis. An interesting study by Bloomston et al. has recently demonstrated distinct patterns of expression associated with pancreatic adenocarcinoma, chronic pancreatitis, and normal pancreatic tissue with identification of miRNA markers associated with short- versus long-term survival (*255*, *256*). These findings are intriguing in terms of potential diagnostic and risk-stratification tools. In addition, modulation of these miRNAs and identification of their targets may give much insight into the complex process of pancreatic oncogenesis.

3 Conclusion

Pancreatic adenocarcinoma is a disease that carries a significant societal burden in terms of incidence and mortality, and one for which our current therapies are still inadequate. Over the last several year new insights into theories of basic cancer formation such as the role of morphogenic gradients, tissue microarchitecture, and 3D structure on the subsequent activity of cancer cells in their tissue milieu are now better understood. The field of cancer research has expanded from its earlier focus solely on the cancer cell to a broader perspective, which includes the local tumor environment or tumor cell niche in models of cancer formation. It has become more and more clear that the local environment plays a modulatory role in tumor cell behavior, eventual tissue invasion, and metastasis.

The signaling pathways involved in pancreatic cancer initiation and progression are also now better understood. Signaling proteins, such as K-ras, PI3K, and INK4a/ARF, were historically the focus of signaling research. Recently there has been an emphasis on new pathways, in particular on various developmental pathways, which are currently experiencing a resurgence of interest due to their role in oncogenesis and stem cell maintenance in various organ systems. The Wnt, Notch, and Hedgehog signaling pathways are only a few examples of these embryologic pathways. There are many intriguing findings suggesting key roles for these and other growth factor signaling pathways in directing local cellular behavior and oncogenic transformation. A further understanding of these cascades may facilitate the eventual design of more focused therapeutics for this malignancy. The end goal of all these studies is the eventual translation of this information into treatment of this dire disease, which carries such a poor prognosis. There are many trials currently underway targeting various signaling pathways, and we anticipate many new and novel approaches to the care and treatment of patients with pancreatic adenocarcinoma.

References

1. Frazier ML. 1999, Gene expression in pancreatic adenocarcinoma. Ann N Y Acad Sci 880:1–4.
2. Bardeesy N, DePinho RA. 2002, Pancreatic cancer biology and genetics. Nat Rev Cancer 2:897–909.
3. Yeo TP, Hruban RH, Leach SD, et al. 2002, Pancreatic cancer. Curr Probl Cancer 26:176–275.
4. Iacobuzio-Donahue CA, Hruban RH. 2003, Gene expression in neoplasms of the pancreas: applications to diagnostic pathology. Adv Anat Pathol 10:125–134.
5. Hruban RH, Wilentz RE, Maitra A. 2005, Identification and analysis of precursors to invasive pancreatic cancer. Methods Mol Med 103:1–13.
6. Hezel AF, Kimmelman AC, Stanger BZ, et al. 2006, Genetics and biology of pancreatic ductal adenocarcinoma. Genes Dev 20:1218–1249.
7. Feldmann G, Beaty R, Hruban RH, et al. 2007, Molecular genetics of pancreatic intraepithelial neoplasia. J Hepatobiliary Pancreat Surg 14:224–232.

8. Menke A, Adler G. 2002, TGFbeta-induced fibrogenesis of the pancreas. Int J Gastrointest Cancer 31:41–46.
9. Ellenrieder V, Schneiderhan W, Bachem M, et al. 2004, Fibrogenesis in the pancreas. Rocz Akad Med Bialymst 49:40–46.
10. Jaster R. 2004, Molecular regulation of pancreatic stellate cell function. Mol Cancer 3:26.
11. Truty MJ, Urrutia R. 2007, Transforming growth factor-beta: what every pancreatic surgeon should know. Surgery 141:1–6.
12. Yeo CJ, Cameron JL. 1996, Pancreatic nodal metastases: biologic significance and therapeutic considerations. Surg Oncol Clin N Am 5:145–157.
13. Hermanek P. 1998, Pathology and biology of pancreatic ductal adenocarcinoma. Langenbecks Arch Surg 383:116–120.
14. Hirai I, Kimura W, Ozawa K, et al. 2002, Perineural invasion in pancreatic cancer. Pancreas 24:15–25.
15. Nakao A, Fujii T, Sugimoto H, et al. 2006, Oncological problems in pancreatic cancer surgery. World J Gastroenterol 12:4466–4472.
16. Berlin JD. 2007, Adjuvant therapy for pancreatic cancer: to treat or not to treat? Oncology (Williston Park) 21:712–718, discussion 20, 25–26, 30.
17. Mulcahy MF. 2007, Adjuvant therapy for pancreas cancer: advances and controversies. Semin Oncol 34:321–326.
18. Hruban RH, Adsay NV, Albores-Saavedra J, et al. 2001, Pancreatic intraepithelial neoplasia: a new nomenclature and classification system for pancreatic duct lesions. Am J Surg Pathol 25:579–586.
19. Kloppel G, Luttges J. 2001, WHO-classification 2000: exocrine pancreatic tumors. Verh Dtsch Ges Pathol 85:219–228.
20. Klein WM, Hruban RH, Klein-Szanto AJ, et al. 2002, Direct correlation between proliferative activity and dysplasia in pancreatic intraepithelial neoplasia (PanIN): additional evidence for a recently proposed model of progression. Mod Pathol 15:441–447.
21. Biankin AV, Kench JG, Dijkman FP, et al. 2003, Molecular pathogenesis of precursor lesions of pancreatic ductal adenocarcinoma. Pathology 35:14–24.
22. Adsay NV, Basturk O, Cheng JD, et al. 2005, Ductal neoplasia of the pancreas: nosologic, clinicopathologic, and biologic aspects. Semin Radiat Oncol 15:254–264.
23. Laghi L, Orbetegli O, Bianchi P, et al. 2002, Common occurrence of multiple K-RAS mutations in pancreatic cancers with associated precursor lesions and in biliary cancers. Oncogene 21:4301–4306.
24. Hingorani SR, Petricoin EF, Maitra A, et al. 2003, Preinvasive and invasive ductal pancreatic cancer and its early detection in the mouse. Cancer Cell 4:437–450.
25. Lohr M, Kloppel G, Maisonneuve P, et al. 2005, Frequency of K-ras mutations in pancreatic intraductal neoplasias associated with pancreatic ductal adenocarcinoma and chronic pancreatitis: a meta-analysis. Neoplasia 7:17–23.
26. Heek NT, van Meeker AK, Kern SE, et al. 2002, Telomere shortening is nearly universal in pancreatic intraepithelial neoplasia. Am J Pathol 161:1541–1547.
27. Hermanova M, Lukas Z, Nenutil R, et al. 2004, Amplification and overexpression of HER-2/neu in invasive ductal carcinomas of the pancreas and pancreatic intraepithelial neoplasms and the relationship to the expression of p21(WAF1/CIP1). Neoplasma 51:77–83.
28. Hustinx SR, Leoni LM, Yeo CJ, et al. 2005, Concordant loss of MTAP and p16/CDKN2A expression in pancreatic intraepithelial neoplasia: evidence of homozygous deletion in a non-invasive precursor lesion. Mod Pathol 18:959–963.
29. Qian J, Niu J, Li M, et al. 2005, In vitro modeling of human pancreatic duct epithelial cell transformation defines gene expression changes induced by K-ras oncogenic activation in pancreatic carcinogenesis. Cancer Res 65:5045–5053.
30. Abe K, Suda K, Arakawa A, et al. 2007, Different patterns of p16INK4A and p53 protein expressions in intraductal papillary-mucinous neoplasms and pancreatic intraepithelial neoplasia. Pancreas 34:85–91.

31. Maitra A, Hruban RH. 2005, A new mouse model of pancreatic cancer: PTEN gets its Akt together. Cancer Cell 8:171–172.
32. Stanger BZ, Dor Y. 2006, Dissecting the cellular origins of pancreatic cancer. Cell Cycle 5:43–46.
33. Friess H, Yamanaka Y, Buchler M, et al. 1993, Enhanced expression of the type II transforming growth factor beta receptor in human pancreatic cancer cells without alteration of type III receptor expression. Cancer Res 53:2704–2707.
34. Chaudhry A, Oberg K, Gobl A, et al. 1994, Expression of transforming growth factors beta 1, beta 2, beta 3 in neuroendocrine tumors of the digestive system. Anticancer Res 14:2085–2091.
35. Di Renzo MF, Poulsom R, Olivero M, et al.1995, Expression of the Met/hepatocyte growth factor receptor in human pancreatic cancer. Cancer Res 55:1129–1138.
36. Furukawa T, Duguid WP, Kobari M, et al.1995, Hepatocyte growth factor and Met receptor expression in human pancreatic carcinogenesis. Am J Pathol 147:889–895.
37. Kiehne K, Herzig KH, Folsch UR. 1997, c-met expression in pancreatic cancer and effects of hepatocyte growth factor on pancreatic cancer cell growth. Pancreas 15:35–40.
38. Liu N, Furukawa T, Kobari M, et al.1998, Comparative phenotypic studies of duct epithelial cell lines derived from normal human pancreas and pancreatic carcinoma. Am J Pathol 153:263–269.
39. Venkatasubbarao K, Ahmed MM, Mohiuddin M, et al. 2000, Differential expression of transforming growth factor beta receptors in human pancreatic adenocarcinoma. Anticancer Res 20:43–51.
40. Zhang L, Yuan SZ. 2002, Expression of c-erbB-2 oncogene protein, epidermal growth factor receptor, and TGF-beta1 in human pancreatic ductal adenocarcinoma. Hepatobiliary Pancreat Dis Int 1:620–623.
41. Nio Y, Omori H, Hashimoto K, et al. 2005, Immunohistochemical expression of receptor-tyrosine kinase c-kit protein and TGF-beta1 in invasive ductal carcinoma of the pancreas. Anticancer Res 25:3523–3529.
42. Ijichi H, Chytil A, Gorska AE, et al.2006, Aggressive pancreatic ductal adenocarcinoma in mice caused by pancreas-specific blockade of transforming growth factor-beta signaling in cooperation with active Kras expression. Genes Dev 20:3147–3160.
43. Winter JP, de Roelen BA, ten Dijke P, et al. 1997, DPC4 (SMAD4) mediates transforming growth factor-beta1 (TGF-beta1) induced growth inhibition and transcriptional response in breast tumour cells. Oncogene 14:1891–1899.
44. Goggins M, Shekher M, Turnacioglu K, et al. 1998, Genetic alterations of the transforming growth factor beta receptor genes in pancreatic and biliary adenocarcinomas. Cancer Res 58:5329–5332.
45. Dai JL, Schutte M, Bansal RK, et al. 1999, Transforming growth factor-beta responsiveness in DPC4/SMAD4-null cancer cells. Mol Carcinog 26:37–43.
46. Izeradjene K, Combs C, Best M, et al. 2007, Kras(G12D) and Smad4/Dpc4 haploinsufficiency cooperate to induce mucinous cystic neoplasms and invasive adenocarcinoma of the pancreas. Cancer Cell 11:229–243.
47. Cowgill SM, Muscarella P. 2003, The genetics of pancreatic cancer. Am J Surg 186:279–286.
48. Schneider G, Schmid RM. 2003, Genetic alterations in pancreatic carcinoma. Mol Cancer 2:15.
49. Friedenson B. 2005, BRCA1 and BRCA2 pathways and the risk of cancers other than breast or ovarian. MedGenMed 7:60.
50. Soto JL, Barbera VM, Saceda M, et al. 2006, Molecular biology of exocrine pancreatic cancer. Clin Transl Oncol 8:306–312.
51. Stanger BZ, Stiles B, Lauwers GY, et al. 2005, Pten constrains centroacinar cell expansion and malignant transformation in the pancreas. Cancer Cell 8:185–195.
52. Ohuchida K, Mizumoto K, Murakami M, et al. 2004, Radiation to stromal fibroblasts increases invasiveness of pancreatic cancer cells through tumor-stromal interactions. Cancer Res 64:3215–3222.

53. Micke P, Ostman A. 2005, Exploring the tumour environment: cancer-associated fibroblasts as targets in cancer therapy. Expert Opin Ther Targets 9:1217–1233.

54. Haraguchi N, Utsunomiya T, Inoue H, et al. 2006, Characterization of a side population of cancer cells from human gastrointestinal system. Stem Cells 24:506–513.

55. Lou H, Dean M. 2007, Targeted therapy for cancer stem cells: the patched pathway and ABC transporters. Oncogene 26:1357–1360.

56. Neuzil J, Stantic M, Zobalova R, et al. 2007, Tumour-initiating cells vs. cancer 'stem' cells and CD133: what's in the name? Biochem Biophys Res Commun 355:855–859.

57. Cullingworth J, Hooper ML, Harrison DJ, et al. 2002, Carcinogen-induced pancreatic lesions in the mouse: effect of Smad4 and Apc genotypes. Oncogene 21:4696–4701.

58. Miyamoto Y, Maitra A, Ghosh B, et al. 2003, Notch mediates TGF alpha-induced changes in epithelial differentiation during pancreatic tumorigenesis. Cancer Cell 3:565–576.

59. Thayer SP, di Magliano MP, Heiser PW, et al. 2003, Hedgehog is an early and late mediator of pancreatic cancer tumorigenesis. Nature 425:851–856.

60. Thayer S. 2004, The emerging role of the hedgehog signaling pathway in gastrointestinal cancers. Clin Adv Hematol Oncol 2:17, 20, 63.

61. Dessimoz J, Bonnard C, Huelsken J, et al. 2005, Pancreas-specific deletion of beta-catenin reveals Wnt-dependent and Wnt-independent functions during development. Curr Biol 15:1677–1683.

62. Lee KM, Yasuda H, Hollingsworth MA, et al.2005, Notch 2-positive progenitors with the intrinsic ability to give rise to pancreatic ductal cells. Lab Invest 85:1003–1012.

63. Lewis BC. 2006, Development of the pancreas and pancreatic cancer. Endocrinol Metab Clin North Am 35:397–404, xi.

64. Nakashima H, Nakamura M, Yamaguchi H, et al. 2006, Nuclear factor-kappaB contributes to hedgehog signaling pathway activation through sonic hedgehog induction in pancreatic cancer. Cancer Res 66:7041–7049.

65. Pasca di Magliano M, Sekine S, Ermilov A, et al. 2006, Hedgehog/Ras interactions regulate early stages of pancreatic cancer. Genes Dev 20:3161–3173.

66. Kimura K, Satoh K, Kanno A, et al. 2007, Activation of Notch signaling in tumorigenesis of experimental pancreatic cancer induced by dimethylbenzanthracene in mice. Cancer Sci 98:155–162.

67. Liu MS, Yang PY, Yeh TS. 2007, Sonic hedgehog signaling pathway in pancreatic cystic neoplasms and ductal adenocarcinoma. Pancreas 34:340–346.

68. Morton JP, Mongeau ME, Klimstra DS, et al. 2007, Sonic hedgehog acts at multiple stages during pancreatic tumorigenesis. Proc Natl Acad Sci U S A 104:5103–5108.

69. Ripka S, Konig A, Buchholz M, et al. 2007, WNT5A—target of CUTL1 and potent modulator of tumor cell migration and invasion in pancreatic cancer. Carcinogenesis 28:1178–1187.

70. Strobel O, Dor Y, Alsina J, et al. In vivo lineage tracing defines the role of acinar-to-ductal transdifferentiation in inflammatory ductal metaplasia. Gastroenterology 2007, in press.

71. Strobel O, Dor Y, Stirman A, et al. 2007, Beta cell transdifferentiation does not contribute to preneoplastic/metaplastic ductal lesions of the pancreas by genetic lineage tracing in vivo. Proc Natl Acad Sci U S A 104:4419–4424.

72. Potter JD. 2007, Morphogens, morphostats, microarchitecture and malignancy. Nat Rev Cancer 7:464–474.

73. Den Brink GR, Van Bleuming SA, Hardwick JC, et al. 2004, Indian Hedgehog is an antagonist of Wnt signaling in colonic epithelial cell differentiation. Nat Genet 36:277–282.

74. Den Brink GR, Van Peppelenbosch MP. 2006, Expression of hedgehog pathway components in the adult colon. Gastroenterology 130:619.

75. Thiery JP. 2003, Epithelial-mesenchymal transitions in development and pathologies. Curr Opin Cell Biol 15:740–746.

76. Bates RC, Pursell BM, Mercurio AM. 2007, Epithelial-mesenchymal transition and colorectal cancer: gaining insights into tumor progression using LIM 1863 cells. Cells Tissues Organs 185:29–39.

77. Moustakas A, Heldin CH. 2007, Signaling networks guiding epithelial-mesenchymal transitions during embryogenesis and cancer progression. Cancer Sci 98:1512–1520.

78. Bakin AV, Tomlinson AK, Bhowmick NA, et al. 2000, Phosphatidylinositol 3-kinase function is required for transforming growth factor beta-mediated epithelial to mesenchymal transition and cell migration. J Biol Chem 275:36803–36810.
79. Nakajima S, Doi R, Toyoda E, et al. 2004, N-cadherin expression and epithelial-mesenchymal transition in pancreatic carcinoma. Clin Cancer Res 10:4125–4133.
80. Nawshad A, Lagamba D, Polad A, et al. 2005, Transforming growth factor-beta signaling during epithelial-mesenchymal transformation: implications for embryogenesis and tumor metastasis. Cells Tissues Organs 179:11–23.
81. Gotzmann J, Fischer AN, Zojer M, et al. 2006, A crucial function of PDGF in TGF-beta-mediated cancer progression of hepatocytes. Oncogene 25:3170–3185.
82. Yang AD, Camp ER, Fan F, et al. 2006, Vascular endothelial growth factor receptor-1 activation mediates epithelial to mesenchymal transition in human pancreatic carcinoma cells. Cancer Res 66:46–51.
83. Guo Y, Zi X, Koontz Z, et al. 2007, Blocking Wnt/LRP5 signaling by a soluble receptor modulates the epithelial to mesenchymal transition and suppresses met and metalloproteinases in osteosarcoma Saos-2 cells. J Orthop Res 25:964–971.
84. Kranenburg O. 2005, The KRAS oncogene: past, present, and future. Biochim Biophys Acta 1756:81–82.
85. Cho KN, Lee KI. 2002, Chemistry and biology of Ras farnesyltransferase. Arch Pharm Res 25:759–769.
86. Bos JL. 1989, ras oncogenes in human cancer: a review. Cancer Res 49:4682–4689.
87. Tsukuda K, Tanino M, Soga H, et al. 2000, A novel activating mutation of the K-ras gene in human primary colon adenocarcinoma. Biochem Biophys Res Commun 278:653–658.
88. Hongyo T, Buzard GS, Palli D, et al.1995, Mutations of the K-ras and p53 genes in gastric adenocarcinomas from a high-incidence region around Florence, Italy. Cancer Res 55:2665–2672.
89. Talar-Wojnarowska R, Malecka-Panas E. 2006, Molecular pathogenesis of pancreatic adenocarcinoma: potential clinical implications. Med Sci Monit 12:RA186–193.
90. Kern S, Hruban R, Hollingsworth MA, et al. 2001, A white paper: the product of a pancreas cancer think tank. Cancer Res 61:4923–4932.
91. Aguirre AJ, Bardeesy N, Sinha M, et al.2003, Activated Kras and Ink4a/Arf deficiency cooperate to produce metastatic pancreatic ductal adenocarcinoma. Genes Dev 17:3112–3126.
92. Friess H, Berberat P, Schilling M, et al. 1996, Pancreatic cancer: the potential clinical relevance of alterations in growth factors and their receptors. J Mol Med 74:35–42.
93. Campbell PM, Groehler AL, Lee KM, et al. 2007, K-Ras promotes growth transformation and invasion of immortalized human pancreatic cells by Raf and phosphatidylinositol 3-kinase signaling. Cancer Res 67:2098–2106.
94. Shields JM, Pruitt K, McFall A, et al. 2000, Understanding Ras: 'it ain't over 'til it's over'. Trends Cell Biol 10:147–154.
95. Norman KL, Hirasawa K, Yang AD, et al. 2004, Reovirus oncolysis: the Ras/RalGEF/p38 pathway dictates host cell permissiveness to reovirus infection. Proc Natl Acad Sci U S A 101:11099–11104.
96. Maekawa M, Nishida E, Tanoue T. 2002, Identification of the Anti-proliferative protein Tob as a MAPK substrate. J Biol Chem 277:37783–37787.
97. Hirano T, Shino Y, Saito T, et al. 2002, Dominant negative MEKK1 inhibits survival of pancreatic cancer cells. Oncogene 21:5923–5928.
98. Xing HR, Campodonico L, Kolesnick R. 2004, The kinase activity of kinase suppressor of Ras1 (KSR1) is independent of bound MEK. J Biol Chem 279:26210–26214.
99. Xing HR, Cordon-Cardo C, Deng X, et al. 2003, Pharmacologic inactivation of kinase suppressor of ras-1 abrogates Ras-mediated pancreatic cancer. Nat Med 9:1266–1268.
100. Dillon RL, White DE, Muller WJ. 2007, The phosphatidyl inositol 3-kinase signaling network: implications for human breast cancer. Oncogene 26:1338–1345.
101. Song G, Ouyang G, Bao S. 2005, The activation of Akt/PKB signaling pathway and cell survival. J Cell Mol Med 9:59–71.

102. Samuels Y, Ericson K. 2006, Oncogenic PI3K and its role in cancer. Curr Opin Oncol 18:77–82.
103. Vivanco I, Sawyers CL. 2002, The phosphatidylinositol 3-Kinase AKT pathway in human cancer. Nat Rev Cancer 2:489–501.
104. Schonleben F, Qiu W, Ciau NT, et al. 2006, PIK3CA mutations in intraductal papillary mucinous neoplasm/carcinoma of the pancreas. Clin Cancer Res 12:3851–3855.
105. Der CJ, Dyke T. Van 2007, Stopping ras in its tracks. Cell 129:855–857.
106. Gupta S, Ramjaun AR, Haiko P, et al. 2007, Binding of ras to phosphoinositide 3-kinase p110alpha is required for ras-driven tumorigenesis in mice. Cell 129:957–968.
107. Crespo P, Schuebel KE, Ostrom AA, et al. 1997, Phosphotyrosine-dependent activation of Rac-1 GDP/GTP exchange by the vav proto-oncogene product. Nature 385:169–172.
108. Takai Y, Sasaki T, Matozaki T. 2001, Small GTP-binding proteins. Physiol Rev 81:153–208.
109. Rodriguez-Viciana P, Warne PH, Khwaja A, et al. 1997, Role of phosphoinositide 3-OH kinase in cell transformation and control of the actin cytoskeleton by Ras. Cell 89:457–467.
110. Crowell JA, Steele VE, Fay JR. 2007, Targeting the AKT protein kinase for cancer chemoprevention. Mol Cancer Ther 6:2139–2148.
111. Semba S, Moriya T, Kimura W, et al. 2003, Phosphorylated Akt/PKB controls cell growth and apoptosis in intraductal papillary-mucinous tumor and invasive ductal adenocarcinoma of the pancreas. Pancreas 26:250–257.
112. Parcellier A, Tintignac LA, Zhuravleva E, et al. PKB and the mitochondria: AKTing on apoptosis. Cell Signal 2007.
113. Yamamoto S, Tomita Y, Hoshida Y, et al. 2004, Prognostic significance of activated Akt expression in pancreatic ductal adenocarcinoma. Clin Cancer Res 10:2846–2850.
114. Leslie NR, Downes CP. 2002, PTEN: The down side of PI 3-kinase signalling. Cell Signal 14:285–295.
115. Ebert MP, Fei G, Schandl L, et al. 2002, Reduced PTEN expression in the pancreas overexpressing transforming growth factor-beta 1. Br J Cancer 86:257–262.
116. Asano T, Yao Y, Zhu J, et al. 2004, The PI 3-kinase/Akt signaling pathway is activated due to aberrant Pten expression and targets transcription factors NF-kappaB and c-Myc in pancreatic cancer cells. Oncogene 23:8571–8580.
117. Li AG, Piluso LG, Cai X, et al. 2006, Mechanistic insights into maintenance of high p53 acetylation by PTEN. Mol Cell 23:575–587.
118. Ito D, Fujimoto K, Mori T, et al. 2006, In vivo antitumor effect of the mTOR inhibitor CCI-779 and gemcitabine in xenograft models of human pancreatic cancer. Int J Cancer 118:2337–2343.
119. Wislez M, Spencer ML, Izzo JG, et al. 2005, Inhibition of mammalian target of rapamycin reverses alveolar epithelial neoplasia induced by oncogenic K-ras. Cancer Res 65:3226–3235.
120. Friday BB, Adjei AA. 2005, K-ras as a target for cancer therapy. Biochim Biophys Acta 1756:127–144.
121. Bruyn KM, de Rooij J, de Wolthuis RM, et al. 2000, RalGEF2, a pleckstrin homology domain containing guanine nucleotide exchange factor for Ral. J Biol Chem 275:29761–29766.
122. Gonzalez-Garcia A, Pritchard CA, Paterson HF, et al. 2005, RalGDS is required for tumor formation in a model of skin carcinogenesis. Cancer Cell 7:219–226.
123. Hamad NM, Elconin JH, Karnoub AE, et al. 2002, Distinct requirements for Ras oncogenesis in human versus mouse cells. Genes Dev 16:2045–2057.
124. Lim KH, Baines AT, Fiordalisi JJ, et al. 2005, Activation of RalA is critical for Ras-induced tumorigenesis of human cells. Cancer Cell 7:533–545.
125. Ji Z, Mei FC, Xie J, et al. 2007, Oncogenic KRAS activates hedgehog signaling pathway in pancreatic cancer cells. J Biol Chem 282:14048–14055.
126. He XC, Yin T, Grindley JC, et al. 2007, PTEN-deficient intestinal stem cells initiate intestinal polyposis. Nat Genet 39:189–198.
127. Clevers H. 2006, Wnt/beta-catenin signaling in development and disease. Cell 127:469–480.
128. Liebmann C. 2001, Regulation of MAP kinase activity by peptide receptor signalling pathway: paradigms of multiplicity. Cell Signal 13:777–785.

129. Parise LV, Lee J, Juliano RL. 2000, New aspects of integrin signaling in cancer. Semin Cancer Biol 10:407–414.
130. Kinbara K, Goldfinger LE, Hansen M, et al. 2003, Ras GTPases: integrins, friends or foes? Nat Rev Mol Cell Biol 4:767–776.
131. Hackel PO, Zwick E, Prenzel N, et al. 1999, Epidermal growth factor receptors: critical mediators of multiple receptor pathways. Curr Opin Cell Biol 11:184–189.
132. Heldin CH. 1995, Dimerization of cell surface receptors in signal transduction. Cell 80:213–223.
133. Lemmon MA, Schlessinger J. 1994, Regulation of signal transduction and signal diversity by receptor oligomerization. Trends Biochem Sci 19:459–463.
134. Korc M. 1998, Role of growth factors in pancreatic cancer. Surg Oncol Clin North Am 7:25–41.
135. Korc M, Chandrasekar B, Yamanaka Y, et al. 1992, Overexpression of the epidermal growth factor receptor in human pancreatic cancer is associated with concomitant increases in the levels of epidermal growth factor and transforming growth factor alpha. J Clin Invest 90:1352–1360.
136. Zhu Z, Kleeff J, Friess H, et al. 2000, Epiregulin is Up-regulated in pancreatic cancer and stimulates pancreatic cancer cell growth. Biochem Biophys Res Commun 273:1019–1024.
137. 137. Frolov A, Schuller K, Tzeng CW, et al. ErbB3 expression and dimerization with egfr influence pancreatic cancer cell sensitivity to erlotinib. Cancer Biol Ther 2007, 6.
138. Yu Y, Rishi AK, Turner JR, et al. 2001, Cloning of a novel EGFR–related peptide: a putative negative regulator of EGFR. Am J Physiol Cell Physiol 280:C1083–1089.
139. Kuang C, Xiao Y, Liu X, et al. 2006, In vivo disruption of TGF-beta signaling by Smad7 leads to premalignant ductal lesions in the pancreas. Proc Natl Acad Sci U S A 103:1858–1863.
140. Wei D, Le X, Zheng L, et al.2003, Stat3 activation regulates the expression of vascular endothelial growth factor and human pancreatic cancer angiogenesis and metastasis. Oncogene 22:319–329.
141. Sharif S, Ramanathan RK, Potter D, et al. NER2/neu gene amplification by fluorescence in situ hybridization (FISH) in resected pancreatic cancer specimens. In: 2005 Gastrointestinal Cancers Symposium, 2005: ASCO Abstract No. 155, 2005.
142. Buchler P, Reber HA, Buchler MC, et al. 2001, Therapy for pancreatic cancer with a recombinant humanized anti-HER2 antibody (Herceptin). J Gastrointest Surg 5:139–146.
143. Sandgren EP, Luetteke NC, Palmiter RD, et al.1990, Overexpression of TGF alpha in transgenic mice: induction of epithelial hyperplasia, pancreatic metaplasia, and carcinoma of the breast. Cell 61:1121–1135.
144. Greten FR, Wagner M, Weber CK, et al. 2001, TGF alpha transgenic mice. A model of pancreatic cancer development. Pancreatology 1:363–368.
145. Freeman JW, Mattingly CA, Strodel WE. 1995, Increased tumorigenicity in the human pancreatic cell line MIA PaCa-2 is associated with an aberrant regulation of an IGF-1 autocrine loop and lack of expression of the TGF-beta type RII receptor. J Cell Physiol 165:155–163.
146. Alberts SR, Schroeder M, Erlichman C, et al. 2004, Gemcitabine and ISIS-2503 for patients with locally advanced or metastatic pancreatic adenocarcinoma: a North Central Cancer Treatment Group phase II trial. J Clin Oncol 22:4944–4950.
147. Brummelkamp TR, Bernards R, Agami R. 2002, Stable suppression of tumorigenicity by virus-mediated RNA interference. Cancer Cell 2:243–247.
148. Cutsem E, Van Velde H, van de Karasek P, et al.2004, Phase III trial of gemcitabine plus tipifarnib compared with gemcitabine plus placebo in advanced pancreatic cancer. J Clin Oncol 22:1430–1438.
149. Gjertsen MK, Buanes T, Rosseland AR, et al. 2001, Intradermal ras peptide vaccination with granulocyte-macrophage colony-stimulating factor as adjuvant: clinical and immunological responses in patients with pancreatic adenocarcinoma. Int J Cancer 92:441–450.
150. Wallace JA, Locker G, Nattam S, et al. 2007 2007 ASCO annual meeting proceedings. J Clin Oncol 25:4608.
151. Rinehart J, Adjei AA, Lorusso PM, et al. 2004, Multicenter phase II study of the oral MEK inhibitor, CI-1040, in patients with advanced non-small-cell lung, breast, colon, and pancreatic cancer. J Clin Oncol 22:4456–4462.

152. Gold LI. 1999, The role for transforming growth factor-beta (TGF-beta) in human cancer. Crit Rev Oncog 10:303–360.

153. Rane SG, Lee JH, Lin HM. 2006, Transforming growth factor-beta pathway: role in pancreas development and pancreatic disease. Cytokine Growth Factor Rev 17:107–119.

153a. Bardeesy N, Cheng KH, Berger JH, et al. 2006, Smad4 is dispensable for normal pancreas development yet critical in progression and tumor biology of pancreas cancer. Genes Dev 20:3130–3146.

154. Coffey RJ, McCutchen CM, Graves-Deal R, et al.1992, Transforming growth factors and related peptides in gastrointestinal neoplasia. J Cell Biochem Suppl 16G:111–118.

155. Moses HL, Arteaga CL, Alexandrow MG, et al.1994, TGF beta regulation of cell proliferation. Princess Takamatsu Symp 24:250–263.

156. Sakorafas GH, Tsiotou AG, Tsiotos GG. 2000, Molecular biology of pancreatic cancer, oncogenes, tumour suppressor genes, growth factors, and their receptors from a clinical perspective. Cancer Treat Rev 26:29–52.

157. Sun L. 2004, Tumor-suppressive and promoting function of transforming growth factor beta. Front Biosci 9:1925–1935.

158. Zavadil J, Bottinger EP. 2005, TGF-beta and epithelial-to-mesenchymal transitions. Oncogene 24:5764–5774.

159. Schniewind B, Groth S, Sebens Muerkoster S, et al. 2007, Dissecting the role of TGF–beta type I receptor/ALK5 in pancreatic ductal adenocarcinoma: Smad activation is crucial for both the tumor suppressive and prometastatic function. Oncogene 26:4850–4862.

160. Siegel PM, Massague J. 2003, Cytostatic and apoptotic actions of TGF-beta in homeostasis and cancer. Nat Rev Cancer 3:807–821.

161. Teicher BA. 2001, Malignant cells, directors of the malignant process: role of transforming growth factor-beta. Cancer Metastasis Rev 20:133–143.

162. Bhowmick NA, Moses HL. 2005, Tumor-stroma interactions. Curr Opin Genet Dev 15:97–101.

163. Bardeesy N, Aguirre AJ, Chu GC, et al.2006, Both p16(Ink4a) and the p19(Arf)-p53 pathway constrain progression of pancreatic adenocarcinoma in the mouse. Proc Natl Acad Sci U S A 103:5947–5952.

164. Schwarte-Waldhoff I, Volpert OV, Bouck NP, et al.2000, Smad4/DPC4-mediated tumor suppression through suppression of angiogenesis. Proc Natl Acad Sci U S A 97:9624–9629.

164a. Hua Z, Zhang YC, Hu XM, et al. 2003, Loss of DPC4 expression and its correlation with clinicopathological parameters in pancreatic carcinoma. World J Gastroenterol 9:2764–2767.

164b. Villanueva A, Garcia C, Paules AB, et al. 1998, Disruption of the antiproliferative TGF-beta signaling pathways in human pancreatic cancer cells. Oncogene 17:1969–1978.

165. Schwarte-Waldhoff I, Schmiegel W. 2002, Smad4 transcriptional pathways and angiogenesis. Int J Gastrointest Cancer 31:47–59.

166. Duda DG, Sunamura M, Lefter LP, et al. 2003, Restoration of SMAD4 by gene therapy reverses the invasive phenotype in pancreatic adenocarcinoma cells. Oncogene 22:6857–6864.

167. Ellenrieder V, Hendler SF, Boeck W, et al. 2001, Transforming growth factor beta1 treatment leads to an epithelial-mesenchymal transdifferentiation of pancreatic cancer cells requiring extracellular signal-regulated kinase 2 activation. Cancer Res 61:4222–4228.

168. Rowland-Goldsmith MA, Maruyama H, Matsuda K, et al. 2002, Soluble type II transforming growth factor-beta receptor attenuates expression of metastasis-associated genes and suppresses pancreatic cancer cell metastasis. Mol Cancer Ther 1:161–167.

169. Stella MC, Comoglio PM. 1999, HGF: a multifunctional growth factor controlling cell scattering. Int J Biochem Cell Biol 31:1357–1362.

170. Ma PC, Maulik G, Christensen J, et al. 2003, c-Met: structure, functions and potential for therapeutic inhibition. Cancer Metastasis Rev 22:309–325.

171. Ohnishi T, Daikuhara Y. 2003, Hepatocyte growth factor/scatter factor in development, inflammation and carcinogenesis: its expression and role in oral tissues. Arch Oral Biol 48:797–804.

172. Kermorgant S, Parker PJ. 2005, c-Met signalling: spatio-temporal decisions. Cell Cycle 4:352–355.
173. Kemp LE, Mulloy B, Gherardi E. 2006, Signalling by HGF/SF and Met: the role of heparan sulphate co-receptors. Biochem Soc Trans 34:414–417.
174. Peruzzi B, Bottaro DP. 2006, Targeting the c-Met signaling pathway in cancer. Clin Cancer Res 12:3657–3660.
175. Birchmeier W, Brinkmann V, Niemann C, et al. 1997, Role of HGF/SF and c-Met in morphogenesis and metastasis of epithelial cells. Ciba Found Symp 212:230–240, discussion 40–46.
176. Perugini RA, McDade TP, Vittimberga FJ Jr, et al.1998, The molecular and cellular biology of pancreatic cancer. Crit Rev Eukaryot Gene Expr 8:377–393.
177. Otte JM, Kiehne K, Schmitz F, et al. 2000, C-met protooncogene expression and its regulation by cytokines in the regenerating pancreas and in pancreatic cancer cells. Scand J Gastroenterol 35:90–95.
178. Tomioka D, Maehara N, Kuba K, et al. 2001, Inhibition of growth, invasion, and metastasis of human pancreatic carcinoma cells by NK4 in an orthotopic mouse model. Cancer Res 61:7518–7524.
179. Betsholtz C. 2004, Insight into the physiological functions of PDGF through genetic studies in mice. Cytokine Growth Factor Rev 15:215–228.
180. Jones AV, Cross NC. 2004, Oncogenic derivatives of platelet-derived growth factor receptors. Cell Mol Life Sci 61:2912–2923.
181. Ostman A. 2004, PDGF receptors-mediators of autocrine tumor growth and regulators of tumor vasculature and stroma. Cytokine Growth Factor Rev 15:275–286.
182. Hwang RF, Yokoi K, Bucana CD, et al. 2003, Inhibition of platelet-derived growth factor receptor phosphorylation by STI571 (Gleevec) reduces growth and metastasis of human pancreatic carcinoma in an orthotopic nude mouse model. Clin Cancer Res 9:6534–6544.
183. Zucker S, Cao J, Chen W-T. 2000, Critical appraisal of the use of matrix metalloproteinare inhibitors in Cancer treatment. Oncogene 19:6642–6650.
184. Brantjes H, Barker N, Es J, van et al. 2002, TCF: Lady Justice casting the final verdict on the outcome of Wnt signalling. Biol Chem 383:255–261.
185. Reya T, Clevers H. 2005, Wnt signalling in stem cells and cancer. Nature 434:843–850.
186. Giles RH, Es JH, van Clevers H. 2003, Caught up in a Wnt storm: Wnt signaling in cancer. Biochim Biophys Acta 1653:1–24.
187. Crosnier C, Stamataki D, Lewis J. 2006, Organizing cell renewal in the intestine: stem cells, signals and combinatorial control. Nat Rev Genet 7:349–359.
188. Wells JM, Esni F, Boivin GP, et al. 2007, Wnt/beta-catenin signaling is required for development of the exocrine pancreas. BMC Dev Biol 7:4.
189. Murtaugh LC, Law AC, Dor Y, et al. 2005, Beta-catenin is essential for pancreatic acinar but not islet development. Development 132:4663–4674.
190. Rulifson IC, Karnik SK, Heiser PW, et al. 2007, Wnt signaling regulates pancreatic beta cell proliferation. Proc Natl Acad Sci U S A 104:6247–6252.
191. Al-Aynati MM, Radulovich N, Riddell RH, et al. 2004, Epithelial-cadherin and beta-catenin expression changes in pancreatic intraepithelial neoplasia. Clin Cancer Res 10:1235–1240.
192. Zeng G, Germinaro M, Micsenyi A, et al. 2006, Aberrant Wnt/beta-catenin signaling in pancreatic adenocarcinoma. Neoplasia 8:279–289.
193. Pandur P, Maurus D, Kuhl M. 2002, Increasingly complex: new players enter the Wnt signaling network. Bioessays 24:881–884.
194. Katoh M. 2005, WNT/PCP signaling pathway and human cancer (review). Oncol Rep 14:1583–1588.
195. Widelitz R. 2005, Wnt signaling through canonical and non-canonical pathways: recent progress. Growth Factors 23:111–116.
196. Kim HJ, Schleiffarth JR, Jessurun J, et al. 2005, Wnt5 signaling in vertebrate pancreas development. BMC Biol 3:23.
197. Aleksic T, Bechtel M, Krndija D, et al. 2007, CUTL1 promotes tumor cell migration by decreasing proteasome-mediated Src degradation. Oncogene 26:5939–5949.

198. Michl P, Ramjaun AR, Pardo OE, et al. 2005, CUTL1 is a target of TGF(beta) signaling that enhances cancer cell motility and invasiveness. Cancer Cell 7:521–532.
199. Michl P, Downward J. 2006, CUTL1: a key mediator of TGFbeta-induced tumor invasion. Cell Cycle 5:132–134.
200. Miele L, Golde T, Osborne B. 2006, Notch signaling in cancer. Curr Mol Med 6:905–918.
201. Buchler P, Gazdhar A, Schubert M, et al. 2005, The Notch signaling pathway is related to neurovascular progression of pancreatic cancer. Ann Surg 242:791–800, discussion –1.
202. Hart A, Papadopoulou S, Edlund H. 2003, Fgf10 maintains notch activation, stimulates proliferation, and blocks differentiation of pancreatic epithelial cells. Dev Dyn 228:185–193.
203. Norgaard GA, Jensen JN, Jensen J. 2003, FGF10 signaling maintains the pancreatic progenitor cell state revealing a novel role of Notch in organ development. Dev Biol 264:323–338.
204. Wang Z, Zhang Y, Li Y, et al. 2006, Down-regulation of Notch-1 contributes to cell growth inhibition and apoptosis in pancreatic cancer cells. Mol Cancer Ther 5:483–493.
205. Wang Z, Banerjee S, Li Y, et al. 2006, Down-regulation of notch-1 inhibits invasion by inactivation of nuclear factor-kappaB, vascular endothelial growth factor, and matrix metalloproteinase-9 in pancreatic cancer cells. Cancer Res 66:2778–2784.
206. Wang Z, Sengupta R, Banerjee S, et al. 2006, Epidermal growth factor receptor–related protein inhibits cell growth and invasion in pancreatic cancer. Cancer Res 66:7653–7660.
207. Aramata S, Han SI, Yasuda K, et al. 2005, Synergistic activation of the insulin gene promoter by the beta-cell enriched transcription factors MafA, Beta2, and Pdx1. Biochim Biophys Acta 1730:41–46.
208. Babu DA, Deering TG, Mirmira RG. 2007, A feat of metabolic proportions: Pdx1 orchestrates islet development and function in the maintenance of glucose homeostasis. Mol Genet Metab 92:43–55.
209. Hale MA, Kagami H, Shi L, et al. 2005, The homeodomain protein PDX1 is required at mid–pancreatic development for the formation of the exocrine pancreas. Dev Biol 286:225–237.
210. Johnson JD, Ahmed NT, Luciani DS, et al. 2003, Increased islet apoptosis in Pdx1+/– mice. J Clin Invest 111:1147–1160.
211. Zhou Q, Law AC, Rajagopal J, et al. 2007, A multipotent progenitor domain guides pancreatic organogenesis. Dev Cell 13:103–114.
212. Guerra C, Schuhmacher AJ, Canamero M, et al. 2007, Chronic pancreatitis is essential for induction of pancreatic ductal adenocarcinoma by K-Ras oncogenes in adult mice. Cancer Cell 11:291–302.
213. Koizumi M, Doi R, Toyoda E, et al. 2003, Increased PDX-1 expression is associated with outcome in patients with pancreatic cancer. Surgery 134:260–266.
214. Okamoto A, Demetrick DJ, Spillare EA, et al.1994, Mutations and altered expression of p16INK4 in human cancer. Proc Natl Acad Sci U S A 91:11045–11049.
215. Attri J, Srinivasan R, Majumdar S, et al. 2005, Alterations of tumor suppressor gene p16INK4a in pancreatic ductal carcinoma. BMC Gastroenterol 5:22.
216. Goldstein AM, Fraser MC, Struewing JP, et al. 1995, Increased risk of pancreatic cancer in melanoma-prone kindreds with p16INK4 mutations. N Engl J Med 333:970–974.
217. Hu YX, Watanabe H, Ohtsubo K, et al. 1997, Frequent loss of p16 expression and its correlation with clinicopathological parameters in pancreatic carcinoma. Clin Cancer Res 3:1473–1477.
218. Gerdes B, Ramaswamy A, Ziegler A, et al. 2002, p16INK4a is a prognostic marker in resected ductal pancreatic cancer: an analysis of p16INK4a, p53, MDM2, an Rb. Ann Surg 235:51–59.
219. vos tot Nederveen Cappel WH, de Offerhaus GJ, et al. 2003, Pancreatic carcinoma in carriers of a specific 19 base pair deletion of CDKN2A/p16 (p16-leiden). Clin Cancer Res 9:3598–3605.
220. Ohtsubo K, Watanabe H, Yamaguchi Y, et al. 2003, Abnormalities of tumor suppressor gene p16 in pancreatic carcinoma: immunohistochemical and genetic findings compared with clinicopathological parameters. J Gastroenterol 38:663–671.
221. Rosty C, Geradts J, Sato N, et al. 2003, p16 Inactivation in pancreatic intraepithelial neoplasias (PanINs) arising in patients with chronic pancreatitis. Am J Surg Pathol 27:1495–1501.

222. Kim WY, Sharpless NE. 2006, The regulation of INK4/ARF in cancer and aging. Cell 127:265–275.
223. Serrano M, Lee H, Chin L, et al. 1996, Role of the INK4a locus in tumor suppression and cell mortality. Cell 85:27–37.
224. Sharpless NE, Bardeesy N, Lee KH, et al. 2001, Loss of p16Ink4a with retention of p19Arf predisposes mice to tumorigenesis. Nature 413:86–91.
225. Sharpless NE, Ramsey MR, Balasubramanian P, et al. 2004, The differential impact of p16(INK4a) or p19(ARF) deficiency on cell growth and tumorigenesis. Oncogene 23:379–385.
226. Whelan AJ, Bartsch D, Goodfellow PJ. 1995, Brief report: a familial syndrome of pancreatic cancer and melanoma with a mutation in the CDKN2 tumor-suppressor gene. N Engl J Med 333:975–977.
227. Rizos H, Scurr LL, Irvine M, et al. 2007, p14ARF regulates E2F-1 ubiquitination and degradation via a p53-dependent mechanism. Cell Cycle 6:1741–1747.
228. Bardeesy N, Morgan J, Sinha M, et al. 2002, Obligate roles for p16(Ink4a) and p19(Arf)-p53 in the suppression of murine pancreatic neoplasia. Mol Cell Biol 22:635–643.
229. Gartel AL, Serfas MS, Tyner AL. 1996, p21-negative regulator of the cell cycle. Proc Soc Exp Biol Med 213:138–149.
230. O'Connor PM. 1997, Mammalian G1 and G2 phase checkpoints. Cancer Surv 29:151–182.
231. Winters ZE. 2002, P53 pathways involving G2 checkpoint regulators and the role of their subcellular localisation. J R Coll Surg Edinb 47:591–598.
232. Maddika S, Ande SR, Panigrahi S, et al. 2007, Cell survival, cell death and cell cycle pathways are interconnected: implications for cancer therapy. Drug Resist Updat 10:13–29.
234. Dotto GP. 2000, p21(WAF1/Cip1): more than a break to the cell cycle? Biochim Biophys Acta 1471:M43–56.
235. Paunesku T, Mittal S, Protic M, et al. 2001, Proliferating cell nuclear antigen (PCNA): ringmaster of the genome. Int J Radiat Biol 77:1007–1021.
236. Bokoch GM. 1998, Caspase-mediated activation of PAK2 during apoptosis: proteolytic kinase activation as a general mechanism of apoptotic signal transduction? Cell Death Differ 5:637–645.
237. Roig J, Traugh JA. 2001, Cytostatic p21 G protein–activated protein kinase gamma-PAK. Vitam Horm 62:167–198.
233. Biankin AV, Kench JG, Morey AL, et al. 2001, Overexpression of p21(WAF1/CIP1) is an early event in the development of pancreatic intraepithelial neoplasia. Cancer Res 61:8830–8837.
234. Hermanova M, Lukas Z, Kroupova I, et al. 2003, Relationship between K-ras mutation and the expression of p21WAF1/CIP1 and p53 in chronic pancreatitis and pancreatic adenocarcinoma. Neoplasma 50:319–325.
235. Vousden KH, Lu X. 2002, Live or let die: the cell's response to p53. Nat Rev Cancer 2:594–604.
236. Moskaluk CA, Hruban RH, Kern SE. 1997, p16 and K-ras gene mutations in the intraductal precursors of human pancreatic adenocarcinoma. Cancer Res 57:2140–2143.
237. Chu TM. 1997, Molecular diagnosis of pancreas carcinoma. J Clin Lab Anal 11:225–231.
238. Stewart SA, Weinberg RA. 2006, Telomeres: cancer to human aging. Annu Rev Cell Dev Biol 22:531–557.
239. Moon IK, Jarstfer MB. 2007, The human telomere and its relationship to human disease, therapy, and tissue engineering. Front Biosci 12:4595–4620.
240. Gisselsson D, Hoglund M. 2005, Connecting mitotic instability and chromosome aberrations in cancer—can telomeres bridge the gap? Semin Cancer Biol 15:13–23.
241. Gisselsson D, Jonson T, Petersen A, et al. 2001, Telomere dysfunction triggers extensive DNA fragmentation and evolution of complex chromosome abnormalities in human malignant tumors. Proc Natl Acad Sci U S A 98:12683–12688.
242. Desmaze C, Soria JC, Freulet-Marriere MA, et al. 2003, Telomere-driven genomic instability in cancer cells. Cancer Lett 194:173–182.
243. Mathieu N, Pirzio L, Freulet-Marriere MA, et al. 2004, Telomeres and chromosomal instability. Cell Mol Life Sci 61:641–656.

also lead to sticky chromosomes. Certain genetic mutations such as mutations in the DNA repair genes BRCA2 and Fanconi anemia pathway genes and probably as yet unidentified mutations in DNA repair genes also likely fuel the development of chromosomal instability (8). Environmental causes of DNA damage such as cigarette smoking are also predicted to influence the development of CIN. In addition, cellular folate deficiency has been postulated as a cause of DNA damage, because anti-folates cause DNA breakages and folate sensitive fragile sites, and there is evidence that genetic alterations in the folate pathway could facilitate chromosomal losses in pancreatic cancers (9).

DNA damage culminates in widespread chromosomal alterations in pancreatic cancers. These chromosomal alterations have been characterized in genome-wide studies characterizing pancreatic cancer deletions using hundreds of microsatellite markers (10). Using a similar strategy patterns of LOH have been identified in familial pancreatic cancers (200). More recently, similar results have been noted using SNP microarrays that have also revealed the extensive chromosomal duplications present in these cancers (11). Array CGH studies have also been used to accurately define genetic deletions and amplifications that occur in these cancers (12–16). The second form of genetic instability, microsatellite instability (MIN) is found in only a small percentage (~3%) of pancreatic cancers (17), but unlike CIN, the mechanism of MIN, inactivation of mismatch repair genes, is well understood. Mitochondrial DNA mutations occur during the development of pancreatic and other cancers but their functional significance is uncertain (18).

Taking advantage of our expanding knowledge of pancreatic cancer genomics in the clinical setting is only beginning to occur. Understanding the genetics of familial pancreatic cancer can be rapidly translatable into patient care. For example, patients with a family history of pancreatic cancer and a germline *BRCA2* mutation can undergo genetic counseling and may benefit from screening for evidence of pancreatic neoplasia. It has recently been determined that individuals with multiple relatives with pancreatic cancer can benefit from pancreatic screening using a combination of endoscopic ultrasound and computed tomography (19). Approximately ten percent of appropriately selected patients have significant precursor lesions in their pancreas such as intraductal papillary mucinous neoplasms and high-grade PanINs treatable with surgical resection. As our knowledge of familial pancreatic cancer susceptibility genes grows, so too will our ability to target the most at-risk individuals for screening. At the same time, screening of the pancreas using imaging identifies many subtle nonspecific alterations of uncertain significance. Accurate diagnostic markers of pancreatic neoplasia could aid in the diagnosis of suspicious pancreatic lesions identified by screening (19, 20, 21).

Genetic markers of pancreatic cancer have the potential to be useful for molecular diagnostic assays. Although most genetic alterations are not suitable as diagnostic markers, sensitive markers such as mutant K-ras or and specific alterations such as p53 mutation have been evaluated using a variety of assays in an attempt to improve the diagnosis of patients suspected of having the disease. Mutant K-ras can be detected in sources distant from the cancer such as pancreatic juice, duodenal fluid, stool and blood using sensitive mutation assays (22–24). Unfortunately, K-ras mutations are not specific for invasive pancreatic cancer; mutant K-ras is found in pancreatic tissue among asymptomatic smokers and patients with chronic pancreatitis (23, 25, 26). Circulating mutant K-ras can be detected in serum in only a minority of patients with resectable pancreatic cancer (27, 28). Although these studies have limited the enthusiasm for mutant K-ras as a diagnostic marker, recently a sensitive assay have been developed that can quantify levels of mutant K-ras in blood and pancreatic juice (29).

Similarly, improvements in assay performance could permit the use of mutant *p53* and *p16* to be used as a marker of pancreatic cancer. In this regard, recently described assay approaches such as "heteroduplex analysis of limiting dilution PCRs" (30) and other approaches may make this feasible (31). Finally, it is widely believed that certain genetic patterns in pancreatic cancer will ultimately be used for clinical decision making because their ability to predict outcome, particularly responses to therapies. In this regard, it is known that pancreatic cancers with inactivation of the *BRCA2/Fanconi* pathway are sensitive to mitomycin C in vitro, analogous to the DNA repair defect in patients with Fanconi anemia (32), and the significance of this observation is being tested in a clinical trial.

3   Epigenetics

Epigenetic alterations, including DNA hypermethylation and hypomethylation, and the associated transcriptional changes of the affected genes are central to the evolution and progression of various human cancers, including pancreatic cancer (33, 34). In human cells, methylation of DNA is restricted to the cytosines at CG dinucleotides. CG dinucleotides (often referred to as CpGs) are often found in regions of DNA rich in CG dinucleotides known as CpG islands. CpG islands are commonly located in the 5' regulatory regions of genes, and most CpG islands are normally unmethylated. With the use of genome-wide screening technologies as well as conventional candidate gene approaches, many genes have been identified that are affected by aberrant DNA methylation in pancreatic cancer. Importantly, the detection of DNA methylation alterations have been proposed for cancer risk assessment, the early detection of cancer, as well as for tumor classification, prognostication, and as therapeutic targets (35–40). Despite advances in our characterizing of cancer DNA methylation alterations, the etiology of these alterations is not well understood.

3.1   *The Etiology of Aberrant DNA Methylation in Human Cancer*

Multiple mechanisms are likely to be responsible for the full spectrum of methylation alterations associated with cancer. Overall, we and others hypothesize that alterations in methylation in cancers likely reflect the combined effects of aging,

showing that global DNA hypomethylation can lead to tumor formation in mice raises a question about the rationale for the use of demethylating agents for cancer. Thus, these questions need to be further investigated before DNA methylation and HDAC inhibitors are moved into clinical use for patients with pancreatic cancer.

4   RNA Alterations in Pancreatic Cancer

The expression of hundreds of genes is altered during pancreatic cancer development, and knowledge of such alterations has been used to identify upstream genetic and epigenetic alterations and downstream protein alterations in pancreatic cancer (73, 114, 115). Identifying the protein products of these overexpressed genes may identify suitable targets for protein-based diagnostic tests. In addition, the direct assaying of pancreatic specimens for changes in specific RNA levels has the potential to assist in diagnosis. Such an approach is important because many of the proteins overexpressed in pancreatic and other cancers are not secreted proteins and therefore are not likely to be found in the circulation. Messenger RNA levels in samples to be screened can be quantified with the use of quantitative reverse transcriptase PCR or global gene expression profiling using chip-based assays.

The promise of discovery using gene expression profiling has led to many publications describing differentially expressed genes in primary neoplastic pancreatic tissues compared with normal pancreas (114, 116–122). However, many tissue gene expression studies are fundamentally flawed because investigators fail to accommodate in their experiments the fact that many of the RNA profiles of a pancreatic cancer arise from expression changes in non-neoplastic stromal cells and normal pancreatic tissue is largely composed of acinar cells and not ductal epithelial cells. Many of the apparent gene expression differences identified are simply the result of comparing two different cell types. For this reason, it is critical to determine the cell of origin of genes tentatively identified as overexpressed in pancreatic cancer. Assays that can evaluate cell morphology, such as immunohistochemistry or in situ hybridization are helpful in this regard, and have been used to identify expression alterations that are unique to the peritumoral compartments (123). Tissue microarrays have been used to efficiently characterize genetic and protein changes of pancreatic and other cancers in a high throughput manner (124–132). Direct microdissection of individual neoplastic and normal ductal epithelium using laser capture techniques can largely overcome the confounding effects of mixed cell populations in tumor masses. Since the limited amounts of RNA from microdissected tissues requires additional amplification prior to array analysis that can lead to amplification bias, validation of RNA expression differences using independent methods is important.

Many of the gene expression differences identified in pancreatic cancer have been evaluated for their potential diagnostic use. Perhaps the best-studied RNA-based marker to date has been the human telomerase reverse transcriptase gene (hTERT). About 90% of cancers express the telomerase subunit hTERT, and ~90% of patients with pancreatic cancer have detectable telomerase activity in their pancreatic juice (*133*). Although the detection of telomerase enzymatic activity or the *hTERT* subunit may be helpful in differentiating pancreatic cancer from benign pancreatic diseases, telomerase is also expressed in inflammatory cells limiting its use in routine clinical practice.

The use of gene expression profiling coupled with confirmatory analysis of expression changes in the tissues has led to the identification of hundreds of genes that are overexpressed in pancreatic cancer cells relative to normal pancreas. Examples of such genes include *mesothelin, prostate stem cell antigen (PSCA), 14-3-3 sigma, S100P, S100A4, osteopontin, MMP-7, Muc4, kallikrein 10, fascin,* and *keratin 17* (*84, 117–119, 134–138*). The protein products of some of these genes have been evaluated as serum markers of pancreatic cancer including MIC-1, osteopontin, gp-39, HIP, TIMP-1 (*139–145*). For example, mesothelin and PSCA are expressed in most pancreatic cancers, and immunolabeling for mesothelin and PSCA has been evaluated as an aid in the interpretation of diagnostically challenging pancreatic biopsies (*146, 147*). It is likely that the expression patterns of other overexpressed genes in cytologic specimens, identified with the use of such approaches as immunohistochemistry, quantitative reverse transcriptase PCR, and gene chip profiling, could be used to distinguish FNAs of pancreatic cancers from noncancerous aspirates. Overall, only a minority of the protein products of overexpressed genes are generally suitable for use in serologic diagnosis. In addition, although some genes may be abundantly expressed in pancreatic cancer cells relative to the normal pancreas, in other tissues, the expression of such genes may be normal. Finally, many genes that are overexpressed in pancreatic cancer cells are also overexpressed in chronic pancreatitis tissues (*120*). Therefore, a careful characterization of the genes whose overexpression is most sensitive and specific for cancer is needed when assays to detect the protein products of overexpressed genes are designed. Ideally, a serum-based marker of pancreatic cancer should be a secreted protein overexpressed in pancreatic cancers, not expressed in non-neoplastic pancreas, and having a restricted pattern of expression in other organs and tissues.

Despite the extensive characterization of pancreatic cancer gene expression profiles, no ideal candidate overexpressed gene has emerged as a suitable marker. One gene that fulfills some of these criteria is macrophage inhibitory cytokine (MIC-1). MIC-1 is overexpressed in pancreatic cancer cells relative to normal pancreas, and the protein product of MIC-1 is secreted. We have found serum MIC-1 to be more sensitive than CA19-9 for patients with resectable pancreatic cancer, although it is not more specific than CA19-9 (*140*). These characteristics could make serum MIC-1 helpful in the early detection of pancreatic cancer in high-risk populations such as those undergoing pancreatic screening with endoscopic ultrasound (EUS) and computed tomography (CT) (*20, 148*), who have a modest pretest probability of disease. Since these patients are undergoing regular pancreatic evaluation, the consequences of an initial false-positive test are less than for an average risk person. In principle, in the absence of other diseases that elevate MIC-1, elevated MIC-1 levels could be used to prioritize subjects to further evaluation using more specific pancreatic imaging tests. Of interest, the combination of serum CA19-9 and MIC-1 measurements better predicted patients with pancreatic cancer than the use of CA19-9 alone (*140,*

143). Another potential marker identified through gene expression profiling is oste-opontin. Osteopontin is expressed in peritumoral macrophages and is usually increased in the serum of patients with pancreatic cancer (*142*).

Infiltrating pancreatic cancer cells also induce changes in adjacent peritumoral cells. These peritumoral cells such as fibroblasts and acinar cells can obscure the specific expression changes that arise in pancreatic cancer cells when bulk pancreatic tissues are profiled. However, investigators have also sought to identify molecular alterations in peritumoral cells that could be useful markers and also determine how peritumoral cells influence tumor progression. Gene expression studies of microdissected peritumoral acinar cells indicate that several acinar derived proteins (HIP/PAP and gp39) are elevated in the serum of patients with pancreatic cancer (*144*). Similarly acinar derived proteins have been identified using direct proteomics approaches (*144*, *145*). Direct characterization of cancer associated fibroblasts is more difficult because they are not easily microdissected, but in vitro studies of primary cancer fibroblast cultures have provided insights into how fibroblasts may influence tumor progression (*149*). More recently pancreatic cancer investigators have moved from expression profiling pancreatic neoplasms to investigating the transcriptional changes associated with specific pathways or genetic alterations such as K-ras mutations (*150*).

4.1   Gene Expression Alterations in Pancreatic Cancer Stroma

Cancer-associated stroma is thought to have a net tumor-promoting effect (*151*, *152*). Pat Brown and colleagues have demonstrated that the gene expression phenotype of cancer associated fibroblasts helps predict outcome of patients with certain cancers (*153–155*). Recent studies by Polyak et al. indicate a role for epigenetic alterations in breast cancer fibroblasts (*149*). SPARC is associated with outcome among patients undergoing surgical resection for pancreatic cancer (*85*). We previously identified *SPARC* (secreted protein acidic and rich in cysteine, or osteonectin/BM40) as a gene that is frequently epigenetically silenced in pancreatic cancers (*83*). SPARC is a calcium-binding protein that interacts with extracellular matrix and influences cell migration, proliferation, angiogenesis (especially during wound healing), matrix cell adhesion, and tissue remodeling (*156*). SPARC is regarded as a marker of activated fibroblasts (*157*). SPARC knockout mice grow cancers faster than mice expressing SPARC highlighting its growth inhibitory functions (*158*, *159*). When evaluating SPARC expression in primary pancreatic cancers, we observed different stromal SPARC expression patterns.

4.2   microRNA Alterations in Pancreatic Cancer

MicroRNAs are small 22 nucleotide noncoding RNAs that function as post-transcriptional regulators. Impressively, ~20% of all genes are microRNA targets. MicroRNAs are formed from larger hairpin RNA transcripts that are degraded by an the RNA enzyme DICER, then associate with an RNA-induced silencing complex (RISC) and bind to the 3′ untranslated regions of many genes thereby inducing RNA degradation or translational repression. Over 400 hundred microRNAs have been identified and widespread alterations in these microRNAs have been identified in various types of cancer including pancreatic cancer (*160–164*). MicroRNA alterations in cancers can be classified according to the developmental origin of the tissue (*165*). While the expression of most microRNAs appear to be reduced in cancer, several microRNAs are overexpressed. The mechanism of these microRNA alterations in human cancers is largely unknown, although epigenetic suppression of microRNA has been described (*166*).

5   Proteomics Alterations of Pancreatic Cancer

Proteomics is the large-scale analysis of unknown proteins in biologic fluids or cells. Proteomics studies are studies that use direct characterization of proteins in contrast to global gene expression profiling, which can be used to prioritize protein expression studies. Direct proteomics strategies have certain advantages. First, there may be significant dissociation between overexpressed transcripts and overexpressed proteins; indeed such discordance has been reported in comparisons of global transcriptomic and proteomic analyses of other human cancers (*17*). Second, because most expression techniques use "bulk" homogenates of cell lines and/or tissues, there is no preferential enrichment for the secreted class of proteins (i.e., the cancer "secretome") (*18*), the portion of the proteome expected to harbor the most promising biomarkers. Indeed, the analysis of bulk tissues that contain mixtures of different cell types can lead to incorrect assignment of the expression status of RNAs or proteins (*167*). Furthermore, although global gene expression profiling of human tissues has led to the identification of important protein alterations in pancreatic cancer, only a few such proteins show promise as biomarkers. A major goal for investigators attempting to identify pancreatic cancer diagnostic markers is to identify the equivalent of a "PSA test" for pancreatic cancer. Although gene expression profiling has been a useful tool for identifying proteins overexpressed in pancreatic cancers such as mesothelin, PSCA, MIC-1, and osteopontin, the direct analysis of unknown proteins in pancreatic cancer tissues is important because many novel cancer protein alterations are post-transcriptional alterations that would not be evident from RNA analysis. Direct and large-scale analysis of proteins using proteomics approaches has the potential to overcome some of the limitations of relying on gene expression analysis, although these approaches come with their own limitations. Proteomics strategies are considered particularly useful for characterizing tissue samples that can not be characterized using gene expression approaches such as secondary fluids like serum, plasma or pancreatic juice. RNA profiling approaches do not readily distinguish secreted from nonsecreted proteins.

A variety of proteomics approaches have also been utilized in an attempt to identify protein markers of pancreatic cancer (*167–183*). Proteomics studies identify hundreds of proteins and protein fragments. With this in mind, the Human Protein Reference Database (HPRD) (http://www.hprd.org) was developed to serve as a comprehensive collection of protein features, post-translational modifications and protein–protein interactions.

Several groups have identified protein fragments in serum using the mass spectrometry technique known as surface enhanced laser desorption ionization (SELDI) and some of these protein fragments appear to perform as well or better than serum CA19–9 as a diagnostic marker (*141, 184*). Several peptides we identified as diagnostically promising have also been identified by others (*185, 186*). There can be problems with assay reproducibility using SELDI unless appropriate technical and analytical measures are taken (*186–189*), in part reflecting the complexity of the proteome and their sensitivity to alterations (*188, 189*). Another mass spectrometry approach utilizes matrix associated laser desorption ionization (MALDI) and has been used to identify pancreatic cancer proteins in serum. One interesting approach utilizes stable isotope labeling with amino acids in cell culture (SILAC) to compare the proteins secreted pancreatic cancer cells from non-neoplastic pancreatic ductal cells (*182*). Antibody microarrays are a promising discovery strategy for profiling serum proteins and have the potential to profile hundreds of protein in sera simultaneously (*190*). Another approach has been to selectively characterize serum glycoproteins (*170*). Pancreatic juice has also been investigated as a source of pancreatic cancer markers. For example, investigators have used one-dimensional gel electrophoresis followed by liquid chromatography tandem mass spectrometry as well as SELDI to identify potential markers of pancreatic cancer (*191, 192*). Several groups have applied proteomics approaches to pancreatic cancer cells rather than secondary sources such as serum and compared them with normal and inflamed pancreas (*193, 194*). This approach has the advantage of evaluating proteins from the source tissue, but since primary tissues reflect a mixture of multiple cell types, determining the relative abundance of proteins in one tissue versus another can be a challenge. On the other hand, many of the proteins identified from serum proteomics studies are high-abundance proteins, and many of the differentially expressed proteins identified are not suitable for diagnostic use. Thus, despite much effort by proteomics investigators to identify markers of pancreatic and other cancers by profiling proteins, only limited success has been achieved to date in identifying markers that will ultimately be useful as diagnostic tests. This limited success highlights the challenge of interrogating the large numbers of proteins in the proteome (hundreds of thousands of proteins and protein modifications), their complex biology, the vexing chemical properties of proteins that can make them hard to separate, and the influence of physiologic states, sample collection, and sample handling can have on protein profiles (*195, 196*). For example, proteolysis of serum and other samples can continue after collection, ex vivo due to the continued activity of circulating proteolytic enzymes (*197*). Another problem that may arise when undertaking marker discovery studies is bias, wherein markers are identified that purport to reflect differences between patients with disease versus those without, but merely reflect trivial differences in the study populations such as patient age, or differences that arise from differences in sample handling or data interpretation (*198*). The problem of bias has been prominent in proteomics studies, which uses a highly sensitive discovery technology that does not easily distinguish artefactual and nonspecific alterations from biologically relevant ones. Despite these problems, recent proteomics studies have identified novel proteins and have also led to a greater understanding of the "peptidome," the small peptides of many proteins found in the circulation and in other compartments that result from protease digestion that arise in inflammatory and neoplastic states (*199*).

6   Conclusion

In conclusion, the molecular profiles of pancreatic cancer continue to be elucidated. In particular, comprehensive sequencing of the pancreatic cancer genome and continued characterization of epigenetic and proteomic profiles of pancreatic cancer is helping scientists to better understand the biology of this devastating disease. Perhaps more importantly, these discoveries are forming the basis of a new generation of studies evaluating molecular diagnostic markers of pancreatic neoplasia. Accurate markers of preinvasive pancreatic neoplasms can be used to help predict future cancer risk among individuals undergoing pancreatic screening. It is also likely that we will also see advances in our understanding and management of familial pancreatic cancer led by the discovery of additional genes responsible for pancreatic cancer susceptibility. Such discoveries will provide opportunities for genetic counseling and screening. Ultimately, it is expected that the discovery of better molecular markers of pancreatic cancer will be useful to help decide whether a patient's cancer is likely to respond to the novel therapies.

Acknowledgment This work was supported by the National Cancer Institute grant (CA90709, CA120432, CA62924), and the Michael Rolfe Foundation.

References

1. Hansel DE, Kern SE, Hruban RH. 2003, Molecular pathogenesis of pancreatic cancer. Annu Rev Genomics Hum Genet 4:237–256.
2. Wilentz RE, Geradts J, Maynard R, 1998, Inactivation of the p16 (INK4A) tumor-suppressor gene in pancreatic duct lesions: loss of intranuclear expression. Cancer Res 58:4740–4744.
3. Redston MS, Caldas C, Seymour AB, 1994, p53 mutations in pancreatic carcinoma and evidence of common involvement of homocopolymer tracts in DNA microdeletions. Cancer Res 54:3025–3033.
4. Goggins M, Schutte M, Lu J, 1996, Germline BRCA2 gene mutations in patients with apparently sporadic pancreatic carcinomas. Cancer Res 56:5360–5364.
5. Heijden MS, van der Yeo CJ, Hruban RH, Kern SE. 2003, Fanconi anemia gene mutations in young-onset pancreatic cancer. Cancer Res 63:2585–2588.

6. Sjoblom T, Jones S, Wood LD, et al. 2006, The consensus coding sequences of human breast and colorectal cancers. Science 314:268–274.
7. Lengauer C, Kinzler KW, Vogelstein B. 1997, Genetic instability in colorectal cancers. Nature 386:623–627.
8. Gallmeier E, Kern SE. 2007, Targeting Fanconi anemia/BRCA2 pathway defects in cancer: the significance of preclinical pharmacogenomic models. Clin Cancer Res 13:4–10.
9. Matsubayashi H, Skinner H, Iacobuzio-Donahue C, 2005, Pancreaticobiliary cancers with deficient methylenetetrahydrofolate reductase genotypes. Clin Gastro Hepatol 3:752–760.
10. Iacobuzio-Donahue CA, Heijden MS, van der Baumgartner MR, 2004, Large-scale allelotype of pancreaticobiliary carcinoma provides quantitative estimates of genome-wide allelic loss. Cancer Res 64:871–875.
11. Calhoun ES, Hucl T, Gallmeier E, 2006, Identifying allelic loss and homozygous deletions in pancreatic cancer without matched normals using high-density single-nucleotide polymorphism arrays. Cancer Res 66:7920–7928.
12. Mahlamaki EH, Kauraniemi P, Monni O, 2004, High-resolution genomic and expression profiling reveals 105 putative amplification target genes in pancreatic cancer. Neoplasia 6:432–439.
13. Holzmann K, Kohlhammer H, Schwaenen C, 2004, Genomic DNA-chip hybridization reveals a higher incidence of genomic amplifications in pancreatic cancer than conventional comparative genomic hybridization and leads to the identification of novel candidate genes. Cancer Res 64:4428–4433.
14. Aguirre AJ, Brennan C, Bailey G, 2004, High-resolution characterization of the pancreatic adenocarcinoma genome. Proc Natl Acad Sci U S A 101:9067–9072.
15. Bashyam MD, Bair R, Kim YH, 2005, Array-based comparative genomic hybridization identifies localized DNA amplifications and homozygous deletions in pancreatic cancer. Neoplasia 7:556–562.
16. Heidenblad M, Lindgren D, Veltman JA, 2005, Microarray analyses reveal strong influence of DNA copy number alterations on the transcriptional patterns in pancreatic cancer: implications for the interpretation of genomic amplifications. Oncogene 24:1794–1801.
17. Goggins M, Offerhaus GJA, Hilgers W, 1998, Pancreatic adenocarcinomas with DNA replication errors (RER+) are associated with wild-type K-ras and characteristic histopathology: poor differentiation, a syncytial growth pattern, and pushing borders suggest RER+. Am J Pathol 152:1501–1507.
18. Maitra A, Cohen Y, Gillespie SE, 2004, The human MitoChip: a high-throughput sequencing microarray for mitochondrial mutation detection. Genome Res 14:812–819.
19. Canto MI, Goggins M, Hruban RH, 2006, Screening for early pancreatic neoplasia in high-risk individuals: a prospective controlled study. Clin Gastrol Hepatol 4:766–781.
20. Canto MI, Goggins M, Yeo CJ, 2004, Screening for pancreatic neoplasia in high risk individuals. Clin Gastro Hepatol 2:606–621.
21. Brentnall TA, Bronner MP, Byrd DR, 1999, Early diagnosis and treatment of pancreatic dysplasia in patients with a family history of pancreatic cancer. Ann Intern Med 131:247–255.
22. Almoguera C, Shibata D, Forrester K, 1988, Most human carcinomas of the exocrine pancreas contain mutant c-K-ras genes. Cell 53:549–554.
23. Caldas C, Hahn SA, Hruban RH, 1994, Detection of K-ras mutations in the stool of patients with pancreatic adenocarcinoma and pancreatic ductal hyperplasia. Cancer Res 54:3568–3573.
24. Hruban RH, Mansfeld AD, van Offerhaus GJ, 1993, K-ras oncogene activation in adenocarcinoma of the human pancreas. A study of 82 carcinomas using a combination of mutant-enriched polymerase chain reaction analysis and allele-specific oligonucleotide hybridization. Am J Pathol 143:545–554.
25. Tabata T, Fujimori T, Maeda S, 1993, The role of Ras mutation in pancreatic cancer, precancerous lesions, and chronic pancreatitis. Int J Pancreatol 14:237–244.
26. Lohr M, Maisonneuve P, Lowenfels AB. 2000, K-Ras mutations and benign pancreatic disease. Int J Pancreatol 27:93–103.

27. Yamada T, Nakamori S, Ohzato H, 1998, Detection of K-ras gene mutations in plasma DNA of patients with pancreatic adenocarcinoma: correlation with clinicopathological features. Clin Cancer Res 4:1527–1532.

28. Mulcahy HE, Lyautey J, Lederrey C, 1998, A prospective study of K-ras mutations in the plasma of pancreatic cancer patients. Clin Cancer Res 4:271–275.

29. Shi C, Eshleman SH, Jones D, 2004, LigAmp for sensitive detection of single-nucleotide differences. Nat Methods 1:141–147. Epub 2004 Oct 21.

30. Bian YMH, Pin-Li C, Abe T, 2006, Detecting low-abundance p16 and p53 mutations in pancreatic juice using a novel assay: heteroduplex analysis of limiting dilution PCRs. Cancer Biol Ther 5:1392–1399.

31. Yan L, McFaul C, Howes N, 2005, Molecular analysis to detect pancreatic ductal adenocarcinoma in high-risk groups. Gastroenterology 128:2124–2130.

32. Heijden MS, van der Brody JR, Gallmeier E, 2004, Functional defects in the fanconi anemia pathway in pancreatic cancer cells. Am J Pathol 165:651–657.

33. Sato N, Goggins M. 2006, Epigenetic alterations in intraductal papillary mucinous neoplasms of the pancreas. J Hepatobiliary Pancreat Surg 13:280–285.

34. Sato N, Goggins M. 2006, The role of epigenetic alterations in pancreatic cancer. J Hepatobiliary Pancreat Surg 13:286–295.

35. Laird PW. 2005, Cancer epigenetics. Hum Mol Genet 14:R65–76.

36. Laird PW. 2003, The power and the promise of DNA methylation markers. Nat Rev Cancer 3:253–266.

37. Baylin SB, Chen WY. 2005, Aberrant gene silencing in tumor progression: implications for control of cancer. Cold Spring Harb Symp Quant Biol 70:427–433.

38. Baylin SB, Ohm JE. 2006, Epigenetic gene silencing in cancer—a mechanism for early oncogenic pathway addiction? Nat Rev Cancer 6:107–116.

39. Herman JG, Baylin SB. 2003, Gene silencing in cancer in association with promoter hypermethylation. N Engl J Med 349:2042–2054.

40. Egger G, Liang G, Aparicio A, 2004, Epigenetics in human disease and prospects for epigenetic therapy. Nature 429:457–463.

41. Anway MD, Cupp AS, Uzumcu M, 2005, Epigenetic transgenerational actions of endocrine disruptors and male fertility. Science 308:1466–1469.

42. Fraga MF, Ballestar E, Paz MF, 2005, Epigenetic differences arise during the lifetime of monozygotic twins. Proc Natl Acad Sci U S A 102:10604–10609. Epub 2005 Jul 11.

43. Feinberg AP, Ohlsson R, Henikoff S. 2006, The epigenetic progenitor origin of human cancer. Nat Rev Genet 7:21–33.

44. Huusko P, Ponciano-Jackson D, Wolf M, 2004, Nonsense-mediated decay microarray analysis identifies mutations of EPHB2 in human prostate cancer. Nat Genet 36:979–983. Epub 2004 Aug 8.

45. Morgan HD, Sutherland HG, Martin DI, Whitelaw E. 1999, Epigenetic inheritance at the agouti locus in the mouse. Nat Genet 23:314–318.

46. Dolinoy DC, Weidman JR, Waterland RA, 2006, Maternal genistein alters coat color and protects Avy mouse offspring from obesity by modifying the fetal epigenome. Environ Health Perspect 114:567–572.

47. Waterland RA, Jirtle RL. 2003, Transposable elements: targets for early nutritional effects on epigenetic gene regulation. Mol Cell Biol 23:5293–5300.

48. Blewitt ME, Vickaryous NK, Paldi A, 2006, Dynamic reprogramming of DNA methylation at an epigenetically sensitive allele in mice. PLoS Genet 2:e49. Epub 2006 Apr 7.

49. Bachman KE PB, Rhee I, Rajagopalan H, 2003, Histone modifications and silencing prior to DNA methylation of a tumor suppressor gene Cancer Cell 3:89–95.

50. Ishihara K, Oshimura M, Nakao M. 2006, CTCF-dependent chromatin insulator is linked to epigenetic remodeling. Mol Cell 23:733–742.

51. Pruitt K, Zinn RL, Ohm JE, 2006, Inhibition of SIRT1 reactivates silenced cancer genes without loss of promoter DNA hypermethylation. PLoS Genet 2:e40. Epub 2006 Mar 31.

52. Song JZ SC, Harrison J, Melki JR, 2002, Hypermethylation trigger of the glutathione-S-transferase gene (GSTP1) in prostate cancer cells. Oncogene 21:1048–1061.

53. Croce L, Di Raker VA, Corsaro M, 2002, Methyltransferase recruitment and DNA hypermethylation of target promoters by an oncogenic transcription factor. Science 295:1079–1082.
54. Bock C, Paulsen M, Tierling S, 2006, CpG island methylation in human lymphocytes is highly correlated with DNA sequence, repeats, and predicted DNA structure. PLoS Genet 2:e26.
55. Frigola J, Song J, Stirzaker C, 2006, Epigenetic remodeling in colorectal cancer results in coordinate gene suppression across an entire chromosome band. Nat Genet 38:540–549. Epub 2006 Apr 23.
56. Schutte M, Hruban RH, Geradts J, 1997, Abrogation of the Rb/p16 tumor-suppressive pathway in virtually all pancreatic carcinomas. Cancer Res 57:3126–3130.
57. Ueki T, Toyota M, Sohn T, 2000, Hypermethylation of multiple genes in pancreatic adenocarcinoma. Cancer Res 60:1835–1839.
58. Toyota M, Ahuja N, Ohe-Toyota M, 1999, CpG island methylator phenotype in colorectal cancer. Proc Natl Acad Sci U S A 96:8681–8686.
59. Ueki T, Toyota M, Skinner H, 2001, Identification and characterization of differentially methylated CpG islands in pancreatic carcinoma. Cancer Res 61:8540–8546.
60. Weisenberger DJ, Siegmund KD, Campan M, 2006, CpG island methylator phenotype underlies sporadic microsatellite instability and is tightly associated with BRAF mutation in colorectal cancer. Nat Genet 38:787–793. Epub 2006 Jun 25.
61. Jansen M, Fukushima N, Rosty C, 2002, Aberrant methylation of the 5Î CpG island of TSLC1 is common in pancreatic ductal adenocarcinoma and is first manifest in high-grade PanINs. Cancer Biol Ther 1:293–296.
62. Fukushima N, Sato N, Sahin F, 2003, Aberrant methylation of suppressor of cytokine signalling-1 (SOCS-1) gene in pancreatic ductal neoplasms. Br J Cancer 89:338–343.
63. Matsubayashi H, Sato N, Fukushima N, 2003, Methylation of cyclin D2 is observed frequently in pancreatic cancer but is also an age-related phenomenon in gastrointestinal tissues. Clin Cancer Res 9:1446–1452.
64. Kuroki T, Yendamuri S, Trapasso F, 2004, The tumor suppressor gene WWOX at FRA16D is involved in pancreatic carcinogenesis. Clin Cancer Res 10:2459–2465.
65. Xu S, Furukawa T, Kanai N, 2005, Abrogation of DUSP6 by hypermethylation in human pancreatic cancer. J Hum Genet 50:159–167. Epub 2005 Apr 12.
66. Martin ST, Sato N, Dhara S, 2005, Aberrant methylation of the human hedgehog interacting protein (HHIP) gene in pancreatic neoplasms. Cancer Biol Ther 4:728–733.
67. Fukushima N, Sato N, Ueki T, 2002, Preproenkephalin and p16 gene CpG island hypermethylation in pancreatic intraepithelial neoplasia (PanIN) and pancreatic ductal adenocarcinoma. Am J Pathol 160:1573–1581.
68. Hruban RH, Takaori K, Klimstra DS, 2004, An illustrated consensus on the classification of pancreatic intraepithelial neoplasia and intraductal papillary mucinous neoplasms. Am J Surg Pathol 28:977–987.
69. Sato N, Ueki T, Fukushima N, 2002, Aberrant methylation of CpG islands in intraductal papillary mucinous neoplasms of the pancreas increases with histological grade. Gastroenterology 123:1365–1372.
70. Sato N, Parker AR, Fukushima N, 2005, Epigenetic inactivation of TFPI-2 as a common mechanism associated with growth and invasion of pancreatic ductal adenocarcinoma. Oncogene 24:850–858.
71. Sato N, Maitra A, Fukushima N, 2003, Frequent hypomethylation of multiple genes overexpressed in pancreatic ductal adenocarcinoma. Cancer Res 63:4158–4166.
72. Sato N, Fukushima N, Maitra A, 2003, Discovery of novel targets for aberrant methylation in pancreatic carcinoma using high-throughput microarrays. Cancer Res 63:3735–3742.
73. Sato N, Matsubayashi H, Abe T, 2005, Epigenetic down-regulation of CDKN1C/p57KIP2 in pancreatic ductal neoplasms identified by gene expression profiling. Clin Cancer Res 11:4681–4688.
74. Sato N, Fukushima N, Chang R, 2006, Differential and epigenetic gene expression profiling identifies frequent disruption of the RELN pathway in pancreatic cancers. Gastroenterology 130:548–565.

75. Yan PS, Efferth T, Chen HL, 2002, Use of CpG island microarrays to identify colorectal tumors with a high degree of concurrent methylation. Methods 27:162–169.
76. Yan PS, Chen CM, Shi H, 2001, Dissecting complex epigenetic alterations in breast cancer using CpG island microarrays. Cancer Res 61:8375–8380.
77. Wei SH, Chen CM, Strathdee G, 2002, Methylation microarray analysis of late-stage ovarian carcinomas distinguishes progression-free survival in patients and identifies candidate epigenetic markers. Clin Cancer Res 8:2246–2252.
78. Doorn R, van Zoutman WH, Dijkman R, 2005, Epigenetic profiling of cutaneous T-cell lymphoma: promoter hypermethylation of multiple tumor suppressor genes including BCL7a, PTPRG, and p73. J Clin Oncol 23:3886–3896. Epub 2005 May 16.
79. Ballestar E, Paz MF, Valle L, 2003, Methyl-CpG binding proteins identify novel sites of epigenetic inactivation in human cancer. Embo J 22:6335–6345.
80. Shi H, Wei SH, Leu YW, 2003, Triple analysis of the cancer epigenome: an integrated microarray system for assessing gene expression, DNA methylation, and histone acetylation. Cancer Res 63:2164–2171.
81. Kondo Y, Shen L, Yan PS, 2004, Chromatin immunoprecipitation microarrays for identification of genes silenced by histone H3 lysine 9 methylation. Proc Natl Acad Sci U S A 101:7398–7403. Epub 2004 May 3.
82. D'Arcangelo G, Homayouni R, Keshvara L, 1999, Reelin is a ligand for lipoprotein receptors. Neuron 24:471–479.
83. Sato N, Fukushima N, Maehara N, 2003, SPARC/osteonectin is a frequent target for aberrant methylation in pancreatic adenocarcinoma and a mediator of tumor-stromal interactions. Oncogene 22:5021–5030.
84. Sato N, Maehara N, Goggins M. 2004, Gene expression profiling of tumor-stromal interactions between pancreatic cancer cells and stromal fibroblasts. Cancer Res 64:6950–6956.
85. Infante JR MH, Sato N, Tonascia J, et al. 2007, Peritumoral fibroblast SPARC expression and patient outcome with resectable pancreatic adenocarcinoma. J Clin Onc 25:319–325.
86. Akada M, Crnogorac-Jurcevic T, Lattimore S, 2005, Intrinsic chemoresistance to gemcitabine is associated with decreased expression of BNIP3 in pancreatic cancer. Clin Cancer Res 11:3094–3101.
87. Erkan M, Kleeff J, Esposito I, 2005, Loss of BNIP3 expression is a late event in pancreatic cancer contributing to chemoresistance and worsened prognosis. Oncogene 24:4421–4432.
88. Sato N, Matsubayashi H, Fukushima N, et al. 2005, The chemokine receptor CXCR4 is regulated by DNA methylation in pancreatic cancer. Cancer Biol Ther 4:70–76.
89. Feinberg AP, Tycko B. 2004, The history of cancer epigenetics. Nat Rev Cancer 4:143–153.
90. Chen RZ, Pettersson U, Beard C, 1998, DNA hypomethylation leads to elevated mutation rates. Nature 395:89–93.
91. Yamada Y, Jackson-Grusby L, Linhart H, 2005, Opposing effects of DNA hypomethylation on intestinal and liver carcinogenesis. Proc Natl Acad Sci U S A 102:13580–13585. Epub 2005 Sep 8.
92. Gaudet F, Hodgson JG, Eden A, 2003, Induction of tumors in mice by genomic hypomethylation. Science 300:489–492.
93. Eden A, Gaudet F, Waghmare A, 2003, Chromosomal instability and tumors promoted by DNA hypomethylation. Science 300:455.
94. Lin H, Yamada Y, Nguyen S, 2006, Suppression of intestinal neoplasia by deletion of Dnmt3b. Mol Cell Biol 26:2976–2983.
95. Stolzenberg-Solomon RZ, Albanes D, Nieto FJ, 1999, Pancreatic cancer risk and nutrition-related methyl-group availability indicators in male smokers. J Natl Cancer Inst 91:535–541.
96. Stolzenberg-Solomon RZ, Pietinen P, Barrett MJ, 2001, Dietary and other methyl-group availability factors and pancreatic cancer risk in a cohort of male smokers. Am J Epidemiol 153:680–687.
97. Sato N, Fukushima N, Matsubayashi H, 2004, Identification of maspin and S100P as novel hypomethylation targets in pancreatic cancer using global gene expression profiling. Oncogene 23:1531–1538.

98. Goggins M. 2005, Molecular markers of early pancreatic cancer. J Clin Oncol 23:4524–4531.
99. Hruban R KA, Eshleman J, Axilbund JE, et al. Familial pancreatic cancer. Expert Rev Gastroenterol Hepatol 2007, in press.
100. Herman JG, Graff JR, Myohanen S, 1996, Methylation-specific PCR: a novel PCR assay for methylation status of CpG islands. Proc Natl Acad Sci U S A 93:9821–9826.
101. Fukushima N, Walter KM, Ueki T, 2003, Diagnosing pancreatic cancer using methylation specific PCR analysis of pancreatic juice. Cancer Biol Ther 2:78–83.
102. Matsubayashi H, Canto M, Sato N, 2006, DNA methylation alterations in the pancreatic juice of patients with suspected pancreatic disease. Cancer Res 66:1208–1217.
103. Jiao L, Zhu J, Hassan MM, 2007, K-ras mutation and p16 and preproenkephalin promoter hypermethylation in plasma DNA of pancreatic cancer patients: in relation to cigarette smoking. Pancreas 34:55–62.
104. Ohtsubo K, Watanabe H, Yao F, 2006, Preproenkephalin hypermethylation in the pure pancreatic juice compared with p53 mutation in the diagnosis of pancreatic carcinoma. J Gastroenterol 41:791–797.
105. Jiang P, Watanabe H, Okada G, 2006, Diagnostic utility of aberrant methylation of tissue factor pathway inhibitor 2 in pure pancreatic juice for pancreatic carcinoma. Cancer Sci 97:1267–1273. Epub 2006 Sep 5.
106. Watanabe H, Okada G, Ohtsubo K, 2006, Aberrant methylation of secreted apoptosis-related protein 2 (SARP2) in pure pancreatic juice in diagnosis of pancreatic neoplasms. Pancreas 32:382–389.
107. Matsubayashi H, Sato N, Brune K, 2005, Age- and disease-related methylation of multiple genes in non-neoplastic duodenal tissues. Clin Cancer Res 11:573–583.
108. Cubilla AL, Fitzgerald PJ. 1976, Morphological lesions associated with human primary invasive nonendocrine pancreas cancer. Cancer Res 36:2690–2698.
109. Kantarjian HM, O'Brien S, Shan J, 2006, Update of the decitabine experience in higher risk myelodysplastic syndrome and analysis of prognostic factors associated with outcome. Cancer 109:265–273.
110. Garcia-Manero G, Kantarjian HM, Sanchez-Gonzalez B, 2006, Phase 1/2 study of the combination of 5-aza-2Î-deoxycytidine with valproic acid in patients with leukemia. Blood 108:3271–3279. Epub 2006 Aug 1.
111. Marks PA, Jiang X. 2005, Histone deacetylase inhibitors in programmed cell death and cancer therapy. Cell Cycle 4:549–551. Epub 2005 Apr 28.
112. http://www.fda.gov/ohrms/dockets/98fr/84n-0102-lst0101–01.pdf.
113. Arnold NB, Arkus N, Gunn J, 2007, The histone deacetylase inhibitor suberoylanilide hydroxamic Acid induces growth inhibition and enhances gemcitabine-induced cell death in pancreatic cancer. Clin Cancer Res 13:18–26.
114. Iacobuzio-Donahue CA, Ashfaq R, Maitra A, 2003, Highly expressed genes in pancreatic ductal adenocarcinomas: a comprehensive characterization and comparison of the transcription profiles obtained from three major technologies. Cancer Res 63:8614–8622.
115. Li D, Zhu J, Firozi PF, 2003, Overexpression of oncogenic STK15/BTAK/Aurora A kinase in human pancreatic cancer. Clin Cancer Res 9:991–997.
116. Iacobuzio-Donahue CAAM, Shen-Ong GL, Heek T, van 2002, Discovery of novel tumor markers of pancreatic cancer using global gene expression technology. Am J Pathol 160:1239–1249.
117. Iacobuzio-Donahue C, Maitra A, Olsen M, 2003, Exploration of global gene expression patterns in pancreatic adenocarcinoma using cDNA microarrays. Am J Pathol 162:1151–1162.
118. Hustinx SR, Cao D, Maitra A, 2004, Differentially expressed genes in pancreatic ductal adenocarcinomas identified through serial analysis of gene expression. Cancer Biol Ther 3:1254–1261.
119. Sato N, Fukushima N, Maitra A, 2004, Gene expression profiling identifies genes associated with invasive intraductal papillary mucinous neoplasms of the pancreas. Am J Pathol 164:903–914.

120. Logsdon CD, Simeone DM, Binkley C, 2003, Molecular profiling of pancreatic adenocarcinoma and chronic pancreatitis identifies multiple genes differentially regulated in pancreatic cancer. Cancer Res 63:2649–2657.
121. Missiaglia E, Blaveri E, Terris B, 2004, Analysis of gene expression in cancer cell lines identifies candidate markers for pancreatic tumorigenesis and metastasis. Int J Cancer 112:100–112.
122. Prasad NB, Biankin AV, Fukushima N, 2005, Gene expression profiles in pancreatic intraepithelial neoplasia reflect the effects of Hedgehog signaling on pancreatic ductal epithelial cells. Cancer Res 65:1619–1626.
123. Ricci F, Kern SE, Hruban RH, 2005, Stromal responses to carcinomas of the pancreas: juxtatumoral gene expression conforms to the infiltrating pattern and not the biologic subtype. Cancer Biol Ther 4:302–307. Epub 2005 Mar 23.
124. Heek NT, van Meeker AK, Kern SE, 2002, Telomere shortening is nearly universal in pancreatic intraepithelial neoplasia. Am J Pathol 161:1541–1547.
125. Maitra A, Adsay NV, Argani P, 2003, Multicomponent analysis of the pancreatic adenocarcinoma progression model using a pancreatic intraepithelial neoplasia tissue microarray. Mod Pathol 16:902–912.
126. Swierczynski SL, Maitra A, Abraham SC, 2004, Analysis of novel tumor markers in pancreatic and biliary carcinomas using tissue microarrays. Hum Pathol 35:357–366.
127. Cao D, Hustinx SR, Sui G, 2004, Identification of novel highly expressed genes in pancreatic ductal adenocarcinomas through a bioinformatics analysis of expressed sequence tags. Cancer Biol Ther 3:1081–1089, discussion 90–9-1. Epub 2004 Nov 12..
128. Hustinx SR, Cao D, Maitra A, 2004, Differentially expressed genes in pancreatic ductal adenocarcinomas identified through serial analysis of gene expression. Cancer Biol Ther 3:1254–1261. Epub 2004 Dec 14.
129. Cao D, Maitra A, Saavedra JA, 2005, Expression of novel markers of pancreatic ductal adenocarcinoma in pancreatic nonductal neoplasms: additional evidence of different genetic pathways. Mod Pathol 18:752–761.
130. Sato N, Fukushima N, Maitra A, 2004, Gene expression profiling identifies genes associated with invasive intraductal papillary mucinous neoplasms of the pancreas. Am J Pathol 164:903–914.
131. Fukushima N, Sato N, Prasad N, 2004, Characterization of gene expression in mucinous cystic neoplasms of the pancreas using oligonucleotide microarrays. Oncogene 23:9042–9051.
132. Hansel DE, Rahman A, House M, 2004, Met proto-oncogene and insulin-like growth factor binding protein 3 overexpression correlates with metastatic ability in well-differentiated pancreatic endocrine neoplasms. Clin Cancer Res 10:6152–6158.
133. Ohuchida K, Mizumoto K, Ogura Y, 2005, Quantitative assessment of telomerase activity and human telomerase reverse transcriptase messenger RNA levels in pancreatic juice samples for the diagnosis of pancreatic cancer. Clin Cancer Res 11:2285–2292.
134. Cao D, Hustinx SR, Sui G, 2004, Identification of novel highly expressed genes in pancreatic ductal adenocarcinomas through a bioinformatics analysis of expressed sequence tags. Cancer Biol Ther 3:1081–1089.
135. Fukushima N, Sato N, Prasad N, 2004, Characterization of gene expression in mucinous cystic neoplasms of the pancreas using oligonucleotide microarrays. Oncogene 23:9042–9051.
136. Zhou W, Sokoll LJ, Bruzek DJ, 1998, Identifying markers for pancreatic cancer by gene expression analysis. Cancer Epidemiol Biomarkers Prev 7:109–112.
137. Ryu B, Jones J, Hollingsworth MA, 2001, Invasion-specific genes in malignancy serial analysis of gene expression comparisons of primary and passaged cancers. Cancer Res 61:1833–1838.
138. Fukushima N, Koopmann J, Sato N, 2005, Gene expression alterations in the non-neoplastic parenchyma adjacent to infiltrating pancreatic ductal adenocarcinoma. Mod Pathol 18:779–787.

139. Zhou W, Sokoll LJ, Bruzek DJ, et al. 1998, TIMP-1 as a diagnostic marker for pancreatic cancer. Cancer Epi Biomarkers Prev 7:109–112.
140. Koopmann J, Buckhaults P, Brown DA, 2004, Serum macrophage inhibitory cytokine 1 as a marker of pancreatic and other periampullary cancers. Clin Cancer Res 10:2386–2392.
141. Koopmann J, Zhang Z, White N, 2004, Serum diagnosis of pancreatic adenocarcinoma using surface-enhanced laser desorption and ionization mass spectrometry. Clin Cancer Res 10:860–868.
142. Koopmann J, Fedarko NS, Jain A, 2004, Evaluation of Osteopontin as Biomarker for Pancreatic Adenocarcinoma. Cancer Epidemiol Biomarkers Prev 13:487–491.
143. Koopmann J, Rosenweig CN, Zhang Z, 2006, Serum markers in patients with resectable pancreatic adenocarcinoma: MIC-1 vs. CA19-9. Clin Cancer Res 15:442–446.
144. Fukushima N, Koopmann J, Sato N, 2005, Gene expression alterations in the non-neoplastic parenchyma adjacent to infiltrating pancreatic ductal adenocarcinoma. Mod Pathol 18:779–787.
145. Rosty C, Christa L, Kuzdzal S, 2002, Identification of hepatocarcinoma-intestine-pancreas/ pancreatitis-associated protein I as a biomarker for pancreatic ductal adenocarcinoma by protein biochip technology. Cancer Res 62:1868–1875.
146. Argani P, Iacobuzio-Donahue C, Ryu B, 2001, Mesothelin is overexpressed in the vast majority of ductal adenocarcinomas of the pancreas: identification of a new pancreatic cancer marker by serial analysis of gene expression (SAGE). Clin Cancer Res 7:3862–388.
147. McCarthy DM, Maitra A, Argani P, 2003, Novel markers of pancreatic adenocarcinoma in fine-needle aspiration: mesothelin and prostate stem cell antigen labeling increases accuracy in cytologically borderline cases. Appl Immunohistochem Mol Morphol 11:238–243.
148. Brentnall TA, Bronner MP, Byrd DR, 1999, Early diagnosis and treatment of pancreatic dysplasia in patients with a family history of pancreatic cancer. Ann Intern Med 131: 247–255.
149. Hu M, Yao J, Cai L, 2005, Distinct epigenetic changes in the stromal cells of breast cancers. Nat Genet 37:899–905. Epub 2005 Jul 10.
150. Qian J, Niu J, Li M, 2005, In vitro modeling of human pancreatic duct epithelial cell transformation defines gene expression changes induced by K-ras oncogenic activation in pancreatic carcinogenesis. Cancer Res 65:5045–5053.
151. Orimo A, Weinberg RA. 2006, Stromal fibroblasts in cancer: a novel tumor-promoting cell type. Cell Cycle 5:1597–1601. Epub 2006 Aug 1.
152. Orimo A, Gupta PB, Sgroi DC, 2005, Stromal fibroblasts present in invasive human breast carcinomas promote tumor growth and angiogenesis through elevated SDF-1/CXCL12 secretion. Cell 121:335–348.
153. Chang HY, Sneddon JB, Alizadeh AA, 2004, Gene expression signature of fibroblast serum response predicts human cancer progression: similarities between tumors and wounds. PLoS Biol 2:E7. Epub 2004 Jan 13.
154. Chang HY, Chi JT, Dudoit S, 2002, Diversity, topographic differentiation, and positional memory in human fibroblasts. Proc Natl Acad Sci U S A 99:12877–12882. Epub 2002 Sep 24.
155. Iyer VR, Eisen MB, Ross DT, 1999, The transcriptional program in the response of human fibroblasts to serum. Science 283:83–87.
156. Funk SE, Sage EH. 1991, The Ca2(+)-binding glycoprotein SPARC modulates cell cycle progression in bovine aortic endothelial cells. Proc Natl Acad Sci U S A 88:2648–2652.
157. Kalluri R, Zeisberg M. 2006, Fibroblasts in cancer. Nat Rev Cancer 6:392.
158. Puolakkainen PA, Brekken RA, Muneer S, 2004, Enhanced growth of pancreatic tumors in SPARC-null mice is associated with decreased deposition of extracellular matrix and reduced tumor cell apoptosis. Mol Cancer Res 2:215–224.
159. Brekken RA, Puolakkainen P, Graves DC, 2003, Enhanced growth of tumors in SPARC null mice is associated with changes in the ECM. J Clin Invest 111:487–495.
160. Cummins JM, He Y, Leary RJ, 2006, The colorectal microRNAome. Proc Natl Acad Sci U S A 103:3687–3692. Epub 2006 Feb 27.

161. Yanaihara N, Caplen N, Bowman E, 2006, Unique microRNA molecular profiles in lung cancer diagnosis and prognosis. Cancer Cell 9:189–198.
162. Calin GA, Ferracin M, Cimmino A, 2005, A MicroRNA signature associated with prognosis and progression in chronic lymphocytic leukemia. N Engl J Med 353:1793–1801.
163. Lu J, Getz G, Miska EA, 2005, MicroRNA expression profiles classify human cancers. Nature 435:834–838.
164. Calin GA, Liu CG, Sevignani C, 2004, MicroRNA profiling reveals distinct signatures in B cell chronic lymphocytic leukemias. Proc Natl Acad Sci U S A 101:11755–1160. Epub 2004 Jul 29.
165. Xie X, Lu J, Kulbokas EJ, 2005, Systematic discovery of regulatory motifs in human promoters and 3Î UTRs by comparison of several mammals. Nature 434:338–345. Epub 2005 Feb 27.
166. Saito Y, Liang G, Egger G, 2006, Specific activation of microRNA-127 with downregulation of the proto-oncogene BCL6 by chromatin-modifying drugs in human cancer cells. Cancer Cell 9:435–443.
167. Chen R, Yi EC, Donohoe S, 2005, Pancreatic cancer proteome: the proteins that underlie invasion, metastasis, and immunologic escape. Gastroenterology 129:1187–1197.
168. Chen R, Pan S, Cooke K, 2007, Comparison of pancreas juice proteins from cancer versus pancreatitis using quantitative proteomic analysis. Pancreas 34:70–79.
169. Lin Y, Goedegebuure PS, Tan MC, 2006, Proteins associated with disease and clinical course in pancreas cancer: a proteomic analysis of plasma in surgical patients. J Proteome Res 5:2169–2176.
170. Zhao J, Simeone DM, Heidt D, 2006, Comparative serum glycoproteomics using lectin selected sialic acid glycoproteins with mass spectrometric analysis: application to pancreatic cancer serum. J Proteome Res 5:1792–1802.
171. Bloomston M, Zhou JX, Rosemurgy AS, 2006, Fibrinogen gamma overexpression in pancreatic cancer identified by large-scale proteomic analysis of serum samples. Cancer Res 66:2592–2599.
172. Honda K, Hayashida Y, Umaki T, 2005, Possible detection of pancreatic cancer by plasma protein profiling. Cancer Res 65:10613–10622.
173. Crnogorac-Jurcevic T, Gangeswaran R, Bhakta V, 2005, Proteomic analysis of chronic pancreatitis and pancreatic adenocarcinoma. Gastroenterology 129:1454–1463.
174. Gronborg M, Kristiansen TZ, Iwahori A, 2006, Biomarker discovery from pancreatic cancer secretome using a differential proteomic approach. Mol Cell Proteomics 5:157–171. Epub 2005 Oct 8.
175. Yu KH, Rustgi AK, Blair IA. 2005, Characterization of proteins in human pancreatic cancer serum using differential gel electrophoresis and tandem mass spectrometry. J Proteome Res 4:1742–1751.
176. Koomen JM, Li D, Xiao LC, 2005, Direct tandem mass spectrometry reveals limitations in protein profiling experiments for plasma biomarker discovery. J Proteome Res 4:972–981.
177. Mishra GR, Suresh M, Kumaran K, 2006, Human protein reference database—2006 update. Nucleic Acids Res 34:D411–414.
178. Suresh S, Sujatha Mohan S, Mishra G, 2005, Proteomic resources: Integrating biomedical information in humans. Gene 364:13–18. Epub 2005 Oct 3.
179. Ping P, Vondriska TM, Creighton CJ, 2005, A functional annotation of subproteomes in human plasma. Proteomics 5:3506–3519.
180. Crnogorac-Jurcevic T, Gangeswaran R, Bhakta V, 2005, Proteomic analysis of chronic pancreatitis and pancreatic adenocarcinoma. Gastroenterology 129:1454–1463.
181. Chen R, Yi EC, Donohoe S, 2005, Pancreatic cancer proteome: the proteins that underlie invasion, metastasis, and immunologic escape. Gastroenterology 129:1187–1197.
182. Gronborg M, Kristiansen TZ, Iwahori A, 2006, Biomarker discovery from pancreatic cancer secretome using a differential proteomic approach. Mol Cell Proteomics 5:157–171. Epub 2005 Oct 8.
183. Yu KH, Rustgi AK, Blair IA. 2005, Characterization of proteins in human pancreatic cancer serum using differential gel electrophoresis and tandem mass spectrometry. J Proteome Res 4:1742–1751.

184. Bhattacharyya S, Siegel ER, Petersen GM, 2004, Diagnosis of pancreatic cancer using serum proteomic profiling. Neoplasia 6:674–686.
185. Koomen JM, Shih LN, Coombes KR, 2005, Plasma protein profiling for diagnosis of pancreatic cancer reveals the presence of host response proteins. Clin Cancer Res 11:1110–1118.
186. Song J, Patel M, Rosenzweig CN, et al. 2006, Quantification of fragments of human serum inter-{alpha}-trypsin inhibitor heavy chain 4 by a surface-enhanced laser desorption/ionization-based immunoassay. Clin Chem 52:1045–1053.
187. Ransohoff DF. 2005, Lessons from controversy: ovarian cancer screening and serum proteomics. J Natl Cancer Inst 97:315–319.
188. Liotta LA, Lowenthal M, Mehta A, 2005, Importance of communication between producers and consumers of publicly available experimental data. J Natl Cancer Inst 97:310–314.
189. Baggerly KA, Morris JS, Coombes KR. 2004, Reproducibility of SELDI-TOF protein patterns in serum: comparing datasets from different experiments. Bioinformatics 20:777–785. Epub 2004 Jan 29.
190. Baggerly KA, Morris JS, Edmonson SR, 2005, Signal in noise: evaluating reported reproducibility of serum proteomic tests for ovarian cancer. J Natl Cancer Inst 97:307–309.
191. Hamelinck D, Zhou H, Li L, 2005, Optimized normalization for antibody microarrays and application to serum-protein profiling. Mol Cell Proteomics 4:773–784. Epub 2005 Mar 25.
192. Gronborg M, Bunkenborg J, Kristiansen TZ, 2004, Comprehensive Proteomic Analysis of Human Pancreatic Juice. J Proteome Res 3:1042–1055.
193. Rosty C, Christa L, Kuzdzal S, 2002, Identification of hepatocarcinoma-intestine-pancreas/pancreatitis-associated protein I as a biomarker for pancreatic ductal adenocarcinoma by protein biochip technology. Cancer Res 62:1868–1875.
194. Shen J, Person MD, Zhu J, 2004, Protein expression profiles in pancreatic adenocarcinoma compared with normal pancreatic tissue and tissue affected by pancreatitis as detected by two-dimensional gel electrophoresis and mass spectrometry. Cancer Res 64:9018–9026.
195. Shekouh AR, Thompson CC, Prime W, 2003, Application of laser capture microdissection combined with two-dimensional electrophoresis for the discovery of differentially regulated proteins in pancreatic ductal adenocarcinoma. Proteomics 3:1988–2001.
196. Caprioli RM. 2005, Deciphering protein molecular signatures in cancer tissues to aid in diagnosis, prognosis, and therapy. Cancer Res 65:10642–10645.
197. Omenn GS, States DJ, Adamski M, 2005, Overview of the HUPO Plasma Proteome Project: results from the pilot phase with 35 collaborating laboratories and multiple analytical groups, generating a core dataset of 3020 proteins and a publicly-available database. Proteomics 5:3226–3245.
198. Ransohoff DF. 2005, Bias as a threat to the validity of cancer molecular-marker research. Nat Rev Cancer 5:142–149.
199. Villanueva J, Shaffer DR, Philip J, 2006, Differential exoprotease activities confer tumor-specific serum peptidome patterns. J Clin Invest 116:271–284
200. Abe T, Fukushima N, Brune K, Boehm C, Sato N, Matsubayashi H, Canto M, Petersen GM, Hruban RH, Goggins M, 2007, Genome wide allelotypes of familial pancreatic adenocarcinomas and familial and sporadic intraductal papillary mucinous neoplasms. Clin Cancer Res 13:6019–6025.

Section III
Pancreatic Cancer Staging

Chapter 13
Imaging of Pancreatic Adenocarcinoma

Haydee Ojeda-Fournier and K. Ann Choe

Imaging plays a crucial role in the diagnosis, staging, and follow-up of pancreatic adenocarcinoma. In addition to identifying the primary tumor, the goals of imaging in pancreatic cancer include assessment of local and regional invasion, evaluation of lymph nodes and vascular structures, and evaluation for possible metastatic disease. Furthermore, imaging assessment identifies those patients who are candidates for resection—the only known therapy associated with long-term survival—and spares others from unnecessary surgical intervention. There is no indication for plain film evaluation and limited value in using ultrasonography (US) in the evaluation of pancreatic cancer. Because of its invasive nature, angiography has fallen out of favor in the evaluation of pancreatic adenocarcinoma. Cross-sectional imaging, including computed tomography (CT) and MRI, however, meet the stated goals in the assessment of pancreatic cancer. Magnetic resonance cholangiopancreatography (MRCP) can also add valuable information in specific cases. Other important modalities that utilize imaging include EUS, endoscopic retrograde pancreatography (ERCP), and PET are discussed elsewhere in this text.

Ultrasonography (US)

Indication

Sonography is widely available, relatively inexpensive, and noninvasive. It is often used for initial screenings of nonspecific abdominal complaints and evaluation of jaundice. Additional advantages of US include portability, ability to evaluate in real-time and the role it plays in image-guided procedures and intraoperative evaluations. In general, disadvantages of sonography include operator dependence, artifacts—particularly those caused by bowel gas—and limitations caused by patients' body habitus. Because of the location of the pancreas in the retroperitoneum and bowel, neighboring the head and tail of the pancreas, transabdominal US evaluation is inherently limited. The gastric body is anterior to the tail of the pancreas, while

A.M. Lowy et al. (eds.) *Pancreatic Cancer*.
doi: 10.1007/978-0-387-69252-4, © Springer Science+Business Media, LLC 2008

the duodenal loop surrounds the pancreatic head and jejunal loops and splenic flexure are anterior to the tail of the pancreas. As an initial screening study for nonspecific abdominal complaints, one of the best utilizations of US is in the evaluation of liver metastasis and assessment of the common bile and pancreatic ducts. The use of US intraoperatively—either laparoscopically or during a laparotomy—has been described as an additional tool in the evaluation of tumor respectability (*1*).

Technique

The pancreas is evaluated as part of the general abdominal examination. It is best visualized after a 4- to 6-hour fast. This allows for decreased gaseous distention and for the gallbladder and biliary system to distend. Transverse and sagittal midline views, at a slight oblique angle below the level of the xiphoid, provide the best views of the pancreas transabdominally. A curved array detector with lower frequency is utilized to allow evaluation of deeper structures.

In the 1990's, laparoscopic US was reported as an effective tool used for assessing resectability with a reported accuracy of 94% (*2*). Intraoperative sonography has also been used and reported to be useful in the assessment of vascular invasion. In the series by Taylor et al. laparoscopic US prevented unnecessary additional surgery in 53% of their patients. With the new multidetector CT (MDCT) and the use of multiphasic contrast-enhanced protocols, however, the information previously provided by either laparoscopic or intraoperative US is often obsolete.

The use of contrast-enhanced US is also reported in the literature (*3*) as a labor intensive experimental technique that may prove to be of use in the future for the evaluation of small pancreatic tumors; however, US contrast is not available for use in the United States. Again, the new generation CT scanners are superior, and thinner slice protocols can detect small tumors. In a meta-analysis comparing US, CT, and MRI, Bipat and colleagues estimated a sensitivity of 76% and a specificity of 75% for the sonographic diagnosis of pancreatic cancer and for resectability sensitivity and specificity of 83% and of 63%, respectively (*4*). Sonography had the lowest sensitivity and specificity as compared to the other modalities evaluated. Even more recent reports of better staging of resectability by intraoperative US over preoperative CT imaging are flawed by the use of conventional CT data (*1*).

Findings

Characteristic findings of pancreatic cancer during sonography are a hypoechoic mass with ill-defined margins. Unfortunately this is indistinguishable from the sonographic appearance of focal pancreatitis. Associated findings include the presence of dilated common bile and pancreatic ducts (the so called double-duct sign indicating a tumor in the pancreatic head) (see Fig. 13.1), and atrophy of the pancreas. Assessment of lymph node involvement

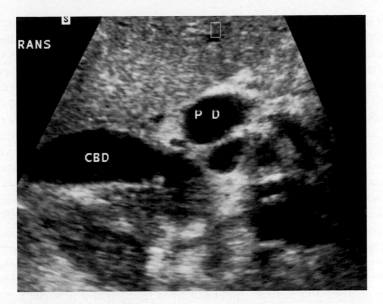

Fig. 13.1 Double duct sign seen by ultrasound. Note marked dilation of the common bile duct. The pancreatic duct which is usually not seen at the time of ultrasound is markedly dilated

by US, as with other modalities, is dependent on size criteria as well as the loss of normal morphologic appearance of the node, including echogenic hilum and smooth hypoechoic cortex. Micrometastasis to the lymph nodes cannot be excluded by the absence of these findings. Evaluation for direct invasion of adjacent organs can be limited by US secondary to location and bowel gas obscuration. Unexplained ascites should raise the suspicion of peritoneal surface metastasis, which is usually too small to resolve by US and other modalities. Evaluation of vessel invasion is better performed by CT. However, although not widely used, power Doppler and color Doppler assessment can prove useful in the assessment of the portal vein, celiac, common hepatic, and superior mesenteric arteries (5-6).

Computed Tomography (CT)

Indication

CT is widely available as a screening tool for nonspecific abdominal complaints. For screening, a 5 mm slice thickness is obtained from the base of the lungs through the pelvis, usually with intravenous contrast during the portal venous phase. With the new helical multislice scanners, single breath hold images of the abdomen can be obtained in seconds. In this manner, CT screening can be used in those patients presenting with painless jaundice, abnormal LFT's, abdominal pain, weight loss, and other nonspecific complaints that may be associated with pancreatic malignancy (7). Findings such as pancreas mass, common bile and pancreatic duct dilation, pancreas atrophy, and abnormalities in the contour of the pancreas should raise the suspicion of pancreatic adenocarcinoma. Suspicion of pancreatic pathology would then lead to targeted study with specialized protocols that can be applied for diagnosis, preoperative assessment of respectability, and post-operative follow-up of pancreatic adenocarcinoma. CT can also be used to guide procedures sometimes needed in the management of complications from the treatment of pancreatic cancer, including anastomotic leaks or abscess formation. In a recent prospective study of preoperative staging and tumor resectability assessment in pancreatic cancer, Soriano and colleagues found CT to have the highest accuracy in assessing the extent of disease, local regional extension, vascular invasion, distant metastases, TNM stage, and resectability, as compared to EUS, US, MRI, and angiography (8). In this study, EUS demonstrated a higher accuracy in assessing tumor size and regional lymph node involvement. Dedicated pancreas CT protocol thus is considered by most to be the study of choice in the initial assessment of pancreatic cancer. CT is widely available, requires little patient preparation, and can be performed in seconds. Abnormal renal function or a previous history of allergic reactions to contrast administration are the major contraindications to performing the contrast-enhanced CT.

Technique

The development of pancreas-specific imaging protocols add specificity to the evaluation of pancreatic cancer and need to be distinguished from CT screening. Table 13.1 outlines the protocols utilized at our institution with the 16- and 64-slice multidetector row scanners. Utilization of a 64-slice scanner adds the capability of isinotropic imaging—the creation of multiplanar reformatted views from the raw data obtained. The coronal reformatted images are particularly helpful in assessing the cranio-caudal extent of lesions (see Fig. 13.2). In addition, a variety of other

Table 13.1 Multiphasic pancreas CT protocol

Patient position:	Supine
Landmarks:	Xiphoid to iliac crest
Oral contrast:	Water
IV contrast:	Isoview
Amount:	150cc
Rate:	2cc/sec
Injection delay:	40, 70, and 90 seconds
Pitch:	1
Slice thickness:	5mm
Interval:	5mm
Reconstruction:	2.5 (through pancreas), 5, 5mm

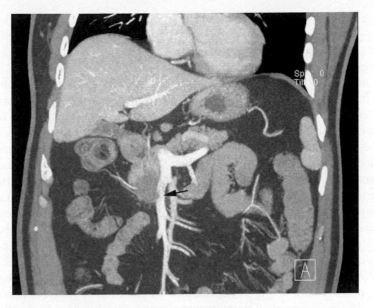

Fig. 13.2 Coronal reformatted CT image demonstrating cranio-caudal extent of pancreatic head mass, as well as invasion of the superior mesenteric vein

post-processing, 3D-imaging capabilities are available that can be applied in specific instances. These advanced technologies include maximum intensity projection (MIP), minimum intensity projection (MIN), volume rendering, and curved reformatting. These techniques are reportedly useful in problem-solving and in providing additional information to clinicians (9-11). MIP is useful in evaluating vessels, and provides a view of the highest-intensity pixels in the data. MIN images utilize the lowest density, and are helpful in evaluating fluid-filled structures such as the pancreatic and common bile ducts. Finally, a curved reformatted image is a technique in which the length of an irregular/curving structure can be "stretched" in a plane for better evaluation. Curved planar reformations can depict the degree of circumferential vascular involvement of the tumor—an important criterion in determining unresectability. In a study by Prokesch and colleges, however, curved planar reformations proved to be equivalent to transverse images in the assessment of tumor involvement along the vessel (10). Although all of these techniques are widely available, they require additional time to process and are often not necessary. At our institution, we reserve the use of these techniques for specific problem-solving situations in which additional imaging helps clarifies specific questions.

The administration of intravenous contrast is of vital importance in the assessment of malignancy, and is optimized to differentiate tissue characteristics. Intravenous contrast is administered as a rapid bolus with a power injector at a rate of 3 to 5 mL/sec. Multiphasic contrast imaging is the accepted modality in evaluating pancreatic adenocarcinoma, although there is no consensus in the number of phases to be obtained (12-15). Specifically, Imbriaco and colleagues found no difference in the accuracy of single-phase versus dual-phase in resectability utilizing the helical

CT technique (*12*). This group has further analyzed the utility of single-phase scanning utilizing MDCT and a delay of 60 seconds. In this study, scanning was performed in a caudal-to-cranial direction and again demonstrated single-phase scanning to be no different than multiphasic evaluation (*16*). In multiphasic evaluation, a noncontrast series is obtained for localization of the pancreas, which is also useful in evaluation of pancreatic calcifications, although calcifications are not a characteristic of adenocarcinoma. The arterial phase (20-30 seconds after the start of contrast infusion) has been reported to be unnecessary in the detection of pancreas adenocarcinoma (*13*), but it is useful in the assessment of arterial anatomy. The pancreatic phase ranges from 40-50 seconds after the initiation of contrast infusion, and is the phase with the greatest tumor-to-gland attenuation difference. During this phase, thin-cut axial images of the pancreas are obtained. Finally, the hepatic phase (60-70 second delay) is obtained throughout the entire abdomen and is necessary in the evaluation of metastatic disease of the liver. Fletcher et al. also demonstrated improved sensitivity for vascular invasion during the hepatic phase; however, there were also false positive cases (*13*). More recently, the combination of multiphasic CT with dedicated thin-cut slices through the pancreas has been shown to be sensitive and highly specific in the detection of pancreas adenocarcinoma, with improvement in detection rate of tumors smaller than 2 cm (*15*).

Findings

Classic appearance of pancreatic adenocarcinoma is that of a low-density mass in the pancreas (see Fig. 13.3). Atrophy of the pancreatic gland, a change in the caliber of the pancreatic and common bile ducts, and contour deformity of the surface of the pancreas are additional findings in CT imaging (see Fig. 13.4). The attenuation appearance of the tumor varies and has been noted to be hypo-attenuating in 83% in one series, and iso-attenuating in 42% in other series (*11*). Most of the tumors (80%) are encountered in the head of the pancreas, and those in the body and tail present in a delayed fashion and have a worse prognosis (*7, 11, 17*). The main differential consideration is chronic pancreatitis, which has several imaging characteristics similar to pancreatic cancer, including atrophy of the gland, pancreatic duct dilation, and fibrotic-type low-density mass (*7, 11, 18, 19*). Chronic pancreatitis is often associated with coarse pancreas calcification, which is not a feature of pancreas cancer.

Once adenocarcinoma of the pancreas is identified, assessment of resectability becomes the next crucial step. It is critical to identify those patients that are not resectable to spare them the morbidity and mortality risk associated with surgical intervention. Table 13.2 summarizes the findings of unresectability. Patients are considered unresectable if there is metastatic disease, local invasion, or involvement of major vessels including superior mesenteric artery, celiac axis. Limited involvement of the superior mesenteric vein/portal vein or hepatic artery may be amenable to resection and surgical reconstruction, therefore the extent of involvement needs to be

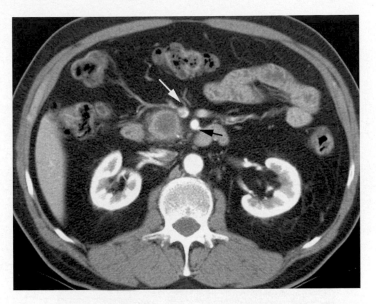

Fig. 13.3 Classic CT appearance of pancreatic cancer, demonstrating a low-density lesion in the head of the pancreas. Note that the superior mesenteric artery and vein have fatty tissue circumferentially and are clear of invasive disease

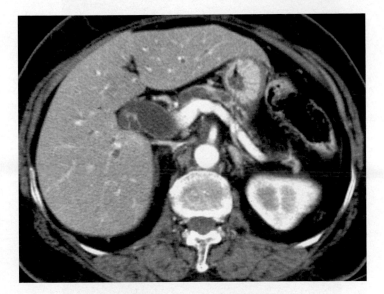

Fig. 13.4 Axial CT image at the level of the pancreas demonstrating pancreatic atrophy, pancreatic and common bile duct dilation, and intrahepatic biliary ductal dilation

Table 13.2 CT criteria for unresectability

Distant metastasis
Extensive Local invasion
Peritoneal involvement
Malignant ascites/pleural effusion
Regional lymphadenopathy
Vessel encasement greater than 50%, occlusion

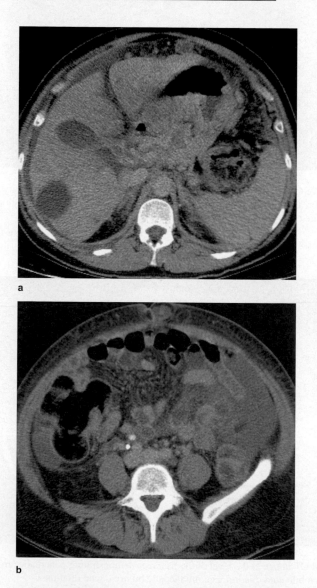

a

b

Fig. 13.5A and B Advanced pancreatic cancer. In Fig. 13.5A, there are liver metastases, peritoneal implants, and malignant ascites. In Fig. 13.5B, at the level of the umbilicus, the Sister Mary Joseph lymph node is visualized. In addition, malignant ascites and peritoneal disease is also noted

carefully described along with the presence or absence of tumor associated thrombus (6, 11, 17). Metastatic disease typically involves the liver and other distant organs, large volume malignant ascites, and peritoneal surfaces (see Fig. 13.5A and B). Classic appearance of liver metastasis is that of a ring-enhancing lesion or low-attenuation lesion in the liver. CT is generally limited in its ability to resolve small peritoneal surface metastasis, small liver metastasis, and micrometastasis to lymph nodes. The stomach, duodenum, and bile ducts are the organs most often involved with local invasion (20). When the tumor is very advanced, invasion of the colon, spleen, kidneys, and spine is possible (ref). An equivocal finding for unresectability includes masses greater than 3cm (11).

Once the presence of distant metastatic disease and local invasion is excluded, it becomes essential to identify vascular involvement as another sign of nonresectability. Vessel involvement—including occlusion, deformation, and encasement—is considered a sign of unresectability (see Figs. 13.6, 13.7A, and 13.7B). Invasion or encasement of the portal vein is not an absolute contraindication to resection, however, as long as less than 2 cm of the vein is involved. There are surgical techniques in which vein grafts and/or patches are utilized in an attempt to achieve curative resection (21). The percent of vascular encasement by the tumor has been shown to be a useful predictor of resectability (20). Lu et al. developed a grading system for tumor involvement based on circumferential involvement, and concluded that tumor with greater than 50% circumferential involvement was a highly specific predictor of unresectability (22). Lu and colleagues consider the following five vessels as critical for nonresectability based on their surgical colleges' operative procedure—celiac artery, hepatic artery, superior mesenteric artery, portal vein, and superior mesenteric vein. The grading

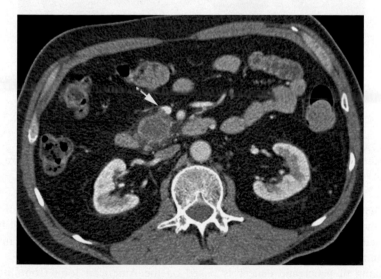

Fig. 13.6 Approximately 50% encasement of the superior vena cava is noted

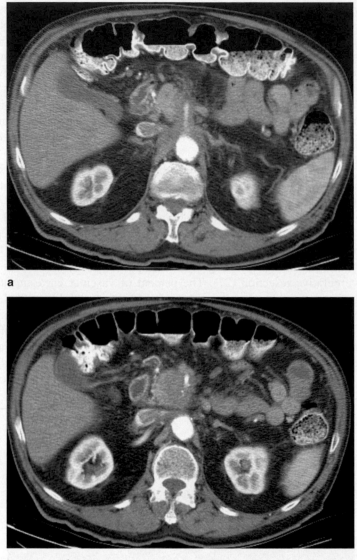

Fig. 13.7A and B: Circumferential encasement of the superior mesenteric artery. In Fig. 13.7A, the proximal SMA is visualized as involved to the level of the origin from the aorta. At a more caudal level, the pancreatic head mass is seen circumferentially encasing the SMA

209 scale that was developed considers a quartile of contiguous involvement of tumor
210 along the vessel as outlined in Table 13.3. These observations have been further
211 validated by others (20), and we include observations regarding vessel involve-
212 ment in the standard evaluation of pancreatic adenocarcinoma.
213   Staging of pancreatic cancer is based on the American Joint Committee on
214 Cancer (AJCC) TNM staging system. Table 13.4 outlines the most recent updated

Table 13.3 Vessel encasement, adapted from Lu (22)

Grade 0	No tumor
Grade 1	Less than 25%
Grade 2	25-50%
Grade 3	50-75%
Grade 4	Greater than 75%

Table 13.4 TNM-staging exocrine pancreas

Primary tumor	
T0	No evidence of primary tumor
Tis	Carcinoma in situ
T1	Tumor limited to pancreas, <=2cm
T2	Tumor limited to pancreas, >2cm
T3	Tumor extends beyond the pancreas but without involvement of the celiac axis or the superior mesenteric artery
T4	Tumor involves the celiac axis or SMA
Tx	Primary tumor cannot be assessed
Regional lymph nodes	
N0	No regional lymph node metastases
N1	Regional lymph node metastases
Nx	Cannot be assessed
Distant metastasis	
M0	No distant metastasis
M1	Distant metastasis
Mx	Cannot be assessed

TNM staging of pancreas cancer definition (23). The use of CT in predicting TNM staging was reported by Zeman and colleagues as effective for tumor and metastasis portion of the TNM staging, but not for the detection of lymph node metastasis (24). In that study, the previous TNM staging was utilized, as well as helical CT. As far as we know, this study has not been replicated utilizing the updated TNM definition and MDCT; however, one can speculate that assessment of lymph node involvement—particularly micrometastasis—will continue to be poor. This assessment may prove to be may be superior by PET/CT.

Magnetic Resonance Imaging (MRI)

Indication

Because of limited availability, cost, and time requirements, MRI has not surpassed CT as the modality of choice in the evaluation of pancreatic adenocarcinoma. Although it has better soft tissue resolution and reports of equal-to-improved sensitivity in the assessment of pancreatic cancer (25), MRI is reserved for those patients with an allergy to iodinated contrast and abnormal renal function, and for those patients in which MRCP is being performed concurrently. Because of the difference in technique and indication, MRCP is described separately. The main advantages of MRI are the increased soft tissue resolution and the ability to image in multiple planes, although this last capability is rivaled by MDCT. Another advantage of MRI includes the ability to perform angiography—either with gad enhancement or utilizing a 2D time-of-flight technique—without intravenous contrast administration. A disadvantage of MRI includes motion degradation secondary to the length of time in acquiring individual sequences, however this is less of an issue with newer, faster sequences utilizing breath hold techniques. Patient factors are also a significant drawback to utilization of MRI and include claustrophobia and patient's body habitus. Claustrophobia can be decreased by the administration of mild sedatives. A scanner table weight limit of 300 lbs precludes the MR imaging of obese patients. The overall accuracy in determining tumor nonresectability, sensitivity, and specificity for MRI was reported to be 85%, 69%, and 95%, respectively, in a prospective study by Lopez Hanninen et al. (26). There are conflicting reports in the literature regarding whether CT or MRI is more accurate in the detection of pancreatic carcinoma (27). Given the wide availability of CT, the short time required to image, and little patient preparation, we consider CT superior but do acknowledge MRI's better soft tissue contrast.

Technique

MRI is contraindicated in patients with indwelling cardiac pacemakers, cochlear implants, certain types of aneurysm clips, and a variety of metals that are susceptible to high magnetic fields. A variety of imaging protocols can be used to evaluate the pancreas and upper abdomen as part of staging with MRI for pancreatic cancer. These protocols vary depending on the equipment being utilized and radiologists' preferences. The sequences most often used include T1 and T1 fat-suppressed sequences, dynamic T1 post contrast sequences, and T2 sequences. The traditional intravenous contrast utilized in MRI is gadolinium, however the new contrast agent mangafodipir trisodium is reported to be taken up by hepatocytes and normal pancreas parenchyma, thus improving lesion detection in both the liver and pancreas (27-28).

Findings

Findings of pancreatic adenocarcinoma are similar to those of CT and include the presence of a pancreatic mass, contour deformity of the surface of the gland, atrophy of the pancreatic gland, and double duct signs. A normal pancreas is lightly hyperintense to the liver in T1 sequences. Pancreatic tumors have lower signal intensity than normal pancreatic parenchyma on both T1 pre- and postgadolinium sequences. As with CT, differentiating chronic pancreatitis from pancreatic adenocarcinoma is problematic because chronic pancreatitis is also hypointense in T1 sequences (25, 29). Staging of pancreatic cancer with MRI is no different than with CT, and the same AJCC TNM staging definitions are applied. Likewise, assessment of major vessel encasement by a tumor is no different than the protocol applied by CT.

Magnetic Resonance Cholangiopancreatography (MRCP)

Indication

MRCP is a noninvasive alternative to ERCP, but as such it lacks the capability for cytology and histology analysis. MRCP images the biliary tract and pancreatic duct using water signals—i.e., T2 signal. One of the main advantages of MRCP over ERCP is the fact that there are no complications associated with this procedure—in addition, operator dependence is less of an issue. Ducts distal to areas of obstruction can also be visualized by MRCP, while this is often not possible with ERCP.

Technique

Water sensitive sequences are prescribed to image the biliary system, hepatic ducts, and pancreatic duct in a noninvasive manner. The study is tailored to each individual patient, and the radiologist at our institution is frequently present to protocol and assess image acquisition.

Findings

Dilation of the pancreatic duct by obstructing lesions is the main imaging finding of MRCP. A useful sign for distinguishing inflammatory process from carcinoma is the "duct penetrating sign," which is seen more often in pancreatitis (85%)—in comparison with pancreatic cancer (4%) (25). The duct penetration sign is defined as the main pancreatic duct—either normal in caliber or smoothly stenotic—"penetrating" a pancreatic mass (30).

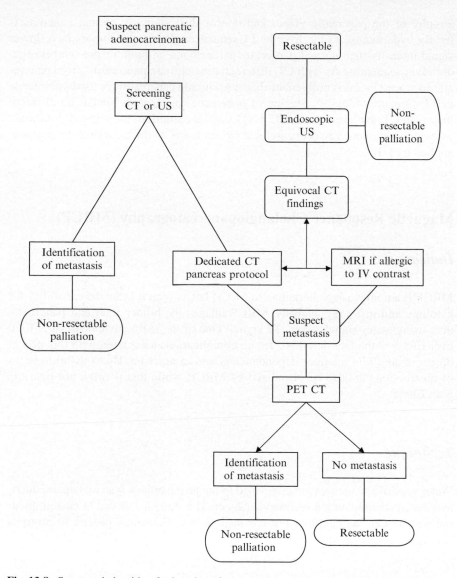

Fig. 13.8 Suggested algorithm for imaging of suspected pancreatic adenocarcinoma

Conclusion

Imaging plays an essential role in the diagnosis, preoperative assessment, and follow-up of pancreatic adenocarcinoma. A number of imaging modalities are available of which CT—because of its availability, relatively low cost, and speed—is regarded as the modality of choice. Unresectability of a tumor has been shown to be accurate using the TNM criteria of distant disease and major vessel involvement. Identification of small liver lesions, peritoneal disease, and lymph node metastasis, however, remains a primary drawback in the accurate assessment of resectability. Differentiation of tumors from chronic pancreatitis also remains a concern. Continued advances in imaging protocols and techniques are to be expected with the goals of improvement in assessing resectability and tumor staging.

References

1. Taylor AM, Roberts SA, Manson JM 2001, Experience with laparoscopic ultrasonography for defining tumour resectability in carcinoma of the pancreatic head and periampullary region. Brit J of Surg 88(8):1077–1083
2. Long EE et al. 2005, Computed tomography, endoscopic, laparoscopic, and intra-operative sonography for assessing resectability of pancreatic cancer. Surg Onc 14(2):105–113
3. Oshikawa O et al. 2002, Dynamic sonography of pancreatic tumors: comparison with dynamic CT. AJR. Am J of Roentgenology 178(5):1133–1137
4. Bipat S et al. 2005, Ultrasonography, computed tomography and magnetic resonance imaging for diagnosis and determining resectability of pancreatic adenocarcinoma: a meta-analysis. J of Comp Asst Tomog 29(4):438–445
5. Kaneko T et al. 2002, Power Doppler ultrasonography for the assessment of vascular invasion by pancreatic cancer. Pancreatology: Off J of the Intl Assoc of Pancreatology (IAP) 2(1):61–68
6. Clarke DL et al. 2003, Preoperative imaging of pancreatic cancer: a management-oriented approach. J of the Am Coll of Surg 196(1):119–129.
7. Katz MH et al. 2005, An evidence-based approach to the diagnosis and staging of pancreatic cancer. Pancreatology: Off J of the Intl Assoc of Pancreatology (IAP) 5(6):576–590
8. Soriano A et al. 2004, Preoperative staging and tumor resectability assessment of pancreatic cancer: prospective study comparing endoscopic ultrasonography, helical computed tomography, magnetic resonance imaging, and angiography. Am J of Gastroenterology 99(3):492–501
9. Tamm E, Charnsangavej C, Szklaruk J 2001, Advanced 3-D imaging for the evaluation of pancreatic cancer with multidetector CT. Intl J of Gastro Cancer 30(1-2):65–71.
10. Prokesch RW et al. 2002, Local staging of pancreatic carcinoma with multi-detector row CT: use of curved planar reformations initial experience. Radiology 225(3):759–765.
11. Smith SL, Rajan PS 2004, Imaging of pancreatic adenocarcinoma with emphasis on multidetector CT. Clin Radiol 59(1):26–38
12. Imbriaco M et al. 2002, Dual-phase versus single-phase helical CT to detect and assess resectability of pancreatic carcinoma. Am J of Roentgenology (AJR) 178(6):1473–1479
13. Fletcher JG et al. 2003, Pancreatic malignancy: value of arterial, pancreatic, and hepatic phase imaging with multi-detector row CT. Radiology 229(1):81–90
14. Valls C et al. 2002, Dual-phase helical CT of pancreatic adenocarcinoma: assessment of resectability before surgeryAm J of Roentgenology (AJR) 178: p. (4)821–6.
15. Bronstein YL et al. 2004, Detection of small pancreatic tumors with multiphasic helical CT. AJR. Am J of Roentgenology (AJR) 182(3):619–623
16. Imbriaco M et al. 2005, Value of the single-phase technique in MDCT assessment of pancreatic tumors. Am J of Roentgenology (AJR) 184(4):1111–1117
17. Balci NC, Semelka RC 2001, Radiologic diagnosis and staging of pancreatic ductal adenocarcinoma. Euro J of Radiol 38(2):105–112
18. Tamm E, Charnsangavej C 2001, Pancreatic cancer: current concepts in imaging for diagnosis and staging. Cancer J 7(4):298–311

19. Leung T-K et al. 2005, Difficulty with diagnosis of malignant pancreatic neoplasms coexisting with chronic pancreatitis. World J of Gastroent (WJG) 11(32):5075–5078

20. O'Malley ME et al. 1999, Adenocarcinoma of the head of the pancreas: Determination of surgical unresectability with thin-section pancreatic-phase helical CT. Am J of Roentgenology (AJR) 173:1513–1518

21. Obuz F et al. 2001, Pancreatic adenocarcinoma: detection and staging with dynamic MR imaging. Eur J of Radiol 38(2):146–150

22. Lu DSK et al. 1997, Local staging of pancreatic cancer: criteria for unresectability of major vessels as revealed by pancreatic-phase, thin-section helical CT. Am J of Roentgenology (AJR) 168:1439–1443

23. Exocrine pancreas. In: American Joint Committee on Cancer: AJCC Cancer Staging Manual, 6th ed. New York, NY: Springer, 2002:157-164

24. Zeman RK et al. 1997, TNM Staging of Pancreatic Carcinoma Using Helical CT. Am J of Roentgenology (AJR) 169:459–464

25. Fayad LM, Mitchell DG 2001, Magnetic resonance imaging of pancreatic adenocarcinoma. Int J of Gastroint Cancer 30(1-2):19–25

26. Lopez Hanninen E et al. 2002, Prospective evaluation of pancreatic tumors: accuracy of MR imaging with MR cholangiopancreatography and MR angiography. Radiology 224(1):34–41

27. Ramsay D et al. 2004, Identification and staging of pancreatic tumours using computed tomography, endoscopic ultrasound and mangafodipir trisodium-enhanced magnetic resonance imaging. Australasian Radiol 48(2):154–161

28. Schima W et al. 2002, Diagnosis and staging of pancreatic cancer: comparison of mangafodipir trisodium-enhanced MR imaging and contrast-enhanced helical hydro-CT. Am J of Roentgenology (AJR) 179(3):717–24

29. Fischer U et al. 2002, Preoperative local MRI-staging of patients with a suspected pancreatic mass. Euro Radiol 12(2):296–303

30. Ichikawa T et al. 2001, Duct-penetrating sign at MRCP: usefulness for differentiating inflammatory pancreatic mass from pancreatic carcinomas. Radiology 221(1):107–116

Chapter 14
The Role of PET Scanning in Pancreatic Cancer

M. Fernandez-Ulloa

1 Introduction

For many years computed tomography (CT) has been the principal imaging modality used for diagnosis and staging of patients with pancreatic cancer. Currently, contrast enhanced multidetector CT (ce MDCT), remains the most commonly used imaging study in the initial evaluation of these patients. Depending on clinical practices and preferences, other modalities, such as magnetic resonance imaging (MRI) and endoscopic ultrasonography (EUS), are also utilized in the diagnosis and staging of pancreatic carcinoma (1, 2).

The use of positron emission tomography (PET) in routine oncology practice has accelerated significantly in the past decade. Oncologic PET imaging is mainly performed with F18-FDG (FDG), a glucose analog that accumulates in cancer cells. This modality is under investigation in the evaluation of patients with pancreatic carcinoma as a diagnostic tool to better define extent of disease and guide treatment. Specifically, the ability of FDG-PET to find metastasis to the liver and elsewhere may be of great value in the management of patients with pancreatic cancer.

2 Principles of Cancer Imaging with F18-FDG

Fluorine-18 belongs to the family of positron emitting radioisotopes. Unstable neutron deficient nuclei in these radioisotopes emit positively charged electrons. These positrons traverse varying distances in tissues depending on their energy but eventually collide with electrons surrounding nuclei and are annihilated. The result of this annihilation is the emission of two gamma rays at a 180-degree angle. This provides the basis for PET imaging. One of the main characteristics of PET is its ability to provide spatial information used for processing and image display in tomographic formats, that is, axial, coronal, and sagittal planes. Other positron emitters include carbon-11, nitrogen-13, and oxygen-15. As opposed to F-18, which has a half-life of 120 minutes, these three have very short half-lives, which

A.M. Lowy et al. (eds.) *Pancreatic Cancer*.
doi: 10.1007/978-0-387-69252-4, © Springer Science+Business Media, LLC 2008

makes them impractical for clinical use. Thus, F-18 is currently the most important PET imaging radioisotope. Substitution of F-18 for the hydroxyl in the carbon 2 of the glucose yields the glucose analog 2-(fluorine-18) fluoro-2-deoxy-D-glucose, or F18-FDG. As a result of this modification to the chemical structure, the metabolic characteristics of F18-FDG differ from those of glucose. Accordingly, F18- FDG is transported into the cells via glucose transporters (Glut) and phosphorylated by the hexokinase enzyme to FDG-6-phosphate, but cannot be metabolized further and is essentially trapped intracellularly since G-6-phosphatase is low in these cells. The unique kinetics of F18-FDG allow for imaging of tumors with PET. The use of F18-FDG for imaging of cancer emerged from the long known concept that cancer cells exist in a hypermetabolic state and concentrate glucose at high levels. Increased accumulation of the glucose analog F18-FDG in cancer cells is caused, to a significant extent, by oncogene-induced increased glucose consumption and activation of glucose transporters (*3*). The uptake of FDG in tumors is also affected by multiple factors, some of which are not well understood. These include the number of viable cells, blood supply, presence of hypoxia, blood sugar and insulin levels, degree of expression of Glut at the cell membrane and the effect of therapeutic interventions such as chemotherapy and radiotherapy. One rationale for the use of FDG-PET imaging in pancreatic cancer rests on evidence of Glut-1 transporter over expression in pancreatic cancer specimens (*4–6*).

The presence or absence of FDG accumulation in pancreatic tumors and other tissues can be assessed well with PET alone. However, since PET lacks the anatomic detail necessary for optimal characterization of normal tissue FDG uptake and precise localization of neoplastic lesions, PET-CT was introduced to overcome these limitations and has largely replaced PET. In these systems the PET and the CT are integrated into one single imaging devise, a design that offers several advantages. The ability to obtain the PET and CT data sets almost simultaneously allows for almost perfect fusion of the two images, resulting in precise localization of PET abnormalities on the anatomic CT images. Also normal accumulation of FDG in the bowel and other intra-abdominal organs can easily be determined, which minimizes false-positive and enhances specificity of the study. Similarly suspicious CT lesions can be evaluated more precisely for the presence of FDG uptake within them. As in any nuclear medicine technique, the effect of tissue attenuation of gamma photons is an important factor that causes loss of resolution and image detail. This problem is dealt with by applying the attenuation maps from the CT data to the PET data during image processing. It should be emphasized that absolute correspondence of the PET and CT images is not always possible, due to the fact that acquisition of the PET and CT data is not simultaneous. Thus, patient and organ movement during and between imaging sessions may result in varying degrees of image misregistration and suboptimal application of the CT derived soft tissue attenuation map to the PET data during image reconstruction. Several brands of PET and PET-CT imaging devices are currently in use, but the clinical imaging performance of these instruments is comparable. This likely will change as various new innovations to the equipment are introduced.

The operation of PET-CT calls for proper tailoring imaging of protocols depending on the clinical situation. The CT portion of any PET-CT study may differ, depending on practice preferences and the clinical question. When the CT is used for anatomic correlation and attenuation correction purposes only, a nondiagnostic low-dose CT is obtained. Although detail and diagnostic content of these CTs are somewhat inferior, most CTs in current PET-CT systems are of very good quality. A diagnostic CT typically is performed with the aid of intravenous contrast media and occasionally oral contrast as well. Acquisition parameters for diagnostic CTs are also modified accordingly.

For the PET images, patients are given the FDG intravenously approximately 1 hour before imaging. The imaging sequence starts with a "scout" CT, followed by the actual CT imaging session and ends with the PET imaging. Prior to the administration of the FDG patients fast for at least 6 hours and are required to avoid strenuous physical activities. The blood sugar ideally should be within normal limits, but levels of up to 150 mg may not affect the kinetics of FDG significantly. Administration of insulin should be avoided for at least 4 hours before the FDG injection.

The use of PET-CT involves radiation exposure to patients. Since combined PET-CT systems are rapidly replacing the dedicated PET system, radiation exposure to patients from both the PET and CT needs to be considered. The effective radiation dose from a standard dose of FDG 370 MBq (10 mCi) is approximately 7 mSv. The addition of a low-dose CT study increases the total effective dose to about 25 mSv (7). Slightly higher radiation exposures are expected if a diagnostic CT study is obtained. As a comparison annual radiation exposure to the general public from background radiation is about 3–4 mSv, depending on geographic location. Thus, the risk-benefit ratio of PET-CT imaging is low and within acceptable levels considering the seriousness of pancreatic cancer.

3   Image Evaluation and Interpretation

Examination of FDG images is performed visually and semiquantitatively from the standard uptake values (SUVs). Usually, the FDG-PET and CT set are evaluated separately followed by examination of the fused images to cross-correlate findings and abnormalities. Analysis of the pattern of FDG uptake when evaluating PET-CT images in patients with pancreatic masses helps determine their malignant or benign etiology. A well-circumscribed focal area of intense uptake is generally indicative of malignancy, whereas FDG uptake that is more diffuse and less intense is suggestive of chronic pancreatitis (8). In addition to the visual inspection of images, SUVs are used in an attempt to provide an objective parameter that estimates the degree of FDG uptake in lesions. SUVs represent a semiquantitative expression of the concentration of FDG in tumors calculated as follows:

$$SUV = \frac{PET\ counts \times calibration\ factor\ (mCi/g)}{Dose\ of\ injected\ FDG\ (mCi)/body\ weight\ (g)}$$

or the percent of injected dose in the lesion normalized for body mass.

To determine the PET counts a volumetric region of interest (ROI) is selected from the axial images encompassing the tumor area with the maximal metabolic activity. Usually two SUV determinations are generated; the average and the maximal. The maximal SUV looks at the highest level of FDG concentration within lesions. The average SUV expresses the differences of distribution of FDG within a tumor and takes into consideration the variation of FDG concentration throughout a lesion due to its heterogeneity of distribution within tumors. Factors that may actually decrease concentration of FDG within a tumor, such as necrosis and blood flow, may affect average SUV values. For this reason, use of maximal SUVs that express the maximal metabolic activity within a tumor is favored. SUVs at various cutoff levels have been proposed as discriminators between cancer and other non-neoplastic processes. There are limitations to the use of SUVs as discriminators, however, as they can be affected by many technical as well as physiologic factors. These include calibration of the PET instruments; selection of ROI, blood sugar level, time elapsed between injection of FDG and imaging, and heterogeneity of FDG uptake in tumors. The effect of these factors can be reduced by proper and detailed attention to patient preparation and imaging techniques. The main limitation, however, is the significant overlap of FDG uptake between cancer and other non-neoplastic processes such as nonspecific inflammation, infection, and granulomatous diseases. In regard to pancreatic cancer, the value of SUVs as tools for diagnosis and evaluation of these patients has not been established. SUVs were found helpful to differentiate pancreas cancer from chronic pancreatitis (8) and improve sensitivity for pancreas cancer detection compared with visual image inspection. In an effort to better refine the usefulness of SUVs, they have been combined with tracer retention indexes (RI). These methods compare the SUV values in tumors at two time (T_1, T_2) intervals, following the injection of the FDG as follows:

$$RI = \frac{SUV2\text{-}SUV1}{SUV1} \times 100\%$$

A common practice is to obtain these SUVs at 1 and 2 hours after injection of FDG. As opposed to benign processes, cancer usually shows higher RIs (9). Disadvantages of this technique include the need for additional imaging of the patient, which makes it impractical in routine clinical practice. The usefulness of SUVs and retention indexes is further limited by the difficulty in defining precise cutoff values that provide the best discriminator function to separate cancer from benign diseases. Moreover, validated SUVs and RIs that differentiate malignant from benign pancreatic lesions that can be interchanged between institutions have not been established. While the implementation of these semiqualitative techniques in clinical practice will need further validation of its usefulness, they mainly remain an important tool of clinical research.

4 Limitations of FDG-PET Imaging

One of the main limitations of FDG imaging is its specificity for cancer. It is a well-known fact that in addition to cancer, uptake of FDG is also observed in various inflammatory and granulomatous processes.

Since F18-FDG commonly concentrates in the bowel as well in the kidneys and urinary tract, evaluation of these regions can be difficult. Physiologic accumulation of FDG in these organs also affects negatively the specificity of PET for cancer. The advent of PET-CT has minimized this problem significantly by reducing the number of false-positives caused by this physiologic FDG uptake.

False-negative results can occur when lesions are <6–8 mm in size and in hyperglycemic patients (*10*).

There are limitations that are unique to imaging with dedicated dual PET-CT instruments as a result of differences in breathing patterns that take place during the PET and CT imaging sessions. As opposed to CT scans, which can be obtained in few seconds during a breath hold, PET images are obtained during tidal breathing and may take 20–30 minutes, and therefore represent an average position of the thoracic cage and upper abdomen. This may lead to misregistration of lesions and failure to detect small lesions in the superior regions of the liver and at the bases of the lungs. This problem can be reduced by obtaining the CT during breath holding in a fixed neutral position such as unforced expiration. Techniques for respiratory gating have been developed that further minimize breathing artifacts and will certainly become routine practice in the future (*11*). It should be remembered that organ movement in the abdomen and pelvis caused by bowel peristalsis and bladder filling during imaging may also result in misregistration of lesions. In addition, fusion of PET and CT images obtained with dual PET-CT may not be perfect due to misregistration of the PET and CT data sets. This is caused by changes of patient position during or between the CT and PET image acquisitions and may lead to anatomical misplacement of lesions.

Dense objects such as pacemakers and orthopedic devises affect the CT generated attenuation maps and may result in "hot spots" in surrounding tissues and falsely elevated SUVs in lesions (*12*). Correction algorithms especially adapted to solve this problem are being developed. Use of low-density oral contrast or water as a negative contrast agent for bowel is helpful to reduce similar problems encountered when dense contrast agents are utilized.

Blood sugar levels have been described to influence the degree of FDG by neoplastic cells. Sugar-induced decreases of FDG uptake by cancer cells of up to 20% have been found in in vitro tumor models (*8, 13*). These negative effects of high sugar levels have also been observed in general oncologic FDG-PET imaging (*14, 15*) as well as in patients with pancreatic cancer (*10*). These negative effects of hyperglycemia have been attributed to competition between glucose and the analog F18-FDG for glucose transporters at the cell membrane level. Therefore, it is important that patients are checked for blood sugar levels prior to FDG-PET imaging. Imaging should be avoided if the glucose levels in blood are >150 mg/dl.

5 Value of FDG-PET Imaging for Detecting Primary Pancreatic Cancer

FDG-PET for the diagnosis of pancreatic carcinoma has been explored in three main clinical situations: at the initial diagnosis in patients with suspicious masses, for differentiating benign pancreatic disease such as chronic pancreatitis from cancer, and in the evaluation of cystic lesions. The majority of pancreatic carcinomas present clinically at a relatively advanced stage and only about 20% of patients are found resectable at the time of diagnosis (16). Imaging with CT and MRI as well as EUS provides the more accurate noninvasive means for confirmation of diagnosis and staging prior to treatment. Use of FDG-PET for evaluation of the primary tumor and pancreatic masses is still controversial, given its limited sensitivity and specificity (17). It should be noted that most published studies report the use of dedicated PET systems. Only recently have new data on FDG imaging with combined PET-CT instruments begun to emerge. However, several studies suggest that FDG-PET may have utility in the diagnosis of cancer in patients with pancreatic masses (9, 10, 18, 19). A study examining the value of FDG-PET to diagnose cancer in 106 suspicious lesions reported a sensitivity and specificity of 85% and 84%, respectively (10). Additionally, comparisons with other diagnostic modalities including CT, EUS, and MRI have found FDG-PET of comparable accuracy (9, 18). In a study of 80 patients, sensitivity and specificity of FDG-PET to detect pancreatic cancer were 88% and 92%, respectively (20). A recent tabulated review of 387 patients demonstrated a weighted average sensitivity of 94% and specificity of 90% for detection of primary pancreatic cancer (21). Thus, there is emerging clinical evidence that FDG-PET is helpful in the evaluation of patients presenting with a pancreatic mass.

The recent emergence of PET-CT has introduced new questions regarding the role and utility of FDG imaging in patients with pancreatic cancer. Because of the simultaneous whole body anatomic and metabolic information that can be obtained in one single imaging session, this technique has the potential to add significant diagnostic value to oncologic FDG imaging. A recent report on the use of digitally fused MDCT and FDG-PET images described an improvement in sensitivity and specificity, as well as positive and negative predictive values in the differential diagnoses between benign and malignant lesions as compared with PET alone (22). A more recent study comparing dual FDG-PET-CT with contrast-enhanced CT in the diagnosis of primary pancreatic carcinoma lesions found sensitivities of 89% and 93%, respectively (23). The specificity for PET-CT and contrast enhanced CT were 93% and 21%, respectively. The positive and negative predictive values for PET-CT were 91% and 64%, respectively. Thus, although in this study combined PET-CT appears to be sensitive and specific, its negative predictive value for detection of pancreatic cancer was low and therefore unreliable. The usefulness and value of combined PET-CT in the evaluation of primary pancreatic lesions is currently unknown; extensive clinical studies will be needed to confirm initial positive results. An important practical question now is how the use of PET-CT will impact the overall value of FDG imaging in difficult clinical situations. Given the usual late clinical presentation of pancreatic carcinoma, the main aim of diagnostic imaging is to separate those patients who have a chance at surgical care from those who do not. In this context PET or PET-CT may not reduce the need for invasive diagnostic procedures in patients with pancreatic masses. This is because from the clinician's point of view, a positive FDG-PET only reaffirms the suspicion of cancer but does not necessarily obviate the need for a tissue diagnosis. Conversely, the imperfect negative predictive value of FDG-PET does not obviate the need for further invasive confirming diagnostic approaches. Similarly, PET is not well suited for evaluation of regional adenopathy and vascular invasion, which are an important determinants of resectability. Reported sensitivity and specificity in detecting lymph node disease is generally suboptimal because the metastases may be below PET resolution of 6–8 mm and varies widely between 46% and 71%, and 63% and 100%, respectively (24, 25). Thus, as discussed in the following, the main role of PET in pancreatic cancer is in the search for otherwise occult metastatic disease, which if present would change management.

6 Detection of Distant Metastases

The presence of radiographically occult distant metastases is common at the time of diagnosis of pancreas cancer. This represents an important clinical problem since radical resections in patients with metastatic disease accomplish nothing and may even result in deleterious outcomes. FDG-PET imaging has been found to be accurate in the detection of hepatic and additional sites of distant metastatic disease (26–28). Although false-positive results may be caused by intrahepatic cholestasis, in some studies, imaging with FDG-PET has shown to be more accurate than CT for detection of metastases to the liver and can detect disease at other distant sites (29, 30) (Figs. 14.1 and 14.2). False-negatives are seen when tumors <8 mm in size are unlikely to be detected.

Using combined PET-CT, the sensitivity and specificity for detection of distant metastasis has been reported as 81% and 100%, respectively (23). Sensitivity and specificity for standard staging were 50% and 95%, respectively. Moreover, dual PET-CT improved detection of distant metastasis compared with standard staging alone (81% versus 56%). Thus, dual PET-CT may emerge as the best tool for detection of distant metastasis in the patient with pancreatic cancer. In this regard, several studies have found that FDG-PET has a significant impact on management of these patients. A change in treatment plan affecting 16–43% of patients has been described in three reports related to the ability of FDG-PET to demonstrate distant metastatic disease and new second primaries (26, 31, 32). Thus, clinical studies strongly suggest an important role of FDG-PET imaging for treatment planning and management of patients with pancreatic cancer. The definite role of FDG-PET in the staging and therapy planning of pancreas carcinoma necessitates further evaluation and properly designed prospective clinical studies (33). It is likely that in the

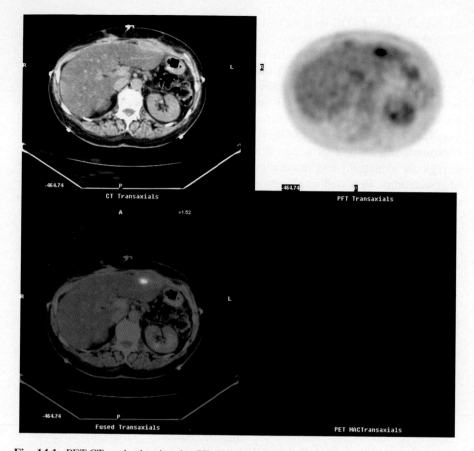

Fig. 14.1 PET-CT study showing the CT *(left upper corner),* the FDG image *(right upper corner),* and fused PET-CT image. Metastatic focus is present in the anterior hepatic margin

near future evaluation of patients with pancreatic carcinoma will continue to include the various established imaging techniques with the addition of FDG-PET, especially in the form of dual PET-CT.

7   PET for Evaluation of Treatment Response and Recurrence

Although histopathologic evaluation of surgical specimens is the gold standard for assessment of response to preoperative therapy in patients with localized pancreas cancer, clinical criteria for determination of response are critical to evaluation of ongoing therapy in patients with localized pancreas cancer. Assessment of response to therapy in routine oncologic practice has traditionally been based on the anatomic

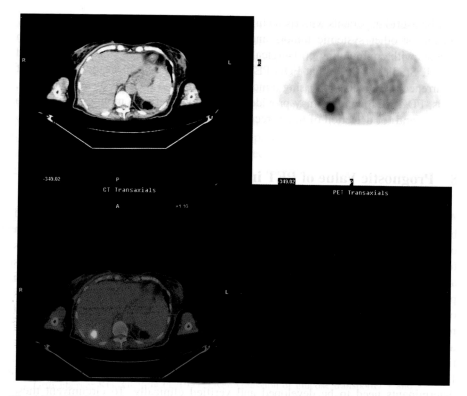

Fig. 14.2 PET-CT study showing the CT, FDG image and fused PET-CT images in a similar format as Fig. 14.1. A lesion is present in the posterior liver not apparent on the CT

changes of tumors and lymph nodes based on size estimates from CT imaging. Because of the desmoplasia associated with pancreatic cancer, changes in tumor size are often minimal, even in the setting of a robust pathologic response. As new treatments for pancreatic cancer are developed and introduced in clinical practice, the need for modalities that assess response to therapy will increase. FDG-PET offers great potential in this area and will certainly become an important and useful tool in this area (*31, 34, 35*). An important question is when to obtain follow-up FDG-PET studies to monitor response to therapy since reactive inflammatory changes are commonly found in tumors that respond to chemotherapy or radiotherapy. These changes result in nonspecific accumulation of FDG that sometimes cannot be readily distinguished from the uptake seen in residual or recurrent tumor. The precise time for a follow-up FDG-PET in pancreatic cancer has not been identified. If extrapolation from experience with other tumors is made, re-evaluation at intervals of 2 to 3 weeks after the completion of chemotherapy and 3 to 4 months after radiotherapy is reasonable. If semiquantitative parameters such as SUVs are used for comparison, close attention should be paid to duplication of conditions of imaging between the studies. This requires close communication among clinicians, imaging department personnel, and radiologists interpreting the studies. FDG-PET

15. Bakkevold KE, Amesjo B, Kambestad B. 1992, Carcinoma of the pancreas and papilla of vater-assessment of respectability and factors influencing respectability in stage I carcinoma. A prospective multicentre trial in 472 patients. Eur J Surg Oncol 18:494–507.

16. Zimny M, Schumpelick V. 2001, (Fluorodeoxyglucose positron emission tomography (FDG-PET) in the differential diagnosis of pancreatic lesions). Chirurgie 72:989–994.

17. Inokuma T, Tamaki N, Torizuka T, 1995, Evaluation of pancreatic tumors with positron emission tomography and F-18 fluorodeoxyglucose: comparison with CT and US. Radiology 195:345–352.

18. Sperti C, Pasquali C, Decet G, 2005, F-18-fluorodeoxyglucose positron emission tomography in differentiating malignant from benign pancreatic cysts: a prospective study. J Gastrointest Surg 9:22–29.

19. Berberat P, Friess H, Kashiwagi M, 1999, Diagnosis and staging of pancreatic cancer by positron emission tomography. World J Surg 23:882–887.

20. Gambhir SS, Czernin J, Schwimmer J, 2001, A tabulated summary of the FDG PET literature. J. Nucl Med 42:1S–93S.

21. Lemke AJ, Nieheus SM, Hosten N, 2004, Retrospective digital image fusion of multidetector CT and ^{18}F-FDG PET: clinical value in pancreatic lesions—a prospective study with 104 patients. J Nucl Med 45(8):1279–1286.

22. Heinrich S, Goerres GW, Schafer M, 2005, Positron emission tomography/computed tomography influences on the management of resectable pancreatic cancer and its cost-effectiveness. Ann Surg 242(2):235–243.

23. Bares R, Klever P, Hauptmann S, 1994, F-18 fluorodeoxyglucose PET in vivo evaluation of pancreatic glucose metabolism for detection of pancreatic cancer. Radiology 192:79–86.

24. Diederichs CG, Staib L, Vogel J, 2000, Values and limitations of 18F-fluorodeoxyglucose-positron-emission tomography with preoperative evaluation of patients with pancreatic masses. Pancreas 20:109–116.

25. Higashi T, Saga T, Nakamoto Y, 2003, Diagnosis of pancreatic cancer using fluorine-18 fluorodeoxyglucose positron emission tomography (FDG-PET): usefulness and limitations in "clinical reality". Ann Nucl Med 17:261–279.

26. Frohlich A, Diederichs CG, Staib L, 1999, Detection of liver metastases from pancreatic cancer using FDG PET. J Nucl Med 40:250–255.

27. Nakamoto Y, Higashi T, Sakahara H, 1999, Contribution of PET in the detection of liver metastases from pancreatic tumours. Clin Radiol 54:248–252.

28. Teffey SA, Hildeboldt CC, Dehashti F, 2003, Detection of primary hepatic malignancy in liver transplant candidates: prospective comparison of CT, MR imaging, US and PET. Radiology 226:533–542.

29. Nishiyama Y, Yamamoto Y, Yokoe K, 2005, Contribution of whole body FDG-PET to the detection of distant metastasis in pancreatic cancer. Ann Nucl Med 19:491–497.

30. Rose DM, Delbeke D, Beauchamp RD, 1999, 18-Fluorodeoxyglucose-positron emission tomography (18FDG-PET) in the management of patients with suspected pancreatic cancer. Ann Surg 229:729–738.

31. Delbeke D, Rose DM, Chapman WC, 1999, Optimal interpretation of FDG PET in the diagnosis, stating and management of pancreatic carcinoma. J Nucl Med 40(11):1784–1791.

32. Orlando LA, Kulasingam SL, Matchar DB. 2004; Meta-analysis the detection of pancreatic malignancy with positron emission tomography. Aliment Pharmacol Ther 20:1063–1070.

33. Higashi T, Sakahara H. Torizuka T, 1999, Evaluation of intraoperative radiation therapy for unresectable pancreatic cancer with FDG PET. J Nucl Med 40:1424–1433.

34. Maisey NR, Webb A, Flux GD, 2000, FDG PET in the prediction of survival of patients with cancer of the pancreas: a pilot study. Br J Cancer 83:287–293.

35. Franke C, Klapdor R, Meyerhoff K, 1999, 18F-positron emission tomography of the pancreas: diagnostic benefit in the follow-up of pancreatic carcinoma. Anticancer Res 19:2437–2442.

36. Nakata B, Chung YS, Nishimura S, 1997, 18F-fluorodeoxyglucose positron emission tomography and the prognosis of patients with pancreatic carcinoma. Cancer 79:695–699.

37. Zimny M, Fass J, Bares R, 2000, Fluorodeoxyglucose positron emission tomography and the prognosis of pancreatic carcinoma. Scand J Gastroenterol 35:883–888.
38. Sperti C, Pasquali C, Chierichetti F, 2003, 18-Fluorodeoxyglucose positron emission tomography in predicting survival of patients with pancreatic carcinoma. J Gastrointest Surg 7:953–960.
39. Lyshchik A, Higashi T, Nakamoto Y, 2005, Dual-phase 18F-fluoro-2-deoxy-D-glucose positron emission tomography as prognostic parameter in patients with pancreatic cancer. Eur J Nucl Med 33:389–397.

Chapter 15
Endoscopic Ultrasound Staging

William R. Brugge

1 Introduction

Preoperative staging of pancreatic cancer determines the therapeutic approach to the malignancy. The major decision point is whether surgical resection will be attempted or nonoperative therapy will be employed. Cross sectional imaging is often used to initially localize the primary site of a pancreatic malignancy. Although staging of the pancreatic malignancy can be assessed with diagnostic CT and MRI scanning, detailed staging is usually performed with specific staging protocols that involve the use of timed administration of intravenous contrast agents. Endoscopic ultrasound (EUS) uses high frequency ultrasound images to provide detailed imaging of the primary malignancy and its relationship to adjacent structures, such as the portal venous system. With accurate staging, inappropriate therapy, such as unsuccessful surgical resection can be avoided and palliative therapy can be provided to patients with advanced disease.

2 Preoperative TNM Staging of Patients with Pancreatic Cancer

The preoperative TNM staging of pancreatic cancer is based on the extent of the invasion by the primary mass, the presence or absence of malignant lymph nodes, and evidence of metastatic disease. The T (tumor) stage of pancreatic cancer is classified as T1–T4 based on the size of the mass and the extent of invasion. The earliest stage, T1, consists of an intrapancreatic mass measuring 2 cm in diameter. Masses that have invaded tissue adjacent to the pancreas, such as the duodenum, stomach, bile duct, and peripancreatic fat are classified as T3 lesions. The most advanced lesions, T4 lesions, have invaded adjacent vessels such as the superior mesenteric vessels, portal vein or celiac artery, and its branches.

Nodal (N) staging of pancreatic cancer attempts to describe whether lymph nodes contain metastasis from the primary, or are benign. With the use of cross sectional imaging, nodal staging is accomplished using the size of the lymph node as an indicator of malignancy. M (metastasis) staging describes the presence of metastatic

A.M. Lowy et al. (eds.) *Pancreatic Cancer.*
doi: 10.1007/978-0-387-69252-4, © Springer Science+Business Media, LLC 2008

disease to tissue remote to the pancreas. The most common location of metastatic lesions is the liver and peritoneum. Cross-sectional imaging detects the presence of liver metastases by the presence of focal low- or high-attenuation lesions within the liver parenchyma. Peritoneal metastases are manifest by the presence of ascites or mass lesions arising in the peritoneal fat.

3   CT Staging

Staging of pancreatic cancer can be performed with spiral or multidetector CT scanning as discussed in Chapter 13. Both techniques use intravenous contrast agents to improve the imaging of the pancreas and the adjacent vessels. Oral contrast is used to delineate the duodenum and stomach.

Spiral CT scanning provides information regarding the TNM staging of pancreatic cancer, but often the information is used to predict whether the primary lesion is "resectable" or not. Generally, T1, 2, and 3 lesions without evidence of nodal or metastatic lesions are considered "resectable." Huang et al. described the accuracy of CT staging in 97 patients who underwent operative staging (1). They found the overall accuracy of predicting resectability was 91%. The positive predictive values were increased from 96% to 100% with the use of triphasic CT scanning, as compared with dual phase CT. However, these high rates of staging accuracy are often achieved only in carefully selected patients who have clear evidence of a pancreatic mass. In other investigations, the diagnostic accuracy of CT staging has been described as low as 74% (2). In a recent study of 89 patients undergoing staging with CT followed by surgical staging, the overall accuracy of spiral CT for prediction of resectability was 81% (3). Vascular staging accuracy was greater, at 91%. More detailed studies of multidetector CT and comparison with intraoperative vascular staging have yielded a series of specific criteria for prediction of vascular invasion. However, the sensitivity remains rather low for venous vessels, despite the use of criteria such as the caliber and contour of the vessel (4). During surgical exploration in the study by Huang, 78 vessels were found to be invaded. With "sign A" (arterial embedment or venous obliteration) as the CT criterion for peripancreatic vascular invasion, the sensitivity of arterial and venous invasion was 66% and 14%, respectively; the specificity of absence of arterial and venous invasion was 100% and 100% (all 100%). In this study, there were 3 superior mesenteric vein (SMV) vessels with a teardrop appearance teardrop (sign E), which were all confirmed to have malignant invasion.

4   EUS Technique

The staging of pancreatic cancer with EUS is performed in a very different manner compared to radiologic cross-sectional imaging. EUS imaging of pancreatic malignancy can be performed with linear or radial EUS instruments during an endoscopic procedure. Traditionally radial EUS was used to provide cross-sectional high frequency ultrasound images of pancreatic masses. The echoendoscope is placed in the duodenum for imaging of head lesions and imaging of the body and tail are obtained from the stomach. Although radial imaging provides high resolution images, the lack of color Doppler decreases the ability to accurately image vessels, particularly small venous structures. Linear EUS imaging provides sector imaging of the pancreas. Although linear echoendoscopes are similar in size and configuration as radial echoendoscopes, linear instruments are often connected to more sophisticated ultrasound processors that provide high-quality images and detailed Doppler functionality. Furthermore, linear EUS can guide fine-needle aspiration (FNA) cytology. FNA enhances the diagnostic ability of EUS and the nodal and metastatic staging.

5   EUS Diagnosis of Pancreatic Cancer

The EUS diagnosis of pancreatic cancer is based on the imaging appearance of the primary pancreatic malignancy. Pancreatic adenocarcinoma appears as a focal hypoechoic mass arising from the bright, hyperechoic parenchyma of the pancreas. Although the borders of the pancreatic malignancy are irregular, there is usually a sharp distinction between malignant and normal pancreas. However, a peritumorous inflammatory response by the pancreas can closely mimic the pancreatic malignancy. The presence of this inflammatory process may result in an overestimation of the size and stage of the primary malignancy.

The appearance of a focal hypoechoic mass in the pancreas is not diagnostic of a malignancy. Chronic inflammatory processes can closely simulate malignancy with a similar echotexture. The most common simulator of pancreatic cancer is focal autoimmune pancreatitis and focal chronic pancreatitis. FNA is often used to differentiate between these lesions and establish the diagnosis of a malignancy. For these reasons, the staging of focal malignancies of the pancreas by EUS may be difficult when the diagnosis of malignancy has not been secured.

EUS fine needle aspiration is often performed during the diagnosis and staging of a pancreatic malignancy. FNA cytology of the primary lesion establishes the diagnosis of the malignancy in a high percentage of patients. FNA is performed using 22- or 25-gauge needles that are passed through the gastric or duodenal wall and into the lesion of interest. With the needle placed in the pancreatic mass, the needle is moved to and fro while aspirating cytologic material. Often several needle passes are required in order to obtain diagnostic material. Similar techniques are used for the diagnosis of liver lesions, ascites, and enlarged lymph nodes.

6   EUS T Staging

EUS staging of pancreatic malignancy may be performed during the initial diagnostic EUS procedure or during a dedicated staging procedure. As stated, radial or linear EUS imaging can be used to obtain serial image of the pancreas and adjacent structures. Image interpretation is usually performed during the examination with live imaging, but reviews of still or video imaging after the procedure can also be used to provide staging information.

Tumor staging by EUS focuses on the primary pancreatic mass lesion. In the first step of staging, the lesion is identified and the location of the lesion is established. The location is usually noted to be in the uncinate, head, neck, body, or tail of the pancreas. Traditionally, EUS staging has focused on the staging of a mass located in the head of the pancreas. The size of the lesion is also documented and this information will be important for differentiating between intrapancreatic and locally invasive lesions. Nodal staging is performed in a similar manner with imaging and sizing of abnormal lymph nodes. Abnormal lymph nodes may be aspirated in order to increase the accuracy of nodal staging. Metastasis staging is performed by examining the liver and perihepatic space for the presence of ascites and masses.

T stage accuracy of EUS has been established in several studies that used the results of surgical exploration as the reference standard. In an initial study, a series of EUS criteria were developed to objectively describe venous invasion (5, 6). Four EUS criteria were studied and the overall accuracy rates were: irregular venous wall (87%), loss of interface (78%), proximity of mass (73%), and size (39%). Although "irregular venous wall" was the most accurate, it suffered from a low sensitivity rate (47%) because of its relative inability to detect superior mesenteric vein invasion (sensitivity of 17%). Angiographic criteria had accuracy rates of 73–90% with low sensitivity rates (20–77%). The R0 resection rate was 86% when all tests were used, 78% if EUS was used without angiography, and 60% if only angiography was used. In a comparison study, Gress et al. compared the accuracy of EUS to traditional CT scanning. EUS accuracy for T staging was as follows: T1 92%, T2 85%, T3 93%; and for N staging: N0 72% and N1 72%. CT accuracy for T staging was as follows: T1 65%, T2 67%, T3 38%; and for N staging : N0 52% and N1 100%. CT failed to detect a mass in 26% of patients with a confirmed tumor at surgery. Overall accuracy for T and N staging was 85% and 72% for EUS and 30% and 55% for CT, respectively. The ability to accurately predict vascular invasion was 93% for EUS and 62% for CT. EUS was 93% accurate for predicting local resectability versus 60% for CT (7).

The EUS criteria for invasion of the portal venous system have remained rather subjective. Rosch confirmed the subjectivity of the EUS image interpretation of a mass and the adjacent venous structures using a blinded interpretation of EUS images (8). The overall sensitivity and specificity of EUS in the diagnosis of venous invasion were 43% and 91%, respectively, when using predetermined parameters (visualization of tumor in the lumen, complete obstruction, or collateral vessels). If the parameter "irregular tumor–vessel relationship" was added to these criteria, the sensitivity rose to 62%, but the specificity fell to 79%. The only vascular system that could be properly visualized by EUS was the portal vein/confluence area. The positive and negative predictive values for the single parameters chosen to diagnose portal venous involvement were as follows: 42% and 33% for irregular tumor–vessel relationship, 36% and 34% for visualization of tumor in the vascular lumen, 80% and 28% for complete vascular obstruction, and 88% and 18% for collateral vessels.

In the context of high-resolution spiral CT scans, the role of EUS has been questioned. In a comparison study of radial EUS and CT, tumor detection, lymph node metastasis, and vascular invasion were compared using the results of surgical exploration in 37 patients (9). Both imaging modalities were reviewed in a blinded fashion and the results compared with pathology and operative reports on all patients. The sensitivity, specificity, positive predictive value, and negative predictive value for tumor detection by EUS were 97%, 33%, 94%, and 50%, respectively, compared with 82%, 66%, 97%, and 25% for CT scan. For lymph nodes the values were 21%, 80%, 57%, and 44%, respectively, for EUS compared with 42%, 73%, 67%, and 50% for CT. For vascular invasion, the values were 20%, 100%, 100%, and 89%, respectively, for EUS, compared with 80%, 87%, 44%, and 96% for CT. In general EUS was found to be superior for detecting tumor and predicting vascular invasion. Therefore, EUS should be used for patients in whom CT does not detect a mass and for those with an identifiable mass on CT in whom vascular invasion cannot be ruled out.

In a study comparing helical CT and EUS in 51 patients with pancreatic cancer, Tierney found both modalities were similar in their specificity for the diagnosis of unresectability (10). Nine patients had surgically confirmed locally unresectable disease, which was accurately predicted by EUS in six patients (sensitivity 67%) and by helical CT in three patients (sensitivity 33%). When only patients with complete EUS examinations were included, the sensitivities of EUS and helical CT for vascular invasion were 100% and 33%, respectively. The specificities of EUS (93%) and helical CT (100%) were similar for predicting resectability.

Linear EUS might provide higher-quality images compared to radial EUS images and enhanced staging accuracy (11). In a unique study using linear EUS staging, patients were evaluated with electronic linear EUS and spiral CT for suspected periampullary malignancies. Surgical/pathology staging results were the reference standard in 48 patients and tumor size, lymph node metastases, and major vascular invasion were assessed. Malignancy was histologically confirmed in 44 patients. EUS was significantly more sensitive (100%), specific (75%), and accurate (98%) than helical CT (68%, 50%, and 67%, respectively) for evaluation of a periampullary mass. In addition, EUS detected regional lymph node metastases in more patients than helical CT. Sensitivity, specificity, and accuracy of EUS were 61%, 100%, and 84%, in comparison with 33%, 92%, and 68%, respectively, with CT. Major vascular involvement was noted in 9 of 44 patients. EUS correctly identified vascular involvement in 100% compared with 45% for CT. This study suggested that high quality electronic linear EUS might be able to provide superior results to the imaging with spiral CT (11).

Recently, EUS was compared with helical CT and MRI staging accuracy in 62 patients with pancreatic cancer (12). A large series of patients with pancreatic carcinoma were studied by EUS, CT, MRI, and angiography. Results of each of the imaging techniques regarding primary tumor, locoregional extension, lymph node involvement, vascular invasion, distant metastases, TNM stage, and tumor resectability were compared with the surgical findings. Univariate, logistic regression, decision, and cost minimization analyses were performed. Helical CT had the

highest accuracy in assessing extent of primary tumor (73%), locoregional extension (74%), vascular invasion (83%), distant metastases (88%), TNM stage (46%),
and tumor resectability (83%), whereas EUS had the highest accuracy in assessing
tumor size ($r = 0.85$) and lymph node involvement (65%). Decision analysis demonstrated that the best strategy to assess tumor resectability was based on CT or
EUS as initial test, followed by the alternative technique in those potentially resectable cases. Cost minimization analysis favored the sequential strategy in which
EUS was used as a confirmatory technique in those patients in whom helical CT
suggested resectability of the tumor.

In a careful pathology-based study, EUS images were compared with a detailed
histologic analysis of portal vein invasion by adjacent pancreatic cancer (13). This
study compared EUS with vascular resection and histologic evidence of vascular
invasion in resected pancreatic masses. Sixty-eight patients with a solid pancreatic
mass who underwent both preoperative EUS and surgery at a single hospital over a
7-year period were identified; 30 of the 68 patients were resectable. Among these
30 patients, vascular adherence was present in eight, including 18% of patients with
an intact echoplane between tumor and adjacent vessels at EUS, 29% of those with
loss of echoplane alone, and 50% of those with additional EUS features of vascular
involvement. Vascular invasion was present in four, including 12% of patients with
an intact echoplane, 0% of those with loss of echoplane alone, and 33% of those
with additional EUS features. Sensitivity, specificity, PPV, and NPV of EUS were
63%, 64%, 43%, and 80% for vascular adherence and 50% 58%, 28%, and 82% for
vascular invasion. NPV rose to 90% for vascular adherence if only the portal confluence vessels were considered.

EUS staging post-neoadjuvant chemotherapy EUS staging is inaccurate due to
local tissue reaction to radiation and pancreatitis, simulating pancreatic malignancy
(14). The most common error after neoadjuvant therapy was overstaging a mass.
The EUS accuracy rate for staging after chemoradiation was 40%. For this single
reason, EUS is usually not indicated after chemotherapy or radiation.

7   Three-Dimensional EUS

Three-dimensional EUS may provide improved accuracy for the staging of pancreatic cancer by enhanced imaging of peripancreatic vessels (15). EUS results of 22
patients with solid pancreatic lesions were compared with surgical histology. FNA-
cytology proved adenocarcinoma in 17 patients and chronic pancreatitis in five.
EUS showed vascular invasion in 10 patients, vascular compression in six, and no
vascular involvement (NVI) in six. Additional 3D evaluation showed vascular invasion in six patients, vascular compression in 10, and NVI in six. Surgery proved
vascular invasion in seven patients, compression in nine, and NVI in six. EUS
showed invasion in 3/5 patients with chronic pancreatitis, 3D showed compression
only, whereas surgery found two patients to have compression and with NVI. In
two patients with pancreatic cancer, invasion was diagnosed on two-dimensional

(2D), but compression on 3D evaluation. Surgery showed compression and invasion in one each. Linear 3D EUS seems feasible for pancreatic evaluation. In addition, linear EUS enhanced the evaluation of vascular involvement of pancreatic lesions, especially in chronic pancreatitis.

Kobayashi has demonstrated similar results with infusion 3D ultrasound (*16*). On the basis of surgical findings, the accuracy rates of 2DUS, fusion 3DUS, DCT, and angiography were 78.6%, 92.9%, 85.3%, and 66.7%, respectively. The kappa values of 2DUS, fusion 3DUS, DCT, and angiography for PV invasion were 0.57, 0.90, 0.63, and 0.49, respectively, being most objective in fusion 3DUS. Fusion 3DUS is useful for diagnosis of PV invasion by pancreatic cancer.

An alternative to the use of specific criteria for the diagnosis of finding of an unresectable pancreatic mass is to look at multiple factors (*17*). In one study patients with pancreatic head cancer underwent EUS. Each patient was examined and each EUS finding was analyzed as a possible prognostic predictor, including heterogeneity of internal echo, irregularity of peripheral echo, clarity of boundary echo, dilatation of the main pancreatic duct (MPD), dilatation of the common bile duct, lymph node swelling, vessel invasion, and the presence of ascites, by univariate and multivariate analysis for survival. Irregular peripheral echo, portal vein invasion, superior mesenteric artery/celiac artery invasion, and the presence of ascites were significant predictors of a poorer prognosis by univariate analysis for survival. In resectable cases, EUS findings of MPD dilatation and portal invasion were significant prognostic predictors by univariate analysis, and MPD dilatation was an independent prognostic predictor by multivariate analysis.

8 Intravenous Ultrasonography

More advanced pancreatic cancer staging has been made possible with the recent introduction of intraportal venous ultrasonography (*18*). Intraportal endovascular ultrasound (IPEUS) has been reported to be the most precise diagnostic procedure for the accurate diagnosis of portal vein/superior mesenteric vein (PV/SMV) invasion in patients with pancreatic cancer. In this study, they evaluated the clinical significance of the length of PV/SMV invasion measured by IPEUS. Twenty-six consecutive patients, who underwent the pancreatic resection and IPEUS using an auto pull-back device between January, 1997 and September, 2000 were retrospectively evaluated. The length of PV/SMV invasion was measured by reviewing the videotapes recorded during the operation. Clinicopathologic data and survival were analyzed. The percentage of PV/SMV invasion was 46%, all of which were treated by PV/SMV resection. The cases without PV/SMV invasion showed significantly longer survival rate. The cases with 18 mm PV/SMV invasion, however, achieved a comparable 2-year survival rate of 28% whereas no patient with >18 mm PV/SMV invasion survived >18 months after the resection. Involvement of the PV/SMV by pancreatic carcinoma seems to be related to the extent of the disease and the PV/SMV involvement >18 mm is associated with a poor prognosis due to high rate of tumor positive margin even with radical operation.

9   Summary of EUS T Staging

In a large retrospective analysis of studies of the accuracy of EUS and CT, DeWitt et al. have compared the two imaging modalities. It is uncertain whether computed tomography (CT) or endoscopic ultrasound (EUS) is superior for the detection, staging, and resectability of pancreatic cancer. A systematic literature review was carried out to determine which test is more accurate. They identified relevant studies from MEDLINE (1986–2004) and evaluated study quality, which was measured on the basis of guidelines for assessing studies of diagnostic tests. Quantitative outcomes data were abstracted from the studies. Eleven studies with 678 patients satisfied inclusion criteria. Nine studies assessed tumor detection, all of which concluded that the sensitivity of EUS was superior to CT. Four of five studies that assessed tumor staging accuracy and five of eight that assessed nodal staging accuracy concluded that EUS was superior to CT. Among the four studies that assessed resectability, two showed no difference between EUS and CT, and one favored each modality. Three of 11 studies met all but one of the quality criteria. The most important and frequent study limitations were lack of a consecutive series of patients and biased patient selection for surgery. Quantitative comparisons among studies were precluded by differences in tumor staging classifications, surgical selection, CT and EUS techniques, and reporting of operating characteristics. The published literature comparing EUS and CT for preoperative assessment of pancreatic cancer is heterogeneous in study design, quality, and results. All studies have methodologic limitations that potentially affect validity. Prospective studies with state-of-the-art imaging are needed to further define the role of each test.

10   EUS Lymph Node Staging

EUS has generally excelled in its ability to detect malignant peripancreatic adenopathy. In a study of 160 patients, 78 had peripancreatic lymph nodes (49%), 25 had celiac lymph nodes (16%), and 14 patients had mediastinal lymph nodes (9%) that were suspicious for malignancy by morphologic criteria (19). In eight of 14 patients with suspicious mediastinal lymph nodes, FNA documented malignancy in 5%. Only one of these eight patients with malignant mediastinal adenopathy had other sites of documented distant metastases by CT and/or positron emission tomography scans. However, seven of eight patients had locally advanced cancers. Malignant mediastinal adenopathy is detected by staging EUS-FNA in 5% of patients with pancreaticobiliary cancer. Because of its important implications, endosonographers should routinely assess for malignant mediastinal adenopathy in patients who undergo staging EUS for pancreaticobiliary malignancy. Lymph node staging with EUS may provide even more important information than tumor staging (*20*). The outcome of pancreatic head cancer after surgical resection is still difficult to predict. In this study of 100 consecutive patients with invasive adenocarcinoma of the head of the pancreas, the results of surgical pathology were retrospectively analyzed to clarify the influence of clinicopathological factors. The overall 1-, 3-, and 5-year survival rates for the 100 patients with pancreatic head cancer were 55%, 16%, and 6%, respectively. Among the 16 clinicopathologic factors, nine were significantly associated with outcome in univariate analysis: tumor type (invasive ductal cancer), poor histologic differentiation, extrapancreatic plexus invasion, bile duct invasion, duodenal invasion, intrapancreatic nerve invasion, lymphatic invasion, venous invasion, and nodal involvement. Multivariate analysis confirmed that nodal involvement and extrapancreatic plexus invasion were significant independent factors for overall survival. Nodal involvement was the strongest predictor of poor survival after pancreatic resection for invasive adenocarcinoma of the head of the pancreas.

11 Conclusions

Preoperative pancreatic cancer staging with EUS provides detailed images of the pancreatic mass and its relationship to the peripancreatic vasculature. The accuracy of EUS staging varies with instrumentation, endoscopists, and patient selection. EUS excels in lymph node staging through the use of EUS. Currently, EUS staging remains a tool for the evaluation of patients with known or suspected pancreatic cancer. EUS has become the preferred method to obtain tissue biopsies in patients with locally advanced disease.

References

1. Huang QJ, Xu Q, Wang XN, 2002, Spiral multi-phase CT in evaluating resectability of pancreatic carcinoma. Hepatobiliary Pancreat Dis Int 1(4):614–619.
2. Agarwal B, Abu-Hamda E, Molke KL, 2004, Endoscopic ultrasound-guided fine needle aspiration and multidetector spiral CT in the diagnosis of pancreatic cancer. Am J Gastroenterol 99(5):844–850.
3. Karmazanovsky G, Fedorov V, Kubyshkin V, 2005, Pancreatic head cancer: accuracy of CT in determination of resectability. Abdom Imaging 30(4):488–500.
4. Li H, Zeng MS, Zhou KR, 2005, Pancreatic adenocarcinoma: the different CT criteria for peripancreatic major arterial and venous invasion. J Comput Assist Tomogr 29(2):170–175.
5. Brugge WR, Lee MJ, Kelsey PB, 1996, The use of EUS to diagnose malignant portal venous system invasion by pancreatic cancer. Gastrointest Endosc 43(6):561–567.
6. Brugge WR. 1995, Pancreatic cancer staging. Endoscopic ultrasonography criteria for vascular invasion. Gastrointest Endosc Clin North Am 5(4):741–753.
7. Gress FG, Hawes RH, Savides TJ, 1999, Role of EUS in the preoperative staging of pancreatic cancer: a large single-center experience. Gastrointest Endosc 50(6):786–791.

8. Rosch T, Dittler HJ, Strobel K, 2000, Endoscopic ultrasound criteria for vascular invasion in the staging of cancer of the head of the pancreas: a blind reevaluation of videotapes. Gastrointest Endosc 52(4):469–477.
9. Shoup M, Hodul P, Aranha GV, 2000, Defining a role for endoscopic ultrasound in staging periampullary tumors. Am J Surg 179(6):453–456.
10. Tierney WM, Francis IR, Eckhauser F, 2001, The accuracy of EUS and helical CT in the assessment of vascular invasion by peripapillary malignancy. Gastrointest Endosc 53(2):182–188.
11. Rivadeneira DE, Pochapin M, Grobmyer SR, 2003, Comparison of linear array endoscopic ultrasound and helical computed tomography for the staging of periampullary malignancies. Ann Surg Oncol 10(8):890–897.
12. Soriano A, Castells A, Ayuso C, 2004, Preoperative staging and tumor resectability assessment of pancreatic cancer: prospective study comparing endoscopic ultrasonography, helical computed tomography, magnetic resonance imaging, and angiography. Am J Gastroenterol 99(3):492–501.
13. Aslanian H, Salem R, Lee J, 2005, EUS diagnosis of vascular invasion in pancreatic cancer: surgical and histologic correlates. Am J Gastroenterol 100(6):1381–1385.
14. Bettini N, Moutardier V, Turrini O, 2005, Preoperative locoregional re-evaluation by endoscopic ultrasound in pancreatic ductal adenocarcinoma after neoadjuvant chemoradiation. Gastroenterol Clin Biol 29(6–7):659–663.
15. Fritscher-Ravens A, Knoefel WT, Krause C, 2005, Three-dimensional linear endoscopic ultrasound-feasibility of a novel technique applied for the detection of vessel involvement of pancreatic masses. Am J Gastroenterol 100(6):1296–1302.
16. Kobayashi A, Yamaguchi T, Ishihara T, 2005, Assessment of portal vein invasion in pancreatic cancer by fusion 3Dimensional ultrasonography. J Ultrasound Med 24(3):363–369.
17. Nakata B, Nishino H, Ogawa Y, 2005, Prognostic predictive value of endoscopic ultrasound findings for invasive ductal carcinomas of pancreatic head. Pancreas 30(3):200–205.
18. Tezel E, Kaneko T, Takeda S, 2005, Intraportal endovascular ultrasound for portal vein resection in pancreatic carcinoma. Hepatogastroenterology 52(61):237–242.
19. Agarwal B, Gogia S, Eloubeidi MA, 2005, Malignant mediastinal lymphadenopathy detected by staging EUS in patients with pancreaticobiliary cancer. Gastrointest Endosc 61(7):849–853.
20. Nakagohri T, Kinoshita T, Konishi M, 2006, Nodal involvement is strongest predictor of poor survival in patients with invasive adenocarcinoma of the head of the pancreas. Hepatogastroenterology 53(69):447–451.

Chapter 16
Laparoscopic Staging

Matthew H. Katz, Abdool R. Moossa, and Michael Bouvet

1 Introduction

Although pancreatic cancer currently ranks tenth in cancer incidence, it represents the fourth leading cause of cancer death in the United States among patients of both sexes (*1*). The therapeutic options available to individuals with this disease are primarily determined by disease stage. Patients with small, localized tumors are typically candidates for surgical resection by pancreaticoduodenectomy or distal pancreatectomy, which currently offer the only chance for long-term survival (*2*). In major, specialized centers, median survival of up to 20 months can now be achieved after complete tumor resection (*3–5*), with 5-year survival rates approaching 40–50% in selected patients (*6, 7*). Unfortunately, only 10–15% of patients with pancreatic cancer are found to have resectable tumors at the time of diagnosis, with the remainder harboring either locoregional extension or distant metastases (*8*) which preclude effective surgical therapy. For this overwhelming majority of patients presenting with advanced disease, treatment strategies are currently limited, and patient prognosis is therefore extremely poor—overall, individuals with advanced pancreatic malignancy have a 5-year survival rate less than 1%, with an overwhelming majority dead within 1 year of diagnosis (*9, 10*).

Timely diagnosis and staging thus play a fundamental role in the evaluation of patients with pancreatic cancer. Two goals are paramount. (*1*) diagnosis of the disease early in its natural history, thereby providing patients an opportunity for curative surgical therapy; and (*2*) preoperative discrimination between those patients with early stage tumors in whom tumor resection is warranted, and those with unresectable disease, and consequently limited survival, in whom the morbidity and expense of major surgery should routinely be avoided. Until recently, tissue diagnosis, staging, and assessment of resectability were all accomplished during exploratory laparotomy. Over the past two decades, however, significant advances in diagnostic and staging technologies, such as computed tomography (CT), endoscopic ultrasonography (EUS), and staging laparoscopy, as well as the development of minimally invasive palliative strategies, have permitted a more selective approach to open surgery (*11*).

A.M. Lowy et al. (eds.) *Pancreatic Cancer.*
doi: 10.1007/978-0-387-69252-4, © Springer Science+Business Media, LLC 2008

First performed as early as 1911 at Johns Hopkins on a patient with pancreatic cancer (*12*), staging laparoscopy in the modern era began with Cuschieri (*13*), who described a series of 23 patients with pancreatic cancer in whom a laparoscopic method was found to be effective in both diagnosis of the disease and determination of operability. Since that time, the different techniques used as well as the potential indications for the procedure have been described and expanded upon in numerous reports. In aggregate, the available data clearly indicate that laparoscopic exploration can be used as a supplemental staging procedure to identify small peritoneal or liver metastases in certain patients in whom such advanced disease may have been missed using other preoperative imaging modalities. The technique can therefore obviate the need for open exploration in certain patients. Further reports have demonstrated the potential value of adjunctive methods including extended dissection, laparoscopic ultrasonography, and the analysis of laparoscopically obtained peritoneal cytologic samples to further enhance the utility of laparoscopic exploration. Controversy continues to exist, however, as to whether laparoscopic staging should be offered to all patients with the disease, or selectively to particular subgroups of patients.

In our view, laparoscopic staging can be a safe and effective staging modality that should be offered selectively based on the likelihood that it will influence management in a given clinical scenario. This chapter reviews the current evidence supporting the use of staging laparoscopy in patients with a diagnosis of pancreatic cancer, and discusses its role in the algorithm we use to both stage and treat patients with this devastating disease.

2   American Joint Committee on Cancer Staging System for Pancreatic Cancer

Recently updated, the American Joint Committee on Cancer (AJCC) TNM staging system is used for the uniform staging of pancreatic cancer (Table 16.1) (*14*) and should be well understood prior to analyzing the efficacy of any staging modality. In the AJCC system, disease stage is determined by three factors: (*1*) the size of the primary tumor and its relationship to the celiac axis and superior mesenteric artery (T); (*2*) the presence or absence of regional lymph node involvement (N); and (*3*) the presence or absence of distant metastases (M). Tumors diagnosed in stage I are small and localized to the pancreas, and are therefore routinely resectable. Stage II disease is characterized by a primary tumor that extends into adjacent organs or involves regional lymph nodes, without distant metastases or invasion into the celiac trunk or superior mesenteric artery. Such tumors, even those with isolated portal or superior mesenteric vein involvement, are also often resectable. Patients with stage III disease have locally advanced disease that involves the major arteries, and those with stage IV tumors are found to have distant metastases at the time of diagnosis. Neither group is eligible for surgical resection. Instead, patients with stage III disease are often enrolled in clinical trials utilizing chemoradiation protocols designed to achieve locoregional control; patients with stage IV disease typically do not receive radiation but may be offered palliative chemotherapy. Adjunctive procedures, such

Table 16.1A TNM definitions for the staging of pancreatic cancer

Primary tumor (T)	
TX	Cannot be assessed
T0	No evidence of primary tumor
Tis	Carcinoma in situ
T1	Tumor confined to pancreas, ≤2 cm in diameter
T2	Tumor confined to pancreas, >2 cm in diameter
T3	Extrapancreatic extension, no celiac axis or SMA involvement
T4	Involvement of celiac axis or SMA
Regional lymph nodes (N)	
NX	Cannot be assessed
N0	Regional lymph node metastases absent
N1	Regional lymph node metastases present
Distant metastases (M)	
MX	Cannot be assessed
M0	Distant metastases absent
M1	Distant metastases present

SMA, superior mesenteric artery.

Table 16.1B AJCC TNM staging of pancreatic cancer

Stage 0	Tis, N0, M0
Stage I	
Ia	T1, N0, M0
Ib	T2, N0, M0
Stage II	
IIa	T3, N0, M0
IIb	T1-3, N1, M0
Stage III	T4, N0-1, M0
Stage IV	T1-4, T0-1, M1

as surgical biliary-enteric bypass or endobiliary stenting, may also be employed to palliate symptoms of biliary and duodenal obstruction.

In describing the utility of a staging modality such as laparoscopy in the context of the AJCC system, it is therefore of primary importance to consider the degree to which it can detect mesenteric arterial invasion and the presence of distant metastases, as both of these findings are associated with an upstaging of disease and a consequent change in the strategies available for treatment. When implemented appropriately, a comprehensive staging algorithm incorporating both noninvasive imaging and selective exploratory laparoscopy can be highly effective in this regard.

3 Techniques of Laparoscopic Staging

The laparoscopic techniques used for staging pancreatic malignancy have evolved over the past two decades. The procedure may be an outpatient study performed several days prior to potential open resection or it can be performed under the same general anesthetic as the open operation. Simple and extended techniques have been described (*15, 16*). We prefer a simple exploratory procedure performed under the same general anesthetic as potential resection. Pneumoperitoneum is initially obtained via an open Hasson technique or by using a Veress needle. Peritoneal access is typically through an infraumbilical incision, although a history of previous abdominal operations may necessitate a change in strategy. Once a single trocar has been placed, meticulous inspection of the liver, greater omentum, diaphragm, and abdominal and pelvic peritoneal surfaces is performed. A second 5-mm trochar, typically placed through a right upper quadrant incision, may be placed to manipulate a retracting device. Suspicious nodules are biopsied using a percutaneously inserted Tru-Cut needle. We do not typically perform an extensive dissection or laparoscopic ultrasonography, nor do we routinely obtain peritoneal aspirates for cytologic examination. Patients are considered to have unresectable disease in the presence of peritoneal or liver metastases (Fig. 16.1); those patients in whom these are not identified undergo immediate open exploration with the hope of curative resection. The entire procedure takes approximately 10–15 minutes of operating time.

Extended procedures, such as that advocated by the group at Memorial Sloan-Kettering Cancer Center, are grounded on the belief that the technique of laparoscopic staging should mimic the operative assessment performed at exploratory laparotomy (*15, 17*). A four-trocar setup is typically used. Prior to tumor manipulation, peritoneal washings are obtained for cytologic assessment. The primary tumor is then completely assessed, as are all peritoneal surfaces and the surface of the liver. Inspection of the mesocolon and middle colic vein is followed by division of the gastrohepatic ligament to expose the lesser sac, caudate lobe of the liver, vena cava, and celiac axis. Finally, laparoscopic ultrasound is performed to evaluate the liver and pancreas, with particular attention paid to the relationship of the primary tumor to major vessels. Biopsy of any suspicious nodes or lesions is performed at any point in the procedure. Patients are considered to have unresectable disease if

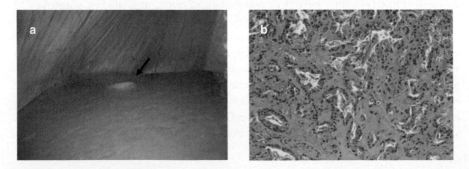

Fig. 16.1 A Surface liver lesion *(arrow)* discovered on laparoscopy in a 73-year-old man who was found on CT scan to have a potentially resectable mass in the head of the pancreas as well as several ambiguous, subcentimeter cystic lesions in the liver. **B** Frozen section biopsy of this liver lesion confirmed metastatic pancreatic cancer and the patient underwent endoscopic palliation of his jaundice

they have histologically confirmed metastases, extrapancreatic extension of tumor, celiac or high portal node involvement, or invasion or encasement of the major visceral vessels. Although it offers the surgeon the ability to more thoroughly evaluate the tumor, this technique takes considerably longer, and the dissection that it requires demands advanced laparoscopic skills.

4   Efficacy and Limitations of Noninvasive Staging

Because staging laparoscopy is an adjunctive staging study, and as such is not intended to replace currently available noninvasive techniques, it is important to consider the strengths and limitations of these existing staging modalities. Today, the diagnostic algorithm for staging pancreatic cancer is based upon abdominal imaging using a high-resolution, multidetector CT scanner. Modern protocols employ helical scanners, with which dual phase cross-sectional imaging of the pancreas and liver in the arterial and portal venous phases can be performed to detect both primary and metastatic disease with high sensitivity. In an evaluation of recent studies assessing helical CT in the diagnosis of pancreatic cancer, Tamm (*18*) found the overall detection rate to be approximately 89% and 71% for cancers >2 cm and <2 cm, respectively.

In addition to its diagnostic role, well-performed, high-quality CT scanning is also the initial, and currently most accurate, step in determining tumor resectability. Preoperative assessment of locoregional tumor extension is facilitated by examination of the tumor–vessel relationship using modern scanning techniques (*19, 20*) (Fig. 16.2 A and B); advances in both scanners and computer software have recently made possible the development of CT angiographic maps that can more accurately and vividly distinguish tumor encasement from tumors that lie adjacent to vessels (*21, 22*). Metastatic disease is also readily apparent (Fig. 16.2C): liver metastases typically appear as low attenuation lesions in the liver parenchyma, whereas peritoneal disease may manifest as low-volume ascites. Both may be missed, particularly when the malignant deposits are <1 cm in size. Nonetheless, the findings of Diehl (*23*), who detected 75% of patients with liver metastases and 80% of patients with peritoneal carcinomatosis using helical CT, are representative of the ability to detect metastatic disease using modern techniques.

In general, the CT criteria for potentially resectable disease can be defined as: (*1*) the absence of extrapancreatic disease, (*2*) the absence of direct tumor extension to the superior mesenteric artery and celiac axis as defined by the presence of a fat plane between the low-density tumor and these arterial structures, and (*3*) a patent superior mesenteric-portal venous confluence (*24*). Using these well-defined criteria for tumor resectability in a study of 145 patients with periampullary malignancies, Fuhrman identified 42 patients with radiographically resectable disease, of whom 88% underwent successful resection. Therefore, although other supplemental techniques, such as EUS, magnetic resonance cholangiopancreatography (MRCP), and positron emission tomography (PET) may be useful in certain

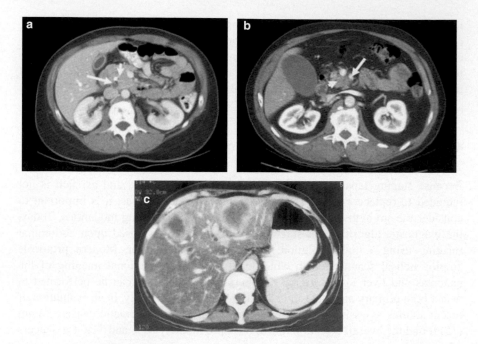

Fig. 16.2 High resolution, multidetector CT scanning is the first step in determining operability in patients with pancreatic cancer. **A** CT findings consistent with resectable stage I disease. A 1.4-cm hypoattenuating mass *(long arrow)* confined to the pancreas is visible just posterior to a previously implanted biliary stent *(short arrow)*. **B** A 2.5-cm hypoattenuating mass in the uncinate process consistent with a stage III tumor. Note the lack of a fat plane between the mass *(short arrow)* and superior mesenteric artery *(long arrow)* suggesting unresectable disease. **C** CT scan of a patient with stage IV disease. Note the multiple hypodense liver metastases

circumstances, a quality CT scan effectively serves as the cornerstone of the diagnostic and staging algorithm for patients with pancreatic malignancy.

5 Laparoscopic Assessment of Resectability

Data such as these and those reported by others (*25–29*) led Pisters (*30*) to determine that, performed properly using modern equipment and objective radiographic criteria, the predictive power of CT to determine resectability reaches 89%. The group therefore argued that progressive advancements in CT diagnostics have not only confounded the growing literature on the subject, but have also rendered the routine use of staging laparoscopy unnecessary. Nonetheless, recent studies using modern equipment continue to demonstrate that although CT is excellent at predicting *unresectability*, it is somewhat limited in its ability to predict *resectability*. Indeed, a substantial population of patients brought to open exploration based on the results of CT scan are still found to be unresectable due to CT-undetected loco-regional extension or metastasis.

Many groups have evaluated the efficacy of staging laparoscopy in detecting occult advanced disease in patients with pancreatic cancer. Much of the initial work in this area was performed at the Massachusetts General Hospital and Memorial Sloan-Kettering Cancer Center. In a prospective study from Memorial (*15*) of 115 patients with radiologically resectable peripancreatic tumors, 90% of whom had pancreatic ductal adenocarcinoma, Conlon identified 41 of 108 evaluable patients to have unresectable disease at staging laparoscopy using an extended technique: Hepatic metastases were found in 20 patients, mesenteric vascular encasement in 14, extrapancreatic/peritoneal involvement in 16, and celiac or portal lymphatic metastases in eight. Of the remaining 67 patients considered to have resectable disease upon completion of the laparoscopic examination, 61 (91%) underwent successful open resection. In aggregate, tumor resection was performed in 76% of patients who underwent open exploration, whereas only 35% of a similar historical cohort with radiographically resectable tumors underwent resection by the same group prior to the use of laparoscopy.

Evidence from the Massachusetts General Hospital also demonstrates the ability of staging laparoscopy to detect radiographically occult metastases and therefore to enhance predictive accuracy for resectability. Fernandez-del Castillo (*31*) laparo-scopically explored 114 patients with pancreatic tumors and no evidence of meta-static disease on preoperative CT and found 24% to have occult intra-abdominal metastases. In a subsequent study of 125 patients with radiographic staged II and III pancreatic cancer, Jimenez (*16*) identified 31% of patients to have unsuspected metastatic disease not evident on preoperative CT scan, in whom open exploration was foregone. Notably, although this group did not utilize an extended approach, they did obtain peritoneal washings as part of their laparoscopic procedure, and 7% of patients had positive peritoneal cytology as their only evidence of metastatic disease. It is also important to recognize that the high rate of occult metastases detected by laparoscopy in these two series is due in no small part to the fact that patients with locally advanced disease were included in the analyses. Nonetheless, these data, as well as those published by other groups (*32–35*), demonstrate that laparoscopy is able to identify radiographically occult metastases and render open operation unnecessary in certain groups of patients. It should be noted that the use of adjuvant techniques, such as the use of laparoscopic ultrasonography (*36–38*) and peritoneal lavage (*39–41*), may be used during laparoscopic exploration with the potential to enhance its diagnostic accuracy.

It is of particular importance to emphasize that for those patients found to have unresectable disease on staging laparoscopy, primary nonoperative therapies can be initiated as expeditiously as possible due to the shorter convalescent period associated with this procedure compared with that after exploratory laparotomy. A retro-spective study of 79 patients found to have various unresectable intraabdominal malignancies upon staging laparoscopy (*n* = 21) or exploratory laparotomy (*n* = 58) by Velanovich (*42*) provides evidence to support this concept. In this study, patients who underwent staging laparoscopy were not only more likely to receive either chemotherapy or radiotherapy (76% versus 43%) than those who underwent laparotomy, but treatment was also initiated more rapidly after exploration (13 versus 35 days).

Finally, as Pisters argues (*30*), the studies supporting the use of staging laparoscopy suffer from the limitation that they do not report the pathologic status of the retroperitoneal margin after attempted curative resection in patients who have undergone such an attempt. Reported as R0 (microscopically and macroscopically negative), R1 (macroscopically negative but microscopically positive), or R2 (macroscopically positive), the status of the retroperitoneal resection margin is of critical importance because patients who have undergone resection and are left with a positive margin have an unfavorable prognosis similar to that of patients with more advanced disease managed nonoperatively. Therefore, the most common endpoint reported in the majority of these analyses, whether or not patients undergo *attempted* curative resection based on the results of a staging protocol employing laparoscopy, may be misleading because incomplete resections are potentially under-reported. A more precise and objective endpoint would be the number of patients in whom an oncologically complete, R0 resection was performed. This important criticism should be kept in mind when analyzing the literature.

6   Factors Increasing the Yield of Selective Laparoscopy

Although laparoscopy may obviate the need for exploration in patients with CT-occult metastases, not all patients staged routinely using laparoscopic exploration would be found to harbor such disease and therefore only some would benefit from the procedure. To put the technique to its best possible use, and to realize its highest yield, we therefore agree with the opinion that laparoscopic exploration should be used only in those patients in whom a high likelihood of radiographically occult advanced disease exists. Several characteristics of otherwise radiographically resectable periampullary tumors have been reported to be associated with a high rate of such disease and may therefore be used as criteria with which patients most likely to benefit from the procedure may be selected.

6.1   Primary Tumor Location

Patients with tumors of the body and tail of the pancreas are at a substantially higher risk for harboring associated intraperitoneal metastases than those with tumors in the head of the gland. This is likely due to the more advanced stage at presentation of these tumors: only 10% of pancreatic tail tumors present with clinically significant biliary obstruction, whereas up to 90% of right-sided tumors do (*43*). It has also been suggested that tumors in the body or tail may harbor a more aggressive biology (*44*). In Jiminez's series (*16*), 36% of tumors in the body or tail were associated with gross metastatic disease, in significant contrast with only 17% of right-sided tumors. Moreover, left-sided tumors were significantly more likely to be associated with positive peritoneal cytologic test results indicative of microme- tastases (36% versus 9%). Similar findings have been documented by others (*44, 45*). Therefore, using the location of the primary tumor as a selection criterion for offering patients staging laparoscopy would increase the diagnostic yield of this procedure.

6.2 *Primary Tumor Size*

Patients with larger tumors are more likely to harbor metastatic disease than those with smaller tumors. In a recent study of 54 patients undergoing exploratory laparotomy after clinical staging with abdominal CT, endoscopic retrograde cholangiopancreatography (ERCP) and abdominal ultrasound, Morganti (*46*) found that no patient with a tumor diameter <30 mm had previously undetected abdomi- nal metastases discovered upon laparotomy, in contrast with 22.2% of patients with tumors >30 mm. Primary tumor size on noninvasive imaging therefore may be used to select high-yield patients for subsequent laparoscopic exploration.

6.3 *Pathologic Diagnosis of Primary Tumor*

It has been well described that patients with nonpancreatic periampullary neo- plasms have a far more favorable prognosis than those with pancreatic ductal aden- ocarcinoma (*47*). These patients are also typically less likely to harbor intra-abdominal metastases than those with pancreatic cancer. Vollmer (*34*) studied 157 patients with peripancreatic and biliary cancers who underwent laparoscopic exploration after more conventional noninvasive staging. Twenty-two patients were diagnosed with adenocarcinoma of the duodenum or ampulla of Vater; among this group, none were found to have occult disease precluding subsequent exploration on staging laparoscopy. In contrast, 31% of patients with cancer of the head of the pancreas were found to have vascular invasion or metastatic disease upon laparoscopy. Similarly, Brooks (*48*) found that patients with distal bile duct tumors benefited from laparoscopic staging both in terms of determining resectability and avoiding unnecessary surgery, but those with known duodenal or ampullary adenocarcino- mas did not. Laparoscopic exploration has also been shown to be of value in patients with nonfunctioning islet cell tumors of the pancreas, in whom high rates of occult metastases have been identified (*49*). The yield of staging laparoscopy therefore appears to be highly dependent on tissue diagnosis. It should be noted, however, that in many centers, particularly those in which neoadjuvant therapy is not routinely advocated, preoperative acquisition of a tissue diagnosis may not be routine prior to either laparoscopic or open exploration. In such centers, such as

ours, tissue diagnosis is obtained only after resection or upon final determination of
unresectability so as to direct subsequent nonoperative therapy.

6.4   Serologic Tumor Marker CA 19-9

Determination of serum levels of the tumor marker CA 19-9 may have a role in the
diagnostic and staging algorithm for patients with pancreatic cancer due to its low
cost and relatively high diagnostic sensitivity (50). Recent studies have also demonstrated that it may be used to select patients in whom staging laparoscopy would
be particularly effective. In a retrospective review of 63 patients, Karachristos correlated serum CA 19-9 levels with intraoperative findings on staging laparoscopy.
Patients with a high serum CA 19-9 antigen level were significantly more likely to
have metastases identified upon laparoscopic exploration. Indeed, no patient with a
CA 19-9 level below 100 U/ml were found to have metastatic disease; the authors
noted that excluding patients from laparoscopy with CA 19-9 levels below this cutoff would have increased its diagnostic yield to 26.7% from 19%. Schlieman (51)
also found serum CA 19-9 levels to be useful in screening patients for subsequent
exploratory laparoscopy, using a serum level of 150 U/ml as a cutoff. Connor
arrived at a similar conclusion in a more recent study (52).

7   Staging Laparoscopy in Patients With
Locally Advanced Disease

Patients with locally advanced pancreatic cancer without evidence of metastatic disease (stage III) are distinctly different from patients with metastatic disease (stage
IV) in terms of both the therapeutic options available to them and their overall prognosis. Those patients with stage III disease are commonly enrolled in clinical trials
typically involving locoregional chemoradiation (53) in either a palliative or neoadjuvant fashion, with a potential for obtaining local control and prolonging survival.
Moreover, due to their more favorable prognosis, some of these patients deemed to
be good risk may be offered surgical procedures designed to palliate symptoms of
biliary and gastric outlet obstruction, which have been shown to provide a longer
symptom-free interval than less-invasive therapies (54–57). In contrast, patients with
stage IV disease, with their severely limited survival, are routinely treated with systemic chemotherapy and minimally invasive palliative procedures.

Accurate discrimination between patients with stage III and stage IV disease is
therefore imperative so as to avoid the potential for understaging, which would lead
to the administration of toxic and expensive therapies to patients who would not
benefit from these treatments. From an outcomes analysis point of view, accurate
discrimination between these groups is also critical to accurately assess response
to various investigational therapies and experimental protocols. The belief that

laparoscopy could be of value in this regard led the group at Massachusetts General Hospital to include patients with advanced stage disease in their early studies of the technique (16, 31). More recently, several groups have studied the use of staging laparoscopy exclusively for this indication. Shoup (58) studied 100 consecutive patients with unresectable disease by CT or magnetic resonance imaging (MRI) but no evidence of distant metastases on preoperative imaging. Exploratory laparoscopy revealed seven patients with both. These upstaged patients were thereby spared the toxicity of local radiation, prompting the authors to conclude that staging laparoscopy should be used for all patients with locally advanced disease prior to their enrollment in clinical trials. A recent analysis by Liu (45) examined 74 patients who similarly were believed to have locally advanced pancreatic cancer without distant metastases based on preoperative imaging; 34% of these patients were found to have occult metastatic disease upon staging laparoscopy. This group utilized peritoneal lavage: 27% of patients had positive cytology (12% had positive cytology as their only evidence of metastatic disease), 16% had occult liver lesions, and 7% were found to have peritoneal implants. The authors therefore emphasized the importance of acquiring peritoneal samples for cytologic analysis in these groups of patients.

8   Cost-Effectiveness

Few data exist concerning the cost-effectiveness of laparoscopic staging in patients with pancreatic cancer. Compared with open exploration alone, laparoscopic exploration is certainly associated with a reduction in hospital stay (15), which has obvious implications for the group of patients in whom findings on laparoscopy preclude open exploration. Indeed, using a decision model to evaluate the cost-effectiveness of various strategies for determining resectability in hypothetical cohorts of patients with pancreatic malignancy, McMahon found that strategies employing laparoscopy and laparoscopic ultrasound were highly cost-effective due to their ability to reduce the number of patients requiring more costly laparotomy (59).

Nonetheless, selective staging laparoscopy may be more cost-effective than routine use. In one study of 180 patients with periampullary malignancies scheduled for open resection based on findings on high-quality CT, Freiss (29) concluded that routine use of laparoscopic staging could not be justified on an economic basis. In this series, preoperative laparoscopy changed the final operative strategy of 30% of patients with radiographically resectable pancreatic ductal adenocarcinoma—14% due to the presence of occult metastases and 17% due to locoregional invasion. Using a simple cost–benefit analysis, the group demonstrated that exploratory laparoscopy would have to be seven times less expensive than open exploration to achieve a cost benefit; however, it should be emphasized that because the identification of local retroperitoneal infiltration by laparoscopic techniques was not considered predictable, the subset of patients with locally advanced disease was not considered in this analysis. In contrast, Andren-Sandberg (60) found that selective use of laparoscopy could reduce hospital costs on the order of 30% in about half of patients with pancreatic malignancy previously assessed with CT scan. Other factors, including whether laparoscopy is performed under the same or separate anesthesia as open exploration, and the efficacy and cost-effectiveness of other staging modalities, must also be taken into account when considering staging laparoscopy from an economic perspective.

9   Position of Staging Laparoscopy in the UCSD Algorithm

Our staging algorithm for pancreatic cancer (*11*) (Fig. 16.3) has been designed to differentiate the small group of patients with potentially resectable cancer from those with locally advanced or disseminated disease as efficiently and as cost-effectively as possible given current technologies. We believe that the existing data support the selective use of staging laparoscopy in patients for whom a high index of suspicion exists for occult advanced disease despite previous imaging studies to the contrary.

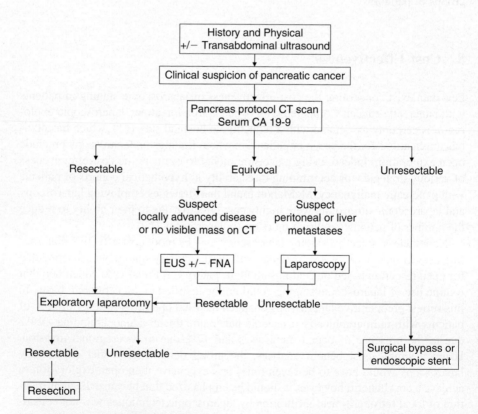

Fig. 16.3 Current algorithm used at University of California, San Diego for the diagnosis and staging of pancreatic tumors

In our institution, laparoscopy is therefore undertaken in patients using the criteria outlined by Pisters (*30*), specifically, in those patients with: (*1*) large but otherwise radiologically resectable tumors, (*2*) CT findings suggestive but not definitive for metastatic disease, (*3*) tumors of the body or tail of the gland, and (*4*) clinical findings consistent with advanced cancer, such as a disproportionate elevation of CA 19-9 to radiographic findings. The remainder of good-risk patients with otherwise radiographically resectable tumors are prepared for open exploratory laparotomy and potential resection with curative intent; those in whom unresectable disease is identified intraoperatively undergo biliary-enteric and gastrojejunal bypass.

10 Conclusion

Diagnostic laparoscopy has become a widely utilized staging modality for pancreatic cancer. There remains variability among pancreatic surgeons as to the use of a simple one- or two-trocar technique versus advanced laparoscopic dissection, the timing of laparoscopy relative to the definitive laparotomy, and which adjunctive modalities such as laparoscopic ultrasound or peritoneal cytology are used. The data clearly indicate that laparoscopy can reduce the number of nontherapeutic laparotomies performed in patients with radiologically resectable pancreatic cancer. The technique may also play an important role in selecting appropriate treatment protocols for patients with advanced, otherwise nonoperative neoplasms, in whom it may be instrumental in discriminating between patients with locally advanced and metastatic disease. We believe that selective use of the procedure in defined groups can maximize both its diagnostic yield and its cost-effectiveness, but given the ongoing evolution in preoperative imaging modalities, studies are needed to continually evaluate the indications and limitations of staging laparoscopy in patients with pancreatic cancer.

References

1. Jemal A, Siegel R, Ward E, 2006, Cancer statistics, 2006. CA Cancer J Clin 56(2):106–130.
2. Stojadinovic A, Brooks A, Hoos A, 2003, An evidence-based approach to the surgical management of resectable pancreatic adenocarcinoma. J Am Coll Surg 196(6):954–964.
3. Bouvet M, Gamagami RA, Gilpin EA, 2000, Factors influencing survival after resection for periampullary neoplasms. Am J Surg 180(1):13–17.
4. Breslin TM, Hess KR, Harbison DB, 2001, Neoadjuvant chemoradiotherapy for adenocarcinoma of the pancreas: treatment variables and survival duration. Ann Surg Oncol 8(2):123–132.
5. Yeo CJ, Cameron JL, Sohn TA, 1997, Six hundred fifty consecutive pancreaticoduodenectomies in the 1990s: pathology, complications, and outcomes. Ann Surg 226(3):248, 57; discussion 257–260.
6. Furukawa H, Okada S, Saisho H, 1996, Clinicopathologic features of small pancreatic adenocarcinoma. A collective study. Cancer 78(5):986–990.

7. Yeo CJ, Cameron JL, Lillemoe KD, 1995, Pancreaticoduodenectomy for cancer of the head of the pancreas. 201 patients. Ann Surg 221(6):721, 31; discussion 731–733.

8. Sener SF, Fremgen A, Menck HR, 1999, Pancreatic cancer: a report of treatment and survival trends for 100,313 patients diagnosed from 1985–1995, using the National Cancer Database. J Am Coll Surg 189(1):1–7.

9. Yeo CJ. 1998, Pancreatic cancer: 1998 update. J Am Coll Surg 187(4):429–442.

10. Lillemoe KD. 1995, Current management of pancreatic carcinoma. Ann Surg 221(2):133–148.

11. Katz MH, Savides TJ, Moossa AR, 2005, An evidence-based approach to the diagnosis and staging of pancreatic cancer. Pancreatology 5(6):576–590.

12. Bernheim B. 1911, Organoscopy: cystoscopy of the abdominal cavity. Ann Surg 53:764–767.

13. Cuschieri A, Hall AW, Clark J. 1978, Value of laparoscopy in the diagnosis and management of pancreatic carcinoma. Gut 19(7):672–677.

14. Exocrine pancreas. In: American Joint Committee on Cancer (AJCC) Cancer Staging Manual, 6th ed. Springer, 2002, 157–164.

15. Conlon KC, Dougherty E, Klimstra DS, 1996, The value of minimal access surgery in the staging of patients with potentially resectable peripancreatic malignancy. Ann Surg 223(2):134–140.

16. Jimenez RE, Warshaw AL, Rattner DW, 2000, Impact of laparoscopic staging in the treatment of pancreatic cancer. Arch Surg 135(4):409, 14; discussion 414–415.

17. Tucker ON, Conlon KC. 2005, Laparoscopic staging. In: Hoff DD, Von Evans DB, Hruban RH (eds.) Pancreatic cancer. Jones and Bartlett, Sudbury, MA, 207 –221.

18. Tamm E, Charnsangavej C. 2001, Pancreatic cancer: current concepts in imaging for diagnosis and staging. Cancer J 7(4):298–311.

19. Loyer EM, David CL, Dubrow RA, 1996, Vascular involvement in pancreatic adenocarcinoma: reassessment by thin-section CT. Abdom Imaging 21(3):202–206.

20. Lu DS, Reber HA, Krasny RM, 1997, Local staging of pancreatic cancer: criteria for unresectability of major vessels as revealed by pancreatic-phase, thin-section helical CT. AJR Am J Roentgenol 168(6):1439–1443.

21. House MG, Yeo CJ, Cameron JL, 2004, Predicting resectability of periampullary cancer with three-dimensional computed tomography. J Gastrointest Surg 8(3):280–288.

22. Horton KM, Fishman EK. 2002, Adenocarcinoma of the pancreas: CT imaging. Radiol Clin North Am 40(6):1263–1272.

23. Diehl SJ, Lehmann KJ, Sadick M, 1998, Pancreatic cancer: value of dual-phase helical CT in assessing resectability. Radiology 206(2):373–378.

24. Fuhrman GM, Charnsangavej C, Abbruzzese JL, 1994, Thin-section contrast-enhanced computed tomography accurately predicts the resectability of malignant pancreatic neoplasms. Am J Surg 167(1):104, 11; discussion 111–113.

25. Spitz FR, Abbruzzese JL, Lee JE, 1997, Preoperative and postoperative chemoradiation strategies in patients treated with pancreaticoduodenectomy for adenocarcinoma of the pancreas. J Clin Oncol 15(3):928–937.

26. Gloor B, Todd KE, Reber HA. 1997, Diagnostic workup of patients with suspected pancreatic carcinoma: the University of California-Los Angeles approach. Cancer 79(9):1780–1786.

27. Holzman MD, Reintgen KL, Tyler DS, 1997, The role of laparoscopy in the management of suspected pancreatic and periampullary malignancies. J Gastrointest Surg 1(3): 236–244.

28. Rumstadt B, Schwab M, Schuster K, 1997, The role of laparoscopy in the preoperative staging of pancreatic carcinoma. J Gastrointest Surg 1(3):245–250.

29. Friess H, Kleeff J, Silva JC, 1998, The role of diagnostic laparoscopy in pancreatic and periampullary malignancies. J Am Coll Surg 186(6):675–682.

30. Pisters PW, Lee JE, Vauthey JN, 2001, Laparoscopy in the staging of pancreatic cancer. Br J Surg 88(3):325–337.

31. Fernandez-del Castillo C, Rattner DW, Warshaw AL, 1995, Further experience with laparoscopy and peritoneal cytology in the staging of pancreatic cancer. Br J Surg 82(8): 1127–1129.
32. Doran HE, Bosonnet L, Connor S, 2004, Laparoscopy and laparoscopic ultrasound in the evaluation of pancreatic and periampullary tumours. Dig Surg 21(4):305–313.
33. Velasco JM, Rossi H, Hieken TJ, 2000, Laparoscopic ultrasound enhances diagnostic laparoscopy in the staging of intra-abdominal neoplasms. Am Surg 66(4):407–411.
34. Vollmer CM, Drebin JA, Middleton WD, 2002, Utility of staging laparoscopy in subsets of peripancreatic and biliary malignancies. Ann Surg 235(1):1–7.
35. Maire F, Sauvanet A, Trivin F, 2004, Staging of pancreatic head adenocarcinoma with spiral CT and endoscopic ultrasonography: an indirect evaluation of the usefulness of laparoscopy. Pancreatology 4(5):436–440.
36. Nieveen van Dijkum EJ, Romijn MG, Terwee CB, 2003, Laparoscopic staging and subsequent palliation in patients with peripancreatic carcinoma. Ann Surg 237(1):66–73.
37. Taylor AM, Roberts SA, Manson JM, 2001, Experience with laparoscopic ultrasonography for defining tumour resectability in carcinoma of the pancreatic head and periampullary region. Br J Surg 88(8):1077–1083.
38. Thomson BN, Parks RW, Redhead DN, 2006, Refining the role of laparoscopy and laparoscopic ultrasound in the staging of presumed pancreatic head and ampullary tumours. Br J Cancer 94(2):213–217.
39. Jimenez RE, Warshaw AL, Fernandez-Del Castillo C, 2000, Laparoscopy and peritoneal cytology in the staging of pancreatic cancer. J Hepatobiliary Pancreat Surg 7(1):15–20.
40. Merchant NB, Conlon KC, Saigo P, 1999, Positive peritoneal cytology predicts unresectability of pancreatic adenocarcinoma. J Am Coll Surg 188(4):421–426.
41. Fernandez-del Castillo CL, Warshaw AL. 1998, Pancreatic cancer. Laparoscopic staging and peritoneal cytology. Surg Oncol Clin North Am 7(1):135–142.
42. Velanovich V, Wollner I, Ajlouni M, 2000, Staging laparoscopy promotes increased utilization of postoperative therapy for unresectable intra-abdominal malignancies. J Gastrointest Surg 4(5):542–546.
43. Bouvet M, Binmoeller KF, Moossa AR. 2001, Diagnosis of adenocarcinoma of the pancreas. In: Cameron JL (ed.) American Cancer Society atlas of clinical oncology: pancreatic cancer. Decker, Hamilton, ON.
44. Karachristos A, Scarmeas N, Hoffman JP. 2005, CA 19-9 levels predict results of staging laparoscopy in pancreatic cancer. J Gastrointest Surg 9(9):1286–1292.
45. Liu RC, Traverso LW. 2005, Diagnostic laparoscopy improves staging of pancreatic cancer deemed locally unresectable by computed tomography. Surg Endosc 19(5):638–642.
46. Morganti AG, Brizi MG, Macchia G, 2005, The prognostic effect of clinical staging in pancreatic adenocarcinoma. Ann Surg Oncol 12(2):145–151.
47. Katz MH, Bouvet M, Al-Refaie W, 2004, Non-pancreatic periampullary adenocarcinomas: an explanation for favorable prognosis. Hepatogastroenterology 51(57):842–846.
48. Brooks AD, Mallis MJ, Brennan MF, 2002, The value of laparoscopy in the management of ampullary, duodenal, and distal bile duct tumors. J Gastrointest Surg 6(2):139, 45; discussion 145–146.
49. Hochwald SN, Weiser MR, Colleoni R, 2001, Laparoscopy predicts metastatic disease and spares laparotomy in selected patients with pancreatic nonfunctioning islet cell tumors. Ann Surg Oncol 8(3):249–253.
50. Katz MH, Moossa AR, Bouvet M, 2005, Serologic diagnosis of pancreatic cancer. In: Von Hoff DD, Evans DB, (eds.) Pancreatic cancer. Jones and Bartlett, Boston, 235–249.
51. Schlieman MG, Ho HS, Bold RJ. 2003, Utility of tumor markers in determining resectability of pancreatic cancer. Arch Surg 138(9):951, 5; discussion 955–956.
52. Connor S, Bosonnet L, Alexakis N, 2005, Serum CA19-9 measurement increases the effectiveness of staging laparoscopy in patients with suspected pancreatic malignancy. Dig Surg 22(1–2):80–85.
53. Moertel CG, Frytak S, Hahn RG, 1981, Therapy of locally unresectable pancreatic carcinoma: a randomized comparison of high dose (6000 rads) radiation alone, moderate dose radiation

(4000 rads + 5-fluorouracil), and high dose radiation + 5-fluorouracil: the Gastrointestinal Tumor Study Group. Cancer 48(8):1705–1710.

54. Lillemoe KD, Cameron JL, Hardacre JM, 1999, Is prophylactic gastrojejunostomy indicated for unresectable periampullary cancer? A prospective randomized trial. Ann Surg 230(3):322, 8; discussion 328–330.

55. Nieveen van Dijkum EJ, Romijn MG, Terwee CB, 2003, Laparoscopic staging and subsequent palliation in patients with peripancreatic carcinoma. Ann Surg 237(1):66–73.

56. Van den Bosch RP, van der Schelling GP, Klinkenbijl JH, 1994, Guidelines for the application of surgery and endoprostheses in the palliation of obstructive jaundice in advanced cancer of the pancreas. Ann Surg 219(1):18–24.

57. Van Wagensveld BA, van Coene PP, van Gulik TM, 1997, Outcome of palliative biliary and gastric bypass surgery for pancreatic head carcinoma in 126 patients. Br J Surg 84(10):1402–1406.

58. Shoup M, Winston C, Brennan MF, 2004, Is there a role for staging laparoscopy in patients with locally advanced, unresectable pancreatic adenocarcinoma? J Gastrointest Surg 8(8): 1068–1071.

59. McMahon PM, Halpern EF, Fernandez-del Castillo C, 2001, Pancreatic cancer: cost-effectiveness of imaging technologies for assessing resectability. Radiology 221(1):93–106.

60. Andren-Sandberg A, Lindberg CG, Lundstedt C, 1998, Computed tomography and laparoscopy in the assessment of the patient with pancreatic cancer. J Am Coll Surg 186(1):35–40.

Section IV
Surgery for Pancreatic Cancer

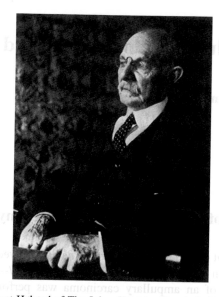

Fig. 17.1 William Stewart Halsted of The Johns Hopkins Hospital. (Reprinted with permission from Schulick RD, Yeo CJ. Whipple procedure: 1935 to present. In: Evans DB, Pisters PWT, Abbruzzese JL (eds.) Pancreatic cancer. New York, Springer-Verlag, 2002, 126)

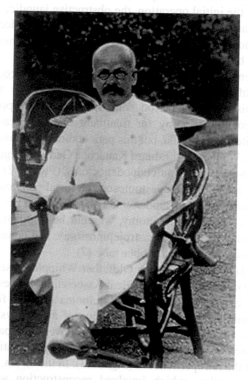

Fig. 17.2 Walther Carl Eduard Kausch.

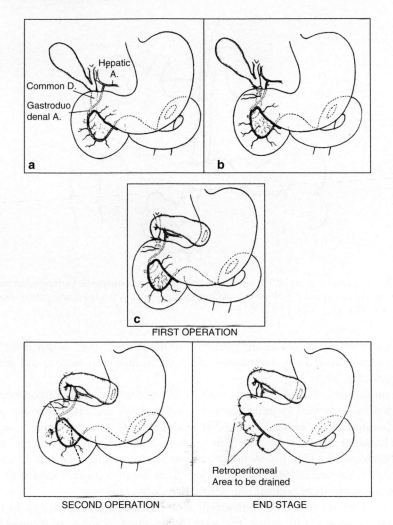

Fig. 17.3 Illustration of the two-stage pancreaticoduodenectomy performed by Whipple. (Reprinted with permission from Whipple AO, Parson WB, Mullins CR. Treatment of carcinoma of the ampulla of Vater. Ann Surg 1935, 102:763–779)

choledochojejunostomy, an end-to-side pancreaticojejunostomy, and an end-to-side gastrojejunostomy. All anastomoses were to the proximal jejunum and all were retrocolic (9, 10). In all, Whipple reported performing 37 pancreaticoduodenectomies in his career (Fig. 17.4).

In 1937, Brunschwig, from the University of Chicago and later Memorial Sloan-Kettering Cancer Center, reported extending the indication for pancreaticoduodenectomy to also include cancer of the head of the pancreas (11). He resected a 4-cm mass from the head of the pancreas in a 69-year-old man in a two-stage procedure. The first stage included the creation of a cholecystojejunostomy,

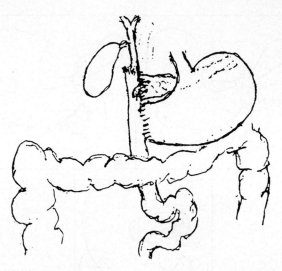

Fig. 17.4 Freehand drawing by Whipple of the one-stage reconstruction he performed on patients starting in 1942. (Reprinted with permission from Whipple AO. A reminiscence: pancreaticoduodenectomy. Rev Surg 1963, 20:221–225)

gastroenterostomy, and enteroenterostomy. In the second stage he performed the pancreaticoduodenectomy, oversewing the pylorus, distal duodenum, and pancreatic neck (Fig. 17.5).

In the decades that followed the work of these surgeons, pancreaticoduodenectomics were performed in limited numbers, with variable and often poor outcomes. This continued even as late as the 1960s and early 1970s, with mortality rates at some hospitals approaching 25%. This led some authors to suggest that the operation be abandoned (*12, 13*). A notable exception to this high mortality rate was reported by Howard in 1968, who reported 41 consecutive patients treated by pancreaticoduodenectomy without one hospital mortality (*14*).

Outcomes have improved dramatically over the last 20 years (*15–18*). In 1990, Trede et al. reported 118 consecutive resections without an operative death (*19*). In 1993, surgeons at Johns Hopkins described 145 consecutive pancreaticoduodenectomies without one mortality (*20*). A more recent study, also from Johns Hopkins, reviewed 650 cases between 1990 and 1996, showing 190 consecutive Whipple procedures performed without one mortality (*21*). Currently, many centers report operative mortalities <4% (15–18, 21).

2 Current Operative Techniques

Upon gaining entrance to the abdominal cavity, the initial maneuvers are to assess the extent of disease and resectability of the mass. First, the entire liver is examined for metastases not seen on preoperative imaging. The celiac axis

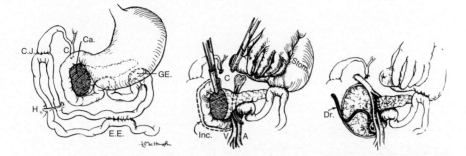

Fig. 17.5 Three steps in the two-stage pancreaticoduodenectomy performed by Brunschwig for adenocarcinoma of the head of the pancreas. A, superior mesenteric artery; C, common bile duct; Ca, pancreatic cancer; CJ, cholecystojejunostomy; Dr, drain; EE, enteroenterostomy; GE, gastroenterostomy; V, superior mesenteric vein. (Reprinted with permission from Brunschwig A. A one stage pancreaticoduodenectomy. Surg Gynecol Obstet 1937, 65:681–684)

is inspected for lymphadenopathy. The omentum, ligament of Treitz, entire visceral and parietal peritoneum, and entire small intestine and intra-abdominal large intestine are examined for tumor involvement. Next, an extensive Kocher maneuver is performed, lifting the duodenum from the retroperitoneum, allowing examination of the superior mesenteric vein and palpation of the superior mesenteric artery pulse in its retropancreatic position (Fig. 17.6). The porta hepatis is assessed by mobilizing the gallbladder off the gallbladder fossa and dissecting the cystic duct down to the junction of the common hepatic duct and common bile duct (Fig. 17.7). In favorable cases, the tumor is localized to the head, neck, or uncinate process, so that all gross disease is within the resection zone.

If the intraoperative assessment suggests that the resection margins will be well free of tumor, the procedure may be performed in the standard manner. However, if the tumor seems to encroach on the resection margins, the sequence of the procedure should be modified. If this is the case, the easiest portions of the dissection should be performed first, with the more difficult parts saved for later. In this manner, it has been found that tumors first judged to be unresectable may instead be removed successfully.

After the gallbladder is dissected from its fossa, the distal common hepatic duct (or common bile duct) is divided. This allows the common bile duct to be retracted caudally, opening a plane of dissection along the anterior surface of the portal vein. At this time, the portal structures should be assessed for a replaced right hepatic artery coming from the superior mesenteric artery or any other arterial anomalies. If a replaced right hepatic artery is discovered, it should be carefully dissected and protected from subsequent damage. Next, the gastroduodenal artery is identified and clamped atraumatically. This confirms that the hepatic artery is not being supplied solely by collateralization from the superior mesenteric artery, such as in

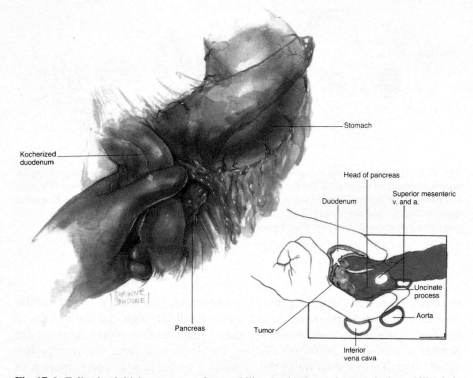

Fig. 17.6 Following initial assessment of resectability, the duodenum is extensively mobilized via a Kocher maneuver. This maneuver is important to be certain that the tumor has not extended beyond the uncinate process and into the superior mesenteric artery. When performed properly, the superior mesenteric artery can be palpated, indicating a normal uncinate process is adjacent to it *(inset)*. (Reprinted with permission from Cameron JL. Atlas of surgery, vol 1. Toronto, ON, BC Decker, 1990, 387)

cases of celiac artery occlusion or stenosis. Once this is proven, the gastroduodenal artery is triply ligated and divided.

Attention is next paid to the most proximal region of GI tract to be resected. We typically favor pylorus preservation. If such preservation is desired, the proximal GI tract should be divided 2 to 3 cm distal to the pylorus with a linear stapling device. The right gastric artery is routinely sacrificed to allow better mobilization of the duodenum. Alternatively, if the pylorus is not to be preserved, then up to a 30–40% distal gastrectomy is performed. Next, the distal GI tract resection is performed, by identifying a proximal region of mobile jejunum, usually 10–20 cm from the ligament of Treitz, and dividing it with a linear stapling device. The mesenteric vessels to the proximal jejunal specimen are clamped, divided, and ligated. Once the proximal jejunum is separated from its mesenteric attachments, it can be delivered dorsal to the superior mesenteric vessels from left to right,

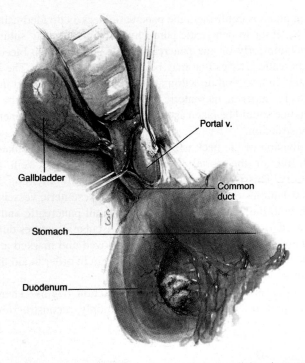

Fig. 17.7 A direct route to expose the portal vein is to dissect medial to the extrahepatic biliary tree and lateral to the proper hepatic artery. A combination of both blunt and sharp dissection usually quickly exposes the anterior surface of the portal vein. (Reprinted with permission from Cameron JL. Atlas of surgery, vol 1. Toronto, ON, BC Decker, 1990, 389)

allowing for easier dissection of the uncinate process off the right lateral aspect of the superior mesenteric vein and artery.

Next, the dissection of the pancreas off of the superior mesenteric vein–portal vein confluence is performed. The superior mesenteric vein is identified running anterior to the third portion of the duodenum, surrounded by adipose tissue. The vein receives tributaries from the uncinate process and neck of the pancreas, the greater curve of the stomach, and the transverse mesocolon. In this location, the vein can be identified by dissecting the fatty tissue of the transverse mesocolon away from the uncinate process of the pancreas. The tributaries emptying into the anterior surface of the superior mesenteric vein are divided, allowing continued cephalad dissection. Under direct vision, the plane anterior to the superior mesenteric vein is developed in a cephalad direction, carefully avoiding branches and tumor involvement. Dissection cephalad to the pancreatic neck will allow exposure of the portal vein. Care should be taken to avoid injury to the splenic vein, as it joins the superior mesenteric vein posterior to the neck of the pancreas. Once dissection of this plane is completed, a Penrose drain can be looped under the neck of the pancreas in order to elevate it.

Once a free plane is confirmed, the pancreatic neck is divided using electrocautery (Fig. 17.8). Prior to pancreatic parenchymal division, stay sutures are placed superiorly and inferiorly on the pancreatic remnant to reduce bleeding from the segmental pancreatic arteries that may be located at these sites. The Penrose drain should be pulled in a ventral direction as the neck is being divided in order to prevent injury to the superior mesenteric and portal veins. During the parenchymal transection, notice should be taken as to the position of the main pancreatic duct for the later reconstruction.

Once the division of the neck is performed, the head and uncinate process can be dissected free of the portal vein, superior mesenteric vein, and superior mesenteric artery. This is performed by serially clamping, dividing, and tying the small venous tributaries off the portal and superior mesenteric vessels. This should be done flush with the vessels in order to remove all pancreatic and nodal tissue. Great care is used to avoid injury to these major vascular structures during this time. After this is completed, the specimen can be removed and marked at the bile duct margin, uncinate margin, and pancreatic neck margin in order to aid the pathologist in proper identification (Fig. 17.9).

After the removal of the specimen, reconstruction begins. There are several options for this part of the procedure. Most commonly, reconstruction begins with

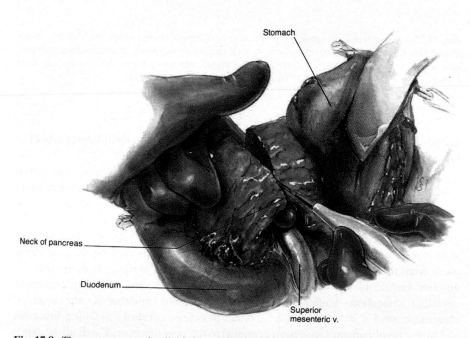

Fig. 17.8 The pancreas may be divided by electrocautery. Note that the surgeon's finger is shown underneath the pancreatic neck to prevent damage to the superior mesenteric and portal veins. A Penrose drain can also be used to elevate the neck during this part of the operation. (Reprinted with permission from Cameron JL. Atlas of surgery, vol 1. Toronto, ON, BC Decker, 1990, 393)

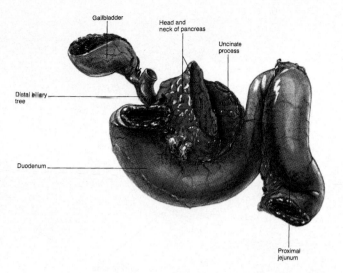

Fig. 17.9 This is a depiction of the pylorus-preserving pancreaticoduodenectomy specimen. It includes the distal portion of the first portion of the duodenum; all of the second, third, and fourth portions of the duodenum; and several centimeters of the proximal jejunum. In addition, all of the head, neck, and uncinate process of the pancreas are included, as well as the tumor, gallbladder, and distal biliary tree. (Reprinted with permission from Cameron JL. Atlas of surgery, vol 1. Toronto, ON, BC Decker, 1990, 399)

the pancreatic anastomosis, followed by the biliary anastomosis, and finally the duodenal or gastric anastomosis (Fig. 17.10). The pancreatic-enteric anastomosis is usually performed as an invagination pancreaticojejunostomy, either in an end-to-side or end-to-end fashion. Controversies in creating this anastomosis include the optimal configuration, the importance of using duct-to-mucosal sutures, and the option of using pancreatic duct stents. An alternative to using a jejunal limb for this anastomosis would be to perform a pancreaticogastrostomy (Fig. 17.11). At our institution, this reconstruction is most commonly performed as an end-to-side pancreaticojejunostomy to the upper part of the retained jejunum, pulling the jejunal limb through the transverse mesocolon to the right of the middle colic artery: 2 to 3 cm of the pancreatic remnant should be mobilized for an optimal anastomosis. The anastomosis is performed in two layers; the outer layer using interrupted 3-0 silk sutures to incorporate the pancreatic capsule and the seromuscular layer of the jejunum, and the inner layer using a running absorbable 3-0 suture between the cut edge of the pancreas and capsule and the full thickness of jejunum (Fig. 17.12). This technique allows invagination of the cut surface of the pancreatic neck into the jejunal lumen.

The second anastomosis to be performed is usually the biliary-enteric anastomosis. It is performed in an end-to-side fashion, either as a hepaticojejunostomy or choledochojejunostomy, approximately 10 cm distal to the pancreatic anastomosis. We use a single layer of interrupted absorbable sutures and we do not routinely

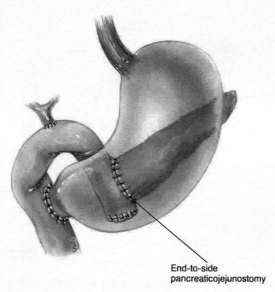

End-to-side
pancreaticojejunostomy

Fig. 17.10 The final anatomy after a pylorus-preserving pancreaticoduodenectomy. (Reprinted with permission from Cameron JL. Atlas of surgery, vol 1. Toronto, ON, BC Decker, 1990, 407)

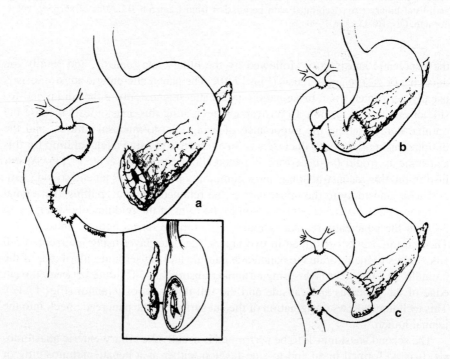

Fig. 17.11 Schematic illustration of (a) pancreaticogastrostomy, (b) end-to-end pancreaticojejunostomy, and (c) end-to-side hepaticojejunostomy. The inset details the posterior gastrotomy. (Reprinted with permission from Yeo CJ, Cameron JL, Maher MM, et al. A prospective randomized trial of pancreaticogastrostomy versus pancreaticojejunostomy after pancreaticoduodenectomy. Ann Surg 1995, 222:580–589)

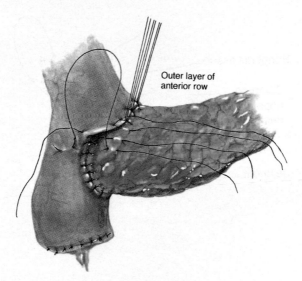

Fig. 17.12 This is a depiction of the final steps in the end-to-side pancreaticojejunostomy, with an outer layer of 3-0 silk suture being placed in the anterior row. (Reprinted with permission from Cameron JL. Atlas of surgery, vol 1. Toronto, ON, BC Decker, 1990, 409)

stent this anastomosis (Fig. 17.13). If the patient has an endoscopically placed biliary prosthesis at the time of the operation, this will be removed with the specimen. However, if the patient has a percutaneous transhepatic biliary drainage catheter, then it is usually left traversing the biliary-enteric anastomosis.

The third and final anastomosis is between the duodenum and the jejunum if pylorus preservation was performed, or between the gastric remnant and jejunum if a distal gastrectomy was performed. We complete a two-layer anastomosis, with an outer layer of interrupted silk and an inner layer of running absorbable suture. This anastomosis is created 10 to 15 cm distal to the hepaticojejunostomy and above the transverse mesocolon. In this way, all three anastomoses are retrocolic. Alternatively, the duodenojejunostomy can be performed in an antecolic fashion, further downstream from the hepaticojejunostomy.

Upon completion of the reconstruction, closed suction drains are placed near the biliary and pancreatic anastomoses. We do not routinely perform a vagotomy or use prophylactic octreotide, nor do we place gastrostomy or jejunostomy tubes.

3 Postoperative Care

After a pancreaticoduodenectomy is performed, patients are routinely transferred to a monitored ICU setting overnight, so that a frequent assessment of their vital signs, oxygen saturation, and fluid status may be completed. Optimally, these patients are

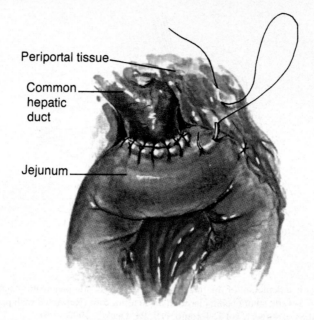

Fig. 17.13 This is the final appearance of the end-to-side hepaticojejunostomy. This anastomosis is performed with a single layer of interrupted sutures. (Reprinted with permission from Cameron JL. Atlas of surgery, vol 1. Toronto, ON, BC Decker, 1990, 403.)

extubated immediately postoperatively, although a small minority remains intubated overnight. In the first 24 hours after the procedure, hemoglobin levels are checked every 2 to 4 hours. Also in the first 24 hours, perioperative IV antibiotics and crystalloid solutions are administered. Patients are also given a proton pump inhibitor and a Patient Controlled Analgesia (PCA) pump for pain control. Prophylaxis for deep vein thrombosis is given in the form of subcutaneous heparin, sequential compression devices, and thigh high Thrombo Embolism Deterrent (TED) hose.

On the first postoperative day, the patient is typically transferred to either a step-down unit or regular floor bed. The nasogastric tube placed intraoperatively is removed and the patient is given sips of clear liquids. The sequential compression devices are removed and the patient is helped out of bed and into a chair. The IV fluids are reduced to 80 cc an hour and antibiotics are discontinued. By postoperative day 2, the patient can usually be started on a clear liquid diet. The Foley catheter is removed, the dressing is removed, and the IV fluid administration is further decreased. If needed, diuresis is commenced with IV furosemide.

By the third postoperative day, most patients are started on a regular diet. IV fluids are further decreased in volume, and if a central venous catheter was placed intraoperatively, it may be removed as long as adequate peripheral access can be obtained. The patient is started on pancrelipase tablets to be taken with each meal. If the pathology report reveals the removal of a malignant process, radiation oncology and medical oncology teams are consulted to provide appropriate outpatient follow-up. Over the following days, the drainage from the closed suction catheters is closely monitored, and the drains are removed if the drainage is serous appearing. If any question exists as to leakage from an anastomosis, the sinister-appearing drain fluid is tested. After patients have tolerated a regular diet, they are started on oral medications. Blood glucose levels are checked at least four times daily and insulin is administered when appropriate. In elderly patients with coronary artery disease, β-blockers are given routinely throughout the hospital course to maintain a heart rate <80 beats per minute.

With this postoperative pathway, patients are targeted for hospital discharge on postoperative day 6 or 7. Patients are given discharge prescriptions for oral pain medications, a proton pump inhibitor, and pancrelipase tablets.

4 Long-Term Outcomes

Several reports from The Johns Hopkins Hospital have analyzed the outcomes of patients undergoing successful pancreaticoduodenectomy. One report reviewed 201 patients undergoing resection for pancreatic cancer between 1970 and 1994 (*18*). Overall, the group had an actuarial 5-year survival of 21% and a median survival of 15.5 months (Fig. 17.14). If the patient had negative surgical margins, the 5-year survival was increased to 26%, whereas positive surgical margins dropped the 5-year survival to 8%. Survival improved depending on the time period, with 3-year

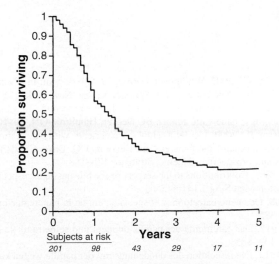

Fig. 17.14 The actuarial survival curve (Kaplan-Meier) for 201 patients undergoing pancreaticoduodenectomy for pancreatic adenocarcinoma. (Reprinted with permission from Yeo CJ, Cameron JL, Lillemoe KD et al. Pancreaticoduodenectomy for cancer of the head of the pancreas: 201 patients. Ann Surg 1995, 221:721–733)

survivals of 14% in the 1970s, 21% in the 1980s, and 36% in the 1990s. The strongest predictors of long-term survival, by multivariate analysis, included tumor diameter >3 cm, negative resected lymph node status, negative resected margins, tumor diploid DNA content, and decade of resection.

A second study from The Johns Hopkins Hospital reviewed 650 pancreaticoduodenectomies performed between January 1990 and July 1996 (21). The patients had a mean age of 63 years, with 54% being male and 91% being white. Two hundred eighty-two patients, or 43%, had resection specimens showing pancreatic ductal adenocarcinoma. Other common pathologic findings included ampullary cancer in 11%, distal common bile duct cancer in 10%, chronic pancreatitis in 11%, neuroendocrine tumors in 5%, and duodenal cancer in 4%. Surgical resection utilized pylorus preservation in 82%, partial pancreatectomy in 95%, and portal or superior mesenteric venous resection in 4%. During this series, 190 consecutive resections were performed without one mortality. Overall, nine deaths occurred in-hospital or within 30 days, yielding a 1.4% operative mortality rate. The postoperative complication rate was 41%, with the most common being early delayed gastric emptying in 19%, pancreatic fistula in 14%, and wound infection in 10%. Twenty-three patients, or 3.5%, required reoperation in the immediate postoperative period, most commonly for bleeding, abscess or dehiscence. A recent update from Johns Hopkins has included all pancreaticoduodenectomies performed through 2005, totaling 1423 patients with pancreatic cancer (22). The addition of the most recent data showed an increase in median age at operation to 66 years, with patients in the current decade averaging 68 years old. This study also showed the postoperative stay declined from 16 days in the 1980s to 8 days in the 2000s. Also, the postoperative mortality declined from 30% in the 1970s to 1% in the 2000s.

References

1. Schulick RD, Yeo CJ. 2002, Whipple procedure: 1935 to present. In: Evans DB, Pisters PWT, Abbruzzese JL (eds.) Pancreatic cancer. Springer-Verlag, New York, 125–138.
2. Yeo CJ. 2001, Surgical management: standard Whipple procedure. In: Cameron JL (ed.) Atlas of clinical oncology: pancreatic cancer. BC Decker, Hamilton, ON, 99–108.
3. Yeo CJ, Cameron JL. 2000, The Johns Hopkins experience with pancreaticoduodenectomy for ductal adenocarcinoma of the pancreas. In: Dervenis CG, Bassi C (eds.) Pancreatic tumors: achievements and prospective. Thieme, Stuttgart, 176–188.
4. Halsted WS. 1899, Contributions to the surgery of the bile passages, especially of the common bile duct. Boston Med Surg J 141:645–654.
5. Sauve L. 1908, Des pancreatectomies et specialement de la pancreatectome cephalique. Rev Chir 37:335–385.
6. Kausch W. 1912, Das carcinoma der papilla duodeni und seine radikale Entfeinung. Beitr Z Clin Chir 78:439–486.
7. Hirschel G. 1914, Die resecktion des duodenums mit der papille wegen karzinoims. Munchen Med Wochenscher 61:1728–1730.
8. Whipple AO, Parson WB, Mullins CR. 1935, Treatment of carcinoma of the ampulla of Vater. Ann Surg 102:763–779.
9. Whipple AO. 1963, A reminiscence: pancreaticoduodenectomy. Rev Surg 20:221–225.

10. Whipple AO. 1946, Observations on radical surgery for lesions of the pancreas. Surg Gynecol Obstet 82:623–631.
11. Brunschwig A. 1937, A one stage pancreaticoduodenectomy. Surg Gynecol Obstet 65:68–684.
12. Crile G Jr.1970, The advantages of bypass operations over radical pancreaticoduodenectomy in the treatment of pancreatic carcinoma. Surg Gynecol Obstet 130:1049–1053.
13. Shapiro TM. 1975, Adenocarcinoma of the pancreas: a statistical analysis of biliary bypass vs Whipple resection on good risk patients. Ann Surg 182:715–721.
14. Howard JM. 1968, Pancreaticoduodenectomy: forty-one consecutive Whipple resections without an operative mortality. Ann Surg 168:629–640.
15. Braasch JW, Rossi RL, Watkins E Jr1986, Pyloric and gastric preserving pancreatic resection. Experience with 87 patients. Ann Surg 204:411–418.
16. Crist DW, Sitzmann Cameron JL. 1987, Improved hospital morbidity, mortality and survival after the Whipple procedure. Ann Surg 206:358–365.
17. Fernandez-del Castillo C, Rattner DW, Warshaw AL. 1995, Standards for pancreatic resection in the 1990's. Arch Surg 130:295–300.
18. Yeo CJ, Cameron JL, Lillemoe KD, et al.1995, Pancreaticoduodenectomy for cancer of the head of the pancreas: 201 patients. Ann Surg 221:721–733.
19. Trede M, Scwall G, Saeger H-D. 1990, Survival after pancreaticoduodenectomy: 118 consecutive resections without an operative mortality. Ann Surg 221:447–458.
20. Cameron JL, Pitt A, Yeo CJ, et al.1993, One hundred and forty five consecutive pancreaticoduodenectomies without mortality. Ann Surg 217:430–438.
21. Yeo CJ, Cameron JL, Sohn TA, et al. 1997, Six hundred fifty consecutive pancreaticoduodenectomies in the 1990's: pathology, complications, outcomes. Ann Surg 226:248–260.
22. Winter JM, Cameron JL, Campbell KA, et al. 2006, Pancreaticoduodenectomies for pancreatic cancer: a single institution experience. J GI Surg, 10:1199–1211.

Chapter 18
Total Pancreatectomy for Treatment of Pancreatic Adenocarcinoma

Thomas Schnelldorfer, Kaye M. Reid Lombardo, Michael B. Farnell, and Michael G. Sarr

1 Introduction

Successful total pancreatectomy was first performed in 1942 by Priestley at the Mayo Clinic in Rochester, Minnesota for an insulinoma (*1*). In 1944, Fallis at the Henry Ford Hospital in Detroit, Michigan undertook the first successful total pancreatectomy for pancreatic carcinoma (*2*). Soon, recommendations were made from several centers for total pancreatectomy in anticipation to cure pancreatic cancer (*3*). In the early 1970s, total pancreatectomy was advocated by several groups as the preferred resection for pancreatic adenocarcinoma. The reasoning for this decision was several-fold. Most surgeons were dissatisfied by survival outcomes after pancreatoduodenectomy and were looking for reasons that might explain the inordinately high recurrence rate (*4*). The option of total pancreatectomy was based on the belief that pancreatic adenocarcinoma was multicentric with undetected foci of neoplasm within the remnant gland (up to 30%) which would be addressed by complete excision. The operation provided a generous pancreatic parenchymal margin with a potentially better oncologic resection (lymphadenectomy and soft tissue clearance), all of which were felt to be advantageous for survival. The absence of need for a pancreaticoenterostomy and its associated morbidity was welcomed by elimination of pancreatic fistulae which at the time were associated with high mortality. The inevitable loss of endocrine and exocrine pancreatic function and the associated splenectomy with its infectious sequelae, although taken into consideration, may not have been appreciated fully. In the mid-1980s, it became evident that total pancreatectomy did not provide a superior outcome compared to other forms of pancreatic resections, and the true incidence of multicentricity has been shown to be quite low (*5, 6*). Currently, the concept of total pancreatectomy as a routine procedure in the management of pancreatic adenocarcinoma is rejected, and only a selected approach is still in use.

A.M. Lowy et al. (eds.) *Pancreatic Cancer*.
doi: 10.1007/978-0-387-69252-4, © Springer Science+Business Media, LLC 2008

2 Morbidity and Mortality After Total Pancreatectomy

In recent years, total pancreatectomy accounts for less than 4 to 8% of all pancreatic resections performed for pancreatic adenocarcinoma in high volume centers (7–10). The perioperative morbidity rate is on average about 45% in patients undergoing total pancreatectomy for pancreatic neoplasms (Table 18.1). The most frequently observed major complication is abdominal sepsis and abscess, followed by fistula from the biliary or gastrointestinal anastomosis and intra-abdominal hemorrhage (5, 9, 11, 12). In contrast to the partial resections of pancreatoduodenectomy and distal pancreatectomy, where intra-abdominal abscesses or sepsis are usually related to pancreatic fistula at the pancreaticoenterostomy or from closure of the pancreatic stump, respectfully, abdominal infections after total pancreatectomy are usually independent of biliary and intestinal fistulae. Although the risk of pancreatic fistula is eliminated after total pancreatectomy, the incidence of overall morbidity is similar when compared to partial pancreatic resections of the head or body/tail (13, 14). The perioperative mortality in series from high-volume centers averages about 14% (see Table 18.1). Two retrospective studies with large numbers of patients found a higher perioperative mortality after total pancreatectomy when compared to subtotal pancreatectomy (5), pancreatoduodenectomy (11), and distal pancreatectomy (11) in patients with pancreatic adenocarcinoma. Comparisons with historic controls, as well as other observational studies, have shown similar operative mortality for total pancreatectomy when compared to pancreatoduodenectomy or distal pancreatectomy (13, 14).

Table 18.1 Large series on total pancreatectomy for pancreatic adenocarcinoma

Source	Years of study	No. of patients	Perioperative morbidity	Perioperative mortality	Median survival	5-year survival
Baumel H et al. (11)	1982–1988	112	41%	17%	12 Months	3%
Sarr MG et al. (13)	1955–1990	99	—	6%	—	10%
Ihse I et al. (5)	1959–1992	89	52%	27%	7 Months	5%
Brooks JR et al. (42)	1970–1986	48	27%	8%	—	14%
Launois B et al. (12)	1968–1986	47	53%	13%	8 Months	8%
Swope TJ et al. (14)	1987–1991	47	39%	8%	17 Months	—
Sohn TA et al. (8)	1984–1999	38	—	—	11 Months	—
Herter FP et al. (43)	1945–1978	34	—	—	9 Months	3%
Karpoff HM et al. (9)	1983–1998	28	61%	9%	8 Months	—
Michelassi F et al. (44)	1946–1987	26	—	24%	—	—
Wagner M et al. (10)	1993–2001	17	56%	—	—	—
Balcom JH et al. (7)	1990–2000	9	18%	0%	—	—
	Total:	594	Mean: 44%	Mean: 14%	Mean: 10 mo	Mean: 7%

3 Does Elimination of the Pancreaticoenterostomy and Its Complications Justify Total Pancreatectomy?

The elimination of complications from the pancreatic anastomosis has always been cited as one of the main advantages of total pancreatectomy for pancreatic adenocarcinoma. Historically, the majority of postoperative deaths after pancreatoduodenectomy were related to fistula from breakdown of the pancreatic anastomosis. Currently, most high-volume centers now perform pancreatoduodenectomy with mortality <5% (7, 8, 15). With recent improvements in experience, early diagnosis, and interventional radiographic drainage, the "fear" of pancreatic fistula which gave pancreatoduodenectomy such a bad name in the past has decreased greatly. Currently, about 90% of pancreatic fistulae have no clinical sequelae and do not affect patient outcome (16, 17). These biochemical, transient, or grade A fistulae usually do not require any further intervention (18). Type B and type C fistulae that affect the clinical condition of the patient can often be controlled with a nonoperative approach via management/manipulation of operative drains and/or by interventional, percutaneous placement of drains if needed. Therefore, the justification of total pancreatectomy as a measure to prevent major "catastrophes" from pancreatic fistula is no longer valid in most patients, because it adds other obligate morbidity.

4 Metabolic Consequences After Pancreatectomy

Although hyperglycemia or recent-onset diabetes mellitus are present in up to 80% of patients with pancreatic cancer, just the presence of preoperative insulin-dependent (type I) or adult-onset (type II) diabetes should not alone be an indication for total resection of the gland (19). Indeed, the added morbidity of hypoglycemia and brittle glycemic control with pancreatogenic or type III diabetes can pose a very real problem for the patient and physician alike. The diabetes mellitus of the apancreatic patient is characterized by the complete absence of insulin and glucagon. The lack of glucagon can lead to a physiologically "unprotected" state of hypoglycemia, as well as subsequent hyperglycemic episodes, which can be at times be very difficult to control (brittle diabetes) because of the complete lack of endogenous insulin. Nevertheless, in most patients under the care of an experienced endocrinologist or internist, the hyperglycemia is usually mild, and clinically important ketoacidosis is rare (20), as reflected by hemoglobin A1c levels being close to normal after total pancreatectomy. With rigorous home monitoring of blood glucose concentrations, the presence of serious, life-threatening hypoglycemia can be minimized. Hospitalization rates secondary to hypoglycemia in patients who understand and practice good self-care can be similar to rates for other insulin-dependent diabetic patients; however, 2–3% of patients will still die from hypoglycemia after total pancreatectomy, thus making the selection of appropriate patients an important criterion when considering total pancreatectomy (*21*, *22*).

In addition to the endocrine insufficiency, exocrine insufficiency plays a substantive negative role. Early metabolic challenges from the maldigestion/malabsorption of the apancreatic state involve control of steatorrhea and weight stabilization. Awareness of these problems, along with intensive postoperative nutritional support, will minimize the postoperative weight loss. Despite use of maximal pancreatic enzyme supplementation, diarrhea continues to occur in up to 10% of patients. In some patients, weight control becomes a long-term problem, despite of control of the steatorrhea. Some studies suggest a nutritional benefit after pylorus-preserving total pancreatectomy as measured by increased body weight at follow-up (*23*, *24*). Deficiencies in fat-soluble vitamins, magnesium, and trace elements should be anticipated and can be prevented with adequate supplementation (*22*).

Another, less well-understood metabolic sequelae of total pancreatectomy is the loss of hepatotrophic factors originating from the pancreas. Numerous experimental studies have shown that the pancreas, in addition to the gut, makes factors that are released into the portal venous system that help to maintain normal hepatic function (*4*). Just how crucial these pancreas-derived hepatotrophic factors are in maintaining normal function and architecture of the liver is unknown. Worrisome, however, is a report by Dressler and colleagues (*22*) who followed long-term survivors of a very aggressive operative approach for pancreatic cancer—the Fortner procedure. Interestingly, several of their patients developed an otherwise unexplained cirrhosis after total pancreatectomy, not explained by alcoholism, suggesting a lack of hepatotrophic factors. This topic remains essentially unexplored in humans.

When examined carefully and comprehensively by appropriate quality-of-life instruments, the overall performance status and global concerns of quality of life, as well as pancreas-specific quality of life, has been reasonable in long-term survivors (*21*, *22*). This important finding indicates that the metabolic consequences of exocrine and endocrine insufficiency are generally well-compensated in the majority of patients, despite the observation that in some patients, deprivation of endocrine function can lead to life-threatening situations. In summary, the ability to control these metabolic changes can justify performing total pancreatectomy if it is felt that the operation would provide better oncologic results and the patient is deemed reliable and has insight into his self-care.

5   Infectious Morbidity from Splenectomy

In contrast to pancreatoduodenectomy, total pancreatectomy for adenocarcinoma always obligates a splenectomy. From a technical aspect, splenic preservation could be feasible in selected patients, but because of putative oncologic considerations of the dorsal resection margin and associated splenic artery nodes, attempts at splenic preservation is not recommended in most cancer patients. Splenectomy does incorporate a small but potential risk for overwhelming post-splenectomy sepsis even in adults; indeed, the lifetime risk in asplenic adults is only 0.3–1.9% and usually manifests within the first 2 years after operation. The high morbidity and mortality associated with overwhelming post-splenectomy infection is largely preventable if appropriate precautions are taken, including appropriate vaccinations against *Meningococcus*, *Haemophilus*, and *Pneumococcus* species (25). Nevertheless, most surgeons believe that the higher rate of intra-abdominal sepsis after total pancreatectomy, despite the absence of a pancreaticoenterostomy, is related to the splenectomy and its nonspecific infectious predisposition even in the early postoperative period. But it is also conceivable in part that patients undergoing total pancreatectomy are selected currently for this operation due to more locally advanced and difficult-to-resect disease causing increased operative blood loss and need for blood transfusion, thereby resulting in an immunocompromised state with a subsequently increased infection rate.

6   Is Total Pancreatectomy the Better Oncologic Resection?

For pancreatic adenocarcinoma, the only chance for cure lies in complete operative resection of localized disease in the absence of distant metastasis outside the realm of resection. To assure the occurrence of not only a gross (R1) but also a microscopic complete resection (R0), adequate tissue margins to the tumor become critical. Although total pancreatectomy would seem to offer wider resection margins, one should be reminded that total pancreatectomy is a resection with a wider longitudinal margin only; the radial margins (retroperitoneal, peri-venous around portal vein structures) are very similar to partial pancreatectomy. The added resection of the remnant gland with its associated nodal basin adds little from an oncologic standpoint, because ductal carcinoma of the pancreas is not multifocal, and metastasis to the nodes on the left side of the mesenteric vessels are involved only rarely (26–28).

7   Is Pancreatic Adenocarcinoma a Multicentric Disease?

The idea of multicentric pancreatic adenocarcinoma was first addressed realistically in the 1960s. Many surgeons believed that because adenocarcinoma is primarily ductal in origin, all ducts were susceptible to malignant transformation when exposed to the "right" stimuli, and therefore they favored a total pancreatectomy to eradicate this risk. This concept was attractive theoretically. In principle, however, substantial differences were found in the rates of multicentric carcinoma or carcinoma in-situ in specimens after total pancreatectomy for adenocarcinoma (see Table 18.2), ranging from as low as 0% to a high of 33%. The problem of such a varied rate of multicentricity was related in great part to the histologic definition of multicentricity of pre-cancer or carcinoma-in-situ. Fairly liberal criteria were used

Table 18.2 Studies reporting the presence of multicentric disease in total pancreatectomy specimens

Source	Year of study	Number of patients	Incidence of "multicentric carcinoma"
Ihse et al. (45)	1977	58	9 (16%)
Tryka et al. (46) *	1979	25	5 (20%)
van Heerden et al. (4)	1988	89	29 (33%)
Kloppel et al. (6)	1987	37	0 (0%)
Michelassi et al. (44)	1989	36	1 (3%)
Launois et al. (12)	1993	47	15 (32%)

*Multicentric disease also included carcinoma-in-situ.

by some groups that, in retrospect, probably were actually ductal hyperplasia which, with our current understanding of the progression of pancreatic intraepithelial neoplasia (PanIN), are not truly premalignant changes (29). Indeed, when sought for by careful, state-of-the-art techniques, Kloppel and colleagues (6) could find no evidence of true multicentric foci of invasive carcinoma or carcinoma-in-situ, and all "positive" margins represented contiguous spread along the main pancreatic duct and not multicentricity. Therefore, the concept of multicentricity is not supported by data or adopted in practice.

Nevertheless, the concept of multicentricity may be relevant in selected individuals. Hereditary pancreatitis and a familial predisposition to pancreatic cancer are becoming recognized with increasing frequency (30). Similarly, certain other acquired disorders (chronic pancreatitis) and an ever increasing number of genetic disorders (familial pancreatitis, von Hippel-Lindau syndrome, Lynch syndrome, BRCA-2 mutations, etc.) predispose to the development of ductal carcinoma of the pancreas. In addition, our understanding of the pathogenesis of intraductal papillary mucinous neoplasm (IPMN) is still in the development stage, raising the question of a global susceptibility to ductal malignant transformation. With a better understanding of germline genetic disorders that predispose to malignant transformation, a select group of familial disorders at a very high risk for pancreatic neoplasia may be identified that may warrant consideration of preemptive pancreatectomy.

8 The Effect of Total Pancreatectomy on Soft-Tissue Clearance

Fully 14 to 32% of partial pancreatic resections have a positive margin for residual microscopic cancer (8, 10, 15, 31, 32). After pancreatic head resection, the most common site for positive margins is the retroperitoneal margin, followed by the pancreatic remnant (8). The latter would be obviated by total pancreatectomy. Advocates of total pancreatectomy have argued that resection of the entire gland will provide improved soft-tissue clearance and thereby decrease the incidence of loco-regional recurrence. In contradistinction, most pancreatic surgeons suggest that the retroperitoneal margin is treated technically in a similar fashion after total pancreatectomy and pancreatoduodenectomy. The same can be true for peripancreatic margins in neoplasms involving the body or tail (*33*). Total pancreatectomy, therefore, does not provide any theoretic advantages over partial resection in actual soft-tissue clearance. Indeed, observational studies have shown that 18% of total pancreatectomy specimens have positive margins (*9*), and local recurrence is equally common after pancreatoduodenectomy compared to total pancreatectomy (*34, 35*).

9   Does Total Pancreatectomy Provide a Better Lymphadenectomy and Does This Make a Difference?

The lymphatic drainage of the pancreas is multidirectional. Adenocarcinoma in the head of the pancreas can spread to lymph nodes in the supra- and infra-pancreatic body and tail region in 10–23% of resectable cases (*26–28*), but the splenic hilum is only involved in 0–1%. Similarly, lymph node involvement of the area around the head of the gland is found in only 5% of patients undergoing resection for carcinoma of the body and tail (*36*). For adenocarcinoma of the head of the gland, pancreatoduodenectomy with extended lymphadenectomy can achieve virtually the same peripancreatic lymph node clearance as total pancreatectomy; the only (theoretic) advantage of total pancreatectomy is removal of lymph nodes along the splenic artery and in the splenic hilum, the importance of which remains unknown and may even be considered a form of distant nodal disease not normally removed. Similarly total pancreatectomy for body/tail lesions will resect right-sided lymph nodes which distal pancreatectomy would not normally remove. But again, the question remains of the importance of this additional extended lymph node resection in terms of any survival benefit, which has never been shown to be advantageous (*32, 37, 38*).

10   Does Total Pancreatectomy Provide Better Survival?

The median survival after total pancreatectomy for pancreatic adenocarcinoma is on average about 10 months with a 5-year survival rate of 7% (see Table 18.1). This survival is slightly less than concurrent patients with adenocarcinoma undergoing partial resection (*39*). Although one study by Swope and colleagues (*14*) suggested an increase in median survival of 5 months after total pancreatectomy compared to pancreatoduodenectomy in a multicenter study of Veteran Administration hospitals, most studies showed shorter median survivals (1–9 months shorter) after total pancreatectomy compared to partial resections (*8, 9, 11, 40*). Even when total pancreatectomy was compared to partial resection with positive margins, survival after total pancreatectomy was not better, and in fact tended to be worse (*9*). Although marked improvements in survival after pancreatoduodenectomy have been reported in the last decade (*41*), the studies of survival after total pancreatectomy primarily in the 1970s to early 1990s failed to provide superior survival rates. Therefore, we conclude that routine use of total pancreatectomy for ductal adenocarcinoma of the pancreas is not indicated over partial pancreatectomy, although we acknowledge that no prospective, randomized, adequately powered study has actually been performed. The question is would it be justified? We believe not.

11   Use of Total Pancreatectomy in Selected Patients

Currently, however, there are rare indications for total pancreatectomy in the treatment of pancreatic adenocarcinoma. The most common indication for total pancreatectomy is the patient with intraoperative histologic evidence of residual neoplasm at the initial surgical margin. Most pancreatic surgeons would advocate a "creeping" extensional resection in this situation with a subtotal further segmental resection. The decision for total pancreatectomy is based both on the ability to preserve a reasonable amount of remnant gland and the patient's ability for self-care in the setting of complete endocrine and exocrine insufficiency. Other indications for total pancreatectomy can arise when a neoplasm in the distal head of the gland extends into the neck and body. In these cases, the oncologic principles of adequate tissue margins and lymphadenectomy may warrant a total pancreatectomy.

Although extremely rare for pancreatic ductal adenocarcinoma, total pancreatectomy is recommended for patients with a synchronous neoplasm within the remnant pancreas. Other potential situations in which total pancreatectomy was advocated in the past were for selected patients with a remnant unsuitable for an anastomosis, i.e., a very soft, normal gland at high risk for anastomotic leak. This "justification" has become exceedingly rare today with the ability to manage most pancreatic fistulae.

A relative indication for total pancreatectomy is the prophylactic or "pre-emptive" resection of the remaining pancreas in patients undergoing proximal or distal resection of a "localized" pancreatic cancer who are a markedly increased risk for metachronous neoplasm. Such patients might include those with a very strong history of familial pancreatic cancer and the presence of pancreatic intraepithelial neoplasia type 3 (PanIN-3) within the remnant (29, 30). Although the concept of "preemptive" surgery is well-accepted for thyroid, colonic, breast, and even gastric cancer, the morbidity, potential mortality, and implications concerning quality of life after total pancreatectomy has not been embraced for hereditary disorders of pancreatic cancer unless a definite established cancer is present or maybe if a screening program suggests markers of malignant transformation.

12   Summary

Although no prospective, randomized trial has compared total pancreatectomy with other partial pancreatic resections for pancreatic adenocarcinoma, historic data suggest no long-term survival advantage after total pancreatectomy. Moreover, the metabolic sequelae and implications concerning quality of life of the apancreatic state make the option of routine total pancreatectomy for ductal carcinoma of the pancreas much less attractive, especially when a solid oncologic justification is unconvincing. Therefore total pancreatectomy cannot be recommended as the standard treatment for pancreatic adenocarcinoma. Total pancreatectomy should be reserved for patients with histologic evidence of neoplasm at the initial surgical margin in whom a further segmental resection is not possible, neoplasm in the head extending into the neck and body, synchronous neoplasm, or the rare situation where the remnant is considered unsuitable for an anastomosis. The idea of "pre-emptive" resection for patients at a markedly increased risk of developing pancreatic cancer secondary to underlying germline mutations predisposing to pancreatic cancer remains undeveloped to date. Similarly, the use of total pancreatectomy for IPMN also remains debatable.

References

1. Priestley JT, Comfort MW, Radcliffe J. 1944, Total pancreatectomy for hyperinsulinism due to an islet-cell adenoma. Ann Surg 119:211–221.
2. Brunschwig A. 1944, The surgical treatment of carcinoma of the body of the pancreas. Ann Surg 120:406–416.
3. Ross DE. 1954, Cancer of the pancreas: a plea for total pancreatectomy. Am J Surg 87:20.
4. Heerden JA, van McIlrath DC, Ilstrup DM, et al. 1988, Total pancreatectomy for ductal adenocarcinoma of the pancreas: an update. World J Surg 12:658–662.
5. Ihse I, Anderson H, Andren-Sandberg A. 1996, Total pancreatectomy for cancer of the pancreas; is it appropriate? World J Surg 20:288–294.
6. Kloppel G, Lohse T, Bosslet K, et al.1987, Ductal adenocarcinoma of the head of the pancreas: incidence of tumor involvement, beyond the Whipple resection line. Histological and immunocytochemical analysis of 37 total pancreatectomy specimens. Pancreas 2:170–175.
7. Balcom JH 4th, Rattner DW, Warshaw AL, et al. 2001, Ten-year experience with 733 pancreatic resections: changing indications, older patients, and decreasing length of hospitalization. Arch Surg 136:391–398.
8. Sohn TA, Yeo CJ, Cameron JL, et al. 2000, Resected adenocarcinoma of the pancreas-616 patients: results, outcomes, and prognostic indicators. J Gastrointest Surg 4:567–579.
9. Karpoff HM, Klimstra DS, Brennan MF, et al. 2001, Results of total pancreatectomy for adenocarcinoma of the pancreas. Arch Surg 136:44–47.
10. Wagner M, Redaelli C, Lietz M, et al. 2004, Curative resection is the single most important factor determining outcome in patients with pancreatic adenocarcinoma. Br J Surg 91:586–594.
11. Baumel H, Huguier M, Manderscheid JC, et al. 1994, Results of resection for cancer of the exocrine pancreas: a study from the French Association of Surgery. Br J Surg 81:102–107.
12. Launois B, Franci J, Bardaxoglou E, et al. 1993, Total pancreatectomy for ductal adenocarcinoma of the pancreas with special reference to resection of the portal vein and multicentric cancer. World J Surg 17:122–126.
13. Sarr MG, Behrns KE, van Heerden JA, et al. 1993, Total pancreatectomy. An objective analysis of its use in pancreatic cancer. Hepatogastroenterology 40:418–421.
14. Swope TJ, Wade TP, Neuberger TJ, et al. 1994, A reappraisal of total pancreatectomy for pancreatic cancer: results from U.S. Veterans Affairs hospitals, 1987–1991. Am J Surg 168:582–585.
15. Christein JD, Kendrick ML, Iqbal CW, et al. 2005, Distal pancreatectomy for resectable adenocarcinoma of the body and tail of the pancreas. J Gastrointest Surg 9:922–927.

16. Kazanjian KK, Hines OJ, Eibl G, et al. 2005, Management of pancreatic fistulas after pancreaticoduodenectomy: results in 437 consecutive patients. Arch Surg 140:849–854.
17. Pratt WB, Maithel SK, Vanounou T, et al. 2007, Clinical and economic validation of the International Study Group of Pancreatic Fistula (ISGPF) Classification Scheme. Ann Surg, 245:443–451.
18. Bassi C, Dervenis C, Butturini G, et al. 2005, Postoperative pancreatic fistula: an international study group (ISGPF) definition. Surgery 138:8–13.
19. Chari ST, Leibson CL, Rabe KG, et al. 2005, Probability of pancreatic cancer following diabetes: a population-based study. Gastroenterology 129:504–511.
20. Slezak LA, Andersen DK. 2001, Pancreatic resection: effects on glucose metabolism. World J Surg 25:452–460.
21. Billings BJ, Christein JD, Harmsen WS, et al. 2005, Quality-of-life after total pancreatectomy: is it really that bad on long-term follow-up? J Gastrointest Surg 9:1059–1066.
22. Dresler CM, Fortner JG, McDermott K, et al. 1991, Metabolic consequences of (regional) total pancreatectomy. Ann Surg 214:131–140.
23. Sugiyama M, Atomi Y. 2000, Pylorus-preserving total pancreatectomy for pancreatic cancer. World J Surg 24:66–70.
24. Wagner M, Z'graggen K, Vagianos CE, et al. 2001, Pylorus-preserving total pancreatectomy. Early and late results. Dig Surg 18:188–195.
25. Lynch AM, Kapila R. 1996, Overwhelming postsplenectomy infection. Infect Dis Clin North Am 10:693–707.
26. Brunner TB, Merkel S, Grabenbauer GG, et al. 2005, Definition of elective lymphatic target volume in ductal carcinoma of the pancreatic head based on histopathologic analysis. Int J Radiat Oncol Biol Phys 62:1021–1029.
27. Ohta T, Nagakawa T, Ueno K, et al. 1993, The mode of lymphatic and local spread of pancreatic carcinomas less than 4.0 cm in size. Int Surg 78:208–212.
28. Cubilla AL, Fortner J, Fitzgerald PJ. 1978, Lymph node involvement in carcinoma of the head of the pancreas area. Cancer 41:880–887.
29. Maitra A, Fukushima N, Takaori K, et al. 2005, Precursors to invasive pancreatic cancer. Adv Anat Pathol 12:81–91.
30. McWilliams RR, Rabe KG, Olswold C, et al. 2005, Risk of malignancy in first-degree relatives of patients with pancreatic carcinoma. Cancer 104:388–394.
31. Ferrone CR, Kattan MW, Tomlinson JS, et al. 2005, Validation of a postresection pancreatic adenocarcinoma nomogram for disease-specific survival. J Clin Oncol 23:7529–7535.
32. Farnell MB, Pearson RK, Sarr MG, et al. 2005, A prospective randomized trial comparing standard pancreatoduodenectomy with pancreatoduodenectomy with extended lymphadenectomy in resectable pancreatic head adenocarcinoma. Surgery 138:618–628.
33. Strasberg SM, Drebin JA, Linehan D, 2003, Radical antegrade modular pancreatosplenectomy. Surgery 133:521–527.
34. Sperti C, Pasquali C, Piccoli A, et al. 1997, Recurrence after resection for ductal adenocarcinoma of the pancreas. World J Surg 21:195–200.
35. Westerdahl J, Andren-Sandberg A, Ihse I, 1993, Recurrence of exocrine pancreatic cancer– local or hepatic? Hepatogastroenterology 40:384–387.
36. Kayahara M, Nagakawa T, Futagami F, et al. 1996, Lymphatic flow and neural plexus invasion associated with carcinoma of the body and tail of the pancreas. Cancer 78:2485–2491.
37. Pedrazzoli S, DiCarlo V, Dionigi R, et al. 1998, Standard versus extended lymphadenectomy associated with pancreatoduodenectomy in the surgical treatment of adenocarcinoma of the head of the pancreas: a multicenter, prospective, randomized study. Ann Surg 228:508–517.
38. Riall TS, Cameron JL, Lillemoe KD, et al. 2005, Pancreaticoduodenectomy with or without distal gastrectomy and extended retroperitoneal lymphadenectomy for periampullary adenocarcinoma - part 3: update on 5-year survival. J Gastrointest Surg 9:1191–1204.
39. Cress RD, Yin D, Clarke L, et al. 2006, Survival among patients with adenocarcinoma of the pancreas: a population-based study (United States). Cancer Causes Control 17:403–409.
40. Grace PA, Pitt HA, Tompkins RK, et al. 1986, Decreased morbidity and mortality after pancreatoduodenectomy. Am J Surg 151:141–149.

41. Nitecki SS, Sarr MG, Colby TV, et al. 1995, Long-term survival after resection for ductal adenocarcinoma of the pancreas. Is it really improving? Ann Surg 221:59–66.
42. Brooks JR, Brooks DC, Levine JD. 1989, Total pancreatectomy for ductal cell carcinoma of the pancreas. An update. Ann Surg 209:405–410.
43. Herter FP, Cooperman AM, Ahlborn TN, et al. 1982, Surgical experience with pancreatic and periampullary cancer. Ann Surg 195:274–281.
44. Michelassi F, Erroi F, Dawson PJ, et al. 1989, Experience with 647 consecutive tumors of the duodenum, ampulla, head of the pancreas, and distal common bile duct. Ann Surg 210:544–554.
44. Strasberg SM, Drebin JA, Linehan D. 2003, Radical antegrade modular pancreatosplenectomy. Surgery 133:521–527.
45. Ihse I, Lilja P, Arnesjo B, Bengmark S. 1977, Total pancreatectomy for cancer. An appraisal of 65 cases. Ann Surg 186:675–680.
46. Tryka AF, Brooks JR. 1979, Histopathology in the evaluation of total pancreatectomy for ductal carcinoma. Ann Surg 190:373–381.

Chapter 19
Distal Pancreatectomy

Andrew S. Resnick and Jeffrey A. Drebin

1 Introduction

Resection of the body and tail of the pancreas is commonly referred to as distal pancreatectomy. Although potentially of benefit to patients with pancreatic adenocarcinoma confined to the body or tail of the pancreas, such tumors commonly metastasize prior to being discovered, and distal pancreatectomy for pancreatic carcinoma is a relatively uncommon procedure even at high volume pancreatic surgery centers. However, a variety of other pancreatic neoplasms that arise in the pancreatic body and tail, including cystic neoplasms, intraductal papillary mucinous neoplasms (IPMNs), and neuroendocrine tumors are being identified with increasing frequency; such lesions are generally amenable to resection with distal pancreatectomy. This chapter briefly reviews the history of distal pancreatectomy, discusses current indications for performing this procedure, compares operative techniques in performing distal pancreatectomy and reviews both early complications seen in patients who have undergone a distal pancreatectomy and the long-term metabolic and oncologic outcomes of these patients.

2 History

As knowledge of pancreatic anatomy increased in the late nineteenth century, initial reports of surgery on the gland began to appear in the literature. Senn wrote in 1889 that when pancreatic tumors were in the tail of the pancreas, conditions for resection were "favorable" (1). Furthermore, he reported that Billroth had attempted resections of both pancreatic head and tail lesions in 1884, but did not mention that Trendelenburg had performed perhaps the first distal pancreatectomy and splenectomy earlier (in 1882) for a spindle cell sarcoma in the tail of the pancreas-perhaps because this first patient died on postoperative day 1 (1).

Even after the ground-breaking work of the 1880s, progress in pancreatic surgery was slow. Von Mickulicz-Radecki blamed the "tardy development" of pancreatic surgery on multiple factors, some of which are relevant to this day. First, the

A.M. Lowy et al. (eds.) *Pancreatic Cancer*.
doi: 10.1007/978-0-387-69252-4, © Springer Science+Business Media, LLC 2008

pancreas was "exceedingly difficult" to reach (*1, 2*). Second, diagnosis of pancreatic disease was extremely difficult and many early laparotomies for pancreatic disease were abandoned due to the advanced nature of the malignant disease encountered (*1*). Discovery of endocrine tumors in the early twentieth century allowed Mayo and others to operate on patients with less aggressive and less advanced lesions than their counterparts in the late nineteenth century, leading to a relatively large increase in pancreatic surgical activity (*1, 3*). Case reports by Finney and Mayo described several distal pancreatectomies in the early twentieth century (*4, 5*). In Finney's review, 9 of 17 patients survived, with all mortalities occurring in those with pancreatic cancer (*4*). The middle of the twentieth century witnessed an increase in the frequency with which distal pancreatectomy was performed, and a period of enthusiasm for performing distal subtotal pancreatectomy for chronic pancreatitis, though enthusiasm for this procedure has waned as more effective and less morbid pancreas preserving drainage procedures have evolved (*6*).

3   Current Indications for Performing Distal Pancreatectomy

Several papers have analyzed the clinical indications for performing distal pancreatectomy at high volume institutions in recent decades. Lillemoe reported on 235 patients who underwent distal pancreatectomy from 1984 through 1997 at the Johns Hopkins Hospital (*7*). Indications were chronic pancreatitis (24%), benign pancreatic cystadenoma (22%), pancreatic adenocarcinoma (18%), neuroendocrine tumor (14%), pseudocyst (6%), cystadenocarcinoma (3%), and others (13%), including papillary cystic and solid neoplasms, nesidioblastosis, and metastatic renal cell carcinoma. Balcom reviewed The Massachusetts General Hospital (MGH) experience, reporting on 10 years of pancreas surgery (1990-2000) in 2001, including 190 distal pancreatectomies during that time period (*8*). Indications for distal pancreatectomy at that institution included cystic tumors (33%), chronic pancreatitis (28%), other (24%), and pancreatic adenocarcinoma (15%). The authors from MGH noted changing indications over the 10-year period. Chronic pancreatitis decreased from 32% to 14% of all distal pancreatectomies, while cystic tumor increased from 26% to 52% (*1*). The increase in diagnosis of IPMNs was particularly significant, as 17% of all distal resections were performed for IPMNs by the end of their study.

Analysis of these two studies allows the reader to draw several conclusions. First, distal pancreatectomy is a relatively uncommon surgical procedure. Even at very high volume institutions, an average of fewer than 20 were performed annually. Three to four times as many pancreaticoduodenectomies (Whipple procedures) were performed at these institutions during the same time spans. Second, the fraction of patients undergoing distal pancreatectomy for cystic neoplasms and IPMNs is increasing, whereas far fewer distal pancreatectomies for the management of chronic pancreatitis are being performed. Finally, in both series pancreatic adenocarcinoma was a relatively uncommon indication for performing distal pancreatectomy, accounting for <20% of these procedures. As noted, this reflects the relative rarity of identifying pancreatic adenocarcinoma while still locoregionally confined to the distal pancreas.

4 Technical Considerations in Performing Distal Pancreatectomy

4.1 The Classic (Retrograde) Approach

The classic approach to distal pancreatectomy involves en bloc splenectomy and the dissection being carried from the spleen medially (9). The steps of the procedure are: (1) the body and tail of the pancreas are exposed in the lesser sac by dividing the short gastric vessels along the greater curve of the stomach and reflecting the stomach superiorly; (2) the inferior border of the pancreas is mobilized from the duodenum, mesocolon and retroperitoneum, dividing vessels as they enter the body of the pancreas; (3) the spleen is mobilized by dividing the lienorenal and lienophrenic attachments; (4) blunt dissection posterior to the spleen and pancreas is used to elevate these structures off Gerota's fascia of the kidney, the adrenal gland, and out of the retroperitoneum; (5) using the spleen as a handle and reflecting the spleen and pancreas body and tail medially, the splenic artery and vein are identified on the superior and posterior surfaces of the pancreas, respectively, and they are divided proximal to the intended site of pancreatic transection; and (6) the pancreas is transected and the specimen is removed from the field.

In experienced hands this approach is straight forward, relatively quick and can be performed with minimal blood loss. However the classic approach compromises standard oncologic principles in bluntly dividing posterior tissue planes without visualizing and optimizing resection margins or ensuring adequate resection of regional lymph nodes. For relatively medially located tumors (i.e., those in the proximal body), this approach can also be problematic with regard to dividing the splenic artery and vein close to their origins and to achieving a negative transection margin.

4.2 Radical Antegrade Modular Pancreatico-Splenectomy

To overcome the limitations of the classic approach to distal pancreatectomy, we have advocated an approach in which medial to lateral dissection is carried out under direct vision (10, 11). The procedure is termed the Radical Antegrade Modular Pancreatico-Splenectomy (RAMPS) procedure, since it combines antegrade dissection with the ability to carry the lateral posterior dissection to varying depths in order to achieve a negative margin in the event that the renal vessels, adrenal gland, or kidney itself are involved by tumor (modular dissection).

The steps of the RAMPS procedure are: (*1*) the lesser sac is entered by dividing the short gastric vessels and reflecting the stomach superiorly. The mobilization of the greater curvature of the stomach is carried to the origin of the right gastroepiploic vessels in order to gain access to the superior mesenteric vein. (*2*) Dissection along the superior mesenteric vein is carried beneath the neck of the pancreas, dividing the middle colic vein at its origin to facilitate exposure. (*3*) The gastroduodenal artery is divided at its origin from the hepatic artery, exposing the portal vein. (*4*) Dissection beneath the neck of the pancreas from the portal vein to the superior mesenteric vein is completed and the pancreatic neck is elevated and transected. (*5*) The splenic artery and splenic vein are identified at their origins and sequentially divided. (*6*) Dissection is carried posterior to the splenic vein onto the anterior surface of the left renal vein and then dissection is carried laterally in the plane anterior to the left renal vein, with all anterior retroperitoneal tissue and lymphatics being mobilized along with the pancreatic body and tail. (*7*) Lateral dissection can be carried anterior to the left adrenal gland if uninvolved by tumor. If tumor is invasive posteriorly in this region the adrenal, and if necessary the renal vessels and kidney can be resected en bloc. (*8*) The spleen is mobilized by dividing the lienorenal and lienophrenic attachments and the specimen is removed.

The RAMPS procedure may permit distal pancreatic resection to be achieved with a better posterior margin and lymphatic clearance. In a relatively small series of patients undergoing the RAMPS procedure, encouraging survival results have been achieved (*11*). However, the procedure has some important limitations. Dissection at the pancreatic neck has the potential for injury to major vascular structures with resultant hemorrhage, particularly in inexperienced hands. Furthermore, RAMPS resection generally involves resection of the entire body and tail of the pancreas, with resultant increased long-term risk of pancreatic endocrine and exocrine insufficiency. For patients with adenocarcinoma of the pancreatic body or tail who are fortunate enough to have their disease identified while still locally confined, the benefits of the RAMPS procedure may justify these risks. For less aggressive lesions such as neuroendocrine tumors or cystic neoplasms, particularly if located at the tail of the pancreas, a more limited resection using the classic approach may be sufficient.

4.3   Splenic Preservation

Resection of the spleen is commonly performed with resection of the pancreatic body and tail, but is not a required component of distal pancreatectomy (*12, 13*). For neoplasms in which lymphatic spread is a consideration, resection of lymphatics in the hilum of the spleen that drain the pancreatic tail will generally require en bloc splenectomy. Furthermore, the splenic artery and vein are located in close proximity to the body and tail of the pancreas and generally must be preserved if splenic preservation is desired. Ligation and division of these vessels leaving the spleen dependent on the short gastric vessels for blood supply, although advocated by some in the past (*13*), is not recommended as it may lead to splenic infarction or the development of gastric varices. While the preservation of the splenic artery and vein with division of branches entering the body and tail of the pancreas can be achieved in many patients, the risk of significant hemorrhage and need for transfusion may be increased, as is the overall time of the procedure.

The advantage of splenic preservation is avoidance of the risk of overwhelming postsplenectomy sepsis. In patients who undergo splenectomy as adults this risk is not high-studies suggest a risk of less than 1 per 1,000 patient years (*14*). As these studies included patients who underwent splenectomy prior to the availability of vaccines against encapsulated bacteria linked to postsplenectomy sepsis such as *S. pneumoniae, H. influenza,* and *N. meningitides,* it is possible (although not proved) that the risk would be even lower in patients who undergo postsplenectomy vaccination. Thus, the lifetime risk of postsplenectomy sepsis in adults who undergo splenectomy as part of a distal pancreatic resection is at most a few percent-certainly not a risk to be encumbered casually but also not sufficient to justify extraordinary operative attempts at spleen preservation or compromising an adequate cancer operation.

4.4 Laparoscopic Distal Pancreatectomy

Multiple studies have demonstrated that laparoscopic distal pancreatectomy can be performed safely (*15-17*). In general these reports represent case series in which distal pancreatectomy has been performed on selected patients, and as with most case series, represent a demonstration of best results in experienced hands. These studies have shown that laparoscopic distal pancreatectomy can be performed with a low incidence of blood loss and a low need for conversion to open surgery. It has also been demonstrated that spleen-preserving distal pancreatectomy can be performed laparoscopically and it has been suggested that spleen preservation may be more easily accomplished via laparoscopic than open technique (*17*).

While laparoscopic resection of pancreatic adenocarcinoma has been reported (*15*), the adequacy of laparoscopic technique with regard to oncologic outcomes has not been established. However, as noted, most distal pancreatectomies are performed for premalignant lesions or lesions of low malignant potential such as cystic neoplasms and neuroendocrine tumors of the pancreas. It is likely that laparoscopic approaches will continue to evolve into the preferred method for the management of such lesions.

4.5 Central Pancreatectomy

The resection of lesions of low malignant potential in the region of the pancreatic neck and proximal body is problematic. If a resection is initiated at the head or tail of the pancreas, performance of either an extended Whipple resection or a subtotal distal pancreatectomy may be necessary to achieve an adequate margin, with a high risk of subsequent endocrine and/or exocrine insufficiency. Since minimal surgical margins are required for such lesions and regional lymphadenectomy is unnecessary, the performance of "central pancreatectomy" with occlusion of the pancreas proximally and internal drainage of the pancreatic duct distally into a Roux-Y jejunal loop or the stomach has been advocated (18-20). The principal advantage of this procedure is not "wasting" pancreatic tissue with more extensive resection, and minimizing endocrine and/or exocrine insufficiency.

Against this must be weighed the potential for greater complications. While some series have suggested a similar overall complication rate to that seen with distal pancreatectomy, others have suggested a markedly higher incidence of pancreatic leakage resulting in a pancreatic fistula (20-22). This is not surprising, since two potential sites of leakage-the occluded pancreatic duct and the pancreaticoenteric anastomosis-are created and located in relatively close proximity in this procedure. Furthermore, it has been suggested that pancreatic leaks in the setting of central pancreatectomy may be particularly likely to generate additional complications and/or require subsequent interventions (22). Thus the decision to perform a central pancreatectomy requires that the surgeon balance the long-term benefits of pancreatic tissue preservation with the potential for greater and potentially more serious early complications.

5 Surgical Complications of Distal Pancreatectomy

5.1 Early Complications

Most serious complications in patients undergoing distal pancreatectomy are uncommon and are similar to complications of other major abdominal surgical procedures (i.e., wound infection, myocardial infarction, pulmonary embolus, pneumonia, etc.) occuiring in 1-5% of patients (7, 8, 23, 24). Perioperative (30-day) mortality rates are generally 1% or less. However, one complication specific to patients undergoing distal pancreatectomy, leakage of pancreatic juice from the divided edge of the pancreas, resulting in a pancreatic fistula, occurs in a significant fraction of patients. As noted by Strasberg and colleagues, this represents a failure of occlusion of the duct, as opposed to the failure of anastomosis of the duct that results in fistula formation after Whipple resections (25). Since there are different definitions of a pancreatic fistula used by different authors (25, 26), the incidence varies in different series, but numbers in the range of 10-40% are commonly noted. Although an annoying complication requiring maintenance of operatively placed drains or placement of new percutaneous drains, pancreatic fistula after distal pancreatectomy rarely results in need for reoperation, major long-term morbidity, or mortality.

Some surgeons believe that the method of dividing the pancreas and occluding the pancreatic duct may contribute to the subsequent development of a pancreatic fistula, with reports suggesting that stapling the pancreas and duct as single step (*27*) or dividing the pancreas sharply and suturing the duct (*28, 29*) result in a lower incidence of pancreatic leakage. However a meta-analysis suggests that the two approaches are not statistically distinct, with a nonsignificant trend favoring a stapled technique (*30*).

Similarly, a variety of adjuncts have been proposed to secure the occlusion of the pancreatic duct after transaction in patients undergoing distal pancreatectomy. The use of fibrin glue or other tissue adhesives has been advocated (*31*), as has the drainage of the pancreatic stump into a Roux-Y jejunal limb (*32*). Recently Hawkins and colleagues observed a very low incidence (<4%) of pancreatic fistula formation when using a stapled technique combined with a bioabsorbable stapler sleeve (*33*). The use of a radiofrequency dissector to occlude the pancreatic duct has also been reported to result in a very low incidence of leakage in experimental models (*34*). As these different approaches have not been studied in prospective randomized trials, it is as yet uncertain which (if any) technique represents the most useful adjunct to minimize the risk of pancreatic fistula in patients undergoing distal pancreatectomy.

5.2   Metabolic Effects

The development of diabetes as a result of the loss of pancreatic endocrine tissue in patients undergoing distal pancreatectomy is not uncommon. Although series are small, often lacking in long-term follow-up and are confounded by the analysis of patients with chronic pancreatitis who have a greater risk of subsequent diabetes regardless of surgical resection, an elevated incidence of diabetes is definitely noted following distal pancreatectomy. The new onset of diabetes in the immediate postoperative period ranges from 8 to 25% (*7, 35, 36*), with a potentially higher incidence with longer-term follow-up. The risk of diabetes is likely related to the amount of pancreatic tissue resected. In a small series of patients Shibata and colleagues found that patients in whom >12 cm of pancreas was resected had a very high incidence of subsequent diabetes, whereas patients undergoing less extensive resections were unlikely to become diabetic (*36*). The use of central pancreatectomy for lesions of low malignant potential may permit preservation of a greater amount of pancreas tissue, at the cost of a higher incidence of early complications, as discussed previously.

6   Oncologic Outcomes

As noted, most patients undergo distal pancreatectomy for management of cystic neoplasms or other tumors of relatively low malignant potential. Such patients are generally cured. However, patients who undergo distal pancreatectomy for adenocarcinoma

of the pancreas have a much more guarded prognosis (*7, 8, 23, 24, 37*). Median survivals of 1-2 years and 5-year survival rates of 10-20% have been noted. As with pancreatic carcinomas involving the head of the pancreas, factors linked to risk of recurrence
after distal pancreatectomy for pancreatic adenocarcinoma include margin positivity,
tumor size and differentiation, and the presence of lymph node metastases. The role of
adjuvant therapy after distal pancreatectomy for tumors of the pancreatic body and tail
has not been formally studied, although such patients have been included (along with
patients undergoing Whipple resection) in studies suggesting a benefit for adjuvant
therapy following resection of pancreatic adenocarcinomas (*38, 39*).

7   Summary

Distal pancreatectomy is a relatively uncommon surgical procedure. Indications
include a broad range of benign and malignant disorders. Several distinct surgical
approaches may be undertaken, including both open and laparoscopic techniques.
Splenectomy, although commonly performed with distal pancreatectomy, can be
avoided in some patients. The development of a pancreatic fistula from the divided
edge of the pancreas is a common early complication, but rarely results in long-
term morbidity or mortality. The development of diabetes, related to the quantity
of pancreas removed, is a significant long-term complication.

References

1. McClusky DA, Skandalakis LJ, Colborn GL, et al. 2002, Harbinger or hermit? Pancreatic
   anatomy and surgery through the ages—part 2. World J Surg 26:1370–1381.
2. Von Mickulicz-Radecki J. 1903, Surgery of the pancreas. Ann Surg 38:1.
3. Wilder RM, Allan FN, Power MH, 1927, Carcinoma of the islands of the pancreas: hyperin-
   sulism and hypoglycemia. JAMA 89:348.
4. Finney JMT. Resection of the pancreas. Trans Am Surg Assoc 1910, 315–330.
5. Mayo WJ. 1913, The surgery of the pancreas. Ann Surg 58:145–150.
6. Izbicki JR, Bloechle C, Knoefel WT, 1995, Duodenum preserving resection of the head of the
   pancreas in chronic pancreatitis. A prospective randomized trial. Ann Surg , 221:350–358.
7. Lillemoe KD, Kaushal S, Cameron JL, 1999, Distal pancreatectomy: indications and outcomes in 235 patients. Ann Sur 229(5):693–700.
8. Balcom JH, Rattner DW, Warshaw AL, 2001, Ten-year experience with 733 pancreatic resections: changing indications, older patients, and decreasing length of hospitalization. Arch Sur
   136:391–398.
9. Cameron JL, 1990, Distal pancreatectomy for tumor. In: Cameron JL (ed.) Atlas of surgery,
   vol 1. BC Decker, Toronto, ON, 428–435.
10. Strasberg SM, Drebin JA, Linehan D, 2003, Radical antegrade modular pancreaticosplenec-
    tomy. Surgery 133:521–527.
11. Strasberg SM, Linehan DC, Hawkins WG, 2007, Radical antegrade modular pancreaticos-
    plenectomy procedure for adenocarcinoma of the body and tail of the pancreas: ability to
    obtain negative tangential margins. J Am Coll Surg 204:244–249.

12. Warshaw AL, 1988, Conservation of the spleen with distal pancreatectomy. Arch Surg 123:550–553.
13. Kimura LS, Inoue T, Futakawa N, 1996, Spleen preserving distal pancreatectomy with conservation of the splenic artery and vein. Surgery 120:885–890.
14. Schwartz PE, Sterioff S, Mucha P, 1982, Postsplenectomy sepsis and mortality in adults. JAMA 248:2279–2283.
15. Gigot J-F, 2005, Laparoscopic pancreatic resection: results of a multicenter European study of 127 patients. Surgery 137:597–6005.
16. Velanovich V, 2006, Case-control comparison of laparoscopic versus open distal pancreatectomy. J Gastrointest Surg 10:95–98.
17. Fernandez-Cruz L, 2004, Laparoscopic distal pancreatectomy combined with preservation of the spleen for cystic neoplasms of the pancreas. J Gastrointest Surg 8:493–501.
18. Rotman N, Sastre B, Fagniez PL, 1993, Medial pancreatectomy for tumors of the neck of the pancreas. Surgery 113:532–535.
19. Warshaw AL, Rattner DW, Fernandez-del Castillo, 1998, Middle segment pancreatectomy: a novel technique for conserving pancreatic tissue. Arch Surg 133:327–331.
20. Efron DT, Lillemoe KD, Cameron JL, 2004, Central pancreatectomy with pancreaticogastrostomy for benign pancreatic pathology. J Gastrointest Surg 8:532–538.
21. Roggin KK, Rudloff U, Blumgart LH, 2006, Central pancreatectomy revisited. J. Gastrointest Surg 10:804–812.
22. Pratt W, Maithel SK, Vanounou T, 2006, Post-operative pancreatic fistulas are not equivalent after proximal, distal and central pancreatectomy. J Gastrointest Surg 10:1264–1279.
23. Christein JD, Kendrick ML, Iqbal CW, 2005, Distal pancreatectomy for resectable adenocarcinoma of the body and tail of the pancreas. J. Gastrointest Surg 9(7):922–927.
24. Brennan MF, Moccia RD, Klimstra D. 1996, Management of adenocarcinoma of the body and tail of the pancreas. Ann Sur 223(5):506–512.
25. Strasberg SM, Linehan DC, Clavien PA, 2007, Proposal for definition and severity grading of pancreatic anastomosis failure and pancreatic occlusion failure. Surgery 141:420–426.
26. Bassi C, 2005, Postoperative pancreatic fistula: an international study group (ISGPF) definition. Surgery 138:8–13.
27. Takeuchi K, 2003, Distal pancreatectomy: is staple closure beneficial? ANZ J Surg 73:922–925.
28. Bilimoria MM, Cormier JN, Mun Y, 2003, Pancreatic leak after left pancreatectomy is reduced following main pancreatic duct ligation. Br J Surg 90:190–196.
29. Kleef J, 2007, Distal pancreatectomy: risk factors for surgical failure in 302 consecutive cases. Ann Surg 245:573–582.
30. Knaebel HP, Diemer MK, Weale MN, 2005, Systematic review and meta-analysis of technique for closure of the pancreatic remnant after distal pancreatectomy. Br J Surg 92:539–546.
31. Suzuki Y, 1995, Fibrin glue sealing for the prevention of pancreatic fistulas following distal pancreatectomy. Arch Surg 130:952–955.
32. Wagner M, 2007, Roux-en Y drainage of the pancreatic stump decreases pancreatic fistula after distal pancreatic resection. J Gastrointest Surg 11:303–308.
33. Thaker RJ, Matthews BD, Linehan DC, 2007, Absorbable mesh reinforcement of a stapled pancreatic transaction line reduces the leak rate with distal pancreatectomy. J Gastrointest Surg 11:59–65.
34. Truty MJ, Sawyer MD, Que FG, 2007, Decreasing pancreatic leak after distal pancreatectomy: saline-coupled radiofrequency ablation in a porcine model. J Gastrointest Surg 11:998–1007.
35. Shoup M, Conlon KC, Klimstra D, 2003, Is extended resection for adenocarcinoma of the body or tail of the pancreas justified? J. Gastrointest Surg 7:946–952.
36. Shibata S, 2004, Outcomes and indications of segmental pancreatectomy: comparison with distal pancreatectomy. Digestive Surg 21:48–53.

37. Shimada K, Sakamoto Y, Sano T, 2006, Prognostic factors after distal pancreatectomy with extended lymphadenectomy for invasive pancreatic adenocarcinoma of the body and tail. Surgery 139:288–295.
38. Chua YJ, Cunningham D, 2005, Adjuvant treatment for respectable pancreatic cancer. J Clin Oncol 23:4532–4537.
39. Oettle H, 2007, Adjuvant chemotherapy with gemcitabine vs observation in patients undergoing curative intent resection of pancreatic cancer. JAMA 297:267–277.

Chapter 20
Vascular Resection for Pancreatic Cancer

Waddah B. Al-Refaie and Jeffrey E. Lee

1 Introduction

Vascular resection for adenocarcinoma of the pancreas is one of the most contro-versial issues in the management of pancreatic cancer (*1*). Pancreaticoduodenectomy (PD) is a complicated and challenging operation; vascular resection and reconstruc-tion adds to this complexity. The potential for high morbidity in patients who undergo PD, the poor prognosis of most patients with pancreatic cancer, and a frequent lack of familiarity with appropriate indications as well as the technical aspects of vascular resection and reconstruction have contributed to making surgeons reluctant to perform this procedure in the context of PD.

Resection and reconstruction of the superior mesenteric vein (SMV) for pan-creatic cancer was first performed in 1951 by Moore at the University of Minnesota (*2*). In 1973, Fortner proposed the concept of "regional pancreatec-tomy," which entailed en bloc pancreatic and peripancreatic resection along with major vascular resection and reconstruction. However, subsequent evaluation of this approach by Fortner and others failed to demonstrate any survival benefit to this radical approach (*3, 4*).

Our experience with vascular resection and reconstruction (*5, 6*) has recently been updated by Tseng et al. (*7*). In our experience, carefully selected patients who require vascular resection as part of PD for adenocarcinoma of the pancreas can undergo this procedure safely, and such patients experience survival duration similar to that of patients who do not require vascular resection. We emphasize three important principles:

1. Appropriate patient selection
2. Careful attention to the retroperitoneal and pancreatic resection margins
3. Meticulous surgical technique

A.M. Lowy et al. (eds.), *Pancreatic Cancer.*
doi: 10.1007/978-0-387-69252-4, © Springer Science+Business Media, LLC 2008

1.1   Patient Selection

Advances in cross-sectional imaging have improved our ability to identify appropriate candidates for PD and exclude those who will not benefit based on the presence of an advanced and unresectable local tumor process or the presence of metastatic disease. To be eligible for PD, patients must meet the following objective radiographic criteria: (*1*) absence of extrapancreatic metastatic disease; (*2*) absence of tumor extension to the superior mesenteric artery (SMA) or celiac axis, as defined radiographically by the presence of a fat plane between the tumor and these arteries; and (*3*) a patent SMPV confluence with a suitable segment of SMV and PV to allow venous reconstruction if necessary (*8*).

1.2   Attention to Resection Margins

Surgeons performing PD must pay close attention to the retroperitoneal (RP) margin and the pancreatic resection margin, as well as the designated residual disease status (R). The RP is defined as the soft tissue margin directly adjacent to the proximal 3–4 cm of the SMA. The importance of this margin has been highlighted in the 2002 revision of The American Joint Commission on Cancer (AJCC) staging system for pancreatic cancer as an appropriate index for margin involvement by disease. Surgeons and radiologists should carefully evaluate preoperative cross-sectional imaging studies for evidence of involvement of the retroperitoneal margin by cancer. Surgeons performing PD should take care to remove the soft tissue (mesenteric tissue) to the right of the SMA during separation of the pancreatic head and uncinate process. Ultimately, the size and location of the tumor, the type and extent of operation performed, and the response to preoperative therapy (if any) will affect the final histologic status of the RP margin (involved versus uninvolved). It is thus imperative that the surgeon at the time of PD, and the pathologist at the time of evaluation of the surgical material, identify the RP margin and include their findings in the operative record and final histopathology report.

Classifying the pancreatic resection margin according to residual disease status, termed the R status, is also important. R status is defined as: R0, no gross or microscopic residual disease; R1, microscopic residual disease (microscopically positive surgical margins with no gross residual disease); and R2, grossly evident residual disease. Differentiation of R1 from R2 resections has significant implications for the conduct of clinical trials that evaluate the potential advantages of nonsurgical adjuvant and neoadjuvant therapies for patients with pancreatic adenocarcinoma (*9*). Determination of R status often can not be made with certainty based on the intraoperative findings and frozen section evaluation of the specimen at the time of surgery; surgeons often (although not always) must await the final histopathology report. For example, if an experienced surgeon determines that the tumor extends to the left of (medial to) the SMA and is not completely removed at the time of surgery, an R2 status can be designated at the conclusion of the procedure based on this finding. On the other hand, if the surgeon performs a grossly complete resection but the RP margin is demonstrated to be involved on final histopathology (when the RP margin has been accurately identified, inked, and examined by the pathologist), then the record should document that an R1 PD was performed.

1.3 Anatomy of the SMV and SMA

Refinement in surgical technique as well as an improved understanding of mesenteric vascular anatomy has resulted in our increased comfort with performance of venous resection and reconstruction as part of PD. Both the SMV and SMA are at risk for tumor extension from pancreatic cancers involving the head, uncinate process, neck, and proximal body of the pancreas, given the close proximity of these portions of the pancreas to these vessels. The SMV and its tributaries are subject to more variation than the arterial system. Therefore, the surgeon performing PD should be familiar with the important venous landmarks and portal venous tributaries. The anterior aspect of the portal vein and SMV are free of tributaries; in the absence of direct tumor involvement of these structures, this usually allows mobilization of the neck of the pancreas by gentle blunt dissection. The SMV drains the mid-gut, courses behind the posterior aspect of the neck of the pancreas, and joins the splenic vein behind the pancreatic neck. Surgeons should be aware that the IMV may drain into either the splenic vein, the SMV, or as a common confluence with the SMV and splenic vein. The middle colic vein and right gastroepiploic vein are early anterior tributaries of the SMV and often share a common trunk (the "gastrocoloic" trunk). This trunk is an important surgical landmark, as its junction with the SMV indicates the lower border of the neck of the pancreas. The first jejunal branch (FJV; which is also called simply the jejunal branch) of the SMV usually runs behind the SMA as it drains the proximal jejunum and then enters the posteromedial aspect of the ileal branch of the SMV to form the main SMV. Rarely, this branch courses anterior to the SMA. The jejunal branch of the SMV may pose unique technical challenges for the surgeon performing PD, as infiltrative tumors of the uncinate process that involve the SMV at the junction of the FJV may prevent separation of the SMV from the uncinate process without division of this branch. Injury to the FJV may lead to excessive hemorrhage caused by a posterior tear in the FJV at its entry into the SMV. There is typically limited exposure for repair of the veins in this situation. In turn, attempted suture repair of the FJV at the level of the uncinate process may result in injury to the SMA if the SMA has not been exposed. Therefore, exposure of the SMA (medial to the SMV) should always be considered early in the operation, especially if SMV involvement is suspected, before proceeding with excessive dissection of the SMV. The FJV can then be approached from the left (medial) aspect of the SMV by transecting the root of the small-bowel mesentery between the SMA and SMV. This permits direct ligation of the FJV proximal to its junction with the SMV when necessary. The small bowel will have adequate venous return if either the ileal or the jejunal branches remain intact; therefore, if either the ileal or jejunal (FJV) branch is resected, but not both, then venous reconstruction is usually not necessary. On the other hand, one is occasionally required to divide the FJV and resect the main SMV extending into the ileal branch; in such cases, the ileal branch must be reconstructed. Attention should also be paid to the coronary (left gastric) vein, which usually (in 59% of patients) drains into the left side of the retroperitoneal portal vein, but may terminate higher (i.e., above the neck of the pancreas) (*10–12*).

The pancreatic head, duodenum, small bowel, and proximal colon derive their blood supply from the celiac truck and SMA. The SMA arises from the aorta and courses caudally, posterior to the pancreas. Early branches of the SMA include the inferior pancreaticoduodenal arteries and tributaries to the uncinate process. Several centimeters distal to its origin, the SMA gives off first jejunal branches. The SMA maintains a relatively constant posteromedial relationship to the SMV. It is uncommon for the SMA to be involved by a pancreatic head tumor without concomitant SMV involvement. Occasionally, however, this can occur; therefore, it is a mistake to assume that if one is able to separate a pancreatic head tumor from the SMPV confluence that it will always be free of the SMA. For example, a posteriorly located tumor arising from the uncinate process can encase the SMA without involving the SMV; such a finding should be apparent on preoperative CT imaging. Similarly, it is rare to have an uninvolved SMA in cases in which the tumor has completely occluded the SMPV confluence because of the close proximity of the SMA and SMV. The SMA is sheathed by autonomic nerves and lymphatic tissue that extend to the celiac ganglia; even when the surgeon performs a complete gross resection of a pancreatic head tumor, a microscopically positive margin may result because of tumor cell infiltration of the perineural plexus surrounding the SMA; this plexus extends into the pancreatic parenchyma and serves as a suitable conduit for microscopic tumor extension back to the SMA and celiac ganglia. For these reasons, we do not generally recommend that PD be performed when the SMPV has been completely encased or occluded by adenocarcinoma.

1.4 Surgical Technique

Our experience with resection and reconstruction of the SMV, portal vein, or SMPV confluence has been restricted to patients in whom tumor adherence to these venous structures prevented the surgeon from mobilizing the SMPV confluence from the pancreatic head and uncinate process. We do not perform elective venous resection in the absence of tumor adherence to a vessel (*9*). The assessment of tumor adherence to the SMPV confluence is a judgment made at the time of surgery; for this reason, final histopathologic evaluation of the surgical specimen will not demonstrate tumor infiltration of the vein wall in all cases (61% histologic tumor involvement in our series). If dissection along the periadventitial plane of the SMV or portal vein does not result in successful separation of the vein from the tumor, venous resection and reconstruction is the only way to accomplish a complete resection. To what extent peritumor inflammation secondary to the neoplastic process or to endoscopic intervention affects the ability of the surgeon to successfully separate the specimen from the SMPV is not known. Similarly, little is known about the effect of chemo-radiation therapy on the tumor–vessel interface. Importantly, venous resection is not performed in an effort to achieve greater lymphatic clearance.

At our institution, tangential or segmental resection of the SMV, portal vein, or SMPV confluence is performed when, in the opinion of the operating surgeon, the pancreatic head and/or uncinate process cannot be dissected free of the SMPV confluence without either leaving gross tumor on the vein or creating a venotomy (9). The traditional technique for segmental venous resection has historically involved transection of the splenic vein. Division of the splenic vein allows complete exposure of the SMA medial to the SMV, thereby providing the needed exposure for separation of the specimen from the SMA, and provides increased SMV and portal vein length (as these structures are no longer tethered by the splenic vein) for a primary venous anastomosis following segmental vein resection. With the splenic vein divided and the SMA dissection completed, the specimen is attached only by the SMPV confluence. Vascular clamps are placed 2–3 cm proximal (on the portal vein) and distal (on the SMV) to the involved venous segment, and the vein is transected, allowing tumor removal. A 2- to 3-cm segment of SMPV confluence generally can be resected without the need for interposition grafting if the splenic vein is divided. At our institution, venous resection is usually performed with inflow occlusion of the SMA to prevent small-bowel edema, which makes pancreatic and biliary reconstruction more difficult. Systemic heparinization (2,500–5,000 U) is employed prior to occluding the SMA. The free ends of the vein are reapproximated using interrupted sutures of 6-0 Prolene.

Splenic vein preservation is possible only when tumor invasion of the SMV or portal vein does not involve the splenic vein confluence. Preservation of the splenic vein–SMPV confluence significantly limits mobilization of the portal vein and prevents primary anastomosis of the SMV following segmental SMV resection unless segmental resection is limited to 2 cm. Therefore, an interposition graft is required in most patients who undergo SMV resection with splenic vein preservation. Our preferred conduit for interposition grafting is the internal jugular vein. Preservation of the splenic vein adds significant complexity to venous resection because it prevents direct access to the most proximal 3–4 cm of the SMA (medial to the SMV). In such cases, venous resection and reconstruction are generally performed either before the specimen is separated from the right lateral wall of the SMA or after complete mesenteric dissection by separating the specimen first from the SMA.

Five types of venous resection can be performed. A tangential resection of the SMPV confluence (VR1) can be performed for tumor adherence that is limited to a small aspect of the lateral or posterior wall of the SMPV confluence and repaired using a patch from the greater saphenous vein. We rarely perform a tangential (nonsegmental) resection of the SMV without a venous patch, the one exception being isolated tumor involvement of the lateral SMPV confluence directly opposite the splenic vein entrance where a pie-shaped defect can be repaired in a transverse fashion (analogous to a pyloroplasty). When tumor involves the SMV–splenic vein–portal vein confluence, splenic vein ligation is usually necessary. If the SMPV confluence can be reapproximated without tension, an end-to-end primary anastomosis can be performed (V2); if the SMPV confluence cannot be reapproximated without tension, autologous internal jugular vein is used for an interposition graft (VR3). When tumor involvement is limited to the SMV or portal vein such that the splenic vein can be preserved, a primary end-to-end anastomosis of the SMV or portal vein is occasionally possible (V4). However, with preservation of the splenic vein, an interposition graft (VR5) is usually necessary because of the limited mobility of the portal vein caused by an intact splenic vein confluence.

An aberrant right hepatic artery may arise from the SMA as an accessory right hepatic artery (type VI, VII, or VIIIb hepatic arterial anatomy), in which case a normal right hepatic artery also arises from the celiac axis; ligation of the accessory artery in such a case would not affect hepatic or bile duct arterial flow. A replaced right hepatic artery arising from the SMA (type III or VIIIa), unlike an accessory right hepatic artery, represents the only direct arterial inflow to the right hepatic lobe. Because the right and left hepatic arteries communicate within the liver, ligation of the right hepatic artery should be tolerated, assuming a normal level of serum bilirubin and normal flow in the portal vein. However, because the proximal bile duct receives virtually all of its arterial supply from the right hepatic artery following interruption of cephalad flow from the GDA, it has been our practice to revascularize this vessel when possible. Although an accessory hepatic artery arising from the SMA is prone to tumor encasement at the posterosuperior border of the pancreatic head, it has been our experience that PD in this situation rarely requires removal of this vessel because most resectable tumors are located more anteriorly in the pancreatic head or uncinate process. Rarely, the entire common hepatic artery arises from the SMA (type IX). Failure to recognize this anatomic variant and inadvertent ligation of the hepatic artery may result in fatal hepatic necrosis.

Celiac axis stenosis with compensatory retrograde flow in the GDA from the SMA may result from atherosclerotic disease, median arcuate ligament syndrome, or inflammatory entrapment. We always assess the hepatic artery pulse at the time of surgery; if the pulse is noted to significantly decreased in intensity or to disappear upon ligation of the GDA, the common hepatic artery is then dissected to its origin at the celiac axis in an attempt to differentiate extrinsic compression from atherosclerotic disease. If flow is not improved, we proceed with placing a reversed saphenous vein interposition graft between the aorta and the hepatic artery at the site of the GDA origin. This event is infrequent; however, a clearly defined strategy for intraoperative management is required.

2   The University of Texas MD Anderson Cancer Center Experience with Vascular Resection and Reconstruction in Pancreas Cancer

In order to determine the perioperative outcome and survival of patients who underwent vascular resection at the time of PD, Tseng et al. (7) analyzed our experience in >500 patients who underwent PD over a 12-year period. In this retrospective analysis, of 572 patients who underwent PD for all histologic diagnoses, 141 (25%) required major vascular resection. Resection of the SMV, portal vein, or SMPV confluence was performed in 126 (89%) of the 141 patients, which included 36 VR1, 24 VR2, 15 VR3, 11 VR4, and 40 VR5. Segmental resection of the hepatic artery, with or without interposition grafting, was performed in 17 (12%) of the 141 patients; seven of these also underwent concomitant venous resection and reconstruction. Resection of a portion of the anterior wall of the inferior vena cava was performed in six patients (4%), one of whom also underwent concomitant venous resection and reconstruction. There were three perioperative deaths, for a mortality rate of 2.1%. Major perioperative complications occurred in 29 patients (21%). Reoperation was necessary in four patients; three of them had intra-abdominal hemorrhage. In the fourth patient, the biliopancreatic and gastrointestinal reconstruction was delayed for approximately 36 hours (necessitating a second laparotomy) because of bowel edema caused by a prolonged period of venous occlusion at the time of venous resection and reconstruction. At reoperation, there was no evidence of intestinal ischemia, and the patient had an uneventful recovery. The median hospital stay was 13 days.

The median overall survival for the 291 patients was 24.9 months. On univariate analysis, the only significant predictor of decreased survival was the presence of lymph node metastases, with a median survival of 21.1 months for patients with N1 disease, compared with 31.9 months for patients with N0 disease ($p = 0.005$). For the 110 patients who required vascular resection, the median survival was 23.4 months compared with 26.5 months for the 181 patients who underwent standard PD ($p = 0.18$). Multivariate analysis of the effect of all potential prognostic factors on survival in patients who underwent PD for pancreatic adenocarcinoma demonstrated that the presence of N1 disease and the occurrence of one or more major perioperative complication(s) were significant predictors of decreased survival (HR 1.50, $p = 0.01$, and HR 1.52, $p = 0.024$, respectively). In contrast, vascular resection was not associated with decreased survival (HR 1.1, $p = 0.499$).

3   Summary

Vascular resection and reconstruction adds complexity to PD, and patients considered potential candidates for this procedure must be carefully selected based on accurate preoperative cross-sectional imaging studies. However, results from our institution suggest that vascular resection can be done safely as part of PD, and that the performance of this procedure in appropriately selected patients with pancreatic adenocarcinoma is not associated with a decreased survival compared with similar patients who undergo PD without vascular resection. Therefore, surgeons experienced in PD should be prepared to perform vascular resection and reconstruction if indicated in order to facilitate complete removal of tumors involving the pancreatic head or uncinate process.

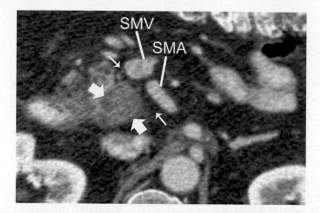

Fig. 20.1 Contrast-enhanced CT scan demonstrating a resectable adenocarcinoma of the pancreatic head. Note the normal fat plane *(narrow arrows)* between the low-density tumor *(wide arrows)* and both the superior mesenteric artery (SMA) and the superior mesenteric vein (SMV). The tumor clearly does not extend to either the superior mesenteric artery or vein.

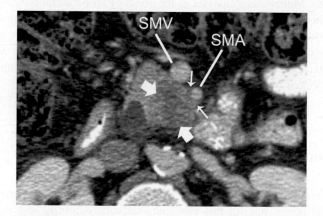

Fig. 20.2 Contrast-enhanced CT scan demonstrating an unresectable adenocarcinoma of the uncinate process of the pancreas. Note the loss of the normal fat plane *(narrow arrows)* between the tumor *(wide arrows)* and the posterior wall of the superior mesenteric artery (SMA). We chose this CT scan image to illustrate relatively limited involvement of the superior mesenteric artery. High-quality scans are needed to demonstrate subtle arterial involvement (as is apparent on this scan), which is of critical importance to the surgeon. This tumor is not amenable to a standard pancreaticoduodenectomy due to tumor extension to the superior mesenteric artery. SMV, superior mesenteric vein.

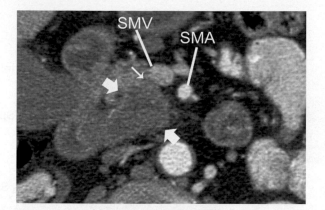

Fig. 20.3 Contrast-enhanced CT scan demonstrating a resectable adenocarcinoma of the pancreatic head *(wide arrows)*, yet with probable focal tumor extension to the lateral wall of the superior mesenteric vein (SMV). Note the area of low density extending to the superior mesenteric vein just posteromedial to the tip of the narrow arrow. This patient may require venous resection and reconstruction at the time of pancreaticoduodenectomy. This subtle finding would not be apparent on a lesser-quality scan. There is a normal fat plane between the low-density tumor and the superior mesenteric artery (SMA).

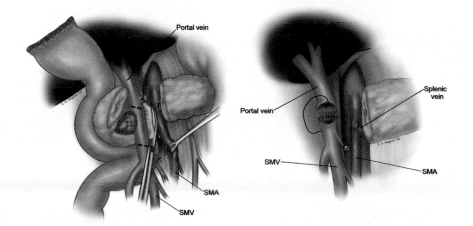

Fig. 20.4 Illustration of the final step in pancreaticoduodenectomy when segmental venous resection is required and the area of venous invasion includes the splenic vein confluence. In preparation for segmental resection of the superior mesenteric vein (SMV), the splenic vein has been divided and the superior mesenteric artery (SMA) identified medial to the SMV and inferior to the divided splenic vein. The retroperitoneal dissection can be completed (following division of the splenic vein) by dissecting the specimen free from the lateral wall of the SMA. The tumor is then attached only by the superior mesenteric–portal vein confluence. Reconstruction is performed (during arterial inflow occlusion) by an end-to-end anastomosis of the portal vein (PV) and the SMV with 6-0 interrupted Prolene sutures.

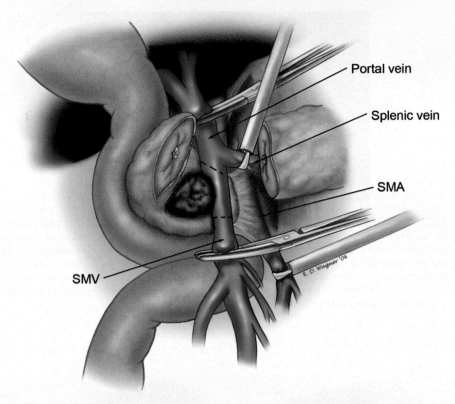

Fig. 20.5 Illustration of resection of the superior mesenteric vein (SMV) with splenic vein preservation. The intact splenic vein tethers the portal vein (PV), making a primary anastomosis impossible in most cases. Our preferred method of reconstruction of the SMV is to use an internal jugular vein interposition graft. With the splenic vein intact, exposure is inadequate to separate the specimen from the lateral aspect of the proximal superior mesenteric artery (SMA). Therefore, the graft can be placed prior to specimen removal, thereby allowing medial retraction of the reconstructed superior mesenteric–portal vein confluence, or after separating the specimen from the SMA posteriorly. Segmental resection of the SMV with splenic vein preservation adds significant complexity to this operation.

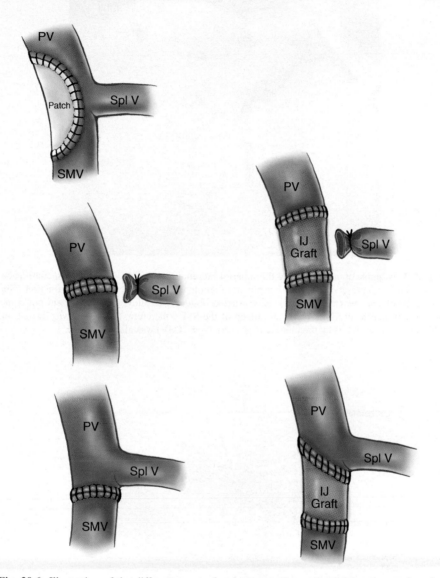

Fig. 20.6 Illustration of the different types of venous resection and reconstruction used at the time of pancreaticoduodenectomy. (From Tseng JF, Raut CP, Lee JE, et al. Pancreaticoduodenectomy with vascular resection: margin status and survival duration. J Gastrointest Surg 2004, 8(8):935–950; used with permission.)

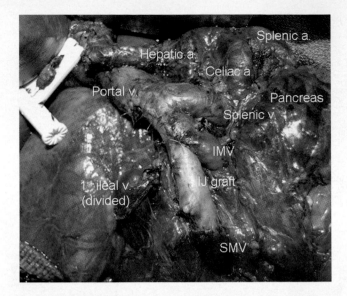

Fig. 20.7 Example of of resection of the superior mesenteric vein (SMV–)portal vein confluence with splenic vein preservation using a segment of autologous jugular vein for reconstruction. The venous confluence was resected and reconstructed obliquely to allow for splenic vein preservation. The tumor involved the first ileal branch of the SMV; therefore, this vessel was ligated. In addition to the splenic vein, the inferior mesenteric vein (IMV) was also preserved.

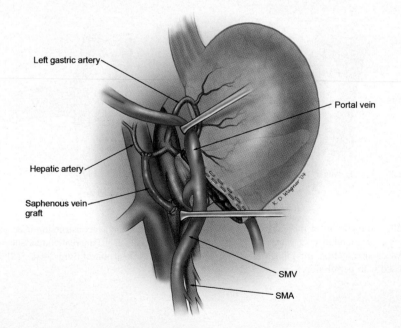

Fig. 20.8 Illustration of our preferred method of celiac revascularization using a reversed saphenous vein graft between the aorta and the origin of the gastroduodenal artery. IVC, inferior vena cava; SMA, superior mesenteric artery; SMV, superior mesenteric vein. (From Evans DB, Lee JE, Leach SD, et al. Vascular resection and intraoperative radiation therapy during pancreaticoduodenectomy: rationale and technique. Adv Surg 1996, 29:235; used with permission.)

References

1. Tseng JF, Tamm EP, Lee JE, et al. 2006, Venous resection in pancreatic cancer surgery. Best Pract Res Clin Gastroenterol 20(2):349–364.
2. Moore GE, Sako Y, Thomas LB. 1951, Radical pancreatoduodenectomy with resection and reanastomosis of the superior mesenteric vein. Surgery 30(3):550–553.
3. Fortner JG, Kim DK, Cubilla A, 1977, Regional pancreatectomy: en bloc pancreatic, portal vein and lymph node resection. Ann Surg 186(1):42–50.
4. Sindelar WF. 1989, Clinical experience with regional pancreatectomy for adenocarcinoma of the pancreas. Arch Surg 124(1):127–132.
5. Leach SD, Lee JE, Charnsangavej C, et al. 1998, Survival following pancreaticoduodenectomy with resection of the superior mesenteric-portal vein confluence for adenocarcinoma of the pancreatic head. Br J Surg 85(5):611–617.
6. Fuhrman GM, Leach SD, Staley CA, et al. 1996, Rationale for en bloc vein resection in the treatment of pancreatic adenocarcinoma adherent to the superior mesenteric-portal vein confluence. Pancreatic Tumor Study Group. Ann Surg 223(2):154–162.
7. Tseng JF, Raut CP, Lee JE, et al. 2004, Pancreaticoduodenectomy with vascular resection: margin status and survival duration. J Gastrointest Surg 8(8):935–949; discussion 49–50.
8. Fuhrman GM, Charnsangavej C, Abbruzzese JL, et al.1994, Thin-section contrast-enhanced computed tomography accurately predicts the resectability of malignant pancreatic neoplasms. Am J Surg 167(1):104–111; discussion 11–13.
9. Scoggins CR, Lee JE, Evans DB. 2005, Pancreaticodenectomy with enbloc vascular resection and reconsruction for localized carcinoma of the pancreas. In; Von Hoff DD, Hruben RH (eds.) Pancreatic cancer. Sudbury, MA, Jones and Bartleh, 321–334.
10. Mackie CR, Moossa AR. 1980, Surgical anatomy of the pancreas. In: Moossa AR (ed.) Tumors of the pancreas. Baltimore, Williams & Wilkns, 1–20
11. Moossa AR. 1980, Tumors of the pancreas, 1st ed. Baltimore, Williams & Wilkins, Baltimore, st ed. .
12. Douglass BE, Baggenstoss AH, Hollinshead WH. 1950, The anatomy of the portal vein and its tributaries. Surg Gynecol Obstet 91(5):562–576.

Chapter 21
Complications of Pancreaticoduodenectomy

Kyla Terhune, Nipun B. Merchant, and Alexander A. Parikh

1 Introduction

Although pancreaticoduodenectomy (PD) was initially performed by Kausch in 1909 and popularized by Allen Whipple in 1935, the operation was traditionally regarded with significant skepticism due to high mortality and morbidity rates. During the past two decades, however, PD has slowly gained acceptance as a safe and effective treatment modality for both malignant and benign diseases of the periampullary region. Due to advances in operative technique and perioperative care, perioperative mortality rates have generally declined from 25–30% to <5% at high-volume centers (1–3). Nevertheless, morbidity rates are still significant— between 30% and 50% in many series (1, 3–5). Given the poor overall survival even in successfully resected patients and the continued need for aggressive and often toxic adjuvant therapy regimens, the impact for postoperative morbidity on the patient's quality of life as well their ability to receive these adjuvant therapies is even more significant. This chapter reviews the most common complications following PD including the diagnosis, risk factors, prevention, and treatment.

2 Incidence and Risk Factors

The most common causes of postoperative morbidity are shown in Table 21.1. In a series of nearly 500 patients undergoing PD at the Massachusetts General Hospital (1), the overall complication rate was 37% and included delayed gastric emptying (DGE) in 12%, pancreatic fistulas in 11%, wound infections in 5%, and other infections in 8% (1). Similarly, in the largest series reported to date of >1,400 patients from Johns Hopkins, the overall complication rate after PD was 38% and most commonly included DGE (15%), wound infections (8%), pancreatic fistulas (5%), and other infections (10%) (3).

Several studies have attempted to identify potential risk factors that may predict adverse outcomes and mortality after PD. In an analysis of 462 patients undergoing PD in the Veterans Affairs National Surgical Quality Improvement

A.M. Lowy et al. (eds.), *Pancreatic Cancer.*
doi: 10.1007/978-0-387-69252-4, © Springer Science+Business Media, LLC 2008

Table 21.1 Complications after pancreaticoduodenectomy

Type of complication	Approximate incidence
Delayed gastric emptying	8–45%
Pancreatic fistula/leak	3–30%
Hemorrhage	2–16%
Intra-abdominal abscess	1–14%
Wound infection	5–10%
Other infections	3–5%
Biliary complications	3–9%
Reoperation	2–4%

Program (6), the overall 30-day mortality rate was 9.3% and morbidity rate was 46%. Significant predictors of mortality included American Society of Anesthesiologists (ASA) classification, preoperative serum albumin, preoperative serum bilirubin >20 mg/dl, and operative time (6). In a study by Adam et al. of 301 patients undergoing PD, the overall mortality and morbidity rates were 3% and 42%, respectively. By multivariate analysis, significant independent risk factors for postoperative complications included impaired renal function (OR 2.7), *absence* of preoperative biliary drainage (OR 1.9), and resection of additional organs (OR 3.2) (7). In a study of 221 patients undergoing PD reported by Boettger et al., the 30-day mortality rate was 3% and morbidity rate was 25% (8). Significant independent risk factors predicting mortality included blood loss, preoperative serum bilirubin, diameter of the pancreatic duct, and development of general or surgical complications. Significant independent risk factors for morbidity included intraoperative blood loss, diameter of the pancreatic duct, age, and sex (8).

2.1 Age of the Patient

As our population continues to age and since the risk of pancreatic cancer increases with age, several studies have attempted to evaluate age as an independent risk factor for increased mortality and morbidity. It has been traditionally thought that patients >70 years undergoing a pancreatic resection have increased complications and mortality. However, this view has been recently challenged by several studies.

In a study from Memorial Sloan Kettering Cancer Center, 138 patients >70 years who underwent a PD had equivalent length of stay, ICU admission rate, overall complication rate and mortality when compared with 350 patients <70 years old (9). Median survival, however, was significantly lower in the elderly group (18 months versus 24 months, $p = 0.03$) (9). In an Italian study of 118 patients undergoing PD, those >70 years old ($n = 33$) had a higher incidence of re-laparotomies and hemorrhagic complications, but equivalent overall complication rate, mortality, and overall survival compared with patients <70 years old ($n = 85$) (10).

In a more recent study comparing >200 patients >80 years old to nearly 2,500 patients <80 years old, the elderly group had a higher incidence of comorbid conditions, including coronary artery disease, HTN, and COPD (11). The overall complication rate (53% versus 42%, $p < 0.05$) and mortality rate (4.1% versus 1.7%, $p < 0.05$) were significantly higher in those aged 80–89 compared with those <80 years old. In addition, pancreatic cancer patients aged 80–89 had a significantly lower median survival when compared with patients <80 years old (11 months versus 18 months, $p = 0.002$) (*11*). Nevertheless, these outcomes are still well within the range of many other studies, even in younger patients, and therefore do not suggest that PD in patients >80 years of age is contraindicated, particularly if the patient is otherwise healthy.

3 Specific Complications

3.1 Delayed Gastric Emptying

Although the precise definition of DGE caused by gastroparesis often varies, most studies agree that it is the most common complication following PD with an incidence between 8% and 45% (*1, 3, 12–14*). The etiology is also unclear, but intra-abdominal infections, resection of the duodenum with interruption of gastrointestinal neural connections, loss of gastrointestinal hormone production, including motilin and local ischemia are all popular theories (*14, 15*). Indeed patients are more likely to suffer from DGE if a complication is present after PD (*16–18*).

It has been suggested that pylorus-preserving pancreaticoduodenectomy (PPPD) is associated with a higher risk of DGE compared to the standard PD (*1, 18–21*). Several trials, both randomized and nonrandomized, have been performed to answer this question, but the results remain unclear. In a small randomized prospective trial of 36 patients by Lin and Lin there were no differences in operative time, blood loss, pancreatic leak, mortality, or overall survival. DGE, however, was more common in the PPPD group (43% versus 0%, $p < 0.05$) (*22*). In contrast, in a much larger randomized trial of 170 patients, operative time, blood loss, mortality, and morbidity, including DGE and median survival were similar between the PPPD and standard PD groups (*23*). Similarly, in a more recent randomized trial of 130 patients, there was no difference in overall morbidity, including DGE, mortality, overall survival, quality of life, or weight gain between the PPPD group and standard PD group (*24*). Without a clear-cut difference in DGE between PPPD and standard PD in randomized trials, the choice of operation therefore should continue to lie with the preference and experience of the surgeon.

3.2 Prevention and Treatment of DGE

Since DGE is such a common problem and as our understanding of the pathophysiology of DGE is still unclear, several technical strategies have been employed to prevent or reduce it. These strategies include pylorotomy and dilatation of the pylorus to prevent pylorospasm (*25, 26*) as well as construction of an antecolic duo-denojejunostomy as part of the reconstruction (*21, 27, 28*). Although results of these strategies appear promising, confirmatory trials and more experience are needed.

The treatment of DGE is nonoperative. Once a mechanical obstruction and intra-abdominal infection is ruled out as a cause of DGE, the treatment is usually conserva-tive. Options for nutrition include enteral feeds via a jejunostomy tube if placed at the time of PD, a nasojejunal feeding tube placed postoperatively, and/or parenteral nutri-tion. Other options include the judicious use of medications that may impair motility including somatostatin (octreotide) which has been shown to suppress plasma motilin level and worsen gastric emptying in a few small studies (*29, 30*).

The use of prokinetic agents such as metoclopramide (Reglan) and erythromycin are also commonly used in the treatment of DGE. Metoclopramide has been shown to improve gastric motility in patients with dyspepsia, critical illness, and diabetic gastroparesis as well as after gastric surgery (*31–36*). The use of erythromycin, meanwhile has been studied in patients having undergone PD and has been shown to reduce the incidence of DGE by 37–75% versus controls in randomized prospec-tive trials (*15, 31–37*).

3.3 Pancreatic Leak and Fistula

The development of a pancreatic leak and fistula is one of the more dreaded compli-cations after PD and occurs in between 3% and 30% in most series (*1, 3, 14, 20, 38–41*). This large range can be explained by a variety of factors, including variabil-ity in defining and reporting a leak. Most of the proposed definitions include the volume of drain output, ranging from 30 cc to >200 cc/day, as well as increased amylase concentration in the drain fluid, ranging from three to five times that of serum to an absolute number. Others additionally add the persistence of amylase-rich fluid over a certain number of days after PD (3–21 days), or radiologic evidence of intra-abdominal fluid collections or the presence of clinical symptoms. Other fac-tors important in helping to explain the difference in incidences include differences in underlying pancreatic disease (soft versus firm pancreatic tissue), individual surgical experience, and different surgical techniques (*1, 3, 14, 20, 38–40*).

A pancreatic anastomotic leak may present in a variety of ways from an overt pancreatic-cutaneous fistula, intra-abdominal abscess in association with a fever, leukocytosis or sepsis, delayed hemorrhage, or associated with another complica-tion, such as DGE. Historically, pancreatic leak contributed significantly to postop-erative death, although in recent years mortality from a pancreatic leak is rare (*1, 3, 14, 20, 38–40*). Increased morbidity secondary to a leak is significant however and includes a higher incidence of intra-abdominal abscesses, wound infections, hem-orrhage, biliary leaks, and cardiac complications (*1, 3, 14, 20, 38–41*). In addition, pancreatic fistulas are associated with increased hospital stays, increased hospital and outpatient costs, and the need for additional invasive or operative procedures (*1, 3, 14, 20, 38–41*).

Many studies have examined potential risk factors in the development of pancreatic fistulas. Although there is considerable variation and some disagreement in these studies, in general, patient characteristics which have been reported to increase pancreatic leak rates include increased age (42) and the presence of comorbidities, including coronary artery disease (CAD) and diabetes mellitus (DM) (40, 43). Perioperative factors which have been associated with an increased leak rate include increased blood loss, transfusion, and operative time (40, 42, 43). Perhaps the most consistent risk factor for an increased leak, however, is the presence of a soft-textured gland (including patients with nonpancreatic cancers) and a small (<3 mm) pancreatic duct (40, 41, 44–47).

A number of strategies have been proposed in hopes of reducing the incidence of pancreatic fistulas after PD. These include different sites of reconstruction (pancreaticogastrostomy versus pancreaticojejunostomy), types of anastomosis (duct-to-mucosa versus invaginated), the use of biologic adhesives, the use of pancreatic stents and the use of somatostatin analogues.

4 Pancreaticogastrostomy versus Pancreaticojejunostomy

One surgical option proposed for decreasing pancreatic fistula rate and subsequent complications after PD is to construct a pancreaticogastrostomy (PG) instead of the traditional pancreaticojejunostomy (PJ). A few retrospective studies have suggested that reconstruction by PG leads to a lower overall morbidity rate and lower pancreatic leak rate compared to PJ reconstruction (48–51). A prospective randomized trial of 145 patients undergoing either a PG or PJ by Yeo et al. however, noted no difference in overall complications including pancreatic leak rate (12.3% versus 11.1%) between the two groups (52). More recently, another prospective randomized trial of 151 patients undergoing PD with either PG or PJ also failed to note any difference in the overall complication rate, including pancreatic leak rate (13% versus 16%) (53). In this study, there was a significantly lower incidence of postoperative biliary collections, DGE and biliary leaks in the PG group, however (53). Since overall experience is limited, however, the method of pancreatic reconstruction should therefore be left to the discretion and experience of the operating surgeon.

5 Type of Anastomosis

The two most common methods of reconstructing pancreatic–intestinal continuity include a duct-to-mucosa anastomosis or invaginated (or intussuscepted end-to-side jejunostomy)—both either with or without stents. There have been several retrospective comparisons of both techniques, but a paucity of randomized trials. Several retrospective studies suggest that there is no difference in the type of anastomosis in regard to the incidence of a leak (40, 42) and a prospective randomized trial from Italy of 144 patients also revealed no difference in leak rates between the two anastomotic techniques (13% versus 15%) (*54*). In light of this, the choice of anastomosis depends on surgeon preference, with most preferring a duct to mucosa anastomosis when possible while reserving an invaginated anastomosis for small duct size.

The use of stents in constructing the pancreatic anastomosis is also controversial. Although a nonrandomized prospective study of 85 patients from Germany suggested an advantage to the use of internal–external pancreatic stent in preventing fistula formation when compared to nonstented patients (7% versus 29%) (*55*), several other studies have failed to show an advantage and have even suggested an increase in complications with the use of stents (*54, 56*). The decision, therefore, should again lie with the surgeon.

The use of bioadhesives around the anastomosis to prevent a leak is also an attractive theoretic option. Nonrandomized retrospective studies have suggested that fibrin glue sealants decrease the incidence of pancreatic fistulas after pancreatic resection (*57, 58*). In addition, a prospective randomized trial in patients undergoing a distal pancreatectomy suggested a decrease in leak rate with the application of fibrin glue (*59*). In prospective randomized trials of patients undergoing both PD and distal pancreatectomy (*59–61*) and of patients undergoing PD considered high risk for a leak (soft gland texture) (*62*); however, no advantage for the use of fibrin glue was noted in preventing pancreatic fistulas or other intraabdominal complications.

6 Prophylactic Use of Octreotide

The use of the native peptide somatostatin was first reported to reduce complications rates after PD in 1979 (*63*). Octreotide is a synthetic octapeptide analog of native somatostatin and has also been used by many in an attempt to prevent as well as to treat pancreatic fistula after PD. There is an ongoing debate as to the effectiveness of prophylactic octreotide in decreasing the incidence of pancreatic anastomotic leaks after pancreatic resection. Multiple randomized control trials have been performed both in the United States and Europe with somewhat conflicting results (Table 21.2). Several European trials suggested a decrease in overall morbidity and/or pancreatic fistula/leak with the use of somatostatin analogues including octreotide (*64–68*), whereas other trials, including those performed in the United States, have failed to show a difference (*69–73*). There are a variety of potential explanations for this discrepancy, including the inconsistent definition of pancreatic leak, varying doses, timing and duration of octreotide administration, different baseline leak rates in the control group, and the inclusion of many types of pancreatic resections (PD, distal pancreatectomies, and enucleations) in the European trials.

Therefore, definitive recommendations are difficult to make. Nevertheless, if prophylactic octreotide is to be used, it most likely will have the largest impact in patient at high risk for leak (soft pancreas, small duct), as was suggested in one prospective trial (*74*), and should be administered starting preoperatively or intraoperatively.

Table 21.2 Prospective randomized trials of the use of octreotide (Oct) for the prevention of overall morbidity, mortality and pancreatic leak after pancreatic resection

Author, year	N	Pancreatic leak %		Morbidity %		Mortality %	
		Control	Oct	Control	Oct	Control	Oct
Buchler, 1992 (*64*)	246	38	18[a]	55	32[a]	6	3
Pederzoli, 1994 (*68*)	252	19	9	29	16[a]	4	2
Montorsi, 1995 (*67*)	218	20	9[a]	36	22[a]	6	8
Friess, 1995 (*65*)	247	22	10[a]	30	16[a]	1	2
Lowy, 1997 (*70*)	110	21	28	25	30	0	2
Yeo, 2000 (*73*)	211	9	11	34	40	0	1
Gouillat, 2001 (*66*)[b]	75	22	5[a,c]	35	21	3	6
Sarr, 2003 (*72*)[d]	275	23	24	26[e]	30[e]	1	0
Shan, 2003 (*126*)	54	7	7	52	26[a]	4	4
Suc, 2004 (*74*)	230	19	17	32[e]	22[e]	7	12
Hesse, 2005 (*127*)	105	8	9	12	11	0	2

[a]$p < 0.05$ versus control.
[b]Somatostatin-14.
[c]Clinical leak.
[d]Somatostatin analogue Vapreotide.
[d]Pancreas-specific complications.
[e]Intra-abdominal complications only.

7 Management of Pancreatic Leaks

Although re-operation was usually necessary for the repair of pancreatic leaks after PD in the past, nonoperative management is now effective in controlling and healing the fistula in the large majority of patients. In a series of 150 patients, Bassi et al. reported a 10.7% (16 patients) pancreatic leak rate. Of these 16 patients, 15 (94%) were successfully managed conservatively (*44*). Similarly, in series of 437 patients undergoing PD reported by Kazanjian et al. a pancreatic fistula developed in 55 (12.6%). Of these, 52 (94%) were also successfully managed conservatively with prolonged drainage (*39*). Median time to removal of drains was 5 weeks (2–14 weeks) with no associated mortality. In addition, the authors note that they did not restrict oral intake, nor did they use parenteral nutrition specifically for the fistula or octreotide in any of those patients (*39*). In the largest series reported to date, 216 patients out of nearly 1,900 (11.4%) developed a pancreatic leak following PD. Conservative management consisting of drainage, parenteral nutrition, and/or octreotide was successful in 92% of the patients and the presence of a fistula did not affect long-term survival (*40*).

For those patients who develop a complication secondary to a fistula, including delayed hemorrhage, intraabdominal abscess not amenable to drainage, wound infections, or ongoing sepsis, operative management will be necessary. Options at the time of re-exploration include repair or revision of the anastomosis with wide drainage, conversion to an isolated Roux-en-y pancreaticojejunostomy with wide drainage, or even completion pancreatectomy (*39*). Not surprisingly, operative mortality can be significant (*39, 43*), especially in the case of hemorrhage, as is discussed in the following.

In a review of 269 patients who underwent pancreaticoduodenectomy, 29 (11%) developed a leak. Of these, eight underwent completion pancreatectomy, and 21 underwent conservative therapy with drainage (*46*). Median hospital stay (55 days versus 74 days) and mortality (0% versus 38%) were significantly lower in those who underwent completion pancreatectomy (*46*). It was unclear, however, the criteria used for resection versus conservative management and the reported 38% mortality in the conservative group is much higher than reported in most studies. In addition, removal of the entire pancreas leads to inherent morbidities associated with the loss of endocrine and exocrine function and should typically be reserved for patients who have failed more conservative measures.

8   Octreotide

The use of octreotide in the *treatment* of established pancreatic fistulas following pancreatic resection has also been studied in at least 10 randomized trials (*69, 75*). The majority of patients in these trials had enterocutaneous fistulas with pancreatic fistulas making up only a minority. Definitive conclusions are therefore difficult to make. Two studies incorporated a crossover design and subjects in both trials experienced a significant reduction in the amount of fistula output, whereas a faster rate of closure was observed in one of them (13.9 days versus 20.4 days) (*76, 77*). The majority of the other eight randomized trials demonstrated a significant decrease in the volume of the fistula output, and three of these trials demonstrated a significant reduction in the time to closure and/or rate of closure (*69, 78, 79*). Since these trials only included a small number of patients with pancreatic fistulas and varying doses and durations of octreotide administration, it is difficult to make definitive recommendations. Nevertheless, it does appear that octreotide reduces fistula output potentially making it easier to manage and may also reduce the time to closure, but probably not the likelihood of eventual closure. The cost of octreotide is significant, however, and must also be taken into account when managing these fistulas.

9   Hemorrhagic Complications

Hemorrhagic complications after PD range from acute bleeding episodes secondary to inadequate hemostasis and/or anticoagulation to delayed hemorrhage, usually from a gastric or marginal ulcer or secondary to a pancreatic leak adjacent to major blood vessels, such as the gastroduodenal artery stump. The majority of studies report an overall bleeding rate of 2–16% after PD with high-volume centers generally reporting rates under 3% (*14, 80–82*). Postoperative bleeding, when it does occur, however, is the most common reason for reexploration and has a mortality rate as high as 30–58% (*4, 80–82*). Hemorrhage can be separated into early versus delayed hemorrhage. Early hemorrhage is usually defined as bleeding within 48–72 hours following PD, whereas delayed hemorrhage usually occurs after the first week (*81–83*).

10 Early Postoperative Hemorrhage

Early hemorrhage is generally the result of technical failure, and can be divided into bleeding into the bowel lumen and extraluminal bleeding into the peritoneal cavity. Although the literature is limited, the incidence appears to vary between 1% and 10% (*80–82*). Similar to the case after other major abdominal surgery, if intraluminal bleeding is suspected (hypotension, tachycardia, a drop in Hgb associated with blood in the nasogastric tube, hematemesis, or melena) upper endoscopy is essential. The usual finding is that of a suture or staple line bleed, rather than a marginal ulcer, and if attempts to stop it endoscopically fail, re-exploration is often necessary (*81, 82*). Re-exploration is also usually necessary if brisk bleeding or clot is seen coming from the afferent limb, suggesting bleeding from the pancreatic anastomosis since this is not amenable to endoscopic control. It is very important to correct any coagulation abnormalities as well. In general, postoperative bleeding requiring more than 2–4 units of PRBC within 24 hours almost always requires relaparotomy and control of the bleeding (*81, 82*).

Suspected extraluminal bleeding in the early postoperative period that requires ongoing transfusion almost always requires relaparotomy (*80–82*). It is important to note than even in patients with intraoperatively placed drains, bleeding may not be evident in these drains (*4*) and that the decision for re-exploration should be based on clinical parameters and a suspicion of bleeding.

At the time of laparotomy, a gastrotomy with oversewing of the suture or staple line usually stops the bleeding in the case of an anastomotic bleed. Careful inspection of the surgical bed, including the retroperitoneal surface and mesentery, must be performed since arterial or venous vessels in these areas are often the source of bleeding (*4, 81*). In the case of a suspected hepaticojejunostomy or pancreaticojejunostomy bleed, the jejunum can be opened opposite the anastomosis or with oversewing of any offending vessel (*80–82*). Occasionally the anastomoses may have to be redone. It is generally hypothesized that bleeding from the pancreatic anastomosis is more common after an invaginated-type anastomosis rather than a duct to mucosa anastomosis due to the lack of tamponade of the pancreatic stump by the jejunum, although supporting data are scant (*4*). It is also important to wash out the jejunal lumen and stomach of any clot that may cause subsequent bowel obstruction (*82*).

11 Delayed Postoperative Hemorrhage

Delayed hemorrhage is generally thought to be more common than early bleeding and often more complicated in diagnosis and treatment (*4, 81–83*). Although the exact mechanism of delayed bleeding is still unclear, most authors agree that a pancreatic leak leading to local sepsis and resultant pseudoaneurysm of an adjacent vessel that had been extensively dissected is the most common etiology (*4, 81–84*). It has also been shown that delayed hemorrhage is associated with other postoperative complications, such as pancreatic fistulae, biliary fistulae, and intra-abdominal abscesses as well as jaundice (*81, 83–85*). Indeed several studies have shown an association between a preceding or concurrent intra-abdominal complication and delayed hemorrhage (*81, 83, 85*).

Immediate and accurate diagnosis is essential to save patients from a massive and life-threatening bleed. Although upper endoscopy has long been used as the diagnostic modality of choice when an intraluminal bleed is suspected, it has several limitations. It is often difficult to discern the exact site of bleeding when the GI tract is filled with clot and blood. Even when found, definite treatment may be difficult. Furthermore, many studies report that delayed intraluminal bleeding is a result of an arterial pseudoaneurysm having eroded into adjacent anastomosis or bowel loop—a problem that usually cannot be repaired endoscopically (*81, 83, 85, 86*).

Angiography is usually the diagnostic and therapeutic modality of choice, as it can often precisely localize the bleeding point and can provide a route for embolization (*81, 83, 85, 86*). In cases when embolization is not possible or unsuccessful, operative re-exploration is required. At the time of exploration, not only must the bleeding source be identified and repaired, but the pancreatic anastomosis should also be carefully inspected for a leak. If present, options include drainage, repair, or revision of the anastomosis or even completion pancreatectomy if needed (*81–83, 86*). Unfortunately, mortality rates after delayed hemorrhage remain significant, as high as 30%, and prompt diagnosis and intervention is therefore paramount (*81–83, 86*).

12 Infectious Complications

12.1 Wound Infections

Wound infections are not uncommon after PD, ranging from 5% to 10% (*1–4, 87*), which is similar to other large clean-contaminated surgical procedures (*88–90*). These are often associated with a concomitant complication, such as intra-abdominal abscesses, pancreatic fistulas, and biliary leaks, as well as preoperative biliary drainage as discussed in the following. Management is similar to that in other gastrointestinal surgical patients and involves opening and cleaning of the wound, antibiotics as needed, and treatment of concomitant infections or complications.

12.2   Intra-abdominal Abscesses

The rate of intra-abdominal abscesses following pancreatic resection has been reported as 1–14% (*1*, *3*, *4*, *6*, *87*, *91*). Despite advances in perioperative care and antimicrobial therapy, the incidence of this complication has remained relatively stable. Several mediating factors have been proposed as potential causal agents including preoperative biliary stenting and intraoperative drain placement (discussed in the following), presence of a pancreatic fistula, intraoperative blood loss and transfusion requirement as well as transient hypotension (*4*, *92–94*). Most abscesses can be managed nonoperatively via percutaneously placed drains; however, ongoing sepsis requires reoperation in approximately 10% and carries a mortality rate near 5% (*4*, *92–94*).

13   Biliary Complications

Biliary complications are relatively uncommon, occurring in 3–9% of patients with PD, with the overall incidence decreasing (*4*, *92*, *93*). These complications include a biliary leak, biliary obstruction, and cholangitis. In a series of 279 patients from the Mayo Clinic, a biliary leak was present in 24 patients (9%), of which three required an operation, whereas the other 21 (87.5%) healed spontaneously (*92*). In a series of 1,061 PD patients from Johns Hopkins, a bile leak was present in 4% and cholangitis in 3%. A total of 39 patients required postoperative intervention— 22 for a leak, five for cholangitis, and six for a clogged t-tube (*93*). In general, biliary complications are relatively rare and most heal spontaneously or with nonsurgical intervention with little or no associated mortality.

14   Other Management Decisions and Outcomes

14.1   Placement of Intraoperative Drains

Operative drains have routinely been placed at the time of PD for the recognition and control of the leakage of blood, bile, lymph, and pancreatic secretions and prevention of intra-abdominal infections. The routine use of these drains has recently been brought into question, however. In an initial retrospective report from MSKCC, 38 patients undergoing PD with no intraabdominal drains were compared to 51 patients who had closed suction drains placed at the time of PD. There was no significant difference in the rate of pancreatic fistula, abscess, need for CT-guided drainage or length of hospital stay between the groups (*95*). This led to the only prospective randomized trial published to date involving 179 patients undergoing PD (139) or distal pancreatectomy (*39*) randomized to closed suction drains in proximity to the biliary and pancreatic anastomoses versus no drains (*96*). There was no difference in overall mortality, complication rates or length of stay between the two groups. In addition the number of patients with intraabdominal fluid collections and fistulas was actually higher in the drain group (*96*), although this may be due to an increased recognition of enterocutaneous and pancreatic fistulas in patients with drains. Nevertheless, it did not appear that the placement of closed suction drains at the time of PD offered any advantage over no drains.

It has also been suggested that the placement of closed suction drains may actually increase the risk of intra-abdominal infections by providing a rout for ascending infections. A recent study of 104 patients undergoing PD suggested that if drains are placed at the time of PD, that they be removed early (*97*). In this study, patients were assigned according to the year of PD to either late (POD 8) or early (POD 4) removal. The rate of pancreatic fistula was significantly lower in the early removal group (4% versus 23%, $p = 0.004$) and the rate of intra-abdominal infections was also significantly lower in the early removal group (8% versus 38%, $p = 0.0003$). Bacterial cultures were also significantly more positive in the late removal group (31% versus 4%, $p = 0.0002$) and the period of drain insertion was the only independent risk factor for the development of intra-abdominal infections (HR 6.7) by multivariate analysis (*97*).

14.2   Preoperative Biliary Drainage

Preoperative biliary drainage (PBD) by either a percutaneously or an ERCP-placed stent is commonly used to relieve jaundice prior to definitive surgical resection. Advantages of PBD include symptomatic relief for the patient, improved digestion, and nutrition, improved immune function as well as the ability to administer neo-adjuvant therapy. Nevertheless, several retrospective reports have suggested an increased risk of complications following PBD, including postoperative infection and pancreatic fistulas (*98–102*). PBD prior to PD therefore remains controversial.

Of the five small randomized control trials (RCT) from 1982 to 1994 comparing preoperative internal and or external biliary drainage versus none in patients undergoing PD, only one trial consisting of 15 patients in each arm reported a benefit (*103*). The other trials failed to show any benefit to PBD and a few showed a deleterious effect (*104–107*). A recent meta-analysis of these trials reported similar perioperative mortality in both groups but a significantly increased *overall* complication rate in the PBD group (57% versus 42%, HR1.99, $p = 0.004$) (*108*). Interestingly, the *post*operative complication rate was significantly *lower* in the PBD group (30% versus 42%, HR 0.59, $p = 0.03$) (*108*).

Several nonrandomized prospective and retrospective studies have also attempted to show a benefit for PBD prior to PD with only a small number suggesting a benefit (*98–102, 109–111*). A meta-analysis of these trials consisting of over 1,800 patients was also reported in 2002. Similar to the meta-analysis of the randomized trials, there was no difference in overall mortality (3.2% versus 4.9%, HR 0.91), but a significant increase in overall complications in the PBD group (59% versus 42%, HR 1.64, $p = 0.002$) (*108*). Unlike the RCT meta-analysis, there was also no difference in post-operative complications (49.3% versus 49.5%, HR 0.96) (*108*).

More recent studies have focused on potential factors of PBD that may increase postoperative complications. It is generally agreed that PBD leads to contamination of the bile with enteric organisms and that patients having undergone PBD have a higher incidence of infected bile, which may explain the higher rate of infectious complications (*98, 112*). In a study of 74 patients having undergone PBD, a positive intraoperative bile culture was the most significant factor predicting postoperative morbidity and mortality after PD. Positive cultures were more common if PD occurred within 6 weeks of PBD and patients without positive bile cultures having undergone PBD had no increase in mortality or morbidity (*113*). In a study from France of 79 patients undergoing PD, preoperative stenting was associated with a higher rate of infected bile as well as postoperative infectious complications and that the organisms responsible for these infections were often those cultured in the bile (*98*). These studies suggested, therefore, that culturing of bile intraoperatively may help predict those patients who are at increased risk of infectious complications and perhaps direct postoperative antibiotic prophylaxis. In addition, a delay of >6 weeks between PBD and PD may be prudent (as in the case of neoadjuvant therapy), if possible.

14.3 Feeding Tubes

The placement of feeding jejunostomy tubes during major abdominal operations including PD is still controversial. Potential benefits include prevention of mucosal atrophy, preservation of normal gut flora, immune competence and potentially less reliance on parenteral nutrition in patients with DGE and other complications (*4*). Nevertheless, the morbidity of j-tube placement can range from 2% to 10% and has predominantly included small bowel obstruction, small bowel necrosis and intraperitoneal leak (*4, 114, 115*). In one study of 125 patients, approximately half of the patients had a jejunostomy tube placed, and 5 (7.4%) had complications, including small bowel obstruction, enteric leaks, or small bowel necrosis. Two of these patients died (*4*).

14.4 Neoadjuvant Therapy

Neoadjuvant chemoradiation has been used by several institutions for the treatment of locally advanced and potentially resectable pancreatic cancer. Nevertheless, very little data exist as to the impact of neoadjuvant therapy on complications after PD. It is important to remember, however, that most patients receiving neoadjuvant therapy will require biliary drainage with its inherent potential complications as discussed in the preceding. Ishikawa et al. first suggested that neoadjuvant chemo-radiation may actually decrease the leak rate after PD (*116*). In their retrospective study, 22 patients who received 50 Gy of preoperative radiation had a 5% (one patient) leak rate compared to while 10 of 54 patients (19%) who did not receive preoperative therapy (*116*). Similarly, a prospective study of 110 PD patients the leak rate in 46 patients who received preoperative 5-FU based chemoradiation had a significantly lower total leak rate than in 64 patients who did not (OR 0.55, $p = 0.02$) (*70*). Finally, in a more recent study of 146 PD patients, the group receiving preoperative 5-FU–based chemoradiation ($n = 79$) had a significantly lower pancreatic leak rate (10% versus 43%, $p < 0.001$) as well as a lower incidence of intra-abdominal abscess (8.8% versus 21%, $p = 0.019$) than those who did not receive preoperative therapy ($n = 67$). Overall morbidity and mortality were similar (*117*). Although these studies are retrospective in nature, they do suggest that neoadjuvant chemoradiation does not increase the complication rate after PD and may in fact be associated with a lower leak rate presumably by causing radiation fibrosis and scarring of the gland.

14.5   Vascular Resection

Portal or superior mesenteric vein resection during PD has been advocated by many when necessary to achieve a margin negative resection for periampullary malignancies. Although vein resection does add complexity, time, and potential blood loss to the operation, multiple studies have failed to show any increase in overall morbidity or mortality (*118–121*).

15   Surgeon and Hospital Experience

As is the case with many other complex procedures, pancreaticoduodenectomy is probably best left in the hands of those who perform the procedure most often. Several studies have suggested that morbidity and mortality rates after PD are significantly related the individual surgeon's experience as well as the hospital's volume, suggesting perhaps that patients should be referred to high-volume centers whenever possible (*122–125*).

16   Conclusions

Pancreaticoduodenectomy remains the only chance of cure in patients with periampullary malignancies. Although now very safe in experienced hands, it is still a procedure fraught with significant complications despite advances in operative technique and perioperative care. Nevertheless, if these complications are recognized and treated in a timely fashion, the impact on overall survival, which is usually relatively short, can be minimized. A complete understanding of the risk factors predicting adverse outcomes as well as prompt recognition and treatment of these complications is crucial in minimizing their impact on the patients overall survival, which is often short. In addition, continued well-designed randomized trials are needed as we discover new therapies and refine old ones in hopes of maximizing survival and minimizing complications after pancreatic resection.

References

1. Balcom JHT, 2001, Ten-year experience with 733 pancreatic resections: changing indications, older patients, and decreasing length of hospitalization. Arch Surg 136(4):391–398.
2. Cameron JL, 2006, One thousand consecutive pancreaticoduodenectomies. Ann Surg 244(1):10–15.
3. Winter JM, 2006, 1423 Pancreaticoduodenectomies for pancreatic cancer: a single-institution experience. J Gastrointest Surg 10(9):1199–1211.
4. Behrman SW, Rush BT, Dilawari RA. 2004, A modern analysis of morbidity after pancreatic resection. Am Surg 70(8):675–682; discussion 682–683.
5. Schmidt CM, 2004, Pancreaticoduodenectomy: a 20-year experience in 516 patients. Arch Surg 139(7):718–725; discussion 725–727.
6. Billingsley KG, 2003, Outcome after pancreaticoduodenectomy for periampullary cancer: an analysis from the Veterans Affairs National Surgical Quality Improvement Program. J Gastrointest Surg 7(4):484–491.
7. Adam U, 2004, Risk factors for complications after pancreatic head resection. Am J Surg 187(2):201–208.
8. Bottger TC, Junginger T, 1999, Factors influencing morbidity and mortality after pancreaticoduodenectomy: critical analysis of 221 resections. World J Surg 23(2):164–171; discussion 171–172.
9. Fong Y, 1995, Pancreatic or liver resection for malignancy is safe and effective for the elderly. Ann Surg 222(4):426–434; discussion 434–437.
10. DiCarlo V, 1998, Pancreatic cancer resection in elderly patients. Br J Surg 85(5):607–610.
11. Makary MA, 2006, Pancreaticoduodenectomy in the very elderly. J Gastrointest Surg 10(3):347–356.
12. Di Carlo V, 1999, Pylorus-preserving pancreaticoduodenectomy versus conventional whipple operation. World J Surg 23(9):920–925.
13. Roder JD, 1992, Pylorus-preserving versus standard pancreatico-duodenectomy: an analysis of 110 pancreatic and periampullary carcinomas. Br J Surg 79(2):152–155.
14. Schafer M, Mullhaupt B, Clavien PA, 2002, Evidence-based pancreatic head resection for pancreatic cancer and chronic pancreatitis. Ann Surg 236(2):137–148.
15. Ohwada S, 2001, Low-dose erythromycin reduces delayed gastric emptying and improves gastric motility after Billroth I pylorus-preserving pancreaticoduodenectomy. Ann Surg 234(5):668–674.
16. Horstmann O, 1999, Is delayed gastric emptying following pancreaticoduodenectomy related to pylorus preservation? Langenbecks Arch Surg 384(4):354–359.
17. Riediger H, 2003, Delayed gastric emptying after pylorus-preserving pancreatoduodenectomy is strongly related to other postoperative complications. J Gastrointest Surg 7(6):758–765.

18. Berge Henegouwen MI, van 1997, Delayed gastric emptying after standard pancreaticoduodenectomy versus pylorus-preserving pancreaticoduodenectomy: an analysis of 200 consecutive patients. J Am Coll Surg 185(4):373–379.
19. Goei TH, 2001, Pylorus-preserving pancreatoduodenectomy: influence of a Billroth I versus a Billroth II type of reconstruction on gastric emptying. Dig Surg 18(5):376–380.
20. Jimenez RE, 2000, Outcome of pancreaticoduodenectomy with pylorus preservation or with antrectomy in the treatment of chronic pancreatitis. Ann Surg 231(3):293–300.
21. Park YC, 2003, Factors influencing delayed gastric emptying after pylorus-preserving pancreatoduodenectomy. J Am Coll Surg 196(6):859–865.
22. Lin PW, 2005, Pancreaticoduodenectomy for pancreatic head cancer: PPPD versus Whipple procedure. Hepatogastroenterology 52(65):1601–1604.
23. Tran KT, 2004, Pylorus preserving pancreaticoduodenectomy versus standard Whipple procedure: a prospective, randomized, multicenter analysis of 170 patients with pancreatic and periampullary tumors. Ann Surg 240(5):738–745.
24. Seiler CA, 2005, Randomized clinical trial of pylorus-preserving duodenopancreatectomy versus classical Whipple resection-long term results. Br J Surg 92(5):547–556.
25. Fischer CP, Hong JC. 2006, Method of pyloric reconstruction and impact upon delayed gastric emptying and hospital stay after pylorus-preserving pancreaticoduodenectomy. J Gastrointest Surg 10(2):215–219.
26. Kim DK, 2005, Is pylorospasm a cause of delayed gastric emptying after pylorus-preserving pancreaticoduodenectomy? Ann Surg Oncol 12(3):222–227.
27. Horstmann O, 2004, Pylorus preservation has no impact on delayed gastric emptying after pancreatic head resection. Pancreas 28(1):69–74.
28. Tani M, 2006, Improvement of delayed gastric emptying in pylorus-preserving pancreaticoduodenectomy: results of a prospective, randomized, controlled trial. Ann Surg 243(3):316–320.
29. Shan YS, 2005, Effects of somatostatin prophylaxis after pylorus-preserving pancreaticoduodenectomy: increased delayed gastric emptying and reduced plasma motilin. World J Surg 29(10):1319–1324.
30. Berge Henegouwen MI, van 1997, The effect of octreotide on gastric emptying at a dosage used to prevent complications after pancreatic surgery: a randomised, placebo controlled study in volunteers. Gut 41(6):758–762.
31. Dumitrascu DL, 1998, The effect of metoclopramide on antral emptying of a semisolid meal in patients with functional dyspepsia. A randomized placebo controlled sonographic study. Rom J Intern Med 36(1–2):97–104.
32. Erbas T, 1993, Comparison of metoclopramide and erythromycin in the treatment of diabetic gastroparesis. Diabetes Care 16(11):1511–1514.
33. Jooste CA, Mustoe J, Collee G, 1999, Metoclopramide improves gastric motility in critically ill patients. Intensive Care Med 25(5):464–468.
34. Malagelada JR, 1980, Gastric motor abnormalities in diabetic and postvagotomy gastroparesis: effect of metoclopramide and bethanechol. Gastroenterology 78(2):286–293.
35. Metzger WH, Cano R, Sturdevant RA, 1976, Effect of metoclopramide in chronic gastric retention after gastric surgery. Gastroenterology 71(1):30–32.
36. Ricci DA, 1985, Effect of metoclopramide in diabetic gastroparesis. J Clin Gastroenterol 7(1):25–32.
37. Yeo CJ, 1993, Erythromycin accelerates gastric emptying after pancreaticoduodenectomy. A prospective, randomized, placebo–controlled trial. Ann Surg 218(3):229–237; discussion 237–238.
38. Buchler MW, 1995, Randomized trial of duodenum-preserving pancreatic head resection versus pylorus-preserving Whipple in chronic pancreatitis. Am J Surg 169(1):65–69; discussion 69–70.
39. Kazanjian KK, 2005, Management of pancreatic fistulas after pancreaticoduodenectomy: results in 437 consecutive patients. Arch Surg 140(9):849–854; discussion 854–856.

40. Lin JW, 2004, Risk factors and outcomes in postpancreaticoduodenectomy pancreaticocutaneous fistula. J Gastrointest Surg 8(8):951–959.
41. Aranha GV, 2006, Current management of pancreatic fistula after pancreaticoduodenectomy. Surgery 140(4):561–568; discussion 568–569.
42. Yeh TS, 1997, Pancreaticojejunal anastomotic leak after pancreaticoduodenectomy—multivariate analysis of perioperative risk factors. J Surg Res 67(2):119–125.
43. Srivastava S, 2001, Determinants of pancreaticoenteric anastomotic leak following pancreaticoduodenectomy. ANZ J Surg 71(9):511–515.
44. Bassi C, 2001, Management of complications after pancreaticoduodenectomy in a high volume centre: results on 150 consecutive patients. Dig Surg 18(6):453–457; discussion 458.
45. Tajima Y, 2006, Risk factors for pancreatic anastomotic leakage: the significance of preoperative dynamic magnetic resonance imaging of the pancreas as a predictor of leakage. J Am Coll Surg 202(5):723–731.
46. Berge Henegouwen MI, van 1997, Incidence, risk factors, and treatment of pancreatic leakage after pancreaticoduodenectomy: drainage versus resection of the pancreatic remnant. J Am Coll Surg 185(1):18–24.
47. Yang YM, 2005, Risk factors of pancreatic leakage after pancreaticoduodenectomy. World J Gastroenterol 11(16):2456–2461.
48. Kim SW, Youk EG, Park YH, 1997, Comparison of pancreatogastrostomy and pancreatojejunostomy after pancreatoduodenectomy performed by one surgeon. World J Surg 21(6):640–643.
49. Oussoultzoglou E, 2004, Pancreaticogastrostomy decreased relaparotomy caused by pancreatic fistula after pancreaticoduodenectomy compared with pancreaticojejunostomy. Arch Surg 139(3):327–335.
50. Schlitt HJ, 2002, Morbidity and mortality associated with pancreatogastrostomy and pancreatojejunostomy following partial pancreatoduodenectomy. Br J Surg 89(10): 1245–1251.
51. Takano S, 2000, Pancreaticojejunostomy versus pancreaticogastrostomy in reconstruction following pancreaticoduodenectomy. Br J Surg 87(4):423–427.
52. Yeo CJ, 1995, A prospective randomized trial of pancreaticogastrostomy versus pancreaticojejunostomy after pancreaticoduodenectomy. Ann Surg 222(4):580–588; discussion 588–592.
53. Bassi C, 2005, Reconstruction by pancreaticojejunostomy versus pancreaticogastrostomy following pancreatectomy: results of a comparative study. Ann Surg 242(6):767–771, discussion 771–773.
54. Bassi C, 2003, Duct-to-mucosa versus end-to-side pancreaticojejunostomy reconstruction after pancreaticoduodenectomy: results of a prospective randomized trial. Surgery 134(5):766–771.
55. Roder JD, 1999, Stented versus nonstented pancreaticojejunostomy after pancreatoduodenectomy: a prospective study. Ann Surg 229(1):41–48.
56. Imaizumi T, 2002, Stenting is unnecessary in duct-to-mucosa pancreaticojejunostomy even in the normal pancreas. Pancreatology 2(2):116–121.
57. Kram HB, 1991, Fibrin glue sealing of pancreatic injuries, resections, and anastomoses. Am J Surg 161(4):479–481; discussion 482.
58. Tashiro S, 1987, New technique for pancreaticojejunostomy using a biological adhesive. Br J Surg 74(5):392–394.
59. Suzuki Y, 1995, Fibrin glue sealing for the prevention of pancreatic fistulas following distal pancreatectomy. Arch Surg 130(9):952–955.
60. D'Andrea AA, 1994, Human fibrin sealant in pancreatic surgery: it is useful in preventing fistulas? A prospective randomized study. Ital J Gastroenterol 26(6):283–286.
61. Suc B, 2003, Temporary fibrin glue occlusion of the main pancreatic duct in the prevention of intra-abdominal complications after pancreatic resection: prospective randomized trial. Ann Surg 237(1):57–65.

62. Lillemoe KD, 2004, Does fibrin glue sealant decrease the rate of pancreatic fistula after pancreaticoduodenectomy? Results of a prospective randomized trial. J Gastrointest Surg 8(7):766–772;discussion 772–774.
63. Klempa I, Schwedes U, Usadel KH. 1979, (Prevention of postoperative pancreatic complications following duodenopancreatectomy using somatostatin). Chirurg 50(7):427–431.
64. Buchler M, 1992, Role of octreotide in the prevention of postoperative complications following pancreatic resection. Am J Surg 163(1):125–130; discussion 130–131.
65. Friess H, 1995, Randomized controlled multicentre study of the prevention of complications by octreotide in patients undergoing surgery for chronic pancreatitis. Br J Surg 82(9):1270–1273.
66. Gouillat C, 2001, Randomized controlled multicentre trial of somatostatin infusion after pancreaticoduodenectomy. Br J Surg 88(11):1456–1462.
67. Montorsi M, 1995, Efficacy of octreotide in the prevention of pancreatic fistula after elective pancreatic resections: a prospective, controlled, randomized clinical trial. Surgery 117(1):26–31.
68. Pederzoli P, 1994, Efficacy of octreotide in the prevention of complications of elective pancreatic surgery. Italian Study Group. Br J Surg 81(2):265–269.
69. Li–Ling J, Irving M. 2001, Somatostatin and octreotide in the prevention of postoperative pancreatic complications and the treatment of enterocutaneous pancreatic fistulas: a systematic review of randomized controlled trials. Br J Surg 88(2):190–199.
70. Lowy AM, 1997, Prospective, randomized trial of octreotide to prevent pancreatic fistula after pancreaticoduodenectomy for malignant disease. Ann Surg 226(5):632–641.
71. Ramos-De la Medina A, Sarr MG. 2006, Somatostatin analogues in the prevention of pancreas-related complications after pancreatic resection. J Hepatobiliary Pancreat Surg 13(3):190–193.
72. Sarr MG, 2003, The potent somatostatin analogue vapreotide does not decrease pancreas-specific complications after elective pancreatectomy: a prospective, multicenter, double-blinded, randomized, placebo-controlled trial. J Am Coll Surg 196(4):556–564; discussion 564–565; author reply 565.
73. Yeo CJ, 2000, Does prophylactic octreotide decrease the rates of pancreatic fistula and other complications after pancreaticoduodenectomy? Results of a prospective randomized placebo-controlled trial. Ann Surg 232(3):419–429.
74. Suc B, 2004, Octreotide in the prevention of intra-abdominal complications following elective pancreatic resection: a prospective, multicenter randomized controlled trial. Arch Surg 139(3):288–294; discussion 295.
75. Martineau P, Shwed JA, Denis R. 1996, Is octreotide a new hope for enterocutaneous and external pancreatic fistulas closure? Am J Surg 172(4):386–395.
76. Nubiola-Calonge P, 1987, Blind evaluation of the effect of octreotide (SMS 201-995), a somatostatin analogue, on small-bowel fistula output. Lancet 2(8560):672–674.
77. Torres AJ, 1992, Somatostatin in the management of gastrointestinal fistulas. A multicenter trial. Arch Surg 127(1):97–99; discussion 100.
78. Gerardo Perez D, Bernardo Acosta M, 1994, (Gastrointestinal fistulas. Treatment with a somatostatin analogue) (SMS 201–995). G E N 48(4):209–218.
79. Hernandez-Aranda JC, 1996, (Treatment of enterocutaneous fistula with or without octreotide and parenteral nutrition). Nutr Hosp 11(4):226–229.
80. Balachandran P, 2004, Haemorrhagic complications of pancreaticoduodenectomy. ANZ J Surg 74(11):945–950.
81. Rumstadt B, 1998, Hemorrhage after pancreatoduodenectomy. Ann Surg 227(2):236–241.
82. Wente MN, 2006, Management of early hemorrhage from pancreatic anastomoses after pancreaticoduodenectomy. Dig Surg 23(4):203–208.
83. Choi SH, 2004, Delayed hemorrhage after pancreaticoduodenectomy. J Am Coll Surg 199(2):186–191.
84. Tien YW, 2005, Risk factors of massive bleeding related to pancreatic leak after pancreaticoduodenectomy. J Am Coll Surg 201(4):554–559.

85. Yoon YS, 2003, Management of postoperative hemorrhage after pancreatoduodenectomy. Hepatogastroenterology 50(54):2208–2212.
86. Berge Henegouwen MI, van 1995, Delayed massive haemorrhage after pancreatic and biliary surgery. Br J Surg 82(11):1527–1531.
87. Sohn TA, 2000, Resected adenocarcinoma of the pancreas—616 patients: results, outcomes, and prognostic indicators. J Gastrointest Surg 4(6):567–579.
88. Barber GR, 1995, Direct observations of surgical wound infections at a comprehensive cancer center. Arch Surg 130(10):1042–1047.
89. Tonelli F, 2002, Amoxicillin/clavulanic acid versus cefotaxime for antimicrobial prophylaxis in abdominal surgery: a randomized trial. J Chemother 14(4):366–372.
90. Wille-Jorgensen P, 2005, Pre-operative mechanical bowel cleansing or not? An updated meta-analysis. Colorectal Dis 7(4):304–310.
91. Cameron JL, 1993, One hundred and forty-five consecutive pancreaticoduodenectomies without mortality. Ann Surg 217(5):430–435; discussion 435–438.
92. Miedema BW, 1992, Complications following pancreaticoduodenectomy. Current management. Arch Surg 127(8):945–949; discussion 949–950.
93. Sohn TA, 2003, Pancreaticoduodenectomy: role of interventional radiologists in managing patients and complications. J Gastrointest Surg 7(2):209–219.
94. Stephens J, 1997, Surgical morbidity, mortality, and long-term survival in patients with peripancreatic cancer following pancreaticoduodenectomy. Am J Surg 174(6):600–603; discussion 603–604.
95. Heslin MJ, 1998, Is intra–abdominal drainage necessary after pancreaticoduodenectomy? J Gastrointest Surg 2(4):373–378.
96. Conlon KC, 2001, Prospective randomized clinical trial of the value of intraperitoneal drainage after pancreatic resection. Ann Surg 234(4):487–493; discussion 493–494.
97. Kawai M, 2006, Early removal of prophylactic drains reduces the risk of intra-abdominal infections in patients with pancreatic head resection: prospective study for 104 consecutive patients. Ann Surg 244(1):1–7.
98. Cortes A, 2006, Effect of bile contamination on immediate outcomes after pancreaticoduodenectomy for tumor. J Am Coll Surg 202(1):93–99.
99. Heslin MJ, 1998, A preoperative biliary stent is associated with increased complications after pancreatoduodenectomy. Arch Surg 133(2):149–154.
100. Hodul P, 2003, The effect of preoperative biliary stenting on postoperative complications after pancreaticoduodenectomy. Am J Surg 186(5):420–425.
101. Pisters PW, 2001, Effect of preoperative biliary decompression on pancreaticoduodenectomy-associated morbidity in 300 consecutive patients. Ann Surg 234(1):47–55.
102. Povoski SP, 1999, Association of preoperative biliary drainage with postoperative outcome following pancreaticoduodenectomy. Ann Surg 230(2):131–142.
103. Smith RC, 1985, Preoperative percutaneous transhepatic internal drainage in obstructive jaundice: a randomized, controlled trial examining renal function. Surgery 97(6):641–648.
104. Hatfield AR, 1982, Preoperative external biliary drainage in obstructive jaundice. A prospective controlled clinical trial. Lancet 2(8304):896–899.
105. Lai EC, 1994, Preoperative endoscopic drainage for malignant obstructive jaundice. Br J Surg 81(8):1195–1198.
106. McPherson GA, 1984, Pre-operative percutaneous transhepatic biliary drainage: the results of a controlled trial. Br J Surg 71(5):371–375.
107. Pitt HA, 1985, Does preoperative percutaneous biliary drainage reduce operative risk or increase hospital cost? Ann Surg 201(5):545–553.
108. Sewnath ME, 2002, A meta-analysis on the efficacy of preoperative biliary drainage for tumors causing obstructive jaundice. Ann Surg 236(1):17–27.
109. Karsten TM, 1996, Preoperative biliary drainage, colonisation of bile and postoperative complications in patients with tumours of the pancreatic head: a retrospective analysis of 241 consecutive patients. Eur J Surg 162(11):881–888.

110. Sewnath ME, 2001, The effect of preoperative biliary drainage on postoperative complications after pancreaticoduodenectomy. J Am Coll Surg 192(6):726–734.
111. Sohn TA, 2000, Do preoperative biliary stents increase postpancreaticoduodenectomy complications? J Gastrointest Surg 4(3):258–267; discussion 267–268.
112. Howard TJ, 2006, Influence of bactibilia after preoperative biliary stenting on postoperative infectious complications. J Gastrointest Surg 10(4):523–531.
113. Jagannath P, 2005, Effect of preoperative biliary stenting on immediate outcome after pancreaticoduodenectomy. Br J Surg 92(3):356–361.
114. Gerndt SJ, Orringer MB, 1994, Tube jejunostomy as an adjunct to esophagectomy. Surgery 115(2):164–169.
115. Tapia J, 1999, Jejunostomy: techniques, indications, and complications. World J Surg 23(6):596–602.
116. Ishikawa O, 1989, Clinical and histopathological appraisal of preoperative irradiation for adenocarcinoma of the pancreatoduodenal region. J Surg Oncol 40(3):143–151.
117. Cheng TY, 2006, Effect of neoadjuvant chemoradiation on operative mortality and morbidity for pancreaticoduodenectomy. Ann Surg Oncol 13(1):66–74.
118. Leach SD, 1998, Survival following pancreaticoduodenectomy with resection of the superior mesenteric-portal vein confluence for adenocarcinoma of the pancreatic head. Br J Surg 85(5):611–617.
119. Riediger H, 2006, Postoperative morbidity and long-term survival after pancreaticoduodenectomy with superior mesenterico-portal vein resection. J Gastrointest Surg 10(8):1106–1115.
120. Shibata C, 2001, Pancreatectomy combined with superior mesenteric–portal vein resection for adenocarcinoma in pancreas. World J Surg 25(8):1002–1005.
121. Tseng JF, 2004, Pancreaticoduodenectomy with vascular resection: margin status and survival duration. J Gastrointest Surg 8(8):935–949; discussion 949–950.
122. Birkmeyer JD, 2003, Surgeon volume and operative mortality in the United States. N Engl J Med 349(22):2117–2127.
123. Gouma DJ, 2000, Rates of complications and death after pancreaticoduodenectomy: risk factors and the impact of hospital volume. Ann Surg 232(6):786–795.
124. Lieberman MD, 1995, Relation of perioperative deaths to hospital volume among patients undergoing pancreatic resection for malignancy. Ann Surg 222(5):638–645.
125. Rosemurgy AS, 2001, Frequency with which surgeons undertake pancreaticoduodenectomy determines length of stay, hospital charges, and in–hospital mortality. J Gastrointest Surg 5(1):21–26.
126. Shan YS, Sy ED, Lin PY, 2003, Role of somatostatin in the prevention of pancreatic stump-related morbidity following elective pancreaticoduodenectomy in high-risk patients and elimination of surgeon-related factors: prospective, randomized, controlled trial. World J Surg 27(6):709–714.
127. Hesse UJ, 2005, Prospectively randomized trial using perioperative low-dose octreotide to prevent organ-related and general complications after pancreatic surgery and pancreaticojejunostomy. World J Surg 29(10):1325–1328.

Chapter 22
Controversies in the Surgical Management of Pancreatic Cancer

Curtis J. Wray and Syed A. Ahmad

1 Overview

Pancreatic ductal adenocarcinoma (PDA) remains the fourth most common cancer in the United States. The National Cancer Institute estimates 33,370 new cases of pancreatic cancer along with 32,300 deaths in the United States in 2006 (*1, 2*). The only hope for cure of PDA is surgical resection of localized disease. Over the past 20 years, significant advances in diagnostic imaging, staging, surgical technique, and perioperative care have led to a clear improvement in the surgical management of these patients (*3*). These advances have also led to decreased morbidity and mortality for patients following potentially curative surgery. Yet controversy remains for several aspects of the multimodality management and surgical care of patients diagnosed with PDA (*4, 5*). This chapter focuses on several topics that at this time remain controversial and are not universally accepted among pancreatic surgeons.

2 Introduction

The nearly equal rates of PDA incidence and mortality demonstrate the virulent nature of this malignancy. The incidence has continued to increase over the last several decades, making it the fourth leading cause of cancer death in the United States. Despite significant advances in the treatment of various solid tumors, a 5-year survival rate of <5% for patients diagnosed with PDA has remained unchanged for decades (*6*). This is due to the inherently aggressive biology of the disease and its late diagnosis in most cases. Unfortunately, although pancreatic cancer is biologically aggressive from the outset, it is most often clinically quiescent and remains so until its latter stages. Operative mortality rates for pancreaticoduodenectomy are now <5% at major centers and the mean length of hospital stay has been reduced to <14 days (*7*). Of those who do undergo potentially curative surgery, most patients eventually relapse and die of their disease. Despite these grim statistics, surgery remains the only hope to cure pancreatic cancer (Table 22.1). Advances in surgical technique, anesthesia, and perioperative care during the last two decades

A.M. Lowy et al. (eds.), *Pancreatic Cancer.*
doi: 10.1007/978-0-387-69252-4, © Springer Science+Business Media, LLC 2008

Table 22.1 Published survival following pancreaticoduodenectomy

Author (year)	*n*	Margin status	Survival
Tseng (2004) (*8*)	45	R1	21 Mos. median
Neoptolemos (2001) (*62*)	101	R1	11 Mos. median
Sohn (2000) (*63*)	184	R1/R2	12 mos. median
Nishimura (1997) (*64*)	70	R1/R2	6 Mos. median
Yeo (1995) (*65*)	58	R1/R2	10 Mos. median
Nitecki (1995) (*66*)	28	R2	Overall actuarial 5-yr survival 6.8%
Willett (1993) (*67*)	37	R1/R2	For R1 patients, median survival 12 mos. There were no survivors past 41 months

R0, microscopically complete resection; R1, positive margins by microscopy; R2, macroscopic tumor at surgical margins.

have significantly improved outcomes for patients undergoing pancreatic cancer surgery. Abundant literature has been devoted to examining technical aspects of pancreaticoduodenectomy, the most common operation for pancreatic cancer. In recent years, surgical investigators have explored more locally aggressive operations, including the use of vascular resection and extended lymphadenectomy, in order to improve patient outcome (*8*). This chapter discusses the current status of surgery for pancreatic cancer, highlighting important controversies and areas of active investigation.

3 Surgery for Pancreatic Cancer

3.1 Historical Considerations

The Italian surgeon Alessandro Codivilla attempted one of the first known one-stage pancreaticoduodenectomy in 1898. Postoperatively, the patient appeared to develop a pancreaticocutaneous fistula, unrelenting diarrhea, severe malnutrition, and eventual death 3 weeks after the operation (*9*). Once Emil Theodor Kocher, a Swiss surgeon, established his classic technique of a more extensive pancreaticoduodenal exposure (the Kocher maneuver) in 1903, several additional attempts were made at pancreatic resection. Walter Kausch initially described the technique of a two-stage pancreaticoduodenal resection in 1912. Two decades later (1935), Allen O. Whipple performed a two-stage pancreaticoduodenectomy, which consisted of biliary diversion and gastrojejunostomy during the initial operation followed by resection of the pancreatic head and duodenum up to 3 weeks later. In 1941, Whipple tailored the procedure to a one-stage pancreaticoduodenectomy with a simultaneous pancreaticojejunostomy (*10*). While major advances have been made in the surgical management of pancreas cancer since the era of Whipple, the principal goal remains the same: Removal of all gross and microscopic disease within the pancreas and draining lymph nodes, a so-called margin-negative or R0 resection.

3.2 Operative Anatomic Approach

The anatomic location of the tumor within the pancreas dictates the type of resection. A lesion confined to the pancreatic head or uncinate process requires pancreaticoduodenectomy (11). Given that 60-70% of pancreatic cancers arise in the head, pancreaticoduodenectomy is the most frequent operation performed for PDA (12). The majority patients with adenocarcinoma of the pancreatic body and tail present with locally advanced disease and/or distant metastases. The delayed presentation of symptoms often precludes surgical therapy. However, for patients with clinically localized disease, a distal pancreatectomy is the appropriate surgical resection. Central pancreatic tumors of the neck and body are rarely resectable, again due to either the presence of metastatic disease or extension to the superior mesenteric or hepatic artery. When resectable, tumors in this location are approached based on their precise anatomic location. If nearer to the head of the gland, an extended pancreaticoduodenectomy may be performed. This has the advantage of sparing pancreatic parenchyma and lessening the risk of postoperative diabetes. For lesions nearer the tail, a distal subtotal pancreatectomy is performed. Central pancreatectomy, which is now often used to resect premalignant and low-grade lesions of the neck and mid-body, has not been adopted for treatment of PDA by most surgeons over concerns regarding adequate lymph node and retroperitoneal soft tissue clearance (13).

3.3 Preoperative Biliary Drainage

In order to alleviate jaundice that accompanies distal biliary tract obstruction, biliary stents are often used in the preoperative setting. In the past, preoperative biliary drainage was almost universally performed due to fears about the morbidity of pancreaticoduodenectomy in the jaundiced patient. Randomized trials have shown these concerns to be unfounded and stenting is now used primarily to palliate symptoms of jaundice, such as pruritus or in the setting of neoadjuvant therapy where surgical resection is intentionally delayed (14–16). The question of whether preoperative stenting contributes to postoperative morbidity has been the subject of controversy in the surgical literature.

Povoski et al. reported the Memorial Sloan Kettering experience with preoperative biliary drainage in 240 consecutive patients undergoing a pancreaticoduodenectomy (17). In this series, 126 patients (53%) underwent preoperative biliary drainage (endoscopic stents, percutaneous drains/stents, or surgical drainage) and 117 were not stented (Table 22.2). The overall postoperative morbidity rate following pancreaticoduodenectomy was 48% (114/240). The most common morbidity was infectious complications, occurring in 34% (81/240) of patients. Among this subset of patients, intra-abdominal abscess occurred in 14% (33/240) of patients. The postoperative mortality rate was 5% (12/240). Preoperative biliary drainage was determined to be the only statistically significant variable associated with complications ($p = 0.025$), infectious complications ($p = 0.014$), intra-abdominal abscess ($p = 0.022$), and most

Table 22.2 Studies of preoperative biliary stenting in pancreatic cancer

Study	n	Percent with infectious complications	Percent with wound infections	Intra-abdominal abscess
Povoski et al. (*17*)	240			
Stented	126	52 (0.41)		24 (0.19)*
Unstented	114	29 (0.25)		9 (0.08)
Sohn et al. (*18*)	567			
Stented	408	131 (0.32)	40 (0.10)*	16 (0. 04)
Unstented	159	35 (0.22)	6 (0.04)	10 (0.06)
Hochwald et al. (*68*)	71			
Stented	42	28 (0.66)*	12 (0.29)	5 (0.12)
Unstented	29	11 (0.38)	4 (0.14)	4 (0.14)
Heslin et al. (*69*)	74			
Stented	39	18 (0.46)		
Unstented	35	4 (0.11)		
Pisters et al. (*19*)	265			
Stented	172	64 (0.37)	23 (0.13)	11 (0.06)
Unstented	93	29 (0.31)	4 (0.04)	10 (0.11)
Hodul et al. (*70*)	212			
Stented	154	43 (0.28)	12 (0.08)*	11 (0.07)
Unstented	58	12 (0.20)	0 (0.0)	3 (0.05)
Mullen et al. (*21*)	272			
No metal stent	243	28 (0.12)	13 (0.05)	9 (0.04)
Metal stent	29	3 (0.10)	2 (0.09)	0

importantly postoperative death ($p = 0.037$). The authors concluded that preoperative biliary drainage, but not preoperative biliary instrumentation alone, was associated with increased morbidity and mortality rates and suggested that preoperative biliary drainage should be avoided whenever possible in patients with potentially resectable pancreatic tumors. The implication of these results were interpreted by some to mean that patients who were symptomatic from their jaundice did not have time to be referred to a tertiary care center and, therefore, should be operated on right away. Because of this, much controversy was generated.

The next major report on this subject was issued by the Johns Hopkins group who evaluated 567 patients that underwent pancreatic resection without prior operative biliary bypass (*18*). Preoperative biliary stenting was performed in 408 patients (72%), whereas the remaining 159 patients (28%) did not undergo biliary stenting. In the stented group, 64% had stents placed via a percutaneous approach and 36% had stents placed endoscopically. Those who had stents placed were more likely to have jaundice (67% versus 38%; $p < 0001$) and fever (5% versus 1%; $p = 0.03$) as presenting symptoms. Patients who had stents placed had a perioperative mortality rate of 1.7% compared with 2.5% in those who did not ($p = 0.3$). Although the overall complication rates were 35% in those who had stents placed and 30% in those who did not ($p = NS$), patients with stents experienced a significantly increased incidence of pancreatic fistula (10% versus 4%; $p = 0.02$) and wound infection (10% versus 4%; $p = 0.02$). The incidence of other postoperative complications was similar between the groups. Eight patients (3%) in the percutaneous stent group developed hemobilia following stent placement, whereas none of the patients undergoing endoscopic stent placement developed hemobilia ($p = 0.03$).

Pisters et al. reviewed the MD Anderson experience in 300 consecutive patients that underwent pancreaticoduodenectomy (19). In this study, 172 had preoperative biliary stenting, 35 had surgical biliary bypass, and 93 did not receive preoperative stenting. In this study, there was no increase in the risk of major postoperative complications or death associated with preoperative stent placement. As demonstrated in other studies, the incidence of wound infection was significantly increased ($p = 0.022$) in the preoperative stent group (13% versus 4%).

Endobiliary metal stents have traditionally been used in those patients deemed unresectable. These metallic stents have been shown to have longer patency than silicone models with fewer episodes of blockage and subsequent biliary sepsis (20). Nonetheless, these metallic stents have been used with success in patients with resectable disease. Currently at MDACC the majority of patients undergoing neoadjuvant chemoradiation receive a metallic stent prior to the initiation of treatment. The MDACC experience was recently reported with encouraging results (21). The rates of perioperative morbidity, mortality, and stent complications in 272 consecutive patients who underwent pancreaticoduodenectomy were analyzed over a 3-year period. Of these 272 patients, 29 (11%) underwent pancreaticoduodenectomy after placement of a metal stent, 141 underwent pancreaticoduodenectomy after placement of a plastic stent, 10 had pancreaticoduodenectomy after biliary bypass without stenting, and 92 had pancreaticoduodenectomy without preoperative biliary decompression. There were no differences observed between the metal stent group and all other patients with regard to median operative time, intraoperative blood loss, or length of hospital stay. There were no perioperative deaths in the metal stent group versus 3 (1.2%) deaths in the other 243 patients. The frequency of major perioperative complications was similar between the two groups, including the rates of pancreatic fistula, intra-abdominal abscess, and wound infection. In addition, there were no statistical differences in the perioperative morbidity or mortality rates between patients who underwent preoperative biliary decompression with a stent of any kind (metal or plastic) and those patients who underwent no biliary decompression at all. Metal stent-related complications occurred in two (7%) of 29 patients during a median preoperative interval of 4.1 months; in contrast, 75 (45%) of the 166 patients who had had plastic stents experienced complications, including 98 stent occlusions, during a median preoperative interval of 3.9 months. The authors concluded that the use of expandable metal stents did not increase PD-associated perioperative morbidity or mortality, and as such an expandable metal stent is their preferred method of biliary decompression in patients with symptomatic malignant distal bile duct obstruction in whom surgery is not anticipated, or in whom there is a significant delay in the time to surgery.

Thus, it appears that stenting may increase the incidence of perioperative infection, likely secondary to bacterial contamination of bile (bactibilia) that results after instrumentation of the biliary tree. Preoperative biliary stenting is safe, but because of the previously mentioned risks, should probably be limited to patients receiving neoadjuvant therapy and those who are severely symptomatic but who will have some delay prior to operation.

3.4   Standard Pancreaticoduodenectomy versus Pylorus-Preserving Pancreaticoduodenectomy

Six decades ago, Watson reported a pancreaticoduodenectomy for ampullary carcinoma, in which the entire stomach and 1 inch of duodenum were preserved, restoring gastrointestinal continuity with a duodenojejunostomy (22). He hypothesized that preservation of the stomach would lead to better digestion, improved nutrition, and that a duodenojejunostomy would prevent marginal ulceration. The modern pylorus-preserving pancreaticoduodenectomy (PPPD) was popularized by Traverso and Longmire (23, 24). Since the reintroduction, concerns have been raised regarding the use of pylorus preservation for pancreatic head tumors with respect to nodal clearance of the suprapyloric and infrapyloric perigastric nodes.

In addition, retrospective series have raised the concern that following PPPD, the incidence of postoperative delayed gastric emptying (DGE) is increased (Table 22.3). One such randomized control trial compared standard pancreaticoduodenectomy ($n = 15$) to PPPD ($n = 16$) for patients with resectable periampullary carcinoma (25). Delayed gastric emptying (DGE) appeared to be more frequent in the PPPD group (6 of 16 patients), than the standard pancreaticoduodenectomy group (one in 15) ($p = 0.08$). Seiler et al. conducted a randomized trial for patients with resectable pancreatic cancer and periampullary tumors to standard pancreaticoduodenectomy ($n = 40$) and PPPD ($n = 37$) (26). The standard pancreaticoduodenectomy was associated with longer operative time; operative blood loss, surgical morbidity (including delayed gastric emptying, bleeding, fistulas, and infections) and mortality, and length of hospitalization were not significantly different between the two trial groups. Sixty-one patients (pancreaticoduodenectomy $n = 33$, PPPD $n = 28$) with histology confirmed pancreatic or periampullary adenocarcinomas were analyzed for long-term follow-up. There were no statistical differences in disease recurrence or overall survival at mean follow-up of 1.1 years. According to Kaplan-Meier analysis, median survival was 16 months for pancreaticoduodenectomy and 24 months for PPPD; however, these

Table 22.3 Selected results of studies comparing standard pancreaticoduodenectomy (PD) to PPPD

Study	Patients	Delayed gastric emptying
Lin et al. (25)	PD ($n = 15$)	1 (0.08)
	PPPD ($n = 16$)	6 (0.38)
Seiler et al. (26)	PD ($n = 40$)	18 (0.45)
	PPPD ($n = 37$)	12 (0.32)
Tran et al. (28)	PD ($n = 83$)	18 (0.23)
	PPPD ($n = 87$)	19 (0.22)

differences were not statistically significant ($p = 0.29$). Zerbi found no significant differences between patients who underwent pancreaticoduodenectomy ($n = 35$) versus PPPD ($n = 37$) for pancreatic cancer, with median survival of 15 months for pancreaticoduodenectomy and 17 months for PPPD (27).

Tran et al. recently reported the results of a prospective randomized multicenter trial ($n = 170$ patients) to assess standard pancreaticoduodenectomy versus PPPD for pancreatic and periampullary tumors (28). In this study, the groups were well matched for age and sex distribution, tumor location, and stage. The authors found no differences in median blood loss, duration of operation, or postoperative DGE between the two techniques. There was a marginal difference in postoperative weight loss, with less seen in the standard pancreaticoduodenectomy. Positive margins of resection were found for 12 patients of the pancreaticoduodenectomy group and 19 patients of the PPPD group ($p < 0.23$). Median disease-free survival was 14 months in the pancreaticoduodenectomy patients and 15 months in PPPD patients ($p = 0.80$). There were no significant statistical differences in overall survival between the two groups ($p < 0.90$). Therefore, the authors concluded that both operations are equally effective for the treatment of pancreatic and periampullary carcinoma.

Tani et al. published the results of a randomized, controlled trial to determine if an antecolic or a retrocolic duodenojejunostomy during PPPD was associated with a lower incidence of DGE (29). Forty patients were enrolled in this trial in which patients were randomly assigned to undergo either an antecolic or a retrocolic duodenojejunostomy. DGE occurred in 5% of patients with the antecolic route for duodenojejunostomy versus 50% with the retrocolic route ($p < 0.05$). The antecolic group had a significantly shorter duration of postoperative nasogastric tube drainage than did those in the retrocolic group (4.2 days versus 18.9 days, respectively, $p = 0.047$). Two weeks postoperation, all patients in the antecolic group were tolerating a regular diet, whereas in the retrocolic group only 55% of the patients could take solid foods ($p = 0.0007$). The length of stay in the hospital was significantly shorter for the antecolic group versus the retrocolic group. Antecolic reconstruction for duodenojejunostomy during PPPD decreases postoperative morbidity and length of hospital stay by decreasing DGE. The authors conclude that a PPPD with antecolic duodenojejunostomy is the safer operation.

Based upon existing retrospective and prospective reports, a standard pancreaticoduodenectomy and PPPD appear to have comparable perioperative morbidity and mortality and there appear to be no major differences in postoperative DGE or nutritional status. To date, no study has demonstrated a difference in recurrence or survival between the pancreaticoduodenectomy and PPPD. Thus, surgeon preference and experience should dictate the type of pancreatic resection and reconstruction.

3.5   Extended Lymphadenectomy

As for nearly all epithelial malignancies, the presence of nodal metastases is a significant prognostic factor in pancreatic cancer. In a standard pancreaticoduodenectomy, peripancreatic, duodenal and subpyloric nodes are generally removed. The high risk of locoregional recurrence following pancreaticoduodenectomy prompted the hypothesis that a more "extensive" lymphadenectomy may favorably impact recurrence and overall survival. These second-echelon nodes are generally removed as a separate specimen and are located along the proximal hepatic artery and/or other celiac axis vessels. One prospective, randomized multicenter trial compared standard ($n = 40$) to extended ($n = 41$) lymphadenectomy during pancreaticoduodenectomy for adenocarcinoma of the pancreatic head (*30*). Overall survival was 12 months for the standard and 15 months for the extended lymphadenectomy groups (Table 22.4). However, there was no significant difference between the two groups in the incidence of positive microscopic resection margins or the number of resected lymph nodes.

A trial from the Johns Hopkins Hospital randomized patients with resectable periampullary adenocarcinoma to a standard pancreaticoduodenectomy ($n = 56$) or pancreaticoduodenectomy with extended lymphadenectomy ($n = 58$) (*31*). In this study, there were a greater number of lymph nodes resected in the extended resection group (27 versus 16 nodes, $p < 0.001$). The 1-year survival for patients with pancreatic adenocarcinoma was 71% and 80% for the standard and radical resection arms , respectively. These findings prompted a larger trial which included 146 patients in the standard pancreaticoduodenectomy group and 148 patients in the extended pancreaticoduodenectomy group (*32*). In this study, extended lymphadenectomy was associated with a longer hospital stay, and an increased incidence of pancreatic fistula, delayed gastric emptying and postoperative complications ($p < 0.05$). In addition, extended pancreaticoduodenectomy was not associated with a survival benefit (median survival, 28 versus 30 months: 3-year survival, 38% versus 36%). These results suggest that extended pancreaticoduodenectomy is associated with an equivalent mortality, but higher morbidity rate. Of note, only one patient had a positive second-echelon lymph node that would not have been resected as part of standard pancreaticoduodenectomy, and no patients had positive second-echelon lymph node without having a positive first-echelon lymph node.

Yang et al. recently published a review that retrospectively analyzed the outcome following extended lymphadenectomy (*33*). Seventy-six patients underwent pancreaticoduodenectomy for adenocarcinoma of the pancreatic head ($n = 20$ standard pancreaticoduodenectomy, $n = 46$ extended pancreaticoduodenectomy). Of the 46 cases in the extended group, 26% had metastatic adenocarcinoma in the

Table 22.4 Selected results of studies comparing standard pancreaticoduodenectomy (PD) to pancreaticoduodenectomy with extended lymphadenectomy (ExPD)

Study	Patients	Results
Pedrazzoli et al. (*30*)	PD ($n = 40$) ExPD ($n = 41$)	Mean overall survival 12 months vs. 15 months ($p = 0.65$)
Yeo et al. (*31*)	PD ($n = 56$) ExPD ($n = 58$)	Median survival 30 months vs. 28 months ($p = 0.60$)
Capussotti et al. (*71*)	PD ($n = 112$) ExPD ($n = 37$)	Trend towards improved survival In first 2 yrs after ExPD

retroperitoneal lymph nodes. The 1-, 2-, and 3-year survival rates were 63%, 32%, and 21%, respectively, in the standard group, and 66%, 38%, and 21% in the radical group (p = NS). Subset analysis of node positive patients demonstrated 1-, 2-, and 3-year survival rates of 42%, 17%, and 8%, respectively, in the standard group, and 65%, 32%, and 16% in the radical group. Improved survival was observed in the first 2 years in the radical group, but no survival differences were seen after 2 years post operation. Study size may limit the authors' conclusions, in which extended lymphadenectomy was associated with an early survival advantage.

Currently there are no convincing data to suggest that an extended lymphadenectomy improves the rates of recurrence or survival. However, the actual feasibility of performing such a study was evaluated at MD Anderson Cancer Center. Pawlik et al. identified 158 patients who underwent pancreaticoduodenectomy for PDA with separate pathologic analysis of second-echelon lymph nodes, defined as lymph nodes along the proximal hepatic artery and/or the great vessels (34). In this study, to estimate the sample size necessary for a randomized trial, a biostatistical model was devised with the following assumptions: extended lymphadenectomy can benefit only patients who: (1) actually have disease removed from second-echelon nodes, (2) have microscopically negative (R0) primary tumor resection margins , and (3) do not have visceral metastatic (M0) disease. Seventy-six patients (48.1%) had negative first- and second-echelon lymph nodes, 65 (41.1%) had positive first-echelon and negative second-echelon lymph nodes, and 17 (10.8%) had positive first- and second-echelon lymph nodes. Patients with positive second-echelon lymph nodes had an R0 resection rate of 47.1%. At a median follow-up of 65.1 months, four patients with positive second-echelon lymph nodes were alive; however, three had recurrent disease. This would imply that only one patient (5.9%) with a positive second-echelon lymph node may have had true M0 disease. As a result, only 0.3% of patients (10.8% with positive second-echelon lymph nodes × 47.1% with R0 resection × 5.9% with M0 disease) may achieve a survival benefit from extended lymphadenectomy. A randomized trial of standard pancreaticoduodenectomy versus pancreaticoduodenectomy with extended lymphadenectomy would require 202,000 patients in each study arm to detect such a small difference. Thus, definitive evaluation of the potential benefits of extended lymphadenectomy would require a prohibitively large sample size.

3.6 Pancreatic Anastomotic Technique

In the preoperative setting, it is imperative that high-quality thin-section CT scanning be used to accurately define the relation of the tumor to the SMV and SMA to detect aberrant anatomy and avoid circumstances of pancreatic division, gastroduodenal artery ligation, and subsequent identification of unresectability (35). The pancreaticoduodenectomy procedure may be divided into several well-defined steps, as described by Tyler and Evans (36). Once the gastrocolic ligament is opened, the transverse and right colon is mobilized, and the duodenum is exposed.

At this point, the infra-pancreatic SMV is exposed by dissection down to the middle colic and gastroepiploic vessels. Following an extended Kocher maneuver, the duodenum is mobilized to expose the left renal vein and aorta. In the next step, the gallbladder is removed, and the common bile duct and the gastroduodenal artery are divided, thus exposing the suprapancreatic PV. Next, the stomach is divided (the duodenum, in cases of pylorus preservation), followed by division and dissection of the proximal jejunum/distal duodenum. The next step involves division of the pancreatic neck over the SMV/PV confluence. The last and most critical step in the extirpation is dissection of the pancreatic head and uncinate process from their attachments to the SMV and artery. The SMA defines the limits of retroperitoneal dissection. Thus, if tumor extends to the SMA or the surgeon does not extend the dissection to this level, a positive margin will result.

The gastrointestinal reconstruction begins with a pancreaticojejunostomy or pancreaticogastrostomy and followed by a choledochojejunostomy and gastrojejunostomy or duodenojejunostomy. A retrocolic pancreatico-jejunal anastomosis is the first step of a standard reconstruction (11). The proximal jejunum is advanced through a mesenteric defect created to the left of the middle colic vessels and a two-layer end-to-side duct-to-mucosa anastomosis is constructed starting approximately 6-8 cm distal to the jejunal staple line. The posterior wall is created by a modified mattress technique using 3-0 Vicryl or silk sutures that are passed full-thickness through the pancreatic parenchyma from anterior to posterior, horizontally through the seromuscular layers of the jejunum, and then back full-thickness through the pancreas from posterior to anterior. Three to four such sutures are placed, being careful to avoid the main pancreatic duct. A duct-to-mucosa anastomosis is fashioned using 6-0 double-armed polydioxanone surgical suture (PDS) placed in a horizontal mattress fashion. The sutures are placed so that knots will be on the outside for the anterior row and inside for the posterior row, which facilitates tying these knots securely. The anastomosis is completed with an anterior row of simple 3-0 Vicryl sutures.

Another common technique of pancreatico-jejunal anastomosis involves a single-layer continuous suture. This technique is often advocated when the main pancreatic duct is small, which may increase the difficulty of performing a duct-to-mucosa anastomosis. In this technique, several interrupted posterior sutures are placed (seromuscular jejunum and pancreatic pseudocapsule). These posterior wall sutures are meant to anchor the jejunum in place. A jejunal enterotomy (2-3 cm) is made with the electrocautery. The edge of the cut pancreatic surface is then sutured in a running, continuous fashion to the jejunal enterotomy. Conceptually, this technique "dunks" the pancreatic edge into the lumen of the jejunum. This technique should be used judiciously in patients with a soft, normal pancreas, as the parenchyma may not securely fix the running suture.

Instead of a standard pancreaticojejunostomy, some surgeons prefer a pancreaticogastrostomy. The technique is performed in much the same manner as a pancreaticojejunostomy, a two-layer duct-to-mucosa anastomosis. Proponents of this technique argue that there is improved exocrine function of the remnant pancreas (37). Data from other institutions suggest that the leak rate following pancreaticogastrostomy is lower than that of pancreaticojejunostomy (*38, 39*). It is possible that gastrointestinal physiology may play a role in the observed lower leak rate following a gastric anastomosis. The advantage of a standard pancreatico-jejunostomy is that exocrine enzymes are activated and absorption is theoretically more normal, whereas after a gastric anastomosis, pancreatic enzymes are not activated, which may result in delayed digestion and absorption. In addition, if there is a leak following a pancreaticogastrostomy, it is postulated that morbidity is lower since the enzymes might not be fully functional (*40*).

A single technique of pancreaticojejunostomy cannot be universally recommended for all patients. Surgeon experience should dictate which type of anastomosis is performed. Currently, there are no data to suggest that one anastomotic technique is better or has a lower leak rate than the other.

3.7 Anastomotic Leak and the Use of Octreotide

A wealth of surgical literature has been devoted to various technical aspects of pancreaticoduodenectomy. Before the 1980s mortality rates of >20% were common and morbidity rates were even higher (*41*). The most frequent source of major morbidity following pancreaticoduodenectomy is leakage at the site of pancreatic anastomosis, most commonly resulting in a peripancreatic fluid collection, abscess, and/or the development of pancreatic fistula. Countless methods have been described to reduce leak rates, including descriptions of various anastomotic techniques, the use of pancreatic duct internal and internal/external stents, and fibrin glue (*42–45*). What is clear from the literature is that numerous techniques may be associated with low rates of leak, and that the occurrence of leak reliably relates to several predominant factors. The texture of the pancreas and size of the pancreatic duct appear to be major risk factors for leak (*46*). A small pancreatic duct and soft pancreatic texture are consistently associated with higher leak rates, presumably because smaller ducts make the anastomosis inherently more technically challenging, and because a soft, more "normal" pancreas cannot hold sutures as well. It is also likely that a more "normal" pancreas has a higher output of pancreatic enzymes. There have been conflicting reports regarding the perioperative use of the somatostatin analogue, octreotide as a means of decreasing pancreatic exocrine secretion, and leak following pancreaticoduodenectomy.

Numerous prospective randomized trials have now examined the use of somatostatin analogues to prevent pancreatic leak following pancreatectomy. Several studies from Europe demonstrated decreased pancreatic fistula rates associated with the use of octreotide. These studies varied somewhat in that some found a decreased incidence of fistula in all patients, whereas others found an effect only in patients with benign disease or only in those undergoing distal pancreatectomy (*47–52*). Two randomized trials from the United States examined the role of octreotide in decreasing the pancreatic fistula rate following pancreaticoduodenectomy. An MD Anderson Cancer Center study by Lowy et al. found no decrease in the pancreatic

leak rates among those patients receiving octreotide after pancreaticoduodenectomy for malignancy (*53*). Yeo and colleagues from Johns Hopkins similarly found
no benefit to the use of octreotide given following pancreaticoduodenectomy (*54*,
55). Another recent study from Saar et al. examined the use of vapreotide, a long-
acting somatostatin analogue in the setting of pancreatectomy (*56*). The authors
found no benefit to vapreotide in reducing pancreas-related leaks or other complications. The most recent study by Suc et al. examined the use of octreotide to
prevent intra-abdominal complications following pancreatectomy (*57*). The authors
found that overall octreotide did not reduce the risk of complications. Of the studies
that have examined the use of somatostatin analogues for the prevention of pancre-
atic-associated complications in the setting of surgery for pancreatic neoplasms,
none have demonstrated a benefit. Each of the European studies that did show some
benefit to octreotide included patients undergoing surgery for chronic pancreatitis.
Since these patients were not stratified for chronic pancreatitis or texture, it remains
unclear if a subset of patients benefit from routine use of octreotide. Thus, on the
basis of available data, there is no clear evidence to recommend the routine use of
octreotide following pancreatectomy for pancreatic cancer.

3.8   Palliative Surgery

A vital principle to pancreatic cancer surgery is that operations should be performed with curative intent only. The use of laparotomy and gastric and biliary
bypass as a routine palliative measure is no longer justified in most pancreatic cancer patients. The ability to palliate patients with endoscopic stenting combined with
the extremely limited survival of patients with advanced pancreatic cancer has
made most palliative surgery obsolete and not in the patients' best interests.
Endoscopic stenting has been shown to be cost-effective and provides equivalent
survival to surgical bypass (*58*). Laparotomy for palliation carries a mortality rate
of 2-5%, a morbidity rate of 20-30%, and a median hospital stay of >10 days in
most series (*59*, *60*). Combined with recovery time from surgery, patients spend a
significant proportion of their remaining life getting over the effects of a palliative
procedure. It can be argued that patients with a good performance status and limited
locally advanced disease whose life expectancy may exceed 1 year are good candidates for palliative operation. Unfortunately, predicting life expectancy is difficult
at best. At the MD Anderson Cancer Center, the current practice is to perform
endoscopic stenting in patients who are not candidates for curative surgery. If
patients cannot be stented internally or they develop stent-related complications
that limit treatment, they are referred for operative bypass. A prospective randomized study by Lillemoe et al. demonstrated that 20% of patients undergoing palliative biliary bypass later require gastric decompression (*61*). Based on these data
and the fact that gastrojejunostomy adds little in the way of morbidity, it is our policy to perform routine gastrojejunostomy along with a Roux-en-y choledochojejunostomy as our preferred palliative operation for pancreatic cancer patients.

4 Summary

Pancreatic cancer remains a lethal disease with overall poor outcome following "curative" surgery. Despite this, surgical resection offers the only possibility of long-term cure. The morbidity and mortality associated with pancreatic surgery has declined significantly in the last two decades. Advances in diagnostic imaging and laparoscopy have contributed to limiting the number of pancreatic cancer patients subjected to nontherapeutic laparotomy. Advances in surgical technique and after-care have made the design and completion of large randomized trials of adjuvant therapy possible in recent years. This is a critical development as it is clear that significant improvements in survival for pancreatic cancer patients await the development and testing of more effective multimodality therapies.

References

1. Petersen GM, Andrade M, de Goggins M. 2006, Pancreatic cancer genetic epidemiology consortium. Cancer Epidemiol Biomarkers Prev 15:704–710.
2. Lowenfels AB, Maisonneuve P. 2006, Epidemiology and risk factors for pancreatic cancer. Best Pract Res Clin Gastroenterol 20:197–209.
3. Lowy AM. 2005, Does size matter most? Reassessing clinical staging for pancreatic cancer. Ann Surg Oncol 12:100–101.
4. Lowy AM. 2004, From bad to worse: prognostic factors in pancreatic cancer. Ann Surg Oncol 11:117–118.
5. Lowy AM. 2006, Putting the chemo in chemoradiation for pancreatic cancer. Ann Surg Oncol 13:135–136.
6. Stojadinovic A, Hoos A, Brennan MF, 2002, Randomized clinical trials in pancreatic cancer. Surg Oncol Clin North Am 11:207–229.
7. Alexakis N, Halloran C, Raraty M, 2004, Current standards of surgery for pancreatic cancer. Br J Surg 91:1410–1427.
8. Tseng JF, Raut CP, Lee JE, 2004, Pancreaticoduodenectomy with vascular resection: margin status and survival duration. J Gastrointest Surg 8:935–949, discussion 949–950.
9. McClusky DA 3rdSkandalakis LJ, Colborn GL, 2002, Harbinger or hermit? Pancreatic anatomy and surgery through the ages—part 2. World J Surg 26:1370–1381.
10. Whipple AO. 1949, An evaluation of radical surgery for carcinoma of the pancreas and ampullary region. Ann Intern Med 31:624–627.
11. Ahmad SA, Lowy AM, McIntyre BC, 2005, Pancreaticoduodenectomy. J Gastrointest Surg 9:138–143.
12. Kalser MH, Barkin J, MacIntyre JM. 1985, Pancreatic cancer. Assessment of prognosis by clinical presentation. Cancer 56:397–402.
13. Warshaw AL, Rattner DW, Fernandez-del Castillo C, 1998, Middle segment pancreatectomy: a novel technique for conserving pancreatic tissue. Arch Surg 133:327–331.
14. Kozarek R, Hovde O, Attia F, 2003, Do pancreatic duct stents cause or prevent pancreatic sepsis? Gastrointest Endosc 58:505–509.
15. Sewnath ME, Birjmohun RS, Rauws EA, 2001, The effect of preoperative biliary drainage on postoperative complications after pancreaticoduodenectomy. J Am Coll Surg 192:726–734.
16. Sewnath ME, Karsten TM, Prins MH, 2002, A meta-analysis on the efficacy of preoperative biliary drainage for tumors causing obstructive jaundice. Ann Surg 236:17–27.

17. Povoski SP, Karpeh MS JrConlon KC, 1999, Association of preoperative biliary drainage with postoperative outcome following pancreaticoduodenectomy. Ann Surg 230:131–142.
18. Sohn TA, Yeo CJ, Cameron JL, 2000, Do preoperative biliary stents increase postpancreaticoduodenectomy complications? J Gastrointest Surg 4:258–267, discussion 267–268.
19. Pisters PW, Hudec WA, Hess KR, 2001, Effect of preoperative biliary decompression on pancreaticoduodenectomy-associated morbidity in 300 consecutive patients. Ann Surg 234:47–55.
20. Maire F, Hammel P, Ponsot P, 2006, Long-term outcome of biliary and duodenal stents in palliative treatment of patients with unresectable adenocarcinoma of the head of pancreas. Am J Gastroenterol 101:735–742.
21. Mullen JT, Lee JH, Gomez HF, 2005, Pancreaticoduodenectomy after placement of endobiliary metal stents. J Gastrointest Surg 9:1094–1104, discussion 1104–1105.
22. McClusky DA 3rdSkandalakis LJ, Colborn GL, 2002, Harbinger or hermit? Pancreatic anatomy and surgery through the ages—part 3. World J Surg 26:1512–1524.
23. Traverso LW, Longmire WP Jr.1978, Preservation of the pylorus in pancreaticoduodenectomy. Surg Gynecol Obstet 146:959–962.
24. Traverso LW, Longmire WP Jr.1980, Preservation of the pylorus in pancreaticoduodenectomy: a follow-up evaluation. Ann Surg 192:306–310.
25. Lin PW, Lin YJ. 1999, Prospective randomized comparison between pylorus-preserving and standard pancreaticoduodenectomy. Br J Surg 86:603–607.
26. Seiler CA, Wagner M, Sadowski C, 2000, Randomized prospective trial of pylorus-preserving versus Classic duodenopancreatectomy (Whipple procedure): initial clinical results. J Gastrointest Surg 4:443–452.
27. Zerbi A, Balzano G, Patuzzo R, 1995, Comparison between pylorus-preserving and Whipple pancreatoduodenectomy. Br J Surg 82:975–979.
28. Tran KT, Smeenk HG, Eijck CH, van 2004, Pylorus preserving pancreaticoduodenectomy versus standard Whipple procedure: a prospective, randomized, multicenter analysis of 170 patients with pancreatic and periampullary tumors. Ann Surg 240:738–745.
29. Tani M, Terasawa H, Kawai M, 2006, Improvement of delayed gastric emptying in pylorus-preserving pancreaticoduodenectomy: results of a prospective, randomized, controlled trial. Ann Surg 243:316–320.
30. Pedrazzoli S, DiCarlo V, Dionigi R, 1998, Standard versus extended lymphadenectomy associated with pancreatoduodenectomy in the surgical treatment of adenocarcinoma of the head of the pancreas: a multicenter, prospective, randomized study. Lymphadenectomy Study Group. Ann Surg 228:508–517.
31. Yeo CJ, Cameron JL, Sohn TA, 1999, Pancreaticoduodenectomy with or without extended retroperitoneal lymphadenectomy for periampullary adenocarcinoma: comparison of morbidity and mortality and short-term outcome. Ann Surg 229:613–622, discussion 622–624.
32. Yeo CJ, Cameron JL, Lillemoe KD, 2002, Pancreaticoduodenectomy with or without distal gastrectomy and extended retroperitoneal lymphadenectomy for periampullary adenocarcinoma, part 2: randomized controlled trial evaluating survival, morbidity, and mortality. Ann Surg 236:355–366, discussion 366–368.
33. Yang YM, Wan YL, Tian XD, 2005, Outcome of pancreaticoduodenectomy with extended retroperitoneal lymphadenectomy for adenocarcinoma of the head of the pancreas. Chin Med J (Engl) 118:1863–1869.
34. Pawlik TM, Abdalla EK, Barnett CC, 2005, Feasibility of a randomized trial of extended lymphadenectomy for pancreatic cancer. Arch Surg 140:584–589, discussion 589–591.
35. Hough TJ, Raptopoulos V, Siewert B, 1999, Teardrop superior mesenteric vein: CT sign for unresectable carcinoma of the pancreas. AJR Am J Roentgenol 173:1509–1512 .
36. Tyler DS, Evans DB. 1994, Reoperative pancreaticoduodenectomy. Ann Surg 219: 211–221.
37. Rault A, SaCunha A, Klopfenstein D, 2005, Pancreaticojejunal anastomosis is preferable to pancreaticogastrostomy after pancreaticoduodenectomy for long-term outcomes of pancreatic exocrine function. J Am Coll Surg 201:239–244.

38. Aranha GV, Hodul PJ, Creech S, 2003, Zero mortality after 152 consecutive pancreaticoduo-denectomies with pancreaticogastrostomy. J Am Coll Surg 197:223–231, discussion 231–232.
39. Takano S, Ito Y, Watanabe Y, 2000, Pancreaticojejunostomy versus pancreaticogastrostomy in reconstruction following pancreaticoduodenectomy. Br J Surg 87:423–427.
40. Takano S, Ito Y, Oishi H, 2000, A retrospective analysis of 88 patients with pancreaticogas-trostomy after pancreaticoduodenectomy. Hepatogastroenterology 47:1454–1457.
41. Crist DW, Sitzmann JV, Cameron JL. 1987, Improved hospital morbidity, mortality, and sur-vival after the Whipple procedure. Ann Surg 206:358–365.
42. Kurosaki I, Hatakeyama K. 2004, Omental wrapping of skeletonized major vessels after pan-creaticoduodenectomy. Int Surg 89:90–94.
43. Muftuoglu MA, Saglam A. 2003, A novel reconstructive procedure after pancreaticoduo-denectomy: J-pouch dunking pancreaticojejunostomy. Hepatogastroenterology 50:2233–2235.
44. Ohwada S, Tanahashi Y, Ogawa T, 2002, In situ vs ex situ pancreatic duct stents of duct-to-mucosa pancreaticojejunostomy after pancreaticoduodenectomy with billroth I-type recon-struction. Arch Surg 137:1289–1293.
45. Lillemoe KD, Cameron JL, Kim MP, 2004, Does fibrin glue sealant decrease the rate of pan-creatic fistula after pancreaticoduodenectomy? Results of a prospective randomized trial. J Gastrointest Surg 8:766–774.
46. Yang YM, Tian XD, Zhuang Y, 2005, Risk factors of pancreatic leakage after pancreaticoduo-denectomy. World J Gastroenterol 11:2456–2461.
47. Buchler M, Friess H, Klempa I, 1992, Role of octreotide in the prevention of postoperative complications following pancreatic resection. Am J Surg 163:125–130, discussion 130–131.
48. Friess H, Beger HG, Sulkowski U, 1995, Randomized controlled multicentre study of the prevention of complications by octreotide in patients undergoing surgery for chronic pancrea-titis. Br J Surg 82:1270–1273.
49. Montorsi M, Zago M, Mosca F, 1995, Efficacy of octreotide in the prevention of pancreatic fistula after elective pancreatic resections: a prospective, controlled, randomized clinical trial. Surgery 117:26–31.
50. Bassi C, Falconi M, Lombardi D, 1994, Prophylaxis of complications after pancreatic surgery: results of a multicenter trial in Italy. Italian Study Group. Digestion 55 Suppl 1:41–47.
51. Presti ME, Burton FR, Niehoff ML, 1998, Effect of octreotide on stimulated insulin release from pancreatic tissue slices. Pancreas 16:141–147.
52. Hesse UJ, DeDecker C, Houtmeyers P, 2005, Prospectively randomized trial using periopera-tive low-dose octreotide to prevent organ-related and general complications after pancreatic surgery and pancreatico-jejunostomy. World J Surg 29:1325–1328.
53. Lowy AM, Lee JE, Pisters PW, 1997, Prospective, randomized trial of octreotide to prevent pancreatic fistula after pancreaticoduodenectomy for malignant disease. Ann Surg 226:632–641.
54. Yeo CJ, Cameron JL, Lillemoe KD, 2000, Does prophylactic octreotide decrease the rates of pancreatic fistula and other complications after pancreaticoduodenectomy? Results of a pro-spective randomized placebo-controlled trial. Ann Surg 232:419–429.
55. Yeo CJ. 1999, Does prophylactic octreotide benefit patients undergoing elective pancreatic resection? J Gastrointest Surg 3:223–224.
56. Sarr MG. 2003, The potent somatostatin analogue vapreotide does not decrease pancreas-specific complications after elective pancreatectomy: a prospective, multicenter, double-blinded, randomized, placebo-controlled trial. J Am Coll Surg 196:556–564, discussion 564–565, author reply 565.
57. Suc B, Msika S, Piccinini M, 2004, Octreotide in the prevention of intra-abdominal complica-tions following elective pancreatic resection: a prospective, multicenter randomized control-led trial. Arch Surg 139:288–294, discussion 295.
58. Profili S, Feo CF, Meloni GB, 2003, Combined biliary and duodenal stenting for palliation of pancreatic cancer. Scand J Gastroenterol 38:1099–1102.

59. Andtbacka RH, Evans DB, Pisters PW. 2004, Surgical and endoscopic palliation for pancreatic cancer. Minerva Chir 59:123–136.
60. Deziel DJ, Wilhelmi B, Staren ED, 1996, Surgical palliation for ductal adenocarcinoma of the pancreas. Am Surg 62:582–588.
61. Lillemoe KD, Cameron JL, Hardacre JM, 1999, Is prophylactic gastrojejunostomy indicated for unresectable periampullary cancer? A prospective randomized trial. Ann Surg 230:322–328, discussion 328–330.
62. Neoptolemos JP, Stocken DD, Dunn JA, 2001, Influence of resection margins on survival for patients with pancreatic cancer treated by adjuvant chemoradiation and/or chemotherapy in the ESPAC-1 randomized controlled trial. Ann Surg 234:758–768.
63. Sohn TA, Yeo CJ, Cameron JL, 2000, Resected adenocarcinoma of the pancreas—616 patients: results, outcomes, and prognostic indicators. J Gastrointest Surg 4:567–579.
64. Nishimura Y, Hosotani R, Shibamoto Y, 1997, External and intraoperative radiotherapy for resectable and unresectable pancreatic cancer: analysis of survival rates and complications. Int J Radiat Oncol Biol Phys 39:39–49.
65. Yeo CJ, Cameron JL, Lillemoe KD, 1995, Pancreaticoduodenectomy for cancer of the head of the pancreas 201 patients. Ann Surg 221:721–731, discussion 731–733.
66. Nitecki SS, Sarr MG, Colby TV, 1995, Long-term survival after resection for ductal adenocarcinoma of the pancreas. Is it really improving? Ann Surg 221:59–66.
67. Willett CG, Lewandrowski K, Warshaw AL, 1993, Resection margins in carcinoma of the head of the pancreas. Implications for radiation therapy. Ann Surg 217:144–148.
68. Hochwald SN, Burke EC, Jarnagin WR, 1999, Association of preoperative biliary stenting with increased postoperative infectious complications in proximal cholangiocarcinoma. Arch Surg 134:261–266.
69. Heslin MJ, Brooks AD, Hochwald SN, 1998, A preoperative biliary stent is associated with increased complications after pancreatoduodenectomy. Arch Surg 133:149–154.
70. Hodul P, Creech S, Pickleman J, 2003, The effect of preoperative biliary stenting on postoperative complications after pancreaticoduodenectomy. Am J Surg 186:420–425.
71. Capussotti L, Massucco P, Ribero D, 2003, Extended lymphadenectomy and vein resection for pancreatic head cancer: outcomes and implications for therapy. Arch Surg 138:1316–1322.

Chapter 23
Laparoscopic Pancreatic Resections

Attila Nakeeb

1 Introduction

Laparoscopic surgery has become the gold standard for the management of gallstones, gastroesophageal reflux disease, and achalasia. It is also the preferred approach for most adrenal and splenic pathology. Laparoscopic colectomy is being offered to an increasing number of patients with both benign and malignant diseases. In the past 15 years significant advances have been made in the application of minimally invasive techniques to the management of pancreatic disorders. However, the utility and indications for laparoscopic pancreatic resection is still under active evaluation and the technical aspects of these procedures remain in evolution.

Initially, laparoscopic pancreatic surgery was limited to diagnostic staging in patients with pancreatic cancer prior to resection. With recent advancements in laparoscopic instrumentation, an increasing number of surgeons are applying minimally invasive techniques to manage both inflammatory and neoplastic disorders of the pancreas. Currently, select patients with necrotizing pancreatitis and pancreatic pseudocysts can be managed with minimally invasive techniques. In addition, laparoscopic techniques to resect both benign and malignant lesions of the pancreas have been described (*1*).

Laparoscopic staging of pancreatic cancer was initially described in 1911 by Dr. Bertram M. Bernheim (*2*) and was reintroduced by Cuscheri and colleagues in 1978 (*3*). The first laparoscopic pancreatic resection was reported by Gagner and Pomp in 1994 (*4*). In recent years, laparoscopic pancreaticoduodenectomies (PD), enucleations (En), and distal pancreatectomies (DP) have all been described in the surgical literature.

2 Indications for Laparoscopic Pancreatic Resections

Potential advantages of laparoscopic surgery include decreased postoperative pain, decreased ileus, preserved immune function, decreased complication rates, shorter hospital stay, and a quicker return to preoperative activity levels. While there have been no randomized prospective trials comparing laparoscopic to open pancreatic

A.M. Lowy et al. (eds.) *Pancreatic Cancer*.
doi: 10.1007/978-0-387-69252-4, © Springer Science+Business Media, LLC 2008

resections in humans, there is evidence from animal studies that laparoscopic pancreatectomy is associated with a decreased stress response and a faster return of gastrointestinal function (5).

Laparoscopic pancreatic resections are complicated procedures and should be undertaken by surgeons with advanced laparoscopic skill sets. Surgeons should be comfortable with intracorporeal suturing, the use of endomechanical staplers, the use of laparoscopic ultrasound, and possess the ability to control intraoperative bleeding. In addition, surgeons should have experience with open pancreatic surgery in case the procedure must be converted to an open pancreatic resection.

Factors important in selecting appropriate patients for laparoscopic resections include the size of the lesion, location of the lesion within the pancreas, involvement of surrounding structures, and the suspected pathology of the lesion.

Conditions that are potentially amenable to a laparoscopic pancreatic resection include benign or premalignant cystic neoplasms, neuroendocrine (islet cell) tumors of the pancreas, chronic pancreatitis with symptomatic ductal obstruction, and pancreatic pseudocysts localized to the distal body and tail of the pancreas (Table 23.1). While there have been a small number of patients with malignant pancreatic tumors that have been resected laparoscopically, it is unclear if a laparoscopic pancreatic resection should be attempted in patients with malignant neoplasms of the pancreas.

Cystic neoplasms of the pancreas that are potentially amenable to laparoscopic pancreatic resections include serous cyst adenomas (SCA), mucinous cystic neoplasms (MCN), and benign intraductal papillary mucinous neoplasms (IPMNs) (6). Serous cystadenomas are benign tumors of the pancreas with a 3:1 female predominance. They have a characteristic microcystic appearance on imaging, often resembling a honeycomb and can have a star burst pattern with a centrally located calcified scar. The majority of patients are asymptomatic and they tend to present with large lesions. Surgical treatment is indicated in symptomatic patients (vague abdominal pain likely related to the mass effect of the cyst) or large tumors (>4 cm) in asymptomatic patients who are acceptable operative candidates (7).

Mucinous cystic neoplasms occur predominantly in the body and tail of the pancreas, have a 2:1 female: male ratio, occur in a younger age group (40–50 years), do not communicate with the pancreatic duct, and microscopically are associated with an

Table 23.1 Indications for laparoscopic pancreatic resection

Solid pancreatic tumors
Functional neuroendocrine tumors
Nonfunctional neuroendocrine tumors
Adenocarcinoma
Cystic pancreatic tumors
Congenital cysts
Serous cystadenoma (SCA)
Mucinous cystadenoma (MCN)
Intraductal papillary mucinous neoplasms (IPMN)
Chronic pancreatitis
Symptomatic ductal obstruction
Persistent pancreatic pseudocyst

ovarian type stroma. Conversely, IPMNs occur more commonly in the head and uncinate process, have a slight male predominance, occur in an older age group (60–80 years), communicate with the pancreatic duct, and do not have an ovarian-like stroma. MCNs and IPMNs have malignant potential; therefore, resection of these lesions is recommended (6).

Neuroendocrine tumors (NETs) of the pancreas may be functional (associated with a clinical syndrome related to hormones secreted by the tumor) or nonfunctional lacking symptoms or hormone production by the tumor). Insulinomas are the most common NET of the pancreas. These tumors secrete insulin, resulting in hypoglycemic symptoms. The vast majority of insulinomas are benign, making them ideally suited for laparoscopic enucleation.

Patients with chronic pancreatitis and isolated strictures of the pancreatic duct limited to the distal body and tail of the pancreas may also be treated with laparoscopic distal pancreatectomy. There is often a dense inflammatory reaction involving the peripancreatic tissues and the splenic vessels in these patients, making a splenectomy more likely.

2.1 Preoperative Evaluation

Currently, helical CT is the preferred noninvasive imaging test for pancreatic diseases (Fig. 23.1). Helical CT can delineate the anatomy of the pancreas and the surrounding organs in considerable detail, and it can easily define pancreatic calcifications, inflammation, necrosis, and masses. A triple-phase intravenous contrast

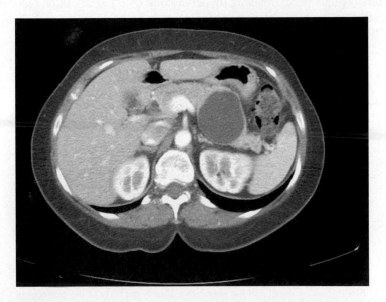

Fig. 23.1 Helical CT scan showing a mucinous cystadenoma of the body of the pancreas

study is ideal for the assessment of pancreatic lesions. Thin cuts are obtained through the pancreas and liver during both the arterial phase and the venous phase after the injection of IV contrast material. Besides being used to determine the primary tumor size, CT is used to look for and evaluate invasion into local structures or metastatic disease. Magnetic resonance imaging (MRI) scanning provides similar information as CT. The addition of magnetic resonance cholangiopancreatography (MRCP) can be quite useful for defining the anatomy and pathology of the bile ducts and pancreatic duct noninvasively.

Endoscopic retrograde cholangiopancreatography (ERCP) allows direct imaging of the pancreatic and bile ducts and is the gold standard for diagnosing chronic pancreatitis. The presence of a long, irregular stricture in an otherwise normal pancreatic duct is highly suggestive of a pancreatic malignancy. The identification of mucin in the pancreatic duct or the communication of a cystic lesion with the pancreatic duct suggests the presence of an IPMN (Fig. 23.2).

Endoscopic ultrasonography (EUS) has begun to play an important role in the evaluation of pancreatic diseases. EUS can diagnose the most common causes of extrahepatic biliary obstruction (e.g., choledocholithiasis and pancreaticobiliary malignancies) with a degree of accuracy equaling or exceeding that of direct cholangiography or ERCP, and is the most sensitive modality for the diagnosis of pancreatic carcinoma. EUS can be combined with fine-needle aspiration biopsy of lesions to obtain a tissue diagnosis. The aspiration of cyst fluid and determination of cyst CEA and mucin levels can help differentiate serous from mucinous cysts (8).

Serum tumor markers, including CEA and CA19–9, are usually measured in patients with both solid and cystic tumors. If a neuroendocrine tumor is suspected by history (symptomatic), imaging (hypervascular on CT scan), or on preoperative biopsy, then serum levels of chromogranins A, insulin, proinsulin, glucagon, gastrin, VIP, or pancreatic peptide (PP) can be measured.

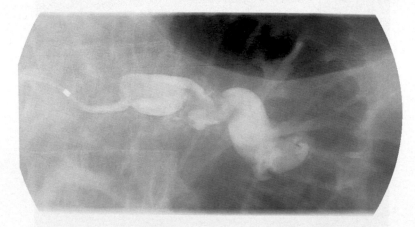

Fig. 23.2 ERCP showing dilation of the pancreatic duct in the body of the pancreas in a patient with IPMN

3   Patient Preparation

Every patient considered for a pancreatic resection needs a full evaluation of cardiac, pulmonary, and renal function. A full array of laboratory tests must be obtained, including a complete blood count, renal panel, and liver panel. A nutritional assessment needs to be made to make sure that the patient can undergo surgery safely, if the patient has severe weight loss or has an albumin of <3 g/dl, strong consideration for supplemental nutrition is indicated.

Patients undergoing distal pancreatectomy or enucleation of lesions in the body or tail of the pancreas should receive vaccinations against encapsulated organisms in case a splenectomy is required. These include *Streptococcus pneumoniae,* *Neisseria meningitidis,* and *Haemophilus influenzae* vaccines. The vaccines should be administered at least 1–2 weeks prior to the operation.

4   Instrumentation

In addition to standard laparoscopic equipment available in most operating rooms, certain specialized equipment is necessary to safely carry out laparoscopic pancreatic surgery (Table 23.2). Intraoperative ultrasound is an invaluable tool during laparoscopic pancreatic resections. Ultrasound can be used to help localize lesions in the pancreas, define the relationship between the lesion and pancreatic duct, assess for vascular invasion by the lesion, assess resection margins, and rule out metastatic disease.

5   Positioning and Room Setup

Following endotracheal intubation and general anesthesia, an orogastric tube and Foley catheter are placed. Sequential compression devices and/or subcutaneous heparin are used for deep venous thrombosis prophylaxis and a first-generation cephalosporin is used for infectious prophylaxis.

Table 23.2 Equipment for laparoscopic pancreatic resection

30° Laparoscope
Flexible laparoscopic ultrasound probe
Ultrasonic dissector
Endo GIA stapler
5- and 10-mm clip applier
Laparoscopic needle holders
Atraumatic graspers
Table mounted retractor

For lesions in the head, uncinate, or neck of the pancreas the patient is positioned supine on a split leg table or in a low lithotomy position. The surgeon stands between the legs and the first assistant to the patient's left. For lesions located in the body and tail of the pancreas, we prefer to position the patient in a semilateral (30°–45°) position with the left side up. The surgeon and camera operator stand on the patient's right side, whereas the first assistant and scrub nurse stand on the patient's left side. Video monitors are placed over both shoulders and the laparoscopic ultrasound monitor is placed on the patient's left side near the video monitor.

3 Laparoscopic Distal Pancreatectomy with or without Splenectomy

Laparoscopic distal pancreatectomy may be performed as a splenic preserving distal pancreatectomy (SPDP) or an en bloc distal pancreatectomy plus splenectomy. Two techniques for splenic preservation have been described (Fig. 23.3). The first involves preservation of the splenic artery and vein and requires a very careful dissection and ligation of the small branches from the splenic artery and vein to the pancreas. The second technique involves the division of the splenic artery and vein proximally; followed by a second division of the vessels as they emerge from the tail of the pancreas. The spleen is vascularized by the short gastric vessels and the left gastroepiploic vessels. Attempts at splenic preservation are appropriate for benign cystic neoplasms and neuroendocrine tumors. Splenectomy is often necessary if the tail of the pancreas extends well into the splenic hilum or there is significant peripancreatic inflammation that makes dissection of the pancreas off of the splenic vessels hazardous. Splenectomy should be performed if the procedure is being done for malignancy or there is left-sided portal hypertension secondary to splenic vein thrombosis.

3.1 Technique

Access to the peritoneal cavity is achieved by either an open technique or via an Optiview technique. Five ports are placed (Fig. 23.4), and a 10-mm 30° laparoscope is used. As in all pancreatic procedures, the peritoneal surfaces, omentum, mesentery, and viscera should all be carefully inspected to rule out metastatic disease. Intraoperative ultrasonography may be employed to evaluate the liver and locate the lesion in the pancreas.

The body and tail of the pancreas are exposed by opening the lesser sac. The gastrocolic omentum is divided and widely mobilized with an ultrasonic dissector (e.g., Harmonic Scalpel; Ethicon Endo-Surgery, Inc., Cincinnati, OH), with care taken to stay outside the gastroepiploic vessels. The short gastric vessels usually do not need

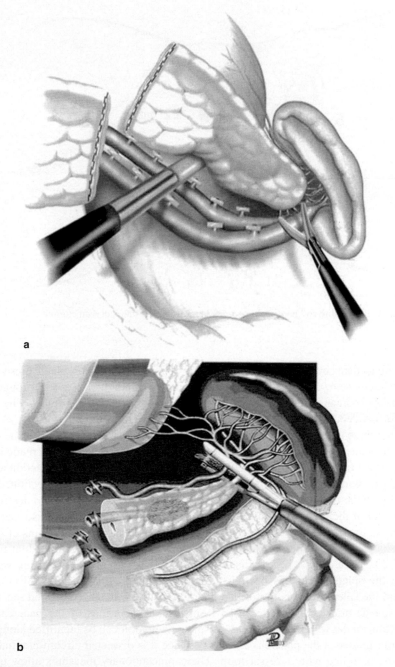

Fig. 23.3 A. Laparoscopic splenic preserving distal pancreatectomy with preservation of the splenic vessels. (From Fernandez-Cruz L, et al. J Gastrointest Surg 2004, 8:493–501.) **B.** Laparoscopic Splenic preserving distal pancreatectomy with ligation of the splenic vessels. The spleen is vascularized by the short gastric vessels and the left gastroepiploic vessel. (From Fernandez-Cruz L, et al. J Gastrointest Surg 2004, 8:493–501.)

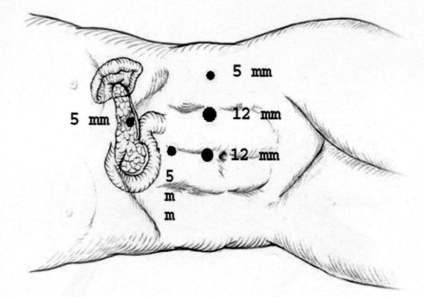

Fig. 23.4 Positioning and port placement for laparoscopic distal pancreatectomy

to be divided and every effort should be made to preserve them if a splenic preserving procedure is being attempted. A retractor is advanced into the lesser sac through the subxiphoid port and used to elevate the stomach anteromedially. The splenocolic ligament is divided, and the splenic flexure of the colon is reflected inferiorly.

After these maneuvers, the inferior pancreatic margin should be exposed. The peritoneum is then incised along the inferior pancreatic border, and the pancreatic body is separated from the retroperitoneum by means of sharp and blunt dissection along its inferior border. Laparoscopic ultrasonography and direct visual inspection, combined with the findings from preoperative imaging, may be employed to determine the extent of the dissection. Initially, the dissection should be directed so that it is medial to the pancreatic lesion. The pancreatic body is elevated by means of blunt and sharp dissection, after which the splenic vein should be easily identifiable (Fig. 23.5). Care must be exercised to prevent inadvertent injury to this vessel. Once the splenic vein has been identified, a careful circumferential dissection around the splenic vein is performed and a vessel loop is placed around the vein. The splenic artery can be identified from the under surface of the pancreas by retracting on the vessel loop around the splenic vein or it can be identified along the superior border of the pancreas anteriorly. Once it is dissected circumferentially it is also controlled with a vessel loop. These precautionary measures allow quick control of bleeding should a vascular tear occur later in the procedure.

Once the pancreatic body has been adequately mobilized from the splenic vessels, the pancreatic parenchyma is divided with the ultrasonic scalpel. Alternatively, an endoscopic stapler can be placed across the body of the pancreas, sparing the main

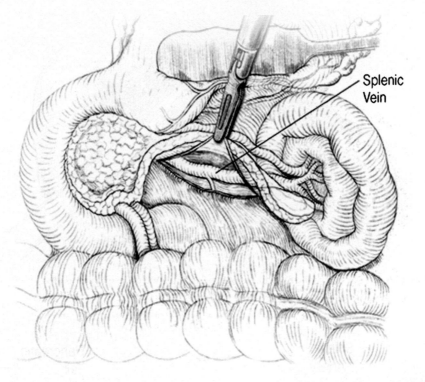

Splenic Vein

Fig. 23.5 Identification of the splenic vein following mobilization of the pancreatic body from the retroperitoneum

splenic vessels (Fig. 23.6). Once the proximal pancreatic tissue is divided, the specimen is grasped and gently retracted anteriorly to allow further dissection of the vessels. The dissection proceeds toward the splenic hilum in a medial-to-lateral direction. The pancreatic branches of the splenic vein are sequentially identified, dissected free with laparoscopic Metzenbaum scissors, and divided with the ultrasonic scalpel (Fig. 23.7). The branches of the splenic artery, which runs just superior to the vein, are treated similarly. Special care must be taken as the dissection approaches the hilum of the spleen.

At the completion of an SPDP, the specimen is placed and removed in a standard endoscopic retrieval bag. The pancreatic remnant is then oversewn with a series of interrupted absorbable horizontal mattress sutures. A single round Jackson Pratt drain is placed near the pancreatic transaction line and brought out through one of the 5-mm lateral ports.

An alternative approach to SPDP (9) involves dividing the splenic vessels proximally and distally while preserving the short gastric and left gastroepiploic vessels to maintain splenic perfusion (see Fig. 23.3). The initial steps of this technique are essentially the same as those already described (see the preceding), up to the division of the pancreas. In the alternative approach to SPDP, after pancreatic transection, the splenic artery and vein are divided with an endovascular stapler.

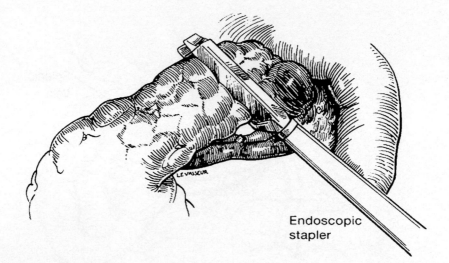

Fig. 23.6 Transection of the body of the pancreas sparing the main splenic vessels

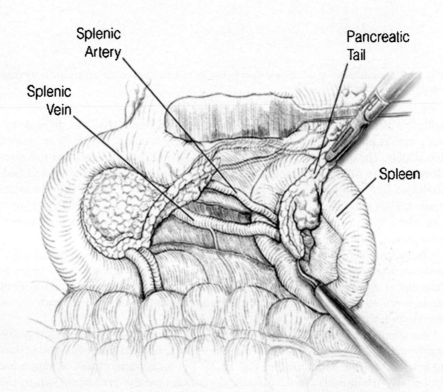

Fig. 23.7 Medial to lateral dissection of the pancreas off of the splenic vessels

The left portion of the pancreas is lifted up and mobilized posteriorly along with the splenic artery and vein, and the vessels are again divided as they emerge from the pancreatic tail to enter the hilum of the spleen. The spleen is then supplied solely by the short gastric vessels and the left gastroepiploic vessels.

If an en bloc distal pancreatectomy with splenectomy is performed, the splenic artery and vein are divided after the pancreas is transected. The distal pancreas is dissected free in a medial-to-lateral direction. The short gastric vessels are divided with the ultrasonic scalpel, with care taken not to injure the stomach wall. The retroperitoneal attachments of the spleen and the tail of the pancreas are divided with the ultrasonic scalpel. The specimen is then placed in a specimen retrieval bag and extracted from a port site that has been enlarged to a size of 3–6 cm. To facilitate extraction of the specimen, the spleen may be morcellated within the bag.

3.2   Results

In the past 5 years it has become clear that laparoscopic distal pancreatectomy can be performed safely by surgeons experienced in both advanced laparoscopic techniques and pancreatic surgery. One large multi-institutional and several smaller single institution series have been published (Table 23.3). In these series the operative time ranged between 3 and 5 hours, the complication rate between 17% and 41%, the pancreatic fistula rate was between 4% and 38%, and the length of stay between 4 and 11 days. In comparison, in a large series of open distal pancreatectomy reported by Lillemoe and colleagues, the mean operative time was 4.7 hours, and the overall morbidity was 31%. The pancreatic fistula rate and abdominal abscess rate was 5% and 4%, respectively. The safety of laparoscopic splenic preserving distal pancreatectomy was demonstrated by Fernandez-Cruz and colleagues (9). In a series of 19 patients with cystic neoplasms of the pancreas, they showed that splenic preservation can be accomplished safely with or without splenic artery and vein ligation (Table 23.4). In their series, the overall conversion rate was 0%; the mean operative

Table 23.3 Comparison of laparoscopic and open distal pancreatectomy

Author	Year	Proc	n	Spleen preservation (%)	Op time (h)	Panc fistula/ abscess (%)	Morbidity (%)	LOS (d)
Marbut (10)	2005	Lap	82	71	3.3	27–38	41	7.0
Park (11)	2002	Lap	23	41	3.7	4	17	4.1
Dulucq (12)	2005	Lap	21	76	4.6	14	23	10.8
Fernandez-Cruz (9)	2004	Lap	19	100	3.7	15	31	5.7
Patterson (13)	2001	Lap	19	37	4.4	16	26	6.0
Edwin (14)	2004	Lap	17	29	4.0	—	38	5.5
Lillemoe (15)	1999	Open	235	16	4.7	9	31	10

Table 23.4 Spleen preserving distal pancreatectomy for cystic neoplasms of the pancreas

	n	Size (cm)	Op time (min)	EML (ml)	Comp (%)	LOS (d)
Splenic vessel preservation	11	5.3	222	496	27	5.5
Splenic vessel ligation	8	5.1	165	275	38	5.6

Adapted from Fernandez-Cruz L. J Gastrointest Surg 2004, 8:493–501.

time was 222 minutes and the overall morbidity 31%. Splenic vessel preservation was associated with a longer operative time and a greater blood loss.

Although there has not been a prospective randomized comparison of laparoscopic and open distal pancreatectomy, it appears that laparoscopic distal pancreatectomy can be accomplished with a similar mortality, morbidity, and pancreatic fistula rate as open pancreatic surgery. However, laparoscopic surgery may be associated with a shorter hospital stay, blood loss, and a higher likelihood of splenic preservation.

4   Laparoscopic Pancreatic Enucleation

Enucleation of benign pancreatic neoplasms has been accepted therapy for small neuroendocrine tumors of the pancreas. More recently, enucleation has been proposed as acceptable therapy for benign cystic tumors of the pancreas. A recent study from the Medical College of Wisconsin (16) compared enucleation with pancreatic resection in 30 patients who underwent surgery for benign cystic pancreatic tumors: 11 patients were managed by enucleation, whereas 19 had pancreatic resection. The two groups were similar with respect to age, gender, and presenting symptoms. According to CT scan measurements cysts that were enucleated were smaller (2.2 versus 4.7 cm, $p < 0.01$). Ten (91%) of 11 enucleated cysts were in the uncinate, head, neck, or body of the pancreas compared to 13 (58%) of 19 resected cysts. Cyst type was similar in the two groups with the majority (53%) being mucinous cystic neoplasms. Both operative time ($p < 0.01$) and blood loss ($p < 0.001$) were less in the enucleated patients. Pancreatic fistula rates (27% versus 26%) and length of hospital stay were similar in the two groups.

Patients may be considered for a pancreatic parenchymal preserving enucleation if the preoperative and intraoperative evaluation strongly suggests a benign MCN, serous cystadenoma, or islet cell tumor. Factors such as cyst size, presence of jaundice, and proximity to the bile duct and major vascular structures also play a role in determining if a lesion is amenable to enucleation. The use of intraoperative ultrasound can be extremely helpful in identifying the relationship of the tumor to these structures as well as the main pancreatic duct (16, 17).

4.1   Technique

Recently, laparoscopic techniques have been applied to the enucleation of benign neuroendocrine tumors of the pancreas. Patient positioning and trocar placement are similar to those for laparoscopic distal pancreatectomy (see the preceding). The body and tail of the pancreas are widely exposed by entering the lesser sac through the gastrocolic omentum. Intraoperative ultrasound is extremely useful for identification of the tumor and further delineation of the relationship to the splenic vessels and pancreatic duct. The lesion can then be dissected out of the pancreatic parenchyma using the ultrasonic shears and electrocautery (Fig. 23.8). The specimen is placed in a specimen retrieval bag and removed. The enucleation bed is then inspected for hemostasis and a closed suction drain placed to control any potential pancreatic leak.

4.2   Results

The largest report of laparoscopic pancreatic enucleations comes from a multi-center European study (Table 23.5). The authors report on successfully completing laparoscopic enucleation in 21 of 22 patients (95%). The mean operative time was 120 minutes and the mean length of stay was 7 days. The pancreatic related (pancreatic

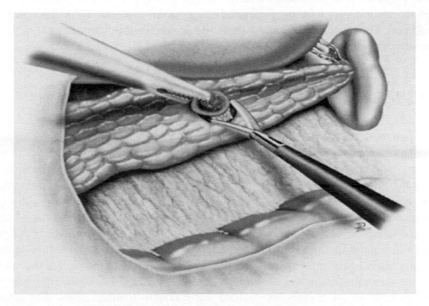

Fig. 23.8 Laparoscopic pancreatic enucleation (From Fernandez-Cruz, et al. World J Surg 2002, 26:1057–1065)

Table 23.5 Results of laparoscopic pancreatic enucleation

Author	Year	n	Op time (min)	Comp (%)	LOS (d)
Marbut (*10*)	2005	21	120	24	7
Fernandez-Cruz (*18*)	2005	7	180	42	5
Edwin (*14*)	2004	6	120	—	5.5
Berends (*19*)	2000	5	180	40	7.0

fistula and/or fluid collection) complication rate was 29%, which is comparable to that reported for open pancreatic enucleation (*10*).

5 Laparoscopic Pancreaticoduodenectomy

In contrast to laparoscopic distal pancreatectomies and laparoscopic enucleations, the role of laparoscopic pancreaticoduodenectomy (PD) is more controversial. Laparoscopic PD is a technically demanding procedure due to the retroperitoneal location of the pancreas, its intimate association with surrounding gastrointestinal and major vascular structures, and the need for three separate anastomoses to complete the reconstruction. In addition, it is unclear whether an adequate cancer operation can be performed with respect to lymph node harvest and margin status in patients with malignancy. Currently, laparoscopic PD is only performed in a handful of specialized centers. Many of the procedures are performed as either hand- or laparoscopic-assisted procedures, with the resection being performed laparoscopically and the reconstruction being completed via a "mini" laparotomy or through the hand port. The technique of laparoscopic PD as described by Dulucq et al. (*20*) is summarized in the following.

5.1 Technique

The patient is placed in the supine in the split leg position. The surgeon stands between the patient's legs, with the first assistant on the left side of the patient. After completing a staging laparoscopy to rule out metastatic disease, the procedure is begun by dividing the gastrocolic ligament with a ligasure or harmonic. The stomach is elevated, and intraoperative laparoscopic ultrasonography of the pancreas is performed. The right colon is completely mobilized off of the head of the pancreas and an extended Kocher maneuver is performed. If necessary, the right gastroepiploic vein and artery are dissected and divided. Next the hepatogastric ligament is opened and the lesser sac entered to visualize the anterior surface of the pancreas. The stomach is retracted anteriorly and the right gastric and gastroduodenal arteries are divided using double titanium clips. The distal stomach is then transected using an endo-GIA stapler. The proximal jejunum is similarly transected with the stapler and the mesentery divided with a ligasure device back toward the superior mesenteric vessels. A 5-mm suction-irrigation probe is used to dissect the posterior pancreas from the portal vein under direct laparoscopic visualization. The neck of the pancreas is then transected with an ultrasonic dissector, beginning inferiorly and moving toward the superior border anteriorly to the portal vein. The posterior area of the portal vein is dissected, and the uncinate process is separated from the mesenteric artery and vein using the ultrasonic dissector and ligasure. Finally, the bile duct is transected approximately 2–3 cm above the pancreatic border.

The reconstruction is performed in a standard fashion. An end-to-end pancreatico-jejunostomy anastomosis is performed in one layer using interrupted absorbable monofilament 4–0 sutures. If the pancreatic duct is dilated, several mucosa-to-mucosa sutures can be placed. The second anastomosis is an end-to-side hepaticojejunos-tomy, usually performed 10–15 cm away from the first anastomosis, with running posterior and anterior 5–0 monofilament absorbable suture lines. The final anastomosis lies 50 cm downstream from the hepaticojejunostomy and consists of an end-to-side mechanical gastrojejunostomy. Alternatively, a small midline laparotomy can be performed and the reconstruction can be completed with an open technique.

5.2   Results

In 1994 Gagner and Pomp (4) described the first laparoscopic PD for chronic pancre-atitis. In 1997, these same authors (21) described 10 patients who had an attempted laparoscopic PD (eight patients for periampullary malignancy and two for chronic pancreatitis) (Table 23.6). The conversion rate was 40% and the mean operative time was 8.5 hours (range 5.5–12 hours). The average length of stay was 22.3 days. The complication rate was 50% in the six patients who completed the laparoscopic proce-dure (one patient each with pancreatic leak, delayed gastric emptying, and splenic hemorrhage). These authors concluded that laparoscopic PD is feasible, but at this time does not provide any significant advantage over the open procedure. More recently, Dulucq et al. (20) describe 25 patients who had an attempted laparoscopic PD with a conversion rate of 12%. Thirteen patients had a laparoscopic reconstruction, whereas nine patients had a mini laparotomy for reconstruction. The complication

Table 23.6 Results of laparoscopic pancreaticoduodenectomy

Author	Year	n	Conv (%)	Lap recon	Op time (min)	Comp (%)	Los (d)	Panc cancer
Gagner (21)	1997	10	40	6	510	30	22.3	4
Dulucq (12)	2005	11	9	6	268	33	13.4	4
Staudacher (22)	2005	7	43	0	416	—	12	1
Dulucq (20)	2006	25	12	13	287	32	16.2	11

rate was 32% and the average length of stay was 16.2 days. These results are comparable to those of open pancreaticoduodenectomy.

Although PD can be performed laparoscopically, it must still be considered an experimental procedure. Its performance should be limited to specialized centers with significant expertise in pancreatic and advanced laparoscopic surgery.

6   Summary

It has become clear that laparoscopic distal pancreatectomy and laparoscopic pancreatic enucleation can be accomplished with acceptable morbidity and a shorter length of stay compared with open procedures. However, laparoscopic pancreatic resections are an advanced minimally invasive procedure and should be performed in carefully selected patients by surgeons with extensive experience in pancreatic surgery with advanced laparoscopic skills. At this time, laparoscopic pancreatectomy is indicated for benign or premalignant pancreatic lesions.

References

1. Nakeeb A. 2005, The role of minimally invasive surgery for pancreatic pathology. Adv Surg 39:455–470.
2. Bernheim BM. 1911, Organoscopy. Cystoscopy of the abdominal cavity. Ann Surg 53:764–767.
3. Cuschieri A, Hall AW, Clark J. 1978, Value of laparoscopy in the diagnosis and management of pancreatic carcinoma. Gut 19:672–677.
4. Gagner M, Pomp A. 1994 Laparoscopic pylorus-preserving pancreatoduodenectomy. Surg Endosc 8:408–410.
5. Naitoh T, Garcia-Ruiz A, Vladisavljevic A, 2002, Gastrointestinal transit and stress response after laparoscopic versus conventional distal pancreatectomy in the canine model. Surg Endosc 16:1627–1630.
6. Nakeeb A, Lillemoe KD, Yeo CJ, 2006, Neoplasms of the exocrine pancreas. In: Mulholland M, Lillemoe K, Doherty (eds.) G, Greenfield's surgery: scientific principles & practice. Lippincott Williams & Wilkins,Philadelphia, 861–879.
7. Tseng FF, Warshaw AL, Sahani DV, 2005, Serous cystadenoma of the pancreas: Tumor growth rates and recommendations for treatment. Ann Surg 242:413–419.
8. Brugge WR, Lauwers GY, Sahani D, 2004, Cystic neoplasms of the pancreas. N Engl J Med 351:1218–1226.
9. Fernandez-Cruz L, Martinez I, Gilabert R, 2004, Laparoscopic distal pancreatectomy combined with preservation of the spleen for cystic neoplasms of the pancreas. J Gastrointest Surg 8:493–501.
10. Mabrut JY, Fernandez-Cruz L, Santiago Azagra J, 2005, Laparoscopic pancreatic resection: results of a multicenter European study of 127 patients. Surgery 137:597–605.
11. Park AE, Heniford BT. 2002, Therapeutic laparoscopy of the pancreas. Ann Surg 236:149–158.
12. Dulucq JL, Wintringer P, Stabilini C, 2005, Are major laparoscopic pancreatic resections worthwhile? Surg Endosc 19:1028–1034.

13. Patterson EJ, Gagner M, Salky B, 2001, Laparoscopic pancreatic resection: single-institution experience of 19 patients. J Am Coll Surg 193:281–287.
14. Edwin B, Mala T, Mathisen O, 2004, Laparoscopic resection of the pancreas: a feasibility study of the short-term outcome. Surg Endosc 18:407–411.
15. Lillemoe KD, Kaushal S, Cameron JL, 1999, Distal pancreatectomy: indications and outcomes in 235 patients. Ann Surg 229:693–698.
16. Kiley JM, Nakeeb A, Komorowski RA, 2003, Cystic pancreatic neoplasms: Enucleate or resect? J Gastrointest Surg 7:890–897.
17. Talamini MA, Moesinger R, Yeo CJ, 1998, Cystadenomas of the pancreas: Is enucleation an adequate operation. Ann Surg 227:896–903.
18. Fernandez-Cruz L, Martinez I, Cesar-Borges G, 2005, Laparoscopic surgery in patients with sporadic and multiple insulinomas associated with multiple endocrine neoplasia type 1. J Gastrointest Surg 9:381–388.
19. Berends FJ, Cuesta MA, Kazemier G, 2000, Laparoscopic detection and resection of insulinomas. Surgery 128:386–391.
20. Dulucq JL, Wintringer P, Mahajna A. 2006, Laparoscopic pancreaticoduodenectomy for benign and malignant diseases. Surg Endosc 20:1045–1050.
21. Gagner M, Pomp A. 1997, Laparoscopic pancreatic resection: Is it worthwhile? J Gastrointest Surg 1:20–26.
22. Staudacher C, Orsengio E, Baccari P, 2005, Laparoscopic assisted duodenopancreatectomy. Surg Endosc 19:352–356.

Chapter 24
Surgical Management of IPMN

Stefano Crippa, Carlos Fernandez-del Castillo, and Andrew L. Warshaw

1 Introduction

Once considered as a "rare" entity, intraductal papillary mucinous neoplasm (IPMN) of the pancreas is nowadays more commonly recognized, thanks to the widespread use of cross-sectioning imaging techniques (*1, 2*). At our institution, IPMN has become the second most common indication for pancreatic resection, following ductal adenocarcinoma.

Since its first description by Ohashi in 1982, knowledge of the clinical, radiologic, and pathologic characteristics of IPMN has increased rapidly (*3*). Several series have documented the prevalence of malignancy and the risk of tumor recurrence after surgical resection among these patients. However, much of the natural history of IPMN still remains unknown.

In 2000 the World Health Organization (WHO) divided IPMN into two different entities: main-duct and branch-duct IPMN. Main-duct IPMNs are characterized by involvement of the main pancreatic duct with or without associated involvement of the branch ducts (combined IPMNs) (*2*). They commonly present with a dilated (≥ 1 cm) main pancreatic duct full of mucus that may extrude through a bulging ampulla. Some have cystic dilation of the main pancreatic duct (*4*). Main-duct IPMNs are usually located in the proximal portion of the gland, but can spread longitudinally along the duct, even to involve the entire main pancreatic duct. Patients affected by main-duct IPMN may present with abdominal pain, pancreatitis, steatorrhea, and weight loss. Diabetes is indicative of late-stage deterioration, and jaundice commonly indicates malignant degeneration (*5–8*).

Branch-duct IPMNs originate in the side branches of the pancreatic ductal system, appearing as a cystic lesion communicating with a nondilated main pancreatic duct. This neoplasm more commonly occurs in the uncinate process, but it can also be seen in the head, neck, and distal pancreas. Multifocal involvement of the gland with two or more branch-duct IPMNs is not an uncommon finding (*1*). Even though patients affected by branch-duct IPMN can present with abdominal pain, pancreatitis, or other symptoms, many are completely asymptomatic and are incidentally detected during radiologic workup performed for other reasons (*9–11*).

A.M. Lowy et al. (eds.) *Pancreatic Cancer.*   419
doi: 10.1007/978-0-387-69252-4, © Springer Science+Business Media, LLC 2008

IPMN occurs more frequently in the seventh and eighth decades of life, which is important when considering the potential treatment. Although pancreatic resection can be safely performed in elderly patients in experienced centers (2), the presence of significant comorbidities must be factored into therapeutic decisions.

Histologically, IPMN encompasses a wide spectrum of epithelial changes ranging from adenoma to invasive carcinoma, with borderline neoplasms and carcinoma-in-situ in between (2, 5–8). Different degrees of dysplasia can be found within the same lesion. Moreover, in our experience the average age of patients with malignant main-duct IPMN is 6.4 years older than that of patients with adenoma or borderline tumor (7). These observations support the theory of a "clonal progression" to malignancy, at least in this variant (13).

In a recent review of the literature, Tanaka et al. found that main-duct and branch-duct IPMN were associated with malignancy in 70% and 25% of the cases, respectively, whereas the rate of invasive carcinoma was 43% for main-duct IPMN and 15% for branch-duct type (2). Because of this lower likelihood of malignancy and because branch-duct IPMN is often asymptomatic (9–11), the International Association of Pancreatology recently proposed to manage asymptomatic patients with small (<30 mm) branch-duct IPMN without nodules with careful observation (2).

2   The Role of Imaging

Different imaging studies are nowadays available for the diagnosis and the characterization of IPMNs: computed tomography (CT), magnetic resonance with or without cholangiopancreatography (MRCP), endoscopic retrograde cholangiopancreatography (ERCP), endoscopic ultrasound (EUS), and positron emission tomography with 18F-fluorodeoxyglucose (FDG-PET) (14). First, it is necessary to differentiate IPMNs from other cystic lesions of the pancreas, which can be nonneoplastic (i.e., pseudocyst) or neoplastic (i.e., mucinous cystic neoplasms, characterized by the absence of a communication with the ductal system and, histologically, by the presence of an ovarian-like stroma). Second, it is important to distinguish between main-duct or combined main-duct/branch-duct IPMNs and branch-duct IPMNs, since the biological behavior of these neoplasms seems to be different. Third, imaging studies should characterize the lesion, evaluating the number and site of the cyst/cysts within the gland, and the presence of those findings suggestive of malignancy such as thick walls and mural nodules, with the goal of differentiating between benign and malignant IPMNs. Furthermore, in the case of malignant neoplasms, an accurate preoperative staging must be performed, including the search for mesenteric or hepatic vascular encasement and distant metastases.

MRCP can adequately indicate the site and the extension of main pancreatic duct dilatation, the presence of a communication between the duct and the cyst lesion, the presence and size of mural nodules, and the presence of multifocal branch-duct IPMNs (1, 4, 15). High-resolution multislice helical CT can provide unique details of the morphologic characteristics IPMNs (16), whereas MRCP seems to be more sensitive in the diagnosis of small branch-duct IPMNs, especially in the setting of a multifocal disease (*1, 17*). If cross-sectional imaging does not provide a definitive diagnosis, additional information can be obtained from EUS (*14*). This is an operator-dependent technique, and EUS alone seems not to significantly improve CT/MRCP results in distinguishing benign from malignant lesions. Fine-needle aspiration cytology and cyst-fluid analysis for amylase, carcinoembryonic antigen (CEA), and other tumor markers may provide further differential diagnostic information. However, cytology may show false-negative and, more often, inconclusive results (*14, 18*); cyst fluid concentrations of CEA is useful for identifying mucinous lesions, but does not differentiate between MCNs and IPMNs or between benign and malignant lesions (*15, 19*). ERCP has been the procedure of choice for the diagnosis of IPMNs for years, allowing brushings or aspiration of the main pancreatic duct contents for cytology (*15*). Nowadays the diagnostic value of ERCP is less, due to the significant improvements in EUS and other radiologic imaging. In addition ERCP carries the risk of inducing acute pancreatitis.

Recently it has been suggested that FDG-PET may play a role in differentiating benign from malignant cystic lesions of the pancreas. In a prospective study of 50 patients with suspected pancreatic cystic tumors or IPMNs, Sperti et al. (*20*) reported that FDG-PET had a specificity and sensitivity of 94% in correctly distinguishing malignant from benign lesions, compared with 65% and 88% for CT. Interestingly, FDG-PET showed increased uptake of FDG even in patients with IPMNs containing carcinoma-in-situ in whom CT did not show any sign of malignancy. Further studies are needed to confirm the validity of this approach.

3 Main-Duct IPMN

3.1 Indications for Surgery

Given the high rate of malignancy among patients affected by main-duct IPMN, the age differences between patients with benign and malignant tumors, which suggests a progression from benign to malignant neoplasm, and the lack of clinical and radiologic parameters that can discriminate between malignant and benign lesions, we advocate that all suspected main-duct and combined IPMNs should be resected, even in asymptomatic patients.

3.2 Surgical Treatment

The surgical management of main-duct IPMN represents a unique challenge to the surgeon. While the preoperative studies for other pancreatic tumors—including CT, MRCP and EUS—can accurately locate the tumor and accordingly indicate a plan for pancreatic resection, the precise localization of a main-duct IPMN may be difficult. Preoperative studies may show only a dilated main pancreatic duct with or without cysts, but not the intraductal mass itself, which is often small. Distinguishing papillary excrescences in the duct from intraluminal mucus may not be possible. Dilation may occur both proximal and distal to the tumor because of overproduction of mucus, making more problematic the localization of the neoplasia. Finally, because main-duct IPMN can spread along the duct and be flat rather than protruding, it may be difficult to ascertain the limits of the neoplastic involvement of the dilated duct without histopathologic proof (Fig. 24.1).

With the information available from the preoperative studies, the surgeon plans the operation but should be prepared to modify the surgical strategy depending on the intraoperative findings, most particularly frozen-section evaluation of the duct at the margin. Since main-duct IPMN most commonly affects the head of the pancreas (60%), in most cases pancreaticoduodenectomy, with or without pylorus preservation, is planned and performed, even when the main duct is dilated in the body and tail (Fig. 24.2). Because of the possible need to extend the surgical resection based on intraoperative findings, even to a total pancreatectomy, it is important to discuss this possibility with patients preoperatively.

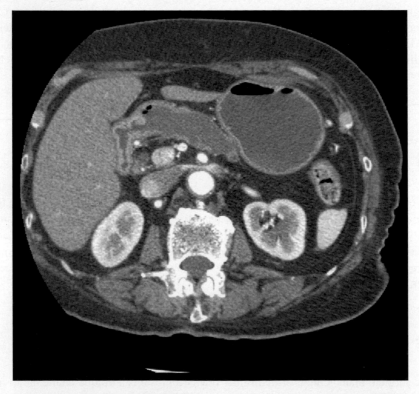

Fig. 24.1 CT scan of a patients affected by a main duct IPMN of the head–neck of the pancreas. It is remarkable the dilatation of the main pancreatic duct

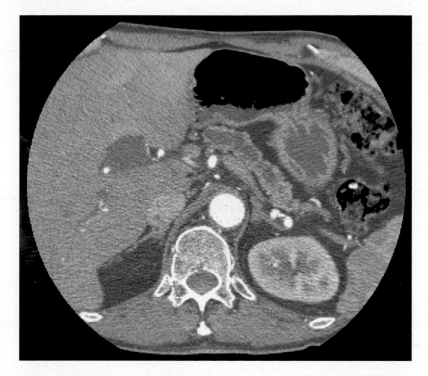

Fig. 24.2 CT scan of a main duct IPMN with significant dilatation of the pancreatic duct and nodules. After Whipple it turned out to be an invasive carcinoma

Intraoperative sonography and pancreatoscopy has been used in uncertain cases to help determine the limits of resection (*21, 22*). In our experience intraoperative ultrasound does not add much to preoperative imaging. Intraoperative pancreatoscopy allows for inspection of the main pancreatic duct of the remnant after resection, and theoretically should be useful to identify missed residual and "skip" lesions in the main duct. We have found, however, that pancreatoscopy may fail to detect areas of flat neoplastic epithelium, including carcinoma-in-situ, and therefore must be considered useful but not definitive.

A formal resection (pancreaticoduodenectomy, left pancreatectomy, total pancreatectomy, according to the site and extension of the disease) with appropriate lymph node dissection is indicated, rather than local excisions or enucleation (Fig. 24.3). Limited resections, such as middle pancreatectomy, provide the advantage of sparing pancreatic parenchyma and maximally preserving exocrine and endocrine function; however, in our experience with middle pancreatectomy we found the rate of positive resection margins and recurrences to be too high when this operation was performed for main-duct IPMN, as also reported by others (*2, 23*). For these reasons we believe that short-segment local resections are probably not suitable for main-duct IPMN. An interesting option for benign main-duct IPMN involving only the duct of Santorini is a complete dorsal pancreatectomy (*24*). Postmortem anatomic

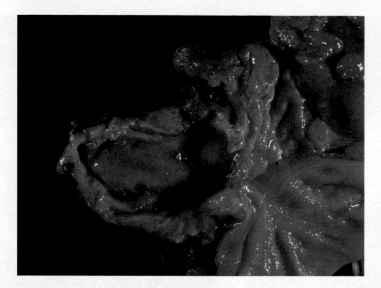

Fig. 24.3 Surgical specimen of a main duct IPMN in the head of the pancreas. There is a significant dilatation (3.5 cm) of the main pancreatic duct to the ampulla of Vater. Mucous and glandular mucosa were evident. The histopathologic diagnosis was carcinoma-in-situ with areas of adenoma and borderline neoplasm

investigations have shown that there is a persistent anatomic fusion plane in the adult between the dorsal (pancreatic neck, body, tail, and anterior segment of the head with the Santorini duct) and ventral (posterior segment of the head with the duct of Wirsung) pancreas, thus allowing a dorsal pancreatectomy with removal of the anterior segment of the pancreatic head but preservation of the posterior segment containing the uncinate process and bile duct. The intraoperative examination of the transection margin is of paramount importance in the management of patients affected by main-duct IPMN (2, 7, 25). Since IPMN extends along the main pancreatic duct, it is important to assess the presence of tumor at the margin so that tumor is not left behind. The pathologic interpretation of the surgical margins must be analyzed with caution: "negative" with normal epithelium in the main duct; mucinous hyperplasia without dysplasia; "positive" for adenoma, varying degrees of dysplasia, or carcinoma. Denuded or de-epithelialized ducts are not uncommon in this entity, possibly due to high-pressure injury, but should not be taken to be a negative margin. Local recurrence can occur in this setting (5), and this phenomenon, we believe, is an important contributing factor to failure of cure in some series in which duct margins have not been adequately evaluated during the operative procedure. The presence of significant neoplasia, high-grade dysplasia, or carcinoma requires an extension of the surgical resection to a negative margin, even if there is need for a total pancreatectomy (2). Low-grade PanIN and mucinous hyperplasia at the resection margin are common, however, and do not require extension of the resection. In our experience with 140 patients affected by main duct IPMN who underwent surgical resection, the surgical margins were negative in 58.5%: The results of the intraoperative frozen section analysis modified the surgical plan, leading to an extension of the resection or total pancreatectomy in 29 patients (20.7%) (7).

Although very uncommon in our experience, recurrence in the pancreatic remnant may occasionally develop even if the transection margin is negative and even in patients with noninvasive disease. In the Mayo Clinic report of 60 patients affected by a benign IPMN who underwent partial pancreatectomy, a negative margin was obtained in 58 cases and, of these, one patient later developed distant metastases and another four local recurrence (8). Similar results have been reported by others (6). Recurrence in the pancreatic remnant after resecting a main-duct IPMN can be related to three different possible reasons:

1. The presence of a "positive" resection margin
2. A multicentric tumor with synchronous "skip" lesions along the main duct
3. A "field defect" leading to metachronous neoplasms

Simultaneous "missed" neoplasms can perhaps be minimized by intraoperative pancreatoscopy of the main duct (21). Gigot et al. suggested intraoperative endoscopic staged biopsies of the main pancreatic duct as a complementary tool (22). More recently, cytologic examination of the pancreatic juice from the remnant has been proposed as an adjunct to detect malignancy or significant dysplasia in the remnant (26).

Some have proposed routine total pancreatectomy in IPMN because of the putative field defect and fear of recurrence in the remnant. In the case of invasive IPMN the frequency of recurrence (local recurrence or distant metastases) has been reported to be similar whether or not total pancreatectomy was performed (27, 28); Chari et al. (8) reported a recurrence rate of 62% after total pancreatectomy and of 67% after partial pancreatectomy for malignant IPMN. Jang et al. (27) reported 37.5% and 32.5% after total and partial pancreatectomy, respectively.

The risks and long-term complications of total pancreatectomy must be balanced against its benefit for prophylaxis. Whereas a total pancreatectomy is clearly an appropriate operation for a young and medically fit patient affected by a malignant main-duct IPMN involving the whole gland, it is not the right operation for an elderly patient with significant comorbidities affected by an adenoma or borderline IPMN. Inasmuch as re-resection for recurrence is usually possible and curative for local recurrences, total pancreatectomy should be utilized selectively for situations when significant neoplasms cannot be eliminated by a more limited resection.

In patients with main-duct IPMN undergoing pancreaticoduodenectomy, pancreaticogastrostomy can be considered instead of pancreaticojejunostomy. Aside from the debate about the relatively safety of the two methods of reconstruction, pancreaticogastrostomy permits greater direct access to the pancreatic stump during follow-up by facilitating pancreatoscopy, pancreatography, and sampling of pancreatic juice for cytologic examination (15, 29).

4   Branch-Duct IPMN

4.1   Indications for Surgery

As indicated, branch-duct IPMN are associated with malignancy in about 25% of
cases. Several studies have shown that patients with malignant branch-duct IPMN
are more likely symptomatic, have bigger lesions (>3 cm), and have mural nodules
(2, 9–11). Thus, whenever these criteria are present, removal is indicated, not only
to alleviate symptoms but also to eliminate a possible malignant neoplasm. On the
other hand, current experience and recommendations (2) hold that asymptomatic
patients with lesions <3 cm without nodules can be safely managed nonoperatively
as long as there is strict follow-up. In this setting, the therapeutic decision can be
guided by patient preferences and willingness to undergo follow-up studies.

4.2   Surgical Treatment

Most branch-duct IPMNs, like main-duct IPMNs, require formal pancreatic resection.
For an asymptomatic patient with a small single lesion of the neck of the pancreas (Fig.
24.4), without any laboratory, clinical, and radiologic suspicion for malignancy, a middle pancreatectomy may be appropriate.

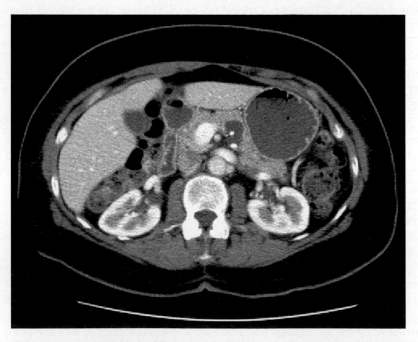

Fig. 24.4 Branch duct IPMN. At CT scan the communication between the cystic lesion and
a nondilated main pancreatic duct is evident

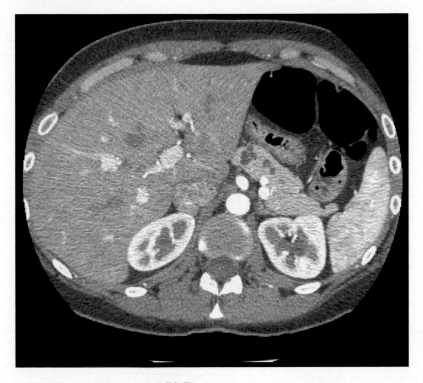

Fig. 24.5 Multifocal branch duct IPMN. The presence of multiple cystic lesions within the pancreatic gland is evident, with a bigger lesion in the head of the pancreas

The incidental diagnosis of branch-duct IPMN is increasing due to the more frequent use of imaging, and the demonstration of multiple branch-duct IPMNs along the gland (multifocal disease) may occur in >25% (Fig. 24.5) (*30*, *31*). Multifocal branch-duct IPMNs require a difficult decision in that an extended resection or total pancreatectomy may be necessary in many cases to clear all of the cystic lesions. We prefer to resect the segment of the gland with the dominant cyst or with cysts >3 cm, especially if those have characteristics suggestive of increased risk of cancer. The remnant with small cysts can be left behind to be followed by periodic imaging, most usually MRCP. In one case with two 3-cm lesions, one in the head and one in the tail, we performed a pancreaticoduodenectomy and a limited resection of the pancreatic tail but preserved the remaining body and tail (Fig. 24.6). The patient did not become diabetic.

Even in patients with multifocal branch-duct IPMN we believe that surgery is appropriate to relieve symptoms (Fig. 24.7), or for those with radiologic findings consistent with malignancy. On the other hand, a careful watchful-waiting policy is preferred for asymptomatic patients with small cysts without nodules, especially if they are elderly. The rate of growth and change of branch-duct IPMNs appear to be very slow, and the majority of patients may never come to

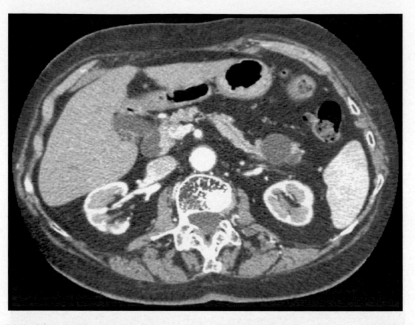

Fig. 24.6 CT scan of a patient affected by a multifocal branch duct IPMN. A pancreaticoduo-denectomy and a limited resection of the pancreatic tail were performed

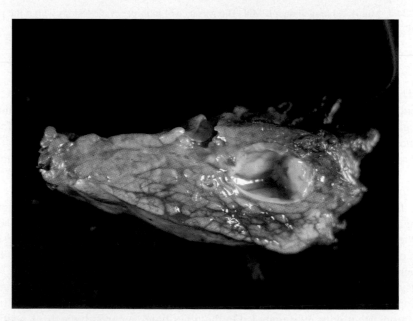

Fig. 24.7 Surgical specimen of a benign branch duct IPMN in the body of the pancreas. The lesion measures 1.5 cm in diameter, without nodules. At final histologic examination it was proved to be an adenoma. In this case surgery was performed because of the presence of abdominal pain

resection. Salvia et al. showed that a nonoperative approach can be safe and effective in a group of 89 asymptomatic patients affected by branch-duct IPMN <3.5 cm without nodules and thick walls. After a median follow-up of 32 months only five patients showed an increase in size of the lesion and underwent resection: The final pathologic examination was adenoma in three and borderline in two (*30*).

It is suggested that nonoperative surveillance, if elected, be carried out in centers with interest in this field, since further experience from large series is still needed to validate this approach (*2*).

Unlike main-duct IPMN, an intraoperative frozen section of the resection margins is less important for branch-duct IPMN, except in the case of a malignant tumor or when there is concern about possible incomplete resection because of proximity of the cyst to the margin or involvement of the main pancreatic duct. At final histopathologic examination it is always important to rule out an extension of the IPMN from the branch-duct system to the main pancreatic duct, because the biological behavior of "combined" main-duct/branch-duct IPMN is more aggressive and resembles the behavior of main-duct lesions.

In the combined experience of Massachusetts General Hospital and University of Verona, Italy, 145 patients underwent surgical resection for branch-duct IPMNs. Of these, 32 (22%) had malignancy, but there was invasive carcinoma in only 11% (16 patients). The majority of the lesions (57%) were located in the head-uncinate process of the pancreas. Thirty-seven (25.5%) of the patients had multifocal lesions at final pathologic examination. In this series from two high-volume centers, there were no perioperative mortality or re-operations; overall morbidity was 51%, with pancreatic fistula occurring in 17%. The median length of postoperative hospitalization was 9 days. Significant factors associated with malignancy were the presence of a thick wall ($p < 0.001$), nodules ($p < 0.001$), and a diameter ≥ 30 mm ($p < 0.001$). All patients with malignancy had symptoms and/or a lesion >3 cm and/or nodules (*31*).

5   The Role of Lymphadenectomy

A standard lymphadenectomy should be performed with resections for IPMN, especially in those cases in which a malignancy is suspected. The rate of lymph-node metastases in patients affected by malignant IPMN ranges from 16% to 46% (*5–8, 27, 32*). Sohn et al. (*6*) and D'Angelica et al. (*33*) showed that lymph-node status was predictive of survival in a univariate model. In our experience 41% of 58 patients with invasive main-duct IPMN had nodal metastases and yet had a respectable 5-year survival rate of 45% (*7*). Similar results were reported also in the Mayo Clinic series, in which positive nodes did not diminish long-term survival (*8*). These findings are in distinct contrast to those in ductal adenocarcinoma, wherein positive nodes markedly diminish the chance for cure.

6   Follow-up and Re-resection

After resection of IPMN, patients should be kept under close follow-up. Our current practice is to perform a clinical and radiologic evaluation by CT or MRCP every 6 months in cases with malignant tumors and yearly for benign IPMNs. Although patients with a malignant IPMN are at higher risk of recurrence, recurrence or new cystic neoplasms do occasionally appear after resection of a benign tumor with negative resection margins. New disease in the remnant is curable by re-resection (2, 5, 6). In our experience with 140 resected patients affected by main-duct IPMN, eight (6%) developed a recurrence in the remnant (7). Of these, seven had invasive carcinoma at initial histology, whereas the remaining had an adenoma with negative resection margin. This patient developed a recurrence 5 years later and underwent a further pancreatectomy for a carcinoma-in-situ of the distal pancreas. Of the seven patients with invasive carcinoma and local recurrence, two also had distant metastases, whereas a further resection was possible in the remaining five; two of these patients are still alive without evidence of cancer after long-term follow-up.

With regard to multifocal branch-duct IPMN who undergo partial pancreatectomy, strict follow-up should be performed to evaluate the remaining lesion or lesions in the remnant and possible development of new ones. MRCP is particularly useful in this setting (17).

7   Prognosis

The survival of patients with IPMN, even when malignant and invasive can be quite good. In our recent experience with follow-up of 137 resected main-duct IPMN, 5- and 10-year disease-specific survival for 80 patients with adenoma, borderline dysplasia, and carcinoma-in-situ was 100%, whereas for 57 patients with invasive carcinoma the survival was 60% and 50%, respectively (7). In other large series the 5-year disease-specific survival for IPMN with invasive carcinoma ranged from 36% to 43% (6, 8, 27, 33). With regard to 145 resected branch-duct IPMN, 5-year disease-specific survival for 129 patients with adenoma, borderline dysplasia and carcinoma-in-situ was 100%; for 16 patients with invasive carcinoma the survival was 60% (7). IPMN is one of the most curable forms of pancreatic cancer.

References

1. Carbognin G, Zamboni G, Pinali L, 2006, Branch duct IPMTs: value of cross-sectional imaging in the assessment of biological behavior and follow-up. Abdom Imaging 31:320–325.
2. Tanaka M, Chari S, Adsay V, 2005, International Consensus guidelines for management of intraductal papillary mucinous neoplasms and mucinous cystic neoplasms of the pancreas. Pancreatology 6:17–32.

3. Ohashi K, Murakami Y, Murayama M, 1982, Four cases of mucus secreting pancreatic cancer. Prog Dig Endoscopy 20:348–351.
4. Lim JH, Lee G, Oh YL, 2001, Radiologic spectrum of intraductal papillary mucinous tumor of the pancreas. Radiographics 21:323–340.
5. Falconi M, Salvia R, Bassi C, 2001, Clinicopathological features and treatment of intraductal papillary mucinous tumour of the pancreas. Br J Surg 88:376–381.
6. Sohn TA, Yeo CJ, Cameron JL, 2004, Intraductal papillary mucinous neoplasms of the pancreas: an updated experience. Ann Surg 239:788–797 .
7. Salvia R, Fernandez-del Castillo C, Bassi C, 2004, Main-duct intraductal papillary mucinous neoplasms of the pancreas: clinical predictors of malignancy and long-term survival following resection. Ann Surg 239:678–685 .
8. Chari ST, Yadav D, Smyrk TC, 2002, Study of recurrence after surgical resection of intraductal papillary mucinous neoplasm of the pancreas. Gastroenterology 123:1500–1507.
9. Kobari M, Egawa S, Shibuya K, 1999, Intraductal papillary mucinous tumors of the pancreas comprise 2 clinical subtypes: differences in clinical characteristics and surgical management. Arch Surg 134:1131–1136 .
10. Terris B, Ponsot P, Paye F, 2000, Intraductal papillary mucinous tumors of the pancreas confined to secondary ducts show less aggressive pathologic features as compared with those involving the main pancreatic duct. Am J Surg Pathol 24:1372–1377.
11. Sugiyama M, Izumisato Y, Abe N, 2003, Predictive factors for malignancy in intraductal papillary-mucinous tumours of the pancreas. Br J Surg 90:1244–1249.
12. Balcom JH, 4thRattner DW, Warshaw AL, 2001, Ten-year experience with 733 pancreatic resections: changing indications, older patients, and decreasing length of hospitalization. Arch Surg 136:391–398.
13. Wada K, Takada T, Yasuda H, 2004, Does "clonal progression" relate to the development of intraductal papillary mucinous tumors of the pancreas? J Gastrointest Surg 8: 289–296.
14. Brugge WR, Lauwers GY, Sahani D, 2004, Cystic neoplasms of the pancreas. N Engl J Med 351:1218–1226.
15. Nichols MT, Russ PD, Chen YK, 2006, Pancreatic imaging. Current and emerging techniques. Pancreas 33:211–220.
16. Sahani DV, Kadavigere R, Blake M, 2006, Intraductal papillary mucinous neoplasm of pancreas: multi-detector row CT with 2D curved reformations—correlation with MRCP. Radiology 238:560–569.
17. Pilleul F, Rochette A, Partensky C, 2005, Preoperative evaluation of intraductal papillary mucinous tumors performed by pancreatic magnetic resonance imaging and correlated with surgical and histopathologic findings. J Magn Reson Imaging 21:237–244.
18. Stelow EB, Stanley MW, Bardales RH, 2003, Intraductal papillary-mucinous neoplasm of the pancreas. The findings and limitations of cytologic samples obtained by endoscopic ultrasound-guided fine-needle aspiration. Am J Clin Pathol 120:398–404.
19. Brugge WR, Lewandrowski K, Lee-Lewandrowski E, 2004, Diagnosis of pancreatic cystic neoplasms: a report of the cooperative pancreatic cyst study. Gastroenterology 126:1330–1336.
20. Sperti C, Pasquali C, Decet G, 2005, F-18-fluorodeoxyglucose positron emission tomography in differentiating malignant from benign pancreatic cysts: a prospective study. J Gastrointest Surg 9:22–28.
21. Kaneko T, Nakao A, Nomoto S, 1998, Intraoperative pancreatoscopy with the ultrathin pancreatoscope for mucin-producing tumors of the pancreas. Arch Surg 133:263–267.
22. Gigot JF, Deprez P, Sempoux C, 2001, Surgical management of intraductal papillary mucinous tumors of the pancreas: the role of routine frozen section of the surgical margin, intraoperative endoscopic staged biopsies of the Wirsung duct, and pancreaticogastric anastomosis. Arch Surg 136:1256–1262.
23. Sauvanet A, Partensky C, Sastre B, 2002, Medial pancreatectomy: a multi-institutional retrospective study of 53 patients by the French Pancreas Club. Surgery 132:836–843.

24. Thayer SP, Fernandez-del Castillo C, Balcom JH, 2002, Complete dorsal pancreatectomy with preservation of the ventral pancreas: a new surgical technique Surgery 131:577–580.
25. Couvelard A, Sauvanet A, Kianmanesh R, 2005, Frozen sectioning of the pancreatic cut surface during resection of intraductal papillary mucinous neoplasms of the pancreas is useful and reliable. A prospective evaluation. Ann Surg 242:774–780.
26. Eguchi H, Ishikawa O, Ohigashi H, 2006, Role of intraoperative cytology combined with histology in detecting continuous and skip type intraductal cancer existence for intraductal papillarymucinous carcinoma of the pancreas. Cancer 107:2567–2575.
27. Jang JY, Kim SW, Ahn YJ, 2005, Multicenter analysis of clinicopathologic features of intraductal papillary mucinous tumor of the pancreas: is it possible to predict the malignancy before surgery? Ann Surg Oncol 12:124–132.
28. Maire F, Hammel P, Terris B, 2002, Prognosis of malignant intraductal papillary mucinous tumours of the pancreas after surgical resection. Comparison with pancreatic ductal adenocarcinoma. Gut 51:717–722.
29. Bassi C, Butturini G, Salvia R, 2006, Open pancreaticogastrostomy after pancreaticoduodenectomy: a pilot study. J Gastrointest Surg 10:1072–1080.
30. Salvia R, Crippa S, Falconi M, 2007, Branch-duct intraductal papillary mucinous neoplasms of the pancreas: to operate or not to operate? Results of a prospective protocol on the management of 109 consecutive patients. Gut 56:1086–1090.
31. Rodriguez JR, Salvia R, Crippa S, 2007, Branch-duct intraductal papillary mucinous neoplasms: observations in 145 patients who underwent resection. Gastroenterology 133:72–79.
32. Wada K, Kozarek RA, Traverso LW, 2005, Outcomes following resection of invasive and noninvasive intraductal papillary mucinous neoplasms of the pancreas. Am J Surg 189:632–637.
33. D'Angelica M, Brennan MF, Suriawinata AA, 2004, Intraductal papillary mucinous neoplasms of the pancreas. Ann Surg 239:400–408.

Section V
Palliation of Pancreatic Cancer

Chapter 25
Cancer Pain and Symptom Management: Drug Therapy

Jane Pruemer and Michelle Rockey

1 Introduction

The symptoms of pancreatic cancer are varied, based upon the location of the disease. However, these symptoms are almost always caused by mass effect of the tumor compressing the vasculature, lymphatics, or other organs rather than disruption of exocrine or endocrine pancreatic function. Classic symptoms of pancreatic cancer include pain, jaundice, and weight loss (Table 25.1) (1). Since early symptoms are usually nonspecific, they may go unrecognized for some time, and most pancreatic cancers are advanced at the time of diagnosis. In addition to the symptoms produced by the tumor itself, pancreatic cancer treatments are associated with significant complications. The following disease- and/or treatment-related symptoms are reviewed, along with strategies for their management: pain, nausea and vomiting, diarrhea, and constipation.

2 Pain Management

Pain due to pancreatic cancer is a complex problem that is the result of many factors. Frequently present in the early stages of the disease, pain is reported by 75–80% of patients at their initial evaluation (2). Pain can be attributed to different mechanisms occurring at the same time. Although it is beyond the scope of this chapter to extensively review the details of the mechanisms of pain and pain perception, an overview of cancer pain syndromes and their management is provided.

Cancer pain can be nociceptive, neuropathic, and/or sympathetic. Causes of cancer pain are varied and may include tumor invasion, inflammation, and necrosis or destruction of soft tissues, bone, and neural structures. Acute and chronic pain also may be related to diagnostic and treatment procedures such as bone marrow biopsy, lumbar puncture, surgery, chemotherapy, or radiation therapy.

Cancer pain can consist of "acute pain," "chronic pain," and "breakthrough" or episodic pain. Acute pain is initiated when nociceptors (primary afferent sensory

A.M. Lowy et al. (eds.) *Pancreatic Cancer*.
doi: 10.1007/978-0-387-69252-4, © Springer Science+Business Media, LLC 2008

435

Table 25.1 Prevalence of pancreatic cancer symptoms

Head of the pancreas		Body and tail of the pancreas	
Symptoms	Patients (%)	Symptoms	Patients (%)
Weight loss	92	Weight loss	100
Jaundice	82	Pain	87
Pain	72	Nausea	43
Anorexia	64	Weakness	42
Dark urine	63	Vomiting	37
Light stool	62	Anorexia	33
Nausea	45	Constipation	27
Vomiting	37	Food intolerance	7
Weakness	35	Jaundice	7

DiMagno EP. Cancer of the pancreas and biliary tract. In: Winawer SJ (ed.) Management of gastrointestinal disease. New York, Gower Medical Publishing, 1992.

neurons) are stimulated by thermal, chemical, or mechanical events. Chronic pain occurs when noxious stimuli are continually present and maintain a background level of pain. Breakthrough pain is defined as a transient increase in pain intensity over background pain. In addition, pain is often described by the mechanism causing the pain (e.g., inflammatory, neuropathic, etc.).

Inflammatory pain is initiated by tissue damage that results in a release of many chemical mediators such as cytokines, growth factors, neurotrophic factors, white blood cells, and platelets. Neuropathic pain results from lesions that arise in the nervous system or via dysfunctions that occur as a result of neurologic deficits (3). Neuropathic pain, unlike inflammatory pain, tends to persist long after the initiating event has healed (4). Patient descriptions of neuropathic pain often include the terms burning, tingling, shooting, electrical, and sharp. Common neuropathic pain syndromes in pancreatic cancer patients include celiac plexus neuropathies, chemotherapy-induced neuropathy, and surgical neuropathy.

Pain management for patients with pancreatic cancer represents a challenge to the clinician, since about 80% of patients present with unresectable disease due to the presence of metastases or local extension (5). The typical pain of locally advanced pancreatic cancer is a dull, fairly constant pain of visceral origin localized to the region of the middle and upper back as a result of invasion of the celiac and mesenteric plexuses. This causes both neuropathic and inflammatory types of pain. Initially, pain associated with unresectable pancreatic cancer can be controlled with nonsteroidal anti-inflammatory drugs (NSAIDs) or oral narcotic combination analgesics. Pain from advanced pancreatic cancer is usually managed with opioid analgesics, radiation therapy, chemotherapy, or celiac plexus neurolysis (i.e., chemical splanchnicectomy of the celiac plexus with alcohol). Celiac plexus neurolysis eases pain without the side effects of opioids and can be administered intraoperatively, percutaneously, or by endoscopic ultrasonography.

2.1 Opioid Use

The mainstay of pain management for pancreatic cancer has been the use of opioid analgesics. Opioids primarily exert their analgesic effect through their action on supraspinal and spinal opioid receptors. Most patients will require a fixed-dose schedule to maintain optimal pain control. There is no evidence to support the selection of one particular opioid over another. However, when selecting an opioid, it is always necessary to establish whether or not the patient has any known drug allergies or past adverse experiences. Comorbid conditions, such as renal insufficiency or liver failure, will influence opioid selection. The 6-glucuronide metabolite of morphine sulfate is increased significantly in patients with decreased renal function, and these patients may exhibit morphine toxicities (6). Therefore, the use of morphine in patients with end-stage renal impairment is usually contraindicated since significant respiratory depression can occur.

The appropriate dosing interval and rate of titration of an opioid is determined largely by the medication and the patient's ability to tolerate the drug. A general rule of thumb is to start at a low dose and titrate upward until good pain relief is achieved or the patient develops intolerable side effects. Opioid agents differ by the subtype of *mu* receptor they bind to, their activity at these receptors, the pharmacokinetic profiles, and the formulations. Table 25.2 provides an example of an equianalgesic dose chart for opioids used in the management of chronic pain (7).

The most common side effects of opioids are constipation, nausea, and sleepiness. The constipation associated with chronic opioid administration is an important cause of nausea; therefore, all patients receiving chronic opioids should be cautioned about the need for daily bowel movements. Almost all patients will need a mild laxative in addition to a stool softener to maintain daily bowel movements. A good guideline for patients is that it is acceptable to miss 1 day of a bowel movement, but should be sure to take a laxative to achieve results by the following day.

The respiratory effects of opioids should be considered in opioid naïve patients, especially when combined with other central nervous system depressant drugs. However, respiratory depression is very rare when opioids are titrated appropriately.

2.2 Adjuvant Agents for Neuropathic Pain

Correct diagnosis of neuropathic pain begins with a thorough history to pinpoint the location, duration, intensity, quality, temporal pattern, and factors that cause and provide relief of the pain. Generally neuropathic pain will follow the anatomic distribution of the affect nerve. Neuropathic pain may be constant, intermittent, or both. It is often evoked by innocuous stimuli and is commonly described as numbness, tingling, or "needles and pins."

When patients with pancreatic cancer present with neuropathic signs and symptoms, an effort should be made to decrease the pain while minimizing toxicities.

Table 25.2 Equianalgesic doses for opioid analgesics used for the treatment of chronic pain

Drug	Dose (mg) equianalgesic to morphine 10 mg IM[a]		Half-life (hrs)	Duration (hr)	Comment
	PO	IM			
Morphine	20–30[b]	10	2–3	2–4	Standard for comparison
Morphine CR	20–30	10	2–3	8–12	Various formulations are not bioequivalent
Morphine SR	20–30	10	2–3	24	
Oxycodone	20		2–3	3–4	
Oxycodone CR	20		2–3	8–12	
Hydromorphone	7.5	1.5	2–3	2–4	Potency may be greater, i.e., IV hydromorphone: IV morphine = 3:1 rather than 6.7:1 during prolonged use
Methadone	20	10	12–19	4–12	Although a 1:1 ratio with morphine was used in a single-dose study, there is a change with repeated administration, and a large dose reduction (75–90%) is needed when switching to methadone
Oxymorphone	10 (rectal)	1	2–3	2–4	Available in rectal and injectable formulations
Levorphanol	4	2	12–15	4–6	
Fentanyl			7–12		Can be administered as a continuous IV or subcut infusion, based on clinical experience, 100 µg/hr is roughly equianalgesic to morphine 4 mg/hr
Fentanyl TS			16–24	48–72	Based on clinical experience, 100 µg/hr is roughly equianalgesic to morphine 4 mg/hr. A recent study indicates a ratio of oral morphine:transdermal fentanyl of 70:1 (the recommended converting ratio was 100:1)

[a] Studies to determine equianalgesic doses of opioids have used morphine by the IM route. The IM and IV routes are considered to be equivalent, and IV is the most common route used in clinical practice.

[b] Although the PO:IM morphine ratio was 6:1 in a single-dose study, other observations indicate a ratio of 2–3:1 with repeated administration.

CR, controlled-release; IM, intramuscular; IV, intravenous; PO, oral; SR, sustained-release; subcut, subcutaneous; TS, transdermal system.

Derby S, Chin J, Portenoy RK. Systemic opioid therapy for chronic cancer pain: practical guidelines for converting drugs and routes of administration. CNS Drugs 1998, 9:99–109.

Today, there are several agents that are considered to be first-line agents in the management of neuropathic pain. Table 25.3 provides a summary of those agents (8). These agents include gabapentin, the lidocaine 5% patch, tramadol, tricyclic antidepressants, and opioid analgesics. Regardless of which agent is initially selected, a standard of care is to introduce one agent at a time with a gradual dose titration based upon patient response. Older agents, such as carbamazepine, phenytoin, and valproic acid, have been used extensively. However, they have many serious side effects, such as agranulocytosis and hepatotoxicity, and their use has fallen out of favor among pain specialists.

A newer agent that has been introduced for the treatment of neuropathic pain associated with diabetic peripheral neuropathy and postherpetic neuropathy is pregabalin. The mechanism of action appears to be the same as that for gabapentin; both exert their effects via inhibition of calcium currents mediated by high-voltage–activated channels, leading to reduced neurotransmitter release and attenuation of postsynaptic excitability (9). The maximum recommended dose of pregabalin is 100 mg three times daily, with dosage adjustment for patients with renal dysfunction.

In summary, the management of the various types of pain syndromes associated with advanced pancreatic cancer can be a challenge for the clinician. Appropriate diagnosis and assessment of the pain is essential to quality patient care, and knowledge of various pharmacologic agents for management of these syndromes is of paramount importance.

3 Nausea and Vomiting

There are many potential causes for nausea and vomiting in a patient with pancreatic cancer. The differential diagnosis should include chemotherapy, radiation, opioids, obstruction, gastroparesis, constipation, hypercalcemia, brain metastases, and anxiety (10). It is well known that chemotherapy and radiation can induce nausea and vomiting. The incidence depends on the chemotherapy agents and the amount and area of radiation. Emesis can be categorized as acute, delayed, anticipatory, and breakthrough.

Chemotherapy- and radiation-induced emesis can affect a patient's quality of life as well as lead to other health-related problems. The key is to prevent nausea and vomiting by assessing the risk of occurrence in each patient as well as prescribing the appropriate antiemetic regimen based on these risks. It is important to determine the emetogenicity level of the chemotherapy regimen or radiation treatment the patient will receive. The emetogenicity of chemotherapy agents can range from minimally to highly emetogenic. There are several patient-related factors that also influence the risk of nausea and vomiting. Generally, women have more nausea and vomiting than men, whereas children have more nausea and vomiting than adults. A history of depression, motion sickness, or pregnancy-induced nausea and vomiting can predispose patients to more nausea and vomiting during chemotherapy.

Table 25.3 First-line medications for neuropathic pain

Medication	Beginning dosage	Titration	Maximum dosage	Duration of adequate trial
Gabapentin	100–300 mg every night or 100–300 mg 3 times daily	Increase by 100–300 mg 3 times daily every 1–7 d as tolerated	3,600 mg/d (1,200 mg 3 times daily); reduce if low creatinine clearance	3–8 wk for titration plus 1–2 wk at maximum tolerated dosage
5% Lidocaine patch	Maximum of 3 patches daily for a maximum of 12 h	None needed	Maximum of 3 patches daily for a maximum of 12 h	2 wk
Opioid analgesics[a]	5–15 mg every 4 h as needed	After 1–2 wk, convert total daily dosage to long-acting opioid analgesic and continue short-acting medication as needed	No maximum with careful titration; consider evaluation by pain specialist at dosages exceeding 120–180 mg/d	4–6 wk
Tramadol hydrochloride	50 mg once or twice daily	Increase by 50–100 mg/d in divided doses every 3–7 d as tolerated	400 mg/d (100 mg 4 times daily); in patients older than 75 y, 300 mg/d in divided doses	4 wk
Tricyclic antidepressants (e.g., nortriptyline hydrochloride or desipramine hydrochloride)	10–25 mg every night	Increase by 10–25 mg/d every 3–7 d as tolerated	75–100 mg/d; if blood level of active drug and its metabolite is <100 ng/ml, continue titration with caution	6–8 wk with at least 1–2 wk at maximum tolerated dosage

[a] Dosages given are for morphine sulfate.
Adapted from Dworkin RH, Backonja M, Rowbotham MC, et al. Advances in neuropathic pain. Arch Neurol 2003; 60:1524–1534.

Poor control of nausea and vomiting during prior chemotherapy increases the risk of nausea and vomiting during subsequent cycles. Patients with a history of chronic alcohol consumption have a decreased risk of emesis (11).

An antiemetic regimen should begin prior to chemotherapy in order to offer the highest protection against chemotherapy-induced nausea and vomiting. Antiemetics can be given via the oral, intravenous, rectal, and intramuscular route. Oral administration of antiemetics is equally effective and safe as other routes of administration (10, 12). Oral agents are also easier to administer and cost less.

Many antiemetic agents are available for the prevention and treatment of chemotherapy- and radiation-induced nausea and vomiting. Antiemetics with the highest therapeutic index include: serotonin receptor antagonists, corticosteroids, and neurokinin-1 receptor antagonists. Adding a corticosteroid to a serotonin receptor antagonist has been shown to increase the efficacy by 20% (13, 14). Head-to-head comparisons to serotonin antagonists have not shown any significant difference in efficacy (15, 16). Dopamine antagonists, butyrophenones, phenothiazines, and cannabinoids have a lower therapeutic index (Table 25.4). Benzodiazepines can also be use adjunctively, mainly in the setting of anticipatory nausea and vomiting.

Several guidelines for the prevention and treatment of chemotherapy- and radiation-induced nausea and vomiting exist (10, 12, 17). Tables 25.5–25.7 summarize the recommended antiemetic regimens for the prevention of both acute and delayed chemotherapy-induced nausea and vomiting as well as for radiation-induced nausea and vomiting. It is easier to prevent nausea and vomiting than it is to treat it once it occurs. Prevention should provide antiemetic coverage through the full period of risk, including the acute emesis period and the delayed emesis period if appropriate. The antiemetic regimen should also include a rescue agent from a different class for the treatment of breakthrough emesis. It is important to evaluate each patient individually and be flexible since many appropriate antiemetic regimens are available. If a patient does not respond to an agent it is still beneficial to try a different agent in the same class before concluding the patient has failed a particular therapy.

Many pancreatic patients experience pain requiring acute and chronic narcotic regimens. Approximately 10–40% of patients will experience nausea and vomiting with the introduction of therapy with opioids (18, 19). Many patients will acclimate to the nausea and vomiting within a week of initiation of opioids but it is reasonable to initially prescribe an antiemetic with the opioid (20). The agents available for the treatment of opioid-induced emesis are similar to the agents for the treatment of chemotherapy-induced emesis. Prescribing prochlorperazine, promethazine, and metoclopramide on an as-needed basis are appropriate initial choices. If this does not control nausea and vomiting, then scheduling the antiemetic around the clock for approximately 1 week should occur next. Other treatment options include switching opioids or adding a coanalgesic to allow reduction of the opioid dose (10). Serotonin antagonists can be utilized but there are no current data to support their use in this setting.

Table 25.4 Dosing and schedule of antiemetic agents in adults

Antiemetic agent (trade name)	Recommended dose and schedule	Therapeutic class
Dolasetron (Anzemet®)	• 100–200 mg orally/day • 100 mg IV/day or 1.8 mg/kg IV/day	Serotonin antagonist
Granisetron (Kytril®)	• 2 mg orally/day or 1 mg BID orally • 1 mg IV/day or 0.01 mg/kg IV/day	
Ondansetron (Zofran®)	• 24 mg orally/day for highly emetogenic 8mg orally/day for moderately emetogenic • 8 mg IV/day or 0.15 mg/kg IV/day	
Palonosetron (Aloxi®)	• 0.25 mg IV × 1 dose only	
Aprepitant (Emend®)	• 125 mg orally on Day 1 followed by 80 mg orally /day on Days 2–3	Neurkininin-1 receptor antagonist
Dexamethasone (Decadron®)	• 12–20 mg orally/day for highly emetogenic 8–10 mg orally/day for moderately emetogenic • 4–8 mg orally BID × 3–4 days for delayed	Corticosteroid
Metoclopramide (Reglan®)	• 1–2 mg/kg orally or IV every 2–4 h • 0.5 mg/kg or 20–30 mg orally or IV every 6 h for delayed	Dopamine receptor antagonist
Prochlorperazine (Compazine®)	• 5–20 mg orally or IV every 6 h • 15–30 mg every 12 h for extended release • 25 mg rectally every 12 h	
Promethazine (Phenergan®)	12.5–25 mg orally, IV, IM, or rectally every 4–6 h	
Haloperidol (Haldol®)	• 1–4 mg orally, IV, or IM every 6–8 h	
Trimethobenzamide (Tigan®)	• 250 mg orally every 6–8 h • 200 mg IM every 6–8 h	
Dronabinol (Marinol®)	• 5-20 mg orally every 3–6 h	Cannabinoid
Diazepam (Valium®)	• 2-10 mg orally or IV every 6–12 h	Benzodiazepine
Lorazepam (Ativan®)	• 0.5–2 mg orally/sublingually or IV every 6–8 h	

Adapted from references *12, 17, 35, 36, 37, 38*.

Table 25.5 Treatment recommendations for the prevention of acute chemotherapy-induced nausea and vomiting

Emetic risk	Antiemetic regimen
High	Serotonin receptor antagonist + dexamethasone + aprepitant
Moderate	Serotonin receptor antagonist + dexamethasone
Low	Dexamethasone
Minimal	None

Adapted from reference *12*.

Table 25.6 Treatment recommendations for the prevention of delayed chemotherapy-induced nausea and vomiting

Emetic risk	Antiemetic regimen
High	Serotonin receptor antagonist + dexamethasone
Moderate	Dexamethasone or serotonin receptor antagonist
Low	None
Minimal	None

Adapted from reference *12*.

Table 25.7 Treatment recommendations for the prevention of radiation-induced nausea and vomiting

Emetic risk	Antiemetic regimen
High	Serotonin receptor antagonist ± dexamethasone
Moderate	Serotonin receptor antagonist
Low	Serotonin receptor antagonist
Minimal	None

Adapted from reference *12*.

4 Bowel Dysfunction

Coordination of motility, mucosal transport, and defecation reflexes is necessary for normal bowel function (*21*). Both constipation and diarrhea can lead to the disruption of normal bowel function in patients with pancreatic cancer.

4.1 Constipation

There are several reasons why patients with cancer may develop constipation. Frequent causes include obstruction, hypercalcemia, bowel surgery, dehydration, and medications. Antidepressants, antiemetics, vinca alkaloids, and opioids are mediations commonly used by cancer patients that can cause constipation (*21*).

Opioid analgesics are commonly used for the treatment of cancer-related pain. Although these agents can effective at controlling pain, constipation can be a concerning adverse effect and is the most common side effect associated with chronic opioid therapy (*22*). Opioid-induced bowel dysfunction is a phrase that represents a collection of symptoms, including hard dry stools, straining, incomplete evacuation, bloating, abdominal distention, and increased gastroesophageal reflux (*23*). Opioid-induced bowel dysfunction occurred in >50% of cancer patients admitted to palliative care units (*24*). Elderly patients experience opioid bowel dysfunction more frequently than younger patients (*25*).

Opioids cause bowel dysfunction via several mechanisms. They decrease gastrointestinal neural activity, reduce propulsive activity, delay transit of contents through the small and large bowel, and enhance absorption of fluids (*23, 25*).

Sequelae of opioid-induced bowel dysfunction include: fecal impaction; pseudo-obstruction of the bowel leading to anorexia, nausea, and vomiting; inadequate absorption of drugs taken orally; urinary retention and incontinence; and confusion (21, 26). Not only does this symptom cause physical discomfort it can affect quality of life. If tolerance to bowel symptoms develops, it occurs slowly (27, 28).

The goal for the management of opioid-induced bowel dysfunction is to prevent the occurrence instead of treating it after it has occurred. Therefore, starting a bowel regimen at initiation of opioid therapy is imperative. It is also very important to assess baseline bowel habits prior to starting opioids. Frequent monitoring of opioid-associated constipation should occur once opioid therapy is initiated.

Common pharmacologic bowel regimens include stool softeners in combination with laxatives (22). Stimulant laxatives, such as bisacodyl and senna, are commonly used for chronic prophylaxis, whereas mineral oil, lactulose, magnesium citrate, and polyethylene glycol-electrolyte solution are frequently used to treat constipation once it occurs. Suppositories and enemas are alternatives to oral therapies but are often limited to short-term management or more severe cases of constipation. Impaction should be ruled out before initiating treatment. Nonpharmacologic approaches consist of increased consumption of fluids and dietary fiber.

4.2   Diarrhea

There are many potential causes of diarrhea in cancer patients, including laxative use, anti-infective agents, surgery, radiation therapy, and chemotherapy (29). Diarrhea occurs more commonly with some chemotherapy treatment than others. It is well known that fluorouracil, irinotecan, and abdominal or pelvic radiation can cause diarrhea (30). Diarrhea can result in fluid and electrolyte depletion, malnutrition, and renal insufficiency (30). Diarrhea associated with cancer treatment can influence a patient's quality of life and in some cases can cause treatment changes (31). Secretory diarrhea is the most common type of diarrhea related to cancer treatments (29). Due to the pancreatic exocrine insufficiency in some pancreatic cancer patients, malabsorption and steatorrhea may occur, which could lead to diarrhea.

Fluid and electrolyte replacement in addition to antidiarrheal agents are the mainstay for the treatment of diarrhea. Several oral agents are available for the practical management of diarrhea. Loperamide, opium, and diphenoxylate are opioid agonists that decrease the release of acetylcholine from gut efferent nerve endings resulting in slower intestinal motility (32). These agents are sufficient for the majority of patients with mild symptoms and are often used as first line treatment of cancer treatment induced diarrhea. These agents should be used cautiously in cancer patients that might have diarrhea caused by infection. Loperamide should be initiated with a single dose of 4 mg followed by 2 mg every 2–4 hours as needed, exceeding the standard limit of 16 mg per day (30). Octreotide, an antisecretory agent, is an intravenous treatment option often reserved for more serious cases of diarrhea or diarrhea unresponsive to oral therapy. Currently, the optimal dose of octreotide has not been established. Data from recent studies indicated that higher doses (500 μg TID) may be more beneficial than lower doses (*30*). Octreotide doses up to 2500 μg TID have been effective in patients experiencing diarrhea with fluorouracil regimens (*33*).

Pelvic radiation can cause diarrhea, and the addition of fluorouracil to pelvic radiation leads to higher rates of severe diarrhea (*34*). Radiation-induced diarrhea can often be managed with continued loperamide as well as with adsorbents such as cholestyramine (*29, 30*).

The American Society of Clinical Oncology has published guidelines for the treatment of cancer treatment–induced diarrhea. These guidelines have categorized diarrhea into two types, uncomplicated and complicated. Their recommendations for treatment are based the type of diarrhea and reflect the necessity for early and aggressive treatment for patients with complicated diarrhea.

5 Summary

The management of symptoms of patients with pancreatic cancer can be challenging for the clinician. Goals for the management of these symptoms should be set by both the patient and clinician to be attainable. It is imperative to balance therapeutic goals with potential side effects of the treatments, and patients must be educated about realistic expectations. The management of pain, nausea and vomiting, constipation, and diarrhea in the patient with pancreatic cancer may be the focus of treatment in patients with advanced disease.

References

1. DiMagno EP. 1992, Cancer of the pancreas and biliary tract. In: Winawer SJ (ed.) Management of gastrointestinal disease. Gower Medical Publishing, New York.
2. Molinari M, Helton WS, Espat NJ. 2001, Palliative strategies for locally advanced unresectable and metastatic pancreatic cancer. Surg Clin North Am 81:651–666.
3. Chong MJ, Bajwa ZH. 2003, Diagnosis and treatment of neuropathic pain. J Pain Symtpm Manage 25(5 Suppl):S4–S11.
4. Woolf CJ, Salter MW. 2000, Neuronal plasticity: increasing the gain in pain. Science 288:1765–1769.
5. Evans DB, Abbruzzese JL, Willett CG. 2001, Cancer of the pancreas. In: DeVita VT, Hellman S, Rosenberg SA (eds.) Cancer: principles and practice of oncology, 6th ed. Philadelphia, Lippincott Williams & Wilkins, 1126–1161.
6. Mercadante S, Arcuri E. 2004, Opioids and renal function. J Pain 5:2–19.
7. Derby S, Chin J, Portenoy RK. 1998, Systemic opioid therapy for chronic cancer pain: practical guidelines for converting drugs and routes of administration. CNS Drugs 9:99–109.
8. Dworkin RH, Backonja M, Rowbotham MC, et al. 2003, Advances in neuropathic pain. Arch Neurol 60:1524–1534.
9. Sills GJ. 2006, The mechanisms of action of gabapentin and pregabalin. Curr Opin Pharmacol 6:108–113.

10. Clinical Practice Guideline in Oncology v.2.2006 Antiemesis. NCCN, 2006 (Accessed 05/20/06).
11. Beckwith M, Mullin S. 2001, Prevention and management of chemotherapy-induced nausea and vomiting, part 1. Hospital Pharmacy 36:67–80.
12. Kris M, Hesketh P, Somerfield M, et al. 2006, American Society of Clinical Oncology guideline for antiemetics in oncology: update 2006. J Clin Oncol 24, epub May 22.
13. Kris M, Baltzer L, Pisters K, et al. 1993, Enhancing the effectiveness of the specifc serotonin antagonists. Cancer 72(Suppl 11):3436 –3642.
14. Kris M, Pendergrass K, Navari R, et al. 1997, Prevention of acute emesis in cancer patients following high-dose cisplatin with the combination of oral dolasetron and dexamethasone. J Clin Oncol 15: 2135–2138.
15. Hesketh P, Navari R, Grote T, et al. 1996, Double-blind, randomized comparison of the antiemetic efficacy of intravenous dolasetron and intravenous ondansetron in the prevention of acute cisplatin-induced emesis in patients with cancer. Dolasetron Comparative Chemotherapy-induced Emesis Prevention Group. J Clin Oncol 14:2242–2249.
16. Navari R, Gandara D, Hesketh P, et al. 1995, Comparative clinical trial of granisetron and ondansetron in the prophylaxis of cisplatin-induced emesis. The Gransistron Study Group. J Clin Oncol 13:1242–1248.
17. Antiemetic Subcommittee of the Multinational Association of Supportive Care in Cancer (MASCC). 1998, Prevention of chemotherapy- and radiotherapy-induced emesis: results of the Perugia consensus conference. Ann Oncol 9: 811–819.
18. Campora E, Merlini L, Pace M, et al. 1991, The incidence of narcotic-induced emesis. J Pain Symptom Manage 6:428–430.
19. Asparasu R, McCoy R, Weber C, et al. 1999, Opioid-induced emesis among hospitalized nonsurgical patients: effect on pain and quality of life. J Pain Symptom Manage 18:280–288.
20. Nicholson B. 2003, Responsible prescribing of opioids for the management of chronic pain. Drugs 63:17–32.
21. Mancini I, Bruera E, 1998, Constipation in advanced cancer patients. Support Care Cancer 6:356–364.
22. Herndon M, Jackson K, Hallin P. 2002, Management of opioid-induced gastrointestinal effects in patients receiving palliative care. Pharmacotherapy 22:240–250.
23. Pappagallo M. 2001, Incidence, prevalence, and management of opioid bowel dysfunction. Am J Surg 182:11S–18S.
24. Grond S, Zech D, Diefenbach C, et al. 1994, Prevalence and pattern of symptoms in patients with cancer pain: a prospective evaluation of 1635 cancer patients referred to a pain clinic. J Pain Symptom Manage 9:372–382.
25. Vanegas G, Ripamonti C, Sbanotto A, et al. 1998, Side of effects of morphine administration in cancer patients. Cancer Nurs 21:289–297.
26. Glare P, Lickiss J. 1992, Unrecognized constipation in patients with advanced cancer: a recipe for therapeutic disaster. J Pain Symptom Manage 7:369–371.
27. Fallon M, Hanks G. 1999, Morphine, constipation and performance status in advanced cancer patients. Palliative Medicine 13:159–160.
28. Sykes N. 1998, The relationship between opioid use and laxative use in terminally ill cancer patients. Palliative Medicine 12:375–382.
29. Ippoliti C. 1998, Antidiarrheal agents for the management of treatment-related diarrhea in cancer patients. Am J Health-Syst Pharm 55:1573–1580.
30. Benson A, Ajani J, Calalano R, et al. 2004, Recommended guidelines for the treatment of cancer treatment-induced diarrhea. J Clin Oncol 22:2918–2926.
31. Arbucle R, Huber S, Zacker C. 2000, The consequences of diarrhea occurring during chemotherapy for colorectal cancer: a retrospective study. Oncologist 5:250–259.
32. Schiller L. 1995, Review article: anti-diarrhoeal pharmacology and therapeutics. Aliment Pharmacol Ther 9:87–106.
33. Wadler S, Haynes H, Wiernik PH. 1995, Phase I trial of the somatostatin analog octreotide acetate in the treatment of fluoropyrimidine-induced diarrhea. J Clin Oncol 13:222–226.

34. Miller R, Martenson J, Sargent D, et al. 1998, Acute treatment-related diarrhea during post-operative adjuvant therapy for high-risk rectal carcinoma. Int J Radiation Oncol Biol Phys 41:593–598.
35. Gralla R, Osoba D, Kris M, et al. 1999, Recommendations for the use of antiemetics: evidence-based clinical practice guidelines. J Clin Oncol 17:2971–2994.
36. American Society of Health-System Pharmacists. 1999, ASHP therapeutic guidelines on the pharmacologic management of nausea and vomiting in adult and pediatric patients receiving chemotherapy or radiation therapy or undergoing surgery. Am J Health-Syst Pharm 56:729–764.
37. Koeller J, Aapro M, Gralla R, et al. 2002, Antiemetic guidelines: creating a more practical treatment approach. Support Care Cancer 10:519–522.
38. Kris M, Hesketh P, Herrstedt J, et al. 2005, Consensus proposals for the prevention of acute and delayed vomiting and nausea following high-emetic-risk chemotherapy. Support Care Cancer 13:85–96.

Chapter 26
Supportive Care: Cachexia, Anorexia Syndrome

Michael John Tisdale

1 Introduction

Patients with pancreatic cancer have a high frequency of cachexia (85%) (*1*), which is characterized by progressive weight loss and depletion of both adipose tissue and skeletal muscle mass. Even at the time of diagnosis, weight loss is apparent (median 14.2% of pre-illness stable weight), and this weight loss is progressive in the absence of effective treatment, increasing to a median of 24.5% over a 6-month period (*2*). Death normally occurs when the weight loss reaches about 30%, and is likely due to impairment of respiratory muscle function through loss of lean body mass, which decreases from 43.4 to 40.1 kg (*2*). There is also a substantive loss of body fat from 12.5 to 9.6 kg. In a study to establish factors influencing survival of cancer patients after diagnosis of terminal cancer of the lung, breast, and GI tract, shorter survival was independently associated with a weight loss of >8.1 kg in the previous 6 months and serum albumin levels of <35 g/L (*3*). In patients with advanced pancreatic cancer there is also a strong inverse relationship between the severity of weight loss and the performance score (*4*). In addition to the poor survival, patients with weight loss have a lower probability of responding to palliative chemotherapy and a lower quality of life as well as problems with pain or fatigue (*5*).

2 Anorexia and Cachexia

Anorexia is common in patients with pancreatic cancer, especially in those with advanced disease. In patients with pancreatic cancer a relationship has been found between caloric intake and survival (*6*). Thus survival was found to be significantly longer for high versus low intake calorie groups (50 versus 32 days). This may reflect the stage of the disease, rather than caloric intake per se, since clinical trials providing extra calories in the form of total parenteral nutrition (TPN) have been shown to have no effect on the median survival time of patients with advanced cancer (*7*). Although anorexia frequently accompanies cachexia, many patients continue to lose weight, even when receiving added calories that would be predicted to

A.M. Lowy et al. (eds.) *Pancreatic Cancer*.
doi: 10.1007/978-0-387-69252-4, © Springer Science+Business Media, LLC 2008

result in weight gain. Cachectic patients who do gain weight by provision of excess calories show an increase only in body fat, without a significant change in total body nitrogen (8). A diminished dietary intake could not account for weight loss in a study of 297 unselected cancer patients with solid tumors, since energy intake in absolute amounts was not different, and intake per kg body weight was actually higher in weight-losing patients compared with weight-stable patients (9). The dietary macro-nutrient composition of weight-losing patients did not differ from the general popu-lation, although the intake of energy and protein were decreased. However, there was no compensation for the weight loss by an increase in food intake.

Cancer anorexia appears to be the result of an imbalance between neuropeptide Y (NPY) (orexigenic) and pro-opiomelanocortin (POMC) (anorexigenic) signals favouring the latter (10). NPY neurons increase parasympathetic output and decrease resting energy expenditure (REE), whereas POMC stimulates sympathetic activity and increases REE.

3 Energy Expenditure

If food intake alone is not responsible for the weight loss in pancreatic cancer patients, then a reduced intake combined with an increased REE could be an important factor. In home-living cachectic patients with advanced pancreatic can-cer REE was found to be increased compared with the predicted values for healthy individuals, while total energy expenditure (TEE) and physical activity level (PAL) were reduced (11). The increase in REE is due to increased operation of futile cycles such as the Cori cycle, whereby lactate produced by tumors by the glycolytic metabolism of glucose is converted back into glucose in the liver. This is an energy consuming process and the Cori cycle may account for a loss of energy of 300 kcal/day (12). Energy can be lost through an increased expression and activity of uncoupling proteins. These are proteins that transport protons across the inner mitochondrial membrane, without being coupled to ADP phos-phorylation, resulting in the energy being released as heat. There are at least three uncoupling proteins (UCPs); UCP-1, -2, and -3. UCP-1 is only found in brown adipose tissue (BAT) mitochondria and is considered to be the main UCP. However, since there is little BAT in adult humans the role of UCP-1 may be taken up by UCP-3, which is also found in skeletal muscle as well as in BAT. Transgenic mice overexpressing UCP-3 in skeletal muscle are hyperphagic, but weigh less than their wild-type littermates, and there is a large reduction in mass of adipose tissue (13). UCP-3 mRNA levels in skeletal muscle have been found to be increased in both rats and mice bearing cachexia-inducing tumors. UCP-3 mRNA levels have also been shown to be five times higher in the skeletal muscle of cancer patients with weight loss compared with controls and with cancer patients who had not lost weight, whereas UCP-2 mRNA levels did not differ significantly between groups (14). This increase in UCP-3 may enhance energy expenditure and this could contribute to tissue catabolism.

The most hypermetabolic pancreatic cancer patients are those with an ongoing hepatic acute phase response (APR) (*15*). Increased serum levels of acute phase proteins (APP), such as fibrinogen and C-reactive protein (CRP), have been associated with a shorter survival time of pancreatic cancer patients (*16*). The link between REE and the APR is not clear, but it could be due to increased APP synthesis in the liver. The cyclo-oxygenase inhibitor ibuprofen has been shown to significantly reduce the high REE and serum CRP levels in patients with pancreatic cancer, suggesting that it may have a role in preventing the catabolic processes that contribute to weight loss (*17*).

4 Tissue Wasting in Cachexia

Depletion of both adipose tissue and skeletal muscle in cancer cachexia results from the combined effect of an increase in catabolism combined with a decrease in anabolism. However, the catabolic effect is probably the most important, since anabolic stimuli alone are unable to reverse the wasting process. An increased lipolysis would result in the higher fasting plasma glycerol levels in weight-losing cancer patients compared with weight-stable individuals (*18*). Muscle atrophy in patients with pancreatic cancer has been attributed to an increased expression of the ubiquitin-proteasome proteolytic pathway for patients with a weight loss of greater than 10% (*19*). Experiments using in vitro and in vivo models of muscle wasting suggest that cachectic factors are remarkably selective in targeting myosin heavy chain, while other core myofibrillar proteins including troponin T, tropomyosin (α and β forms) and α-sarcomeric actin did not change (*20*). In vitro loss of myosin was attributed to an RNA-dependent mechanism, while in vivo, in mice bearing colon-26 tumors, loss of myosin was associated with the ubiquitin-proteasome pathway. Thus it seems that muscle atrophy does not result from a general down-regulation of muscle proteins, but is highly selective as to which proteins are targeted during the wasting state.

In addition to the ubiquitin-proteasome pathway, apoptosis of muscle cells may play a role in skeletal muscle atrophy, although the magnitude of this effect has not been quantitated. Thus apoptosis in skeletal muscle of rabbits implanted with the VX2-tumor was found to be elevated in the early stages of loss of lean body mass (18%), but decreased almost to control levels by the time the loss of lean body mass reached 30% (*21*). In contrast total DNA fragmentation, as a measure of apoptosis, increased with total tumor burden in rats bearing the Yoshida AH-130 ascites hepatoma and in mice bearing the Lewis lung carcinoma (*22*).

Lipolysis in adipose tissue appears to be due to up-regulation of hormone sensitive lipase resulting in an increased release of free fatty acids (*23*). Cancer patients have been shown to have a twofold elevation in serum triacylglycerol and FFA compared with normal controls, without an effect on the mRNA for the synthetic enzyme lipoprotein lipase (LPL). In patients with pancreatic cancer, leptin concentrations, when corrected for body mass index, were lower than levels reported for healthy subjects, reflecting a lower mass of adipose tissue (24). There was no association between patients with increased leptin concentrations and weight loss or anorexia, and leptin does not appear to mediate the metabolic changes of the APR.

There are a number of factors that can be considered as candidates for the induction of tissue wasting in pancreatic cancer patients.

5   Mediators of Cachexia

Although certain tumor types are commonly associated with cachexia, even with the same tumor type there are variations in the extent to which patients become cachectic. Thus even in pancreatic cancer up to 15% of the patients do not become cachectic. This is probably due to variations in tumor phenotype resulting in some tumors producing and releasing circulatory factors that induce atrophy of adipose tissue and skeletal muscle (25). There may also be variations in host genotype, which resist the development of cachexia, although none have been found to date. There are a number of factors produced both by tumor and host tissue that have the potential to induce the wasting process characteristic of cancer cachexia.

5.1   Tumor Necrosis Factor (TNF-α)

Tumor necrosis factor (TNF-α) or cachectin was originally identified as a cachectic factor from studies on the mechanism of weight loss in rabbits chronically infected with *Trypanosoma brucei brucei,* and was also suggested to play a similar role in cancer cachexia (26). Although elevated circulating TNF-α levels have been reported in AIDS patients (27) most studies of patients with cancer cachexia have not been able to detect elevated TNF-α, or if elevated levels were detected this did not correlate with weight loss, but with the stage of the disease. Some of the studies are contradictory. Thus, while Ebrahimi et al. (28) found that circulating levels of TNF-α were not significantly elevated in patients with pancreatic carcinoma, another study (29) found serum levels of TNF-α to be detectable in 36.5% of pancreatic cancer patients, with higher levels in patients with metastatic compared with non-metastatic disease. Serum levels of TNF-α inversely correlated with body weight and body mass index, as well as serum albumin levels. These differences may reflect differences in the sensitivity of the immunoassays used to detect TNF-α, but many more studies have reported an inability to detect TNF-α in cancer cachexia than those reporting an increase. It has been suggested that increases in TNF-α in the serum of cancer patients may be transient, although this would not explain why it has been found in other weight-losing conditions.

Certainly TNF-α has the potential to induce loss of skeletal muscle and adipose tissue in cancer cachexia. Thus implantation of Chinese hamster ovary cells

(CHO) transfected with the human TNF-α gene into nude mice produced a syndrome resembling cancer cachexia with progressive wasting, anorexia and early death (30). A single IV injection of TNF-α increased BAT thermogenesis, as measured by mitochondrial GDP binding as well as producing a significant increase in UCP-2 and UCP-3 gene expression in skeletal muscle (31). This may play a role in the increase in energy expenditure associated with cytokine treatment. Treatment with TNF-α also causes loss of skeletal muscle protein through a depression in protein synthesis and an increase in degradation, which is associated with an increase in gene expression, and higher levels of free and conjugated ubiquitin (32). Loss of adipose tissue after treatment with TNF-α was originally thought to be due to inhibition of the clearing enzyme LPL, which would attenuate lipogenesis (33). However, TNF-α has also been shown to directly stimulate lipolysis in human adipocytes by activation of mitogen-activated protein kinase (MEK) and extracellular signal-related kinase (ERK), producing an increase in cyclic AMP, which would then activate hormone sensitive lipase, as with the lipolytic hormones (34).

5.2 Interleukin-6 (IL-6)

In contrast to TNF-α, IL-6 is generally detectable in serum or plasma of cancer patients. Thus an elevated level of IL-6 and APR has been found in weight losing patients with non-small cell lung cancer, compared with patients with the same tumour, but without weight loss (35). In a study of 28 terminally ill cancer patients IL-6 levels increased gradually during the early stages of cachexia and then showed a sudden and steep rise just before death (36). Circulating levels of IL-6 are also significantly elevated in patients with pancreatic carcinoma, and patients with levels >5.2 pg/ml had a significantly worse survival compared with patients with lower levels. Higher levels were also associated with a poor performance status and/or weight loss (28). IL-6 together with IL-8 are important proinflammatory cytokines involved in the induction of the APR.

IL-6 has the potential to act as a cachectic factor. Atrophy of muscle is observed in IL-6 transgenic mice, which is completely blocked by anti-mouse IL-6 receptor antibody (37). Muscle atrophy was associated with increased mRNA levels for cathepsins B and L, as well as mRNA levels of poly and monoubiquitin, although other studies (32), in which IL-6 was administered IV into rats could not detect any changes in expression of ubiquitin mRNA. An increase in whole body lipolysis and/or fat oxidation was observed after infusion of recombinant human IL-6 in resting humans (38). As with TNF-α this effect could result from inhibition of LPL (33), although IL-6 may also directly increase lipolysis and fat oxidation in adipocytes. Evidence for a role for IL-6 in cancer cachexia has mainly come from the murine colon-26 adenocarcinoma model, although such studies suggest that IL-6 may not act alone to produce cachexia, and that an additional unknown factor may be responsible (39).

5.3 Other Cytokines

A number of other cytokines including interleukin-1 (IL-1) and interferon-γ (IFN-γ) have been implicated in the induction of cachexia in animal models. However, as with TNF-α no correlation has been found between serum levels of IL-1 or IFN-γ and cachexia or anorexia in patients with advanced and terminal cancer (*40*), although both cytokines induced ubiquitin mRNA expression in the skeletal muscle of rats, and thus have the potential to induce protein degradation (*32*). The serum concentration of soluble IL-2 receptor has been found to be highest in cachectic patients and was inversely correlated with the serum concentration of nutritional parameters such as prealbumin and transferrin (*41*). The length of survival of cachectic patients was inversely correlated with the serum concentration of soluble IL-2 receptor.

5.4 Zinc α2-Glycoprotein

The search for a lipid mobilizing factor (LMF), associated with cancer cachexia, led to the isolation of a 43-kDa glycoprotein from the urine of cancer patients with weight loss, which was subsequently shown to be zinc α2-glycoprotein (ZAG) (*42*). LMF/ZAG stimulates lipolysis directly in isolated adipocytes, through stimulation of adenylate cyclase, in a GTP-dependent process, through interaction with the β3-adrenergic receptor (β3-AR) (*43*). ZAG also induces an increase in expression of UCP-1 and -2 in isolated BAT, through interaction with the β3-AR, and an increase in UCP-3 in murine myotubes through activation of mitogen activated protein kinase (*44*). In vivo studies using obese male mice showed ZAG to induce a loss of body weight, without a reduction in food intake, which was attributed entirely to the loss of body fat, without a reduction in food and water intake (*45*). This was attributed to the lipolytic effect of ZAG coupled with an increase in energy expenditure, due to induction of UCP-1 expression in BAT. ZAG is expressed not only by cachexia-inducing tumors, but also by white adipose tissue (WAT) and BAT (*46*). Moreover, ZAG expression in WAT and BAT increased 10- and 3-fold, respectively, in cachectic mice, which had lost 19% of their body weight, and 60% of their adipose tissue. This increase in ZAG expression appears to be induced by glucocorticoids (*47*), and the glucocorticoid receptor antagonist, RU38486, attenuated both the loss of body weight and increase in ZAG expression in WAT in mice bearing a cachexia-inducing tumour. Other anti-cachectic agents such as eicosapentaenoic acid (EPA) also down-regulate ZAG expression in WAT and BAT by opposing the action of glucocorticoids (*48*). There have been no direct measurements of circulating ZAG levels in cachectic cancer patients, although the ability of serum or urine to induce lipolysis in isolated adipocytes was found to be significantly higher (twofold) in cancer patients with weight loss, compared with weight-losing patients with Alzheimer's disease, non–weight-losing cancer patients or healthy controls (*49*).

5.5   Proteolysis-Inducing Factor

Bioassays of serum from cancer patients with a weight loss >10% provided evidence for a circulating factor capable of producing protein degradation in isolated gastrocnemius muscle (50). This factor, named proteolysis-inducing factor (PIF), was subsequently isolated from the urine of cachectic patients with pancreatic cancer, and was shown to be a sulfated glycoprotein of molecular mass 24 kDa, and unlike any of the known cytokines (51). Although PIF has been identified in the urine of weight-losing patients with other types of cancer, it was not detectable in other weight-losing conditions such as sepsis, multiple injuries, surgery, or sleeping sickness (52). Experiments in mice suggest that PIF may be an embryonic protein expressed during the stage of patterning and eventual development of skeletal muscle, and that it may be abnormally expressed in certain tumors (53). Administration of PIF to normal mice caused profound weight loss (about 10% in 24 hours) without a reduction in food and water intake. The major contributor to the loss of body weight was lean body mass, and this was found to arise from a depression in protein synthesis (by 50%) and an increase in protein degradation (by 50%), as occurs in the skeletal muscle of cachectic cancer patients (54). Unlike the cytokines PIF induces protein degradation directly in isolated murine myotubes, and the effect both in vitro and in vivo is due to an increase in activity and expression of the ubiquitin-proteasome proteolytic pathway (55). PIF induces an intracellular signalling pathway in skeletal muscle, which results in the activation of the transcription factor nuclear factor-κB (NF-κB), leading to increased expression of proteasome subunits and ubiquitin conjugating enzyme (56). PIF has been detected in the urine of 80% of patients with pancreatic cancer, and these patients had a significantly greater total weight loss and rate of weight loss than patients whose urine did not contain PIF, but this was not associated with a reduced survival (57). PIF also activates NF-κB and the transcription factor STAT3 in human hepatocytes, resulting in the increased production of IL-6, IL-8, and CRP, and the decreased production of transferrin (53). Thus PIF is likely to be involved in the proinflammatory response in cachexia.

5.6   Angiotensin II

Angiotensin II (Ang II) is capable of causing anorexia and wasting in animal models with a decrease in lean body mass arising from an increased protein breakdown (58). Protein degradation is mediated through the ubiquitin-proteasome proteolytic pathway, since mRNA levels of the ubiquitin-ligases atrogin-1 and muscle ring-finger-1 (MuRF1) were upregulated in skeletal muscle by Ang II (59). Ang II also directly induces protein degradation in vitro, suggesting a direct effect, and the cellular signaling pathway leading to increased proteasome expression and activity appears to be the same as with PIF, through activation of NF-κB (60). Ang II has also been shown to directly inhibit protein synthesis in murine myotubes and the effect is attenuated by insulin-like growth factor 1 (IGF-1) (*61*). There are no reports of Ang II having an effect on adipose tissue.

6   Agents Used in the Treatment of Cachexia

6.1   Progestins

The progestational agents megestrol acetate (Megace) and medroxyprogesterone acetate (MPA) are appetite stimulants and have been evaluated in the treatment of cancer cachexia/anorexia. All studies with Megace report an increase in appetite and weight gain of variable degrees (*62*). However, some studies with MPA, although reporting an improvement in appetite, did not find any weight gain (*63*). Long-term treatment with Megace (>12 weeks) results in side effects, principally hypertension and edema resulting from water retention, as well as thromboembolic events (*62*). For both Megace (*64*) and MPA (*65*) measurements of body composition using dual energy X-ray absorptiometry and tritiated body water at the time of weight gain showed that the majority of the gained weight resulted from an increase in adipose tissue, and some body fluid, but there was no increase in lean body mass. This explains why the performance status (Karnofsky index) was not improved with either agent. MPA has been shown to reduce levels of the cytokines IL-1β, IL-6, and TNF-α produced by peripheral blood mononuclear cells of cancer patients in response to phytohemagglutinin stimulation (*66*). This result may explain the appetite promoting effect of progestational agents.

6.2   Eicosapentaenoic Acid

Animal studies have shown that of the two principal omega-3 fatty acids found in fish oil, only eicosapentaenoic acid (EPA) has an anticachectic effect, whereas DHA is devoid of therapeutic activity in this area (*67*). Despite this the two omega-3 fatty acids are often used in combination in clinical studies and sometimes the dose is calculated as the total omega-3 fatty acids rather than EPA alone. However, there have been promising results in the treatment of cachexia with fish oil, particularly for patients with pancreatic cancer. The optimum dose of EPA is around 2 g per day, or slightly higher, and treatment needs to proceed for at least 3 weeks for a therapeutic benefit to be seen. Treatment with EPA alone stabilizes body weight, whereas the combination of EPA with a caloric and protein enriched nutritional supplement produces an increase in body weight of up to 2 kg after 7 weeks of treatment (*68*). Unlike Megace, the increase in body weight was attributed to an increase in lean body mass, with no change in fat mass, and also unlike Megace there was a statistically significant improvement in Karnofsky performance status.

Patients taking the EPA supplement that gained weight reported an improved quality of life, and this was reflected by an increase in TEE and PAL (*11*). There was a
considerable improvement in the survival of both cachectic and non-cachectic subjects with generalized solid tumors receiving a daily supplement of 18 g omega-3
fatty acids (*69*), and treatment also increased the ratio of T-helper cells to T-sup-
pressor cells in cachectic subjects. Although EPA is thought to work by attenuating
the action of PIF (*70*), which does not induce anorexia, clinical studies have shown
EPA to be as effective as Megace in improving appetite (*71*).

6.3   Thalidomide

Thalidomide has been shown to be effective in attenuating loss of body weight in
patients with advanced pancreatic cancer who had lost at least 10% of their body
weight (*72*). As with EPA thalidomide produced weight stabilization rather than
producing large weight gain and anthropometric measurements suggested that the
effect was on lean body mass. Thalidomide has also been shown to improve lean
body mass in a small uncontrolled study in patients with nonobstructing and inoperable esophageal cancer (*73*). Thalidomide has the potential to reduce production of
TNF-α by increasing the degradation rate of TNF mRNA, but it also blocks NF-κB
regulated genes through suppression of IκB kinase activity (*74*). An effect on TNF-
α production seems unlikely since pentoxifylline, a methylxanthine derivative, also
shown to inhibit TNF-α production, had no effect on appetite or body weight of
cachectic cancer patients (*75*). The most likely mechanism for the effect of thalidomide is due to suppression of protein degradation induced by factors such as PIF
(*56*) and Ang II (*60*) by attenuating activation of NF-κB and the subsequent
increase in proteasome and MuRF1 expression.

6.4   β-Hydroxy-β-Methylbutyrate

β-Hydroxy-β-methylbutyrate (HMB) is formed by transamination of leucine to α-
ketoisocaproate in muscle, followed by oxidation of the α-ketoisocaproate in the
liver cytosol to HMB. HMB, combined with arginine and glutamine, has been
shown to be effective in increasing body weight through an increase in lean body
mass in weight-losing patients with advanced (stage IV) cancer (*76*). No other clinical studies have been reported in cancer cachexia, although HMB has also been
shown to attenuate AIDS-associated wasting. In an experimental model of cancer
cachexia HMB has been shown to attenuate both muscle protein degradation and
the depression in protein synthesis (*77*). The effect on protein degradation was due
to attenuation of the up-regulation of the ubiquitin-proteasome pathway. HMB
appears to act like EPA to inhibit cellular signalling induced by PIF leading to activation of NF-κB (*78*).

6.5   Appetite Stimulants

Dronabinol, the active ingredient in marijuana, at a dose of 5 mg daily caused a subjective improvement in both mood and appetite in patients with unresectable cancer, but all patients showed a progressive loss of body weight (79). In a placebo-controlled trial, the serotonin antagonist cyproheptadine, although having a small effect on appetite, failed to significantly abate progressive weight loss in cancer patients (80). Ghrelin is a brain-gut peptide that stimulates appetite by activating neurons of the arcuate nucleus of the hypothalamus, an area that regulates feeding. When administered to patients with cancer anorexia it increases energy intake by about 30% without any side effects (81). Although there were no reported effects on body weight, in nude mice bearing the SEKI human melanoma, ghrelin suppressed weight loss through an increase in fat mass with no reported increase in muscle mass (82). These results are similar to those reported with the appetite stimulants Megace and MPA. None of the other orexigenic neuropeptides has yet undergone clinical evaluation.

7   Conclusion

Despite the introduction of new treatments cachexia and anorexia still remain formidable clinical problems in the management of cancer patients. Knowledge of the mechanism of this syndrome is important in the future clinical development of new forms of treatment. Unfortunately in the quest to treat the cancer, cachexia and anorexia are often overlooked as being an inevitable consequence of the disease. If treatment is successful, then the syndrome disappears, but at the present time for patients with pancreatic cancer this rarely happens, and anti-cachexia therapy should be a part of the armaments for the treatment of this disease.

References

1. Wys WD, De Begg C, Lowin PT, 1980, Prognostic effect of weight loss prior to chemotherapy in cancer patients. Am J Med 69:491–497.
2. Wigmore SJ, Plester CE, Richardson RA, 1997, Changes in nutritional status associated with unresectable pancreatic cancer. Br J Cancer 75:106–109.
3. Vigano A, Bruera E, Jhangri GS, 2000, Clinical survival predictors in patients with advanced cancer. Arch Int Med 160:861–868.
4. Barber MD, Ross JA, Fearon KCH, 1999, Changes in nutritional, functional and inflammatory markers in advanced pancreatic cancer. Nutr Cancer 35:106–110.
5. Persson C, Glimelius B, 2002, The relevance of weight loss for survival and quality of life in patients with advanced gastrointestinal cancer treated with palliative chemotherapy. Anticancer Res 22:3661–3668.
6. Okusaka T, Okada S, Ishii H, 1998, Prognosis of advanced pancreatic cancer patients with reference to calorie intake. Nutr Cancer 32:55–58.

7. Heber D, Byerley LO, Chi J, 1998, Pathophysiology of malnutrition in the adult cancer patient. Cancer 58:1867–1873.
8. Bozzetti F, 1992, Nutritional support in the adult cancer patient. Clin Nutr 11:167–175.
9. Bosaeus I, Daneryd P, Svanberg E, 2001, Dietary intake and resting energy expenditure in relation to weight loss in unselected cancer patients. Int J Cancer 93:380–383.
10. Davis MP, Dreicer R, Walsh D, 2004, Appetite and cancer-associated anorexia—A review. J Clin Oncol 22:1510–1517.
11. Moses AGW, Slater C, Preston T, 2004, Reduced total energy expenditure and physical activity in cachectic patients with pancreatic cancer can be modulated by an energy and protein dense oral supplement enriched with n-3 fatty acids. Br J Cancer 90:991–1002.
12. Eden E, Edstrom S, Bennegard K, 1984, Glucose flux in relation to energy expenditure in undernourished patients with and without cancer during periods of fasting and feeding. Cancer Res 44:1718–1724.
13. Clapham JC, Arch JRS, Chapman H, 2000, Mice overexpressing human uncoupling protein-3 in skeletal muscle are hyperphagic and lean. Nature 406:415–418.
14. Collins P, Bing C, McColloch P, 2002, Muscle UCP-3 mRNA levels are elevated in weight loss associated with gastrointestinal adenocarcinoma in humans. Br J Cancer 86:372–375.
15. Falconer JS, Fearon KCH, Plester CE, 1994, Cytokines, the acute phase response and energy expenditure in weight-losing patients with pancreatic cancer. Ann Surg 219:325–331.
16. Falconer JS, Fearon KC, Ross JA, 1995, Acute phase protein response and survival duration of patients with pancreatic cancer. Cancer 75:2077–2082.
17. Wigmore SJ, Falconer JS, Plester CE, 1995, Ibuprofen reduces energy expenditure and acute-phase protein production combined with placebo in pancreatic cancer patients. Br J Cancer 72:185–188.
18. Drott C, Persson H, Lundholm K, 1989, Cardiovascular and metabolic response to adrenaline infusion in weight-losing patients with and without cancer. Clin Physiol 9:427–439.
19. Khal J, Hine AV, Fearon KCH, 2005, Increased expression of proteasome subunits in skeletal muscle of cancer patients with weight loss. Int J Biochem Cell Biol 37:2196–2206.
20. Acharyya S, Ladner KJ, Nelsen LL, 2004, Cancer cachexia is regulated by selective targeting of skeletal muscle gene products. J Clin Invest 114:370–378.
21. Ishiko O, Sumi T, Hirai K, 2001, Apoptosis of muscle cells causes weight loss prior to impairment of DNA synthesis in tumor-bearing rabbits. Jpn J Cancer Res 92:30–35.
22. Royen M, van Carbo N, Busquets S, 2000, DNA Fragmentation occurs in skeletal muscle during tumor growth: a link with cancer cachexia? Biochem Biophys Res Commun 270:533–537.
23. Thompson MP, Cooper ST, Parry BR, 1993, Increased expression of the mRNA for hormone-sensitive lipase in adipose tissue of cancer patients. Biochem Biophys Acta 1180:236–242.
24. Brown DR, Berkowitz DE, Breshaw MJ, 2001, Weight loss is not associated with hyperleptinemia in humans with pancreatic cancer. J Clin Endocrinol Metab 86:162–166.
25. Monitto CL, Berkowitz D, Lee KM, 2001, Differential gene expression in a murine model of cancer cachexia. Am J Physiol 281:E289–E297.
26. Beutler B, Cerami A, 1986, Cachectic and tumor necrosis factor as two sides of the same biological coin. Nature 320:584–588.
27. Lahdevirta J, Maury CPJ, Teppo AM, 1988, Elevated levels of circulating cachectin/tumor necrosis factor in patients with the acquired immunodeficiency syndrome. Am J Med 85:289–295.
28. Ebrahimi B, Tuker SL, Li D, 2004, Cytokines in pancreatic carcinoma. Cancer 101:2727–2736.
29. Karayiannakis AJ, Syrigos KN, Polychronidis A, 2001, Serum levels of tumor necrosis factor-α and nutritional status in pancreatic cancer patients. Anticancer Res 21:1355–1358.
30. Oliff A, Defo-Jones D, Boyer M, 1987, Tumours secreting human TNF/cachectin induce cachexia in mice. Cell 50:555–563.

31. Busquets S, Sanchis D, Alvarez B, 1998, In the rat, tumor necrosis factor α administration results in an increase in both UCP-2 and UCP-3 mRNA in skeletal muscle: a possible mechanism for cytokine-induced thermogenesis? FEBS Lett 440:348–350.
32. Llovera M, Carbo N, Lopez-Sorino J, 1998, Different cytokines modulate ubiquitin gene expression in rat skeletal muscle. Cancer Lett 13:83–87.
33. Berg M, Fraker DL, Alexander HR, 1994, Characterisation of differentiation factor/leukaemia inhibitory factor effect on lipoprotein lipase activity and mRNA in 3T3-L1 adipocytes. Cytokine 6:425–432.
34. Zhang HH, Halbleib M, Ahmad R, 2002, Tumor necrosis factor-α stimulates lipolysis in differentiated human adipocytes through activation of extracellular signal-related kinase and elevation of intracellular cyclic AMP. Diabetes 51:2929–2935.
35. Scott HR, McMillan DC, Crilly A, 1996, The relationship between weight loss and interleukin 6 in non-small-cell lung cancer. Br J Cancer 73:1560–1562.
36. Iwase S, Murakami T, Sato Y, 2004, Steep elevation of blood interleukin-6 (IL-6) associated with late stages of cachexia in cancer patients. Eur Cytokine Netw 15:312–316.
37. Tsujinaka T, Fujita J, Ebisui C, 1996, Interleukin 6 receptor antibody inhibits muscle atrophy and modulates proteolytic systems in interleukin 6 transgenic mice. J Clin Invest 97:244–249.
38. Hall G, Van Steensberg A, Sacchetti M, 2003, Interleukin-6 stimulates lipolysis and fat oxidation in humans. J Clin Endocrinol Metab 88:3005–3010.
39. Fujiki F, Mukaida N, Hirose K, 1997, Prevention of adenocarcinoma colon 26-induced cachexia by interleukin 10 gene transfer. Cancer Res 57:94–99.
40. Maltoni M, Fabbri L, Nanni O, 1997, Serum levels of tumour necrosis factor alpha and other cytokines do not correlate with weight loss and anorexia in cancer patients. Support Care Cancer 5:130–135.
41. Shibata M, Takekawa M. 1999, Increased serum concentration of circulating soluble receptor for interleukin-2 and its effect as a prognostic indicator in cachectic patients with gastric and colorectal cancer. Oncology 56:54–58.
42. Todorov PT, McDevitt TM, Meyer DJ, 1998, Purification and characterisation of a tumor-lipid mobilising factor. Cancer Res 58:2353–2358.
43. Russell ST, Hirai K, Tisdale MJ, 2002, Role of β3-adrenergic receptors in the action of a tumour lipid mobilising factor. Br J Cancer 86:424–428.
44. Sanders PM, Tisdale MJ, 2004, Effect of zinc-α2-glycoprotein (ZAG) on expression of uncoupling proteins in skeletal muscle and adipose tissue. Cancer Lett 212:71–81.
45. Russell ST, Zimmerman TP, Domin BA, 2004, Induction of lipolysis in vitro and loss of body fat in vivo by zinc-α2-glycoprotein. Biochim Biophys Acta 1636:59–68.
46. Bing C, Jenkins J, Sanders P, 2004, Zinc-α2-glycoprotein, a lipid mobilising factor, is expressed in adipocytes and is up-regulated in mice with cancer cachexia. Proc Natl Acad Sci U S A 101:2500–2505.
47. Russell ST, Tisdale MJ, 2005, The role of glucocorticoids in the induction of zinc-α2-glycoprotein expression in adipose tissue in cancer cachexia. Br J Cancer 92:876–881.
48. Russell ST, Tisdale MJ, 2005, Effect of eicosapentaenoic acid (EPA) on expression of a lipid mobilising factor in adipose tissue in cancer cachexia. Prostaglandins, Leukotrines, Essential Fatty Acids 72:409–414.
49. Groundwater P, Beck SA, Barton C, 1990, Alteration of serum and urinary lipolytic activity with weight loss in cachectic cancer patients. Br J Cancer 62:816–821.
50. Belizario JE, Katz M, Raw CI, 1991, Bioactivity of skeletal muscle proteolysis-inducing factors in the plasma proteins from cancer patients with weight loss. Br J Cancer 63:705–709.
51. Todorov P, Caruik P, McDevitt T, 1996, Characterisation of a cancer cachectic factor. Nature 379:739–742.
52. Caruik P, Lorite MJ, Todorov PT, 1997, Induction of cachexia in mice by a product isolated from the urine of cachectic cancer patients. Br J Cancer 76:606–613.
53. Watchorn TM, Waddell ID, Dowidar N, 2001, Proteolysis-inducing factor regulates hepatic gene expression via the transcription factors NF-κB and STAT3. FASEB J 15:562–564.

54. Lorite MJ, Caruik P, Tisdale MJ, 1997, Induction of muscle protein degradation by a tumour factor. Br J Cancer 76:1035–1040.
55. Lorite MJ, Smith HJ, Arnold JA, 2001, Activation of ATP-ubiquitin-dependent proteolysis in skeletal muscle in vivo and murine myoblasts in vitro by a proteolysis-inducing factor (PIF). Br J Cancer 85:297–302.
56. Wyke SM, Tisdale MJ, 2005, NF-kB mediates proteolysis-inducing factor induced protein degradation and expression of the ubiquitin-proteasome system in skeletal muscle. Br J Cancer 92:711–721.
57. Wigmore SJ, Todorov PT, Barber MD, 2000, Characteristics of patients with pancreatic cancer expressing a novel cancer cachectic factor. Br J Surg 87:53–58.
58. Brink M, Price SR, Chrast J, 2001, Angiotensin II induces skeletal muscle wasting through enhanced protein degradation and down-regulates autocrine insulin-like growth factor 1. Endocrinology 142:1489–1496.
59. Song Y-H, Li Y, Du J, 2005, Muscle-specific expression of IGF-1 blocks angiotensin-II-induced skeletal muscle wasting. J Clin Invest 115:451–458.
60. Russell ST, Wyke SM, Tisdale MJ, 2006, Mechanism of induction of muscle protein degradation by angiotensin II. Cell Sig 18:1087–1096.
61. Russell ST, Sanders PM, Tisdale MJ, 2006, Angiotensin II directly inhibits protein synthesis in murine myotubes. Cancer Lett 231:290–294.
62. Maltoni M, Nanni O, Scarpi E, 2001, High-dose progestins for the treatment of cancer anorexia-cachexia syndrome: A systematic review of randomised clinical trials. Ann Oncol 12:289–300.
63. Downer S, Joel S, Albright A, 1993, A double blind placebo controlled trial of medroxyprogesterone acetate (MPA) in cancer cachexia. Br J Cancer 67:1102–1105.
64. Loprinzi CL, Schaid DJ, Dose AM, 1993, Body composition changes in patients who gain weight while receiving megestrol acetate. J Clin Oncol 11:152–154.
65. Simms JPFHA, Schols AMJ, Hoefangels JMJ, 1998, Effects of medroxyprogesterone acetate on food intake, body composition and resting energy-expenditure in patients with advanced nonhormone-sensitive cancer. Cancer 82:553–560.
66. Montovani G, Maccio A, Esu S, 1997, Medroxyprogesterone acetate reduces in vitro production of cytokines and serotonin involved in anorexia/cachexia and emesis by peripheral blood mononuclear cells of cancer patients. Eur J Cancer 33:602–607.
67. Beck SA, Smith KL, Tisdale MJ, 1991, Anticachetic and antitumour effect of eicosapentaenoic acid and its effect on protein turnover. Cancer Res 51:6089–6093.
68. Barber MD, Ross JA, Voss AC, 1999, The effect of an oral nutritional supplement enriched with fish oil on weight-loss in patients with pancreatic cancer. Br J Cancer 81:80–86.
69. Gogos CA, Ginopoulos P, Salsa B, 1998, Dietary omega-3 polyunsaturated fatty acids plus vitamin E restore immunodeficiency and prolong survival for severely ill patients with generalised malignancy. Cancer 82:395–402.
70. Smith HJ, Lorite MJ, Tisdale MJ. 1999, Effect of a cancer cachectic factor on protein synthesis/degradation in murine C2. C12 myoblasts: Modulation by eicosapentaenoic acid Cancer Res 59:5507–5513.
71. Jatoi A, Rowland K, Loprinzi Cl, 2004, An eicosapentaenoic acid supplement versus megestrol acetate versus both for patients with cancer-associated wasting: a North Central Cancer Treatment Group and National Cancer Institute of Canada collaborative effort. J Clin Oncol 22:2469–2476.
72. Gordon JN, Trebble TM, Ellis RD, 2005, Thalidomide in the treatment of cancer cachexia: A randomised placebo controlled trial. Gut 54:540–545.
73. Khan ZH, Simpson EJ, Cole AT, 2003, Oesophageal cancer and cachexia. The effect of short-term treatment with thalidomide on weight loss and lean body mass. Aliment Pharmacol Ther 17:677–682.
74. Keifer JA, Guttridge DC, Ashburner BP, 2001, Inhibition of NF-kB kinase activity. J Biol Chem 276:22382–22387.

75. Goldberg RM, Loprinzi CL, Maillard JA, 1995, Pentoxifylline for treatment of cancer cachexia and cachexia? A randomised, double-blind, placebo-controlled trial. J Clin Oncol 13:2856–2859.
76. May PE, Barber A, D'Olimpio JT, 2002, Reversal of cancer-related wasting using oral supplementation with a combination of β-hydroxy-β-methylbutyrate, arginine and glutamine. Am J Surg 183:471–479.
77. Smith HJ, Mukherji P, Tisdale MJ, 2005, Activation of proteasome-induced proteolysis in skeletal muscle by β-hydroxy-β-methylbutyrate in cancer-induced muscle loss. Cancer Res 65:277–283.
78. Smith HJ, Wyke SM, Tisdale MJ, 2004, Mechanism of attenuation of proteolysis-inducing factor stimulated protein degradation in muscle by β-hydroxy-β-methylbutyrate. Cancer Res 64:8731–8735.
79. Wadleigh R, Spaulding GM, Lumbersky B, 1990, Dronabinol enhancement of appetite and cancer patients. Proc Amer Soc Oncol 9:331.
80. Kardinal CG, Loprinzi CL, Schaid DJ, 1990; A controlled trial of cyproheptadine in cancer patients with anorexia and/or cachexia. Cancer 65:2657–62.
81. Neary NM, Small CJ, Wren AM, 2004, Ghrelin increases energy intake in cancer patients with impaired appetite: Acute randomised, placebo-controlled trial. J Clin Endocrinol Metab 89:2832–2836.
82. Hanada T, Toshinai K, Kajimura N, 2003, Anti-cachectic effect of gherlin in nude mice bearing human melanoma cells. Biochem Biophys Res Commun 301:275–279.

Chapter 27
Endoscopic Palliation

Nathan Schmulewitz

1 Introduction

Pancreatic duct adenocarcinoma will be diagnosed in nearly 34,000 persons in the United States this year, and almost the same number will die of their disease (*1*). Pancreatic cancer has an overall survival rate of <4% (*2*), and even in patients with tumors truly limited to the pancreas and without nodal disease, actuarial 5-year survival rates are 18–24% (*3*). In fact, nearly 85% of patients are deemed unsuitable for potentially curative resection at time of diagnosis (*4–6*). Therefore, palliation of symptoms and/or imminent morbidity is the cornerstone of care for most patients with pancreatic cancer. Furthermore, the absence of therapeutic interventions is a predictor of decreased survival (*7*). With these facts as a backdrop, this chapter discusses the role of endoscopic interventions in the management of advanced pancreatic malignancy.

2 Management of Biliary Obstruction

Between 70% and 90% of patients with pancreatic adenocarcinoma present with biliary obstruction (*8*). Left alone, biliary obstruction leads to jaundice, pruritus, cholangitis, liver dysfunction, anorexia, malabsorption, and altered coagulation. These symptoms tend to have a profound effect on quality of life, and so biliary drainage procedures are generally appropriate for patients who are not candidates for resection (*9, 10*). Biliary drainage can be accomplished in two ways, surgical bypass with biliary-enteric anastomosis or placement of an endoprosthesis. Endoprosthetic drainage of the bile duct can be accomplished by percutaneous or transduodenal approaches.

Overall, the most durable therapy for malignant biliary obstruction is surgical bypass. Some studies have shown recurrent biliary obstruction rates as low as 2% (*11, 12*). However, perioperative morbidity and mortality rates run from 20% to 40% and 10% to 24%, respectively (*11, 13–19*). Other concerns with surgical therapy have included prolonged ileus, prolonged hospitalizations, and expense. One

A.M. Lowy et al. (eds.), *Pancreatic Cancer*.
doi: 10.1007/978-0-387-69252-4, © Springer Science+Business Media LLC 2008

recent surgical series only included patients with pancreatic head cancers who were taken to the operating room for potentially curative surgery and examined outcomes of 83 consecutive patients who were found unresectable and underwent both biliary-enteric bypass and gastrojejunostomy (12). In that series, 30-day mortality was 4.8%, perioperative morbidity 27%, delayed gastric emptying occurred in 9%, and the mean hospital stay was 16 days. To try to minimize the morbidity of surgery, there has been some experience with laparoscopic biliary bypass, but this has not been widely used as the morbidity still far surpasses that of nonoperative biliary decompression (20).

For nonoperative biliary decompression, percutaneous, transhepatic placement of drainage tubes and stents is an alternative with a high success rate. Relief of biliary obstruction can be achieved in >97% of patients with this approach (21–24). Self-expanding metallic stents are favored, as they obviate the need for permanent external catheters, thereby decreasing complications of leakage, infection, and hemorrhage, and eliminate concerns of tube dislodgement, migration, or blockage, in addition to improving the patient's psychological condition (25) Metallic-stent mean patency rates range from 129 to 324 days (22, 24, 26). Nevertheless, although metallic stents reduce morbidity and mortality over plastic stents (26), presumedly due to improved patency, 30-day mortality rates range from 7.5% to 36% (24, 26, 27), and complication rates can be significantly higher. There are several other shortcomings to the percutaneous transhepatic approach. First, although biliary access, drainage, and stent placement are usually possible, transpapillary stent placement is not always possible, condemning some patients to lifelong external drainage. Second, even when transpapillary stent placement is successful, the patient usually has to return for several procedural sessions, including dilations prior to metallic stent placement and then for removal of external catheter(s). The temporary presence of external drains can cause significant problems, such as dislodgements, infections, leaking, or bleeding. More recently, efforts have been made to study the feasibility of placing a stent at the initial percutaneous procedure, although a temporary percutaneous catheter is generally still required for hemostatic purposes (28). Nevertheless, the percutaneous approach for biliary drainage remains an important therapeutic option and is particularly important for several patient subsets. These special patient groups include those with acute cholangitis and no immediate access to endoscopic decompression, those failing endoscopic decompression (29), and those with postsurgical anatomy limiting enteric access to the bile duct.

For most unresectable pancreatic cancer patients with biliary obstruction, endoscopic decompression is the procedure of choice. The bile duct is accessed via the major papilla in the duodenum using endoscopic retrograde cholangiography (ERC). During the procedure, a catheter and/or wire is passed across the papilla and into the biliary tree and across the malignant stricture, under fluoroscopy. Thereafter, a stent can be guided over the wire to bridge the stricture, allowing the distal end of the stent to hang into the duodenum. Traditionally, biliary stents have been made of plastic. Plastic stents can be placed with a >93% technical success rate, and do not require biliary sphincterotomy (30). When endoscopic access into the bile duct or across the stricture is unsuccessful, temporary percutaneous drainage with passage of a tube or wire across the stricture and into the duodenum frequently allows for subsequent endoscopic stenting. Once endoscopic stent placement is achieved, any external drain can be removed. Unfortunately, plastic stents have high occlusion rates resulting from development of a biofilm on the internal surface leading to bacterial colonization (31, 32). Bacteria lead to calcium bilirubinate precipitation with sludge accumulation. Bilioduodenal reflux and food may also play a role in stent occlusion (33, 34). Because of such inevitable occlusions, standard 10 French (F) plastic stents generally stay patent for 3–4 months (35, 36). Furthermore, changes in plastic stent composition, surface features, and even use of antibiotics have not significantly affected patency (37–39). As a result, obstructive jaundice recurs in up to 50% of patients, requiring that plastic stents be changed every several months (40).

With the evolution of self-expandable metal stents (SEMS), there has been significant improvement in stent patency. SEMS are made of stainless steel alloy or nickel-titanium alloy. They come packaged within a 7.5- to 10-F sheath and are passed over a wire into the bile duct and across the stricture, after biliary sphincterotomy. Thereafter, the sheath is retracted and the stent expands as it is deployed, up to 10 mm in diameter. As the metal struts press into surrounding tissue, and granulation tissue and tumor grows between the struts, the stent becomes fixed to its surroundings and thereby is usually considered permanent. Having a larger internal bore, these stents can maintain patency for an average of 9 months (41–44). Like the plastic stents, SEMS can be placed with a very high technical success rate. Unfortunately, SEMS are far more expensive than plastic stents. Cost-effectiveness studies have shown that metal stents are only economical and appropriate when the patients are expected to survive 6 months or longer (45–47). Some also advise routine placement of a SEMS after occlusion of a plastic stent. Two other appropriate situations for metal stents include management of a patient who might not comply with medical follow-up and the patient with impending duodenal obstruction (35). The latter scenario is an important one, because endoscopic placement of a biliary stent in a patient with duodenal obstruction or after duodenal enteral stent placement can be exceedingly difficult.

Of course, even metal stents succumb to occlusion via tumor ingrowth, overgrowth at the ends, mucosal hyperplasia, biliary sludge, or food impaction (35). When a SEMS becomes occluded, mechanical "cleaning" can be performed endoscopically, although that process alone is rarely efficacious. More frequently, stent cleaning is followed by placing another metal stent within the first one or by placing a plastic stent within the metal stent (48). Although both of these stent-in-a-stent techniques are successful >90% of the time, deploying a plastic stent within the SEMS tends to be more cost effective (48, 49).

Polyethylene and silicone covers for SEMS have been tried to reduce tissue ingrowth through the wire mesh, generally without significant improvements in patency (50–52). One study of covered versus uncovered nickel-titanium SEMS did show a patency advantage to the covered stents, but the covered stents also led to more complications (53). There are three downsides to covered metals stents. First, covered SEMS are more prone to migration, as a result of poor friction between the polymer surface and the tumor. Second, covered SEMS can predispose to acute cholecystitis or pancreatitis, with incidences as high as 4.2% and 8.7%, respectively, presumably when a portion of the covered section blocks the cystic duct or pancreatic duct orifice (53, 54). Third, unlike wire mesh stents that "dig" into adjacent tissue, facilitating full expansion, covered stents, even when only the internal surface is covered, cannot cut deeply into adjacent tissue, which may occasionally limit full radial deployment (55). Obviously a stent with a narrower lumen will be more prone to occlusion due to biofilm and sludge. Luckily, coated SEMS are usually retrievable, although it can certainly be difficult to place these stents so that the coated portion does not cover the cystic duct or ampulla.

Unfortunately, endoscopic stenting of biliary obstruction in pancreatic cancer is certainly not without complications. Overall complication rates range from 15% to 34% (56), and the range of adverse events is broad. Procedurally related complications can include cardiopulmonary compromise, hemorrhage, cholangitis, pancreatitis, and perforation. Stent placement in malignant biliary obstruction is a significant risk factor for cholangitis (57), particularly if complete drainage cannot be achieved, and all patients should receive periprocedural broad-spectrum antibiotics, if they are not already on antibiotics for their biliary obstruction. Additionally, endoscopic sphincterotomy is needed for metallic stent placement, and sphincterotomy is a risk factor for hemorrhage and perforation (57). Indeed this patient group has the highest 30-day mortality rates of ERC cohorts.

Beyond intraprocedural complications, untoward outcomes in this patient group can include cholangitis, stent migration, recurrent obstruction, and frank failure to adequately drain the bile duct. Although cholangitis is usually of greatest concern prior to therapy for biliary obstruction, it can also occur in patients after therapeutic stenting, even in the context of stent patency. Patients at highest risk are those with a SEMS across the major papilla (58). The mechanism might be related to duodenal contents, food, or digestive juices traveling into the biliary tree. Of course, adequate biliary drainage is the most common short- and long-term concern in biliary obstruction. Although some studies demonstrate ERC to have therapeutic success for stent placement in well over 90% of cases, other studies have shown failure rates as high as 13% or more (29). Percutaneous drainage and attempted stenting is generally the preferred approach in these patients not technically amenable to successful endoscopic drainage.

One other approach to failed biliary cannulation by ERC is biliary access gained through use of endoscopic ultrasound (EUS). The roles of EUS in periampullary neoplasms has traditionally been for staging and tissue acquisition via fine-needle aspiration (FNA). However, with its ability to image the biliary tree in real time, EUS can also be used to gain access into the biliary tree. A FNA needle or needle knife can be passed through the wall of the duodenum directly into the bile duct, or through the wall of the stomach into a distended left intrahepatic duct (59–62). Once access is achieved with a hollow-bore needle, a wire can be passed into the duct, under fluoroscopy. Sometimes the wire can be guided through the stricture and into the duodenum, where it can be captured by a traditional duodenoscope and used to guide transpapillary stenting via ERC (i.e., a "rendezvous" procedure). When transpapillary passage of the wire is not possible, the newly formed cholangioenteric fistula can be dilated over the wire and a drainage catheter or stent can be placed for biliary drainage. The allure of EUS-guided biliary drainage after failed ERC-guided stenting is the avoidance of percutaneous catheter drainage and its associated morbidity. However, the role for this technique in the salvage management of malignant biliary obstruction is yet unclear.

In summary, endoscopic biliary stenting via ERC is the preferred route for palliative management of biliary obstruction in patients with unresectable pancreatic cancer. Despite a higher incidence or recurrent obstruction, endoscopic stenting affords lower morbidity, shorter hospitalization and lower 30-day mortality than surgical bypass with similar technical success and quality of life (47). Endoscopic stenting also has fewer complications than percutaneous stenting (27), in addition to requiring fewer sessions and not obligating patients to have temporary external catheters. Plastic stents tend to remain patent for 3–4 months, whereas the more costly metal stents can be expected to remain patent for up to 9 months, and the latter usually do not require retreatment thereafter (63). Occlusions to either plastic or metal stents can be managed endoscopically. Patients expected to survive >6 months would likely benefit most from SEMS, although some other groups are also appropriate candidates for having metallic stents placed initially. Some covered metal stents might further delay recurrent obstruction, but there are not enough data to recommend their use at this time. Biliary obstruction with failed attempts at ERC stenting is usually best managed percutaneously, although endoscopic and surgical options are also available.

3 Management of Gastric Outlet Obstruction

Traditionally, gastroduodenal obstruction in cases of unresectable malignancy was managed with open surgical gastrojejunostomy. Placement of a surgically deployed plastic prosthesis for palliation of obstructive gastric cancer was first described in 1980 (64). Eventually, use of endoscopically placed self-expanding metallic stents for malignant gastroduodenal obstruction became popularized in the early 1990s. Since then, there have been many published series of patients managed with endoscopic stenting. The procedure can be done in two ways, depending on patient anatomy and available devices. One technique is to pass an endoscope to the level of obstruction and then pass a wire across the stenosis, under fluoroscopy. Typically, the distal or proximal aspect of the stenosis is marked with a radiopaque marker either internally, as with a metallic hemoclip, or externally, as can be done with a paper clip taped to the patient so as to lie over the stricture during fluoroscopy. After the scope is backed out of the patient over the wire, a sheathed SEMS is carefully passed over the wire, using fluoroscopic guidance to deploy the stent across the stenosis. The second technique is to use a through-the-scope SEMS device that can be pushed out of the endoscope channel and visually guided, with or without fluoroscopy, to the appropriate site of deployment.

The largest single series of endoscopically placed SEMS for malignant gastroduodenal obstruction was a retrospective study of 176 patients treated over 7 years at four centers (65). Technical success was achieved in 98% of patients, and procedure-related complications occurred in 14 patients. These complications included stent migration, bowel perforation, intestinal bleeding, and abdominal pain. Another nine patients (6%) developed cholangitis during the follow-up period. Regarding the patients for whom follow-up data was available, 84% resumed oral intake for a median time of 146 days, 22% of patients were restented, and 60% of the patients who died during follow-up were tolerating oral intake up until their deaths. Importantly, the only factor significantly predictive of prolonged oral intake was chemotherapy after stent placement. Another series of 63 patients with malignant gastric outlet obstruction treated endoscopically showed similar results (66). In this study there was 95% technical success, with 92% of patients taking exclusively peroral nutrition and 73% tolerating soft or solid food. Complications occurred in 30% of patients, including two perforations, 13 stent obstructions, and four stent migrations.

One systematic review looked at 32 published case series of gastroduodenal obstruction managed with metallic stents (67). Procedures included fluoroscopy procedures, fluoroscopy with endoscopic guidance, and through-the-scope stent placements in a total of 606 patients. Stents were deployed in 97% of cases and symptoms were relieved in 87%, with almost half of patients achieving a full diet. In those who did not improve after stenting, failure was ascribed to disease progression in 61%, early stent migration in 20%, and poor stent placement/deployment in 15%. Severe complications such as perforation or bleeding occurred in 1.2%. However, minor complications occurred in almost 27% of patients, including stent obstruction or migration in 22%. Stent obstruction can be related to tumor ingrowth, overgrowth, food impaction, stent fracture or collapse, or prolapse of adjacent tissue. Both stent migration and obstruction can generally managed by re-stenting. Data on efficacy of palliative re-stenting are scant, but the practice seems reasonable, if anatomic factors permit, since this patient group as a whole may have even more advanced disease than primary stent candidates, and thus might inspire less enthusiasm for surgical bypass.

Few studies have compared the outcomes of endoscopic stenting with those of surgical bypass. One retrospective study from Boston, of 27 patients with pancreatic cancer and gastric outlet obstruction demonstrated equivalent survival after surgical versus endoscopic palliation, but the endoscopic group had fewer re-hospitalizations and lower costs (68). Another study from Burlington, MA, albeit of only 23 patients, suggested that, in contrast to endoscopically stented patients, surgically bypassed patients had frequent postoperative delayed gastric emptying, longer postprocedural hospitalization, higher 30-day mortality, and shorter overall survival (69). A Swedish study of 36 patients demonstrated that stented patients had shorter hospitalizations, better 30-day survival, and better 30-day solid food tolerance than surgically bypassed patients (70). One Japanese study of 39 patients with malignant gastroduodenal obstruction suggested that surgery and endoscopic stenting had equivalent technical and clinical successes, survival, and complications, but that endoscopic stenting led to much faster resumption of oral intake (1 versus 9 days) and more frequent improvements in performance status (*71*). The largest nonrandomized study was done in Italy and compared 24 SEMS-treated patients with 23 open-surgical bypass patients (*72*). That study also showed the SEMS group to have less morbidity and shorter hospitalizations, as well as improved clinical success, 30-day survival, and overall survival. Indeed one small prospective, randomized trial of open gastrojejunostomy versus endoscopic stenting has been done in patients with malignant antropyloric strictures (*73*). With nine patients in each arm, there were equivalent 3-month outcomes, but shorter mean time to oral intake and shorter hospitalizations in the endoscopic group.

In general, biliary stenting should be done before or at the time of gastroduodenal stenting for two reasons. First, duodenal stent insertion may lead to secondary biliary obstruction in some patients (*65, 74, 75*). Second, biliary stenting through an enteric stent can be technically challenging, especially if the stent is covering the major ampulla, which is commonly the case. In fact, there has been one study where nearly half of patients who had enteral SEMS placed required biliary interventions (*76*). Combined stenting of both the bile duct and the duodenum, in the same session, is successful in 91–94% of cases (*61, 77*). Thereby, in any patient without biliary obstruction who undergoes palliative stenting for malignant duodenal obstruction, biliary stenting should be attempted first. Furthermore, a biliary SEMS should be placed, to minimize the potential need for exchanging a plastic biliary stent, which has higher odds of obstructing sooner. In the patient in whom an enteral stent already exists, and biliary obstruction ensues, percutaneous biliary drainage may be the easiest option. That being said, it is possible to manage this situation endoscopically. One group described successfully placing biliary stents through metallic duodenal stents in 17 of 18 patients (*78*). Obviously these procedures are usually relegated to the most expert biliary endoscopists.

Although endoscopic stenting often provides successful palliation of malignant gastric outlet obstruction, it does not have the durability of surgical bypass and does not address the gastroparesis that often accompanies advanced pancreatic cancer (*77*). Recent advances in endoscopic techniques have allowed for endoscopic facilitation of gastrojejunostomy without the need for an abdominal incision. These procedures require techniques to create apposition of the stomach and a loop of jejunum, as well as their fixation and creation of a fistula. Early techniques included the endoscopic placement of magnets to create apposition, as well as the use of endoscopic ultrasound to direct a needle and traction device to pull a loop of jejunum to the stomach (*80–83*). Once apposition is achieved a tract can be dilated, and different endoscopic suturing devices employed. Finally, there will be a subset of obstructed patients, usually with highly advanced disease, who cannot be properly bypassed or stented, or whose symptoms do not respond to those maneuvers. Such patients have persistent nausea and vomiting with an exceedingly poor quality of life. For these individuals, consideration should be given to placement of a venting gastrostomy, performed endoscopically or otherwise, which usually prevents persistent nausea and vomiting and often allows for some modestly restored oral intake (*84*).

4 Splanchnic Neurolysis

Over 80% of patients with pancreatic cancer present with or develop pain (*85–87*). As most patients are not candidates for curative therapy, and the median survival is approximately 6 months (*84*), pain management is of paramount importance. Furthermore, patients with better pain management may have improved survival (*86*, *88*). Unfortunately, in spite of its prevalence, pain in pancreatic cancer is not well understood, and multiple mechanisms may be at work. Potential causes include pancreatic ductal obstruction, inflammation, increased interstitial pressure, ischemia, and direct nerve infiltration or stretching by primary tumor or adenopathy (*89–94*). Additionally, peritumoral inflammation may sensitize nerves to further stimulation (*89, 95, 96*). As efficacy of therapies directed at these specific mechanisms has not been demonstrated, the usual standard of care for managing pain in unresectable pancreatic cancer involves escalating doses of narcotic analgesics. Unfortunately, narcotics can also impair quality of life when they cause mental status changes, unsteady gait, nausea, constipation, or make it unsafe for the patient to drive a car.

Another means of palliating pain in advanced pancreatic cancer is splanchnic neurolysis. Sympathetic innervation of the pancreas, which includes fibers that mediate pain, arise from the tractus intermediolateralis in the spinal cord and travel along thoracic nerve roots 5 through 11. Afferent fibers from the pancreas, as well as other upper-abdominal viscera, directly enter the celiac plexus and then ascend along splanchnic nerves to the T5-T12 dorsal root ganglia. The celiac plexus itself is composed of a right and left ganglion that are wrapped around the aorta at the level of the celiac trunk, with a mean size of 3.1 × 3.2 × 3.5 centimeters, often lying between the celiac trunk and superior mesenteric artery (*97*), although the celiac trunk is the most reliable landmark (*98*).

Pain fibers passing through the celiac plexus can be ablated chemically or transected with surgical splanchnicectomy. A placebo-controlled trial of intraoperative, chemical splanchnicectomy with 20 ccs of 50% alcohol versus saline in 137 patients with unresectable pancreatic cancer showed that patients with pre-existing pain had: (1) significant diminution of pain for a mean of over 3 months, (2) a 70% reduction in need for narcotics (versus 0% in placebo group), and (3) a prolonged survival (*88*). Furthermore, patients in that study without significant preoperative pain demonstrated a delay in onset of significant pain from 3 months to 7.2 months. A less invasive surgical technique to transect afferent splanchnic innervation is thoracoscopic splanchnicectomy, which can be done unilaterally or bilaterally, with >80% of patients achieving clinical benefit of pain reduction (*99–103*). Interestingly, there is no clear evidence that bilateral splanchnicectomy imparts an advantage over unilateral splanchnicectomy, particularly as an initial intervention, and so a left-sided unilateral technique is common.

Nevertheless, nonoperative chemical splanchnicectomy tends to be the preferred approach in unresectable patients. Percutaneous celiac plexus blocks have been done for >90 years. The most common percutaneous route is a posterior one, where a 15- to 20-cm needle is passed from a position posterolateral to the first lumbar vertebra alongside the vertebral body so that the tip reaches a position just anterior to the spine. There are different posterior approaches, including retrocrural, transcrural, and transaortic ones, and these are accomplished under fluoroscopic or CT guidance. Anterior approaches have also been described, usually with ultrasound or CT guidance, although bowel and solid organ puncture are concerning risks. Although the celiac ganglia are not visible by fluoroscopy or CT, various approaches are effective because liquids spread around the preaortic space when injected nearby within the retroperitoneum, even if injected retrocrurally (*104*, *105*). For patients with cancer pain, celiac plexus neurolysis (CPN) is accomplished by injecting phenol, or, more commonly, alcohol (usually 20 ccs of 98% alcohol), after first injecting bupivacaine, a local anesthetic, to avoid the pain associated with alcohol administration to neural tissue. The traditional technique involved injection of alcohol on the day following an "analgesic test dose" of bupivacaine. More contemporary practice allows for the alcohol injection to immediately follow the local anesthetic test dose and the patient's elicited response to the latter.

A review of 24 studies of percutaneous CPN, in which 63% of patients had pancreatic cancer, demonstrated partial to complete pain relief in about 90% of patients at 3 months, and 70–90% of patients at the time of death (*106*). However, patient selection may be important. Some data suggest that factors predictive for CPN success are tumors in the head of the pancreas, shorter duration of cancer pain, and tumors undergoing chemotherapy and/or radiation (*107–109*). These factors are intuitive because they relate to a lower likelihood of peripancreatic nerve involvements. More specifically, smaller tumors that present earlier, as do lesions in the head that cause jaundice and tumors in general that have been symptomatic for shorter periods tend to have less peripancreatic nervous tissue invasion. Similarly, patients receiving local or systemic therapy may have their tumors shrink away from peripancreatic nerves. Contrarily, large tumors in the body and/or tail may impede the ability of injected liquid to freely "bathe" the area around the celiac ganglia and may involve peripancreatic nerves that do not respond to celiac neurolysis. That being said, CPN later in the disease course still can often be effective (*110*).

The most common side effects of CPN include pain (up to 96%), hypotension (up to 38%), and diarrhea (up to 44%) (*109*). The pain results from alcohol's immediate caustic effects on nerves and lasts for 1–2 days. Hypotension occurs transiently after the procedure and presumably reflects splanchnic vasodilation resulting from acute splanchnic neuronal injury, but the mechanism is not understood. Significant hypotension can often be averted by prophylactic volume expansion during and immediately after the procedure. Diarrhea, when it occurs, usually only lasts a couple of days, and not more than a week. Rare CPN complications include vascular injury, retroperitoneal infection, pneumothorax, chylothorax, chest pain, hematuria, hiccupping, and gastrointestinal motility disruptions such as chronic diarrhea or persistent gastroparesis (*106*, *111–113*). However, the most important potential complication is neurologic injury. Neurologic injuries are the most concerning potential complications of percutaneous CPN, regardless of approach. These injuries include lower-extremity weakness, paresthesias, or paraplegia, the latter occurring in up to 1% of patients, mediated by direct injury to the cord or somatic nerves or cord ischemia from needle injury to the artery of Adamkiewicz (*106*, *114–117*).

CPN practice has changed a bit with the availability of the endoscopic approach, done via EUS. First reported in the mid 1990s, EUS-CPN is now practiced in most centers where EUS is available. Patients are sedated for endoscopy and a linear echoendoscope is passed near the esophagogastric junction, where posterior-wise rotation of the ultrasound probe allows for visualization of the aorta. As the probe is advanced distally, the diaphragm disappears from between the esophageal wall and aorta and the origins of the celiac trunk and superior mesenteric artery below it will come into view. A hollow-gauge needle (19G, 22 G, or the newly available 20 G CPN needle with side holes for expeditious injections) is passed through the posterior gastric wall and the needle tip placed anterior and superior to the celiac trunk takeoff. Here 4–6 ccs of 0.25–0.50% bupivacaine is injected, followed by 20 ccs of 98% alcohol. Some operators choose a single midline injection, whereas others prefer two divided doses injected just laterally to the right and left of the celiac trunk. In one study of EUS-CPN in 30 patients, patients demonstrated a 79–88% reduction in pain scores and a 49% reduction in pain medication usage at 12 weeks (*118*). Another study of 58 patients yielded reduction in pain in 78% of patients but without significant change in narcotic usage (*109*).

The biggest advantage of EUS-CPN is the close proximity of the ultrasound probe in the stomach to the target area adjacent to the celiac trunk, which is usually <2 cm away. This proximity and real-time imaging of the vasculature allows for safe and precise needle tip placement and a short procedure, with endoscopy time (not including sedation) usually lasting <10 minutes. Furthermore, patients are sedated for procedure, sometimes provoking less anxiety regarding the procedure. However, endoscopy also adds the risks related to sedation and potential scope trauma (hemorrhage or perforation). There have been isolated reports of retroperitoneal abscess related to EUS-guided celiac plexus blockade (CPB)/neurolysis (*119, 120*). These reports have been too infrequent to clearly identify risk factors, although acid suppression and resultant gastric bacterial overgrowth has been discussed as a potential infection risk (*121*). Additionally, a case has been reported of retroperitoneal bleeding from an arterial pseudoaneurysm, thought to have developed secondary to direct alcohol causticity to the arterial wall (*122*). This event occurred in a patient with chronic pancreatitis who received CPN after failing to respond to CPB. Last, there has been a case of chylous ascites presumably from trauma to the thoracic duct (personal communication). There have not yet been reports of neurologic injury or mortality associated with EUS-CPB/N technique. There have been no large series of EUS-CPN from which to derive a true overall complication rate. The closest approximation would be the complication rate of 1–2% associated with EUS-FNA of the pancreas (*123*), although the risk would likely be lower for EUS-CPN, as the scope does not need to be passed into the duodenum (with risk for trauma there), there is no risk of pancreatitis, and there is no need for multiple needle passes into sterile, vascularized, parenchymal tissue.

One other advantage of EUS-CPN is the ability to combine the procedure with another endoscopic procedure. For instance, a patient found to be unresectable during EUS staging, or undergoing FNA purely for tissue acquisition, could have a EUS-CPN done in the same session, saving time and money. Similarly, a patient with unresectable pancreatic cancer and jaundice could have a biliary stent placed in the same endoscopic period with a CPN.

Only one trial has compared endoscopic to percutaneous techniques and involved celiac plexus blockade in 22 patients with chronic pancreatitis randomized to EUS- or CT-guided blockade with bupivacaine and triamcinolone (*121*). In that study patients in the EUS arm derived more-frequent persistent benefit at 8 and 24 weeks, and of patients who had undergone both techniques, patients preferred the endoscopic approach. EUS was also the less expensive modality in that study. Given the small sample size and dissimilar patient population, it is unlikely the results of that study can be extrapolated to CPN. To date, there have been no comparative trials of EUS versus percutaneous CPN for patients with cancer. Currently, selecting an approach depends on local expertise, availability, and costs.

References

1. American Cancer Society. Cancer facts and figures 2006. Atlanta, American Cancer Society, 2006.
2. Greenlee RT, Murray T, Bolden S, 2000. Cancer statistics, CA Cancer J Clin 200, 50(1):7–33.
3. Yeo CJ, Abrams RA, Grochow LB, 1997, Pancreaticoduodenectomy for pancreatic adenocarcinoma: postoperative adjuvant chemoradiation improves survival. A prospective, single-institution experience. Ann Surg 225(5):621–633; discussion 633–636.
4. Tan HP, Smith J, Garberoglio CA. 1996, Pancreatic adenocarcinoma: an update. J AM Coll Surg 183:164–184.
5. Warshaw AL, Fernandez-del Castillo C. 1992, Pancreatic carcinoma. N Engl J Med 326:455–465.
6. Yeo CJ. 1998, Pancreatic cancer: 1998 update. J Am Coll Surg 187:429–442.
7. Engelken FJ, Bettschart V, Rahman MQ, 2003, Prognostic factors in the palliation of pancreatic cancer. Eur J Surg Oncol 29:368–373.
8. Bosch RR, va den Schelling GP, va der Klinkenbijl JH, 1994, guidelines for the application of surgery and endoprostheses in the palliation of obstructive jaundice in advanced cancer of the pancreas. Ann Surg 1:18–24.
9. Yan LN, 2001, Complex therapy of malignant obstruction jaundice. Zhongguo Shiyong Waike Zazhi 21: 473.
10. Abraham NS, Barkun JS, Barkun AN. 2002, Palliation of malignant biliary obstruction: a prospective trial examining impact on quality of life. Gastrointest Endosc 56:835–841.
11. Smith AC, Dowsett JF, Russell RC, 1994, Randomized trial of endoscopic stenting versus surgical bypass in malignant low bile duct obstruction. Lancet 344:1655–1660.
12. Lesurtel M, Dehni N, Tiret E, 2006, Palliative Surgery for unresectable pancreatic and periampullary cacner: a reappraisal. J Gastrointest Surg 10:286–291.
13. Sohn TA, Lillemoe KD, Cameron JL, 1999, Surgical palliation of unresectable periampullary adenocarcinoma in the 1990's. J Am Coll surg 188:658–666.
14. Lillemoe KD, Sauter PK, Pitt HA, 1993, Current status of surgical palliation of periampullary carcinoma. Surg Gynecol Obstet 176:1–10.
15. Wagensveld BA, van Coene PP, Gulik TM, van 1997, Outcome of palliative biliary and gastric bypass surgery for pancreatic head carcinoma in 126 patients. Br J Surg 84:1402–1406.
16. Borie F, Rodier JG, Guillon F, 2001, Palliative surgery of pancreatic adenocarcinoma (in French). Gastroenterol Clin Biol 2 Pt 2:C7–C14.

17. Shepherd HA, Royle G, Ross AP, 1988, Endoscopic biliary endoprosthesis in the palliation of malignant obstruction of the distal common bile duct: a randomized trial. Br J Surg 75:1166–1168.

18. Andersen JR, Sorensen M, Kruse A, 1989, Randomized trial of endoscopic endoprosthesis versus operative bypass in malignant obstructive jaundice. Gut 30:1132–1135.

19. Bowman PC, Harries-Jones EP, Tobias R, 1986, Prospective controlled trial of transhepatic biliary endoprosthesis versus bypass surgery for incurable carcinoma of head of pancreas. Lancet 1:69–71.

20. Date RS, Siriwardena AK. 2005, Current status of laparoscopic biliary bypass in the management of non-resectable peri-ampullary cancer. Pancreatology 5: 325–329.

21. Oikarinen H, Leinonen S, Karttunen A, 1999, Patency and complications of percutaneously inserted metallic stents in malignant biliary obstruction. J Vasc Interv Radiol 10:1387–1393.

22. Lee BH, Choe DH, Lee JH, 1997, Mettalic stents in malignant biliary obstruction: prospective long-term clinical results. AJR 168:741–745.

23. Rieber A, Brambs HJ, 1997, Metallic stents in malignant biliary obstruction. Cardiovasc Interv Radiol 20:43–49.

24. Pappas P, Leonardou P, Kurkuni A, 2003, Percutaneous insertion of metallic endoprostheses in the biliary tree in 66 patients: relief of the obstruction. Abdom Imaging 28:678–683.

25. Pasricha P. 1995, Stent or surgery for the palliation of malignant biliary obstruction: is the choice clear now? Gastroenterology 109:1398–1340.

26. Guo YX, Li YH, Chen Y, 2003, (Comparative assessment of clinical efficacy of percutaneous transhepatic metal versus plastic biliary stent implantation for malignant biliary obstruction: a multi–centered investigation.) Di Yi Jun Yi Da Xue Xue Bao 23:1237–1241.

27. Pinol V, Castells A, Bordas JM, 2002, Percutaneous self-expanding metal stents versus endoscopic polyethylene endoprostheses for treating malignant biliary obstruction: randomized clinical trial. Radiology 225:27–34.

28. Yoshida H, Mamada Y, Taniai N, 2006, One-step palliative treatment method for obstructive jaundice caused by unresectable malignancies by percutaneous transhepatic insertion of an expandable metallic stent. World J Gastroenterol 12:2423–2426.

29. Doctor N, Dick R, Rai R, 1999, Results of percutaneous plastic stents for malignant distal biliary obstruction following failed endoscopic stent insertion and comparison with current literature on expandable metallic stents. Eur J Gastroenterol Hepatol 11:775–780.

30. Di Giorgio P, De Luca L, 2004, Comparison of treatment outcomes between biliary plastic stent placements with and without endoscopic sphincterotomy for inoperable malignant common bile duct obstruction. World J Gastroenterol 10:1212–1214.

31. Groen AK, Out T, Hiibregtse KK, 1987, Characterization of the content of occluded biliary endoprosthesis. Endoscopy 19:5759.

32. Sung JY, Leung JW, Shaffer EA, 1993, Bacterial biofilm, brown pigment stone and blockage of biliary stents. J Gastrenterol Hepatol 8:28–34.

33. Berkel AM, van marle J, van Groen AK, 2005, Mechanisms of stent clogging: confocal laser scanning and scanning electron microscopy. Endoscopy 37:729–734.

34. Weichert U, Venzke T, Konig J, 2001, Why do bilioduodenal plastic stents become occluded? A clinical and pathological investigation on 100 consecutive patients. Endoscopy 33:786–790.

35. Levy M, Baron T, Gostout J, 2004, Palliation of malignant extrahepatic biliary obstruction with plastic versus expandable metal stents: an evidence-based approach. Clin Gastroenterol Hepatol 2:273–285.

36. Siegel J, Puillano W, Kodsi B, 1988, Optimal palliation of malignant bile duct obstruction: experience with endoscopic 12 French endoprostheses. Endoscopy 20:137–141.

37. Das A, Sivak MV, 2000, Endoscopic palliation for inoperable pancreatic cancer. Cancer Control 7:452–457.

38. Galandi D, Schwarzer G, Bassler D, 1998, Treatment of malignant biliary obstruction with polyurethane covered Wallstents. AJR 170:403–408.

39. Chan G, Barkun J, Barkun AN, 2005, The role of ciprofloxacin in prolonging polyethylene biliary stent patency: a multicentre double-blinded effectiveness study. J Gastrointest Surg 9:481–488.
40. Huibregste KK, Katon RM, Coene PP, 1986, Endoscopic palliative treatment in pancreatic cacner. Gastrointest Endosc 32:334–338.
41. Davids PH, Fockens P, Groen AK, 1992, A prospective randomized trial of self–expanding metal stents vs polyethylene stents for malignant obstruction: preliminary results. Netherlands J Med 41:A13–14.
42. Knyrim K, Wagner HJ, Pausch J, 1993, A prospective, randomized, controlled trial of metal stents for malignant obstruction of the common bile duct. Endoscopy 25:207–212.
43. Prat F, Chapat O, Ducot B, 1998, A randomized trial of endoscopic drainage methods for inoperable malignant strictures of the common bile duct. Gastrointest Endosc 41:1–7.
44. Kaassis M, Boyer J, Dumas R, 2003, Plastic or metal stents for malignant stricture of the common bile duct? Results of a randomized retrospective study. Gastrointest Endosc 57:178–182.
45. Arguedas MR, Heudebert GH, Sinnett AA, 2002, Biliary stents in malignant obstructive jaundice due to pancreatic carcinoma: a cost effectiveness analysis. Am J Gastroenterol 97:898–904.
46. Yeoh KG, Zimmerman MJ, Cunningham JT, 1999, Comparative costs of metal versus plastic biliary stent strategies for malignant obstructive jaundice by decision analysis. Gastrointest Endosc 49:466–471.
47. Moss AC, Morris E, MacMathuna P, 2006, Palliative biliary stents for obstructing pancreatic carcinoma. Cochrane Database Syst Rev 1:CD004200.
48. Bueno J, Gerdes H, Kurtz R, 2003, Endoscopic management of occluded biliary wallstents: a cancer center experience. Gastrointest Endosc 58:879–884.
49. Tham TC, Carr-Locke DL, Vandervoort J, 1998, Management of occluded wallstents. Gut 42:70–77.
50. Hausegger KA, Thurnher S, Borderdorfer G, 1998, Treatment of malignant biliary obstruction with polyurethane-covered Wallstents. AJR 170:403–408.
51. Soderlund C, Linder S. 2006, Covered metal versus plastic stents for malignant common bile duct stenosis: a prospective, randomized, controlled trial. Gastrointest Endosc 63:986–995.
52. Yoon WJ, Lee KJ, Lee KH, 2006, A comparison of covered and uncovered Wallstents for the management of distal malignant biliary obstruction. Gastrointest Endosc 63:986–995.
53. Isayama H, Komatsu Y, Tsujino T, 2000, A prospective randomized study of covered vs uncovered metallic stent for distal malignant biliary stricture. Gastrointest Endosc 51:AB191.
54. Carr-Locke DL. 2005, Metal stents for distal biliary malignancy: have we got you covered? Gastrointest Endosc 61:534–535.
55. Leung J, Rahim N, 2006, The role of covered self-expandable metallic stents in malignant biliary strictures. Gastrointest Endosc 63:1001–1003.
56. Smilanich RP, Hafner GH, 1994, Complications of biliary stents in obstructive pancreatic malignancies. A case report and review. Dig Dis Sci 39: 2645–2649.
57. Christensen P, Matzen P, Schultze S, 2004, Complications of ERCP: a prospective study. Gastrointest Endosc 60:721–731.
58. Okamoto T, Fujioka Yanagisawa S, 2006, Placement of a metallic stent across the main duodenal papilla may predispose to cholangitis. Gastrointest Endosc 63:792–796.
59. Puspok A, Lomoschitz F, Dejaco C, 2005, Endoscopic ultrasound guided therapy of benign and malignant biliary obstruction. Am J Gastroenterol 100:1743–1747.
60. Burmester E, Niehaus J, Leineweber T, 2003, EUS-cholangio-drainage of the bile duct: report of 4 cases. Gastrointest Endosc 57:246–251.
61. Giovannini M, Moutardier V, Pesenti C, 2001, Endoscopic ultrasound-guided bilioduodenal anastomosis: a new technique for biliary drainage. Endoscoy 33:898–900.
62. Kahaleh M, Yoshida C, Kane L, 2004, Interventional EUS cholangiography: a report of 5 cases. Gastrointest Endosc 60:138–142.

63. Maire F, Hammel P, Ponsot P, 2006, Long-term outcome of biliary and duodenal stents in palliative treatment of patients with unresectable adenocarcinoma of the head of the pancreas. Gastrointest Endosc 101:735–742.
64. Turnbull A, Kussin S, Kurtz RC, 1980, Palliative prosthetic intubation in gastric cancer. J Surg Oncol 15:37–42.
65. Telford J, Carr-Locke DL, Baron TH, 2004, Palliation of patients with malignant gastric outlet obstruction with the enteral wallstent: outcomes from a multicenter study. Gastrointest Endosc 60:916–920.
66. Nassif T, Prat F, Meduri B, 2003, Endoscopic palliation of malignant gastric outlet obstruction using self-expandable metallic stents: results of a multicenter study. Endoscopy 35:483–489.
67. Dormann A, Meisner S, Verin N, 2004, Self-expanding metal stents for gastroduodenal malignancies: systematic review of their clinical effectiveness. Endoscopy 36:543–550.
68. Yim HB, Jacobson BC, Saltzman JR, 2001, Clinical outcome of the use of enteral stents for palliation of patients with malignant upper GI obstruction. Gastrointest Endosc 53:329–332.
69. Wong YT, Brams DM, Munson L, 2002, Gastric outlet obstruction secondary to pancreatic cancer. Surg Endoscopy 16:310–312.
70. Johnsson E, Thune A, Liedman B. 2004, Palliation of malignant gastroduodenal obstruction with open surgical bypass or endoscopic stenting: clinical outcome and health economic evaluation. World J Surg 8:812–817.
71. Maetani I, Tada T, Ukita T, 2004, Comparison of duodenal stent placement with surgical gastrojejunostomy for palliation in patients with duodenal obstructions caused by pancreaticobiliary malignancies. Endoscopy 36:73–78.
72. Del Piano M, Ballare M, Montino F, 2005, Endoscopy or surgery for malignant GI outlet obstruction? Gastrointest Endosc 61:421–426.
73. Fiori E, Lamazza A, Volpino P, 2004, Palliative management of malignant antro pyloric strictures. Gastroenterostomy vs. endoscopic stenting. A randomized prospective trial. Anticancer Res 24:269–271.
74. Adler DG, Baron TH, 2002, Endoscopic palliation of malignant gastric outlet obstruction using self-expanding metal stents: experience in 36 patients. Am J Gastroenterol 97:72–78.
75. Baron TH, Schofl R, Peuspoek A, 2001, Expandable metal stent placement for gastric outlet obstruction. Endoscopy 33:623–628.
76. Mittal A, Windsor J, Woodfield J, 2004, Matched study of three methods for palliation of malignant pyloroduodenal obstruction. Br J Surgery 91:205–209.
77. Kaw M, Singh S, Gagneja H, 2003, Clinical outcome of simultaneous self-expandable metal stents for palliation of malignant biliary and duodenal obstruction. Surg Endosc 17:457–461.
78. Vanbiervliet G, Demarquay J, Dumas R, 2004, Endoscopic insertion of biliary stents in 18 patients with metallic duodenal stents who developed secondary malignant obstructive jaundice. Gastroenterol Clin Biol 28:1209–1213.
79. Barkin JS, Goldberg RI, Sfakianasis GN, Levi J, 1986, Pancreatic carcinoma is associated with delayed gastric emptying. Dig Dis Sci 31:265–267.
80. Ginsberg G, Barthel L, Cope C, 2000, Peroral creation of durable gastroenteric anastomosis with magnetic compression and stenting (abstract). Gastrointest Endosc 51:AB97.
81. Takada H, Kuwayama H, Takehashi N, 2000, Non-invasive gastrointestinal anastomosis with magnet rings (abstract). Gastrointest Endosc 3l:AB104.
82. Swain P, Mukherjee D, Moose A, 2002, A single lumen access anastomosis device for flexible endoscopy (abstract). Gastrointest Endosc 55:AB96.
83. Villaverde A, Cope C, Chopita N, 2004, Long term follow-up of endoscopic gastroenteric anastomoses with magnets (EGAM). (Abstract) Gastrointest Endosc 59:AB92.
84. Brooksbank MA, Game PA, Ashby MA, 2002, Palliative venting gastrostomy in malignant intestinal obstruction. Palliat Med 16:520–526.
85. Kalser MH, Barkin J, MacIntyre JM, 1985, For the Gastrointestinal Study Group, pancreatic cancer: assessment of prognosis by clinical presentation. Cancer 56:397–402.

86. Grahm AL, Andren-Sandberg A, 1997, Prospective evaluation of pain in exocrine pancreatic cancer. Digestion 58:542–549.
87. Trede M, Carter DC 1993, Clinical evaluation and preoperative assessment. In: Trede M, Carter DC (eds.) Surgery of the pancreas. Churchill Livingstone, Edinburgh, 423–431.
88. Lillemoe KD, Cameron JL, Kaufman HS, 1993, Chemical splanchnicectomy in patients with unresectable pancreatic cancer: a prospective randomized trial. Ann Surg 217:447–457.
89. Kayahara M, Nagakawa T, Futagami F, 1996, Lymphatic flow and neural plexus invasion associated with carcinoma of the body and tail of the pancreas. Cancer 78:2485–2491.
90. Bockman DE, Buchler M, Malfertheiner P, et al. Analysis of nerves in chronic pancreattis. Gastroenterology 198, 94:1459–1469.
91. Karanjia ND, Reber HA. 1990, The cause and management of the pain of chronic pancreatitis. Gastroenterol Clin North Am 19:895–904.
92. Keith RG, Keshavjee SH, Kerenyi NR, 1985, Neuropathology of chronic pancreatitis in humans. Can J Surg 28:207–211.
93. Malfertheiner P, Dominguez-Munoz JE, Buchler MW, 1994, Chronic pancreatitis: management of pain. Digestion 55:29–34.
94. Busch EH, Atchison SR, 1989, Steroid celiac plexus block for chronic pancreatitis: results in 16 cases. J Clin Anesth 1:431–433.
95. Vercauteren MP, Coppejans H, Adriaensen HA, 1994, Pancreatitis pain treatment: an overview. Acta Anaesthsiol Belg 45:99–105.
96. Nagakawa T, Mori K, Nakano T, 1993, Perineural invasion of carcinoma of the pancreas and biliary tract. Br J Surg 80:619–621.
97. Paz Z, Rosen A, 1989, The human celiac ganglion and its splanchnic nerves. Acta Anat 136:129–133.
98. Ward EM, Rorie DK, Nauss LA, 1979, The celiac ganglia in man: normal anatomic variations. Anesth Analg 58:461–465.
99. Ihse I, Zoucas E, Gyllstedt E, 1999, Bilateral thoracoscopic splanchnicectomy: effects on pancreatic pain and function. Ann Surg 230:785–790.
100. Pimpec Barthes F, Le Chapuis O, Riquet M, 1998, Thoracoscopic splanchnicectomy for control of intractable pain in pancreatic cancer. Ann Thor Surg 65:810–813.
101. Leksowski K. 2001, Thoracoscopic splanchnicectomy for control of intractable pain due to advanced pancreatic cancer. Surg Endosc 15:129–131.
102. Pietrabissa A, Vistoli F, Carrobi A, 2000, Thoracoscopic splanchnicectomy for pain relief in unresectable pancreatic cancer. Arch Surg 135:332–335.
103. Saenz A, Kuriansky J, Salvador L, 2000, thoracoscopic splanchnicectomy for pain control in patients with unresectable carcinoma of the pancreas. Surg Endosc 14:717–720.
104. Lieberman RP, Walman SD, 1990, Celiac plexus neurolysis with modified transaortic approach. Radiology 175:274–276.
105. Ng KF, Tsui SL, Yang CS, 1999, Unilateral approach to posterior retrocrural celiac plexus block. Chinese Med J 112:89–92.
106. Eisenberg E, Carr DB, Chalmers TC, 1995, Neurolytic celiac plexus block for treatment of cancer pain: a meta-analysis. Anesth Analg 80:290–295.
107. Rykowski J, Hilgier M, 2000, Efficacy of neurolytic celiac plexus block in varying locations of pancreatic cancer: influence on pain relief. Anesthesiology 92:347–354.
108. Ischia S, Ischia A, Polati E, 1992, Three posterior celiac plexus block techniques. Anesthesiology 76:534–540.
109. Gunaratnam NT, sarma AV, Norton ID, 2001, A prospective study of EUS-guided celiac plexus neurolysis for pancreatic cancer pain. Gastrointest Endosc 54:316–324.
110. Oliveira R,de dos reis MP, Prado WA, 2004, The effects of early or late neurolytic sympathetic plexus block on the management of abdominal or pelvic cancer pain. Pain 10:400–408.
111. Caraceni A, Portenoy RK, 1996, Pain management in patients with pancreatic carcinoma. Cancer 44:656–662.

112. Gafanovich I, Shir Y, Tsvang E, 1998, Chronic diarrhea induced by celiac plexus block? J Clin Gastroenterol 26:300–302.
113. Iftikhar S, Loftus EV, 1998, Gastroparesis after celiac plexus block. Am J Gastroenterol 93:2223–2225.
114. Brown DL, Moore DC. 1988, The use of neurolytic celiac plexus block for pancreatic cancer: anatomy and technique. J Pain Symptom Manag 3:206–209.
115. Davies DD, 1993, Incidence of major complication of coeliac plexus block. J R Soc Med 86:264–264.
116. Conno F, De Caraceni A, Aldrighetti L, 1993, Paraplegia following celiac plexus block. Pain 55:383–385.
117. Dongen RT, van Crul BJ, 1991, Paraplegia following celiac plexus block. Anesthesia 46:862–863.
118. Wiersema MJ, Wiersema LM. 1996, Endosonography guided celiac plexus neurolysis. Gastrointest Endosc 44:656–662.
119. Gress F, Schmitt C, Sherman S, 2001, Endoscopic ultrasound guided celiac plexus block for managing abdominal pain associated with chronic pancreatitis: a prospective single center experience. Am J Gastroenterol 96:409–416.
120. Hoffman BJ, 2002, EUS-guided celiac plexus block/neurolysis. Gastrointest Endosc 56(Suppl):S26–28.
121. Gress F, Schmitt C, Sherman S, 1999, A prospective randomized comparison of endoscopic ultrasound and computed tomography-guided celiac plexus block for managing chronic pancreatitis pain. Am J Gastroenterol 94:872–874.
122. Gress F, Ciaccia D, Kiel J, 1997, Endoscopic ultrasound (EUS) guided celiac plexus block (CB) for management of pain due to chronic pancreatitis (CP): a large single center experience (abstract). Gastrointest Endosc 45:AB173.
123. Bhutani MS, 1999, Endoscopic ultrasound guided fine needle aspiration of pancreas. In: Bhutani MS (ed.) Interventional endoscopic ultrasonography. Harwood Academic Publishers, Amsterdam, 65–72.

Section VI
Multimodality Therapy of Pancreatic Cancer

Chapter 28
State of the Art in Radiation Therapy for Pancreas Cancer

Aaron C. Spalding and Edgar Ben-Josef

1 Introduction

Despite an extraordinary tendency for metastatic spread, radiotherapy may have an important role in the management of locally advanced unresectable cancer of the pancreas. Local control remains a significant clinical problem. In patients with unresectable disease, failure to control local disease is virtually uniform, and in patients undergoing curative resection, the rate of local relapse is 50–85% (*1*). Failure to control the primary is associated with symptoms such as pain, gastric outlet, and duodenal obstruction, and upper gastrointestinal ulceration and bleeding. Palliation of symptoms with radiotherapy (as the sole modality) is accomplished in nearly half of patients (*2*). It is almost certain that modern day combined-modality therapy provides even better palliation, but unfortunately solid data on symptom control and quality of life associated with such therapy are not available.

Improved local control not only provides a palliative benefit, but may also impact on survival. Chemotherapy can extend survival of patients with advanced disease by 2–3 months to a median of 5–6 months (*3, 4*) and it has been suggested that radiotherapy can also extend survival (*5*). The Gastrointestinal Tumor Study Group (GITSG) conducted a prospective phase III trial comparing SMF (streptozotocin, mitomycin, and 5-fluorouracil) chemotherapy alone to SMF plus external-beam radiotherapy to a dose of 54 Gy. They reported a significant benefit in median survival (9.7 months versus 7.4 months) in favor of the combined modality arm. Patients with unresectable disease who are rendered resectable by chemoradiotherapy and undergo surgery, appear to have a survival similar to patients who are surgical candidates at presentation (*10*), suggesting that aggressive local therapy may have an impact on survival. Like other fields of oncology (breast cancer and lymphoma, for instance), with the advent of more effective systemic agents, the need for local control and the impact of local control on survival are likely to become more evident.

A number of approaches have been taken to improve efficacy of radiation therapy, including the use of cytotoxic chemotherapy to enhance radiation effects and escalation of the physical radiation dose by means of intraoperative radiotherapy (IORT) or brachytherapy. Unfortunately, delivery of adequate radiation doses to the pancreas is limited by the radiosensitivity of the adjacent uninvolved organs in

A.M. Lowy et al. (eds.) *Pancreatic Cancer*.
doi: 10.1007/978-0-387-69252-4, © Springer Science+Business Media, LLC 2008

the upper abdomen. This chapter focuses on the new methodologies to overcome limitations of external beam radiotherapy.

2 Radiotherapy Targets

Selection of targets for radiotherapy is based on understanding of the pattern of spread of the tumor and on careful analysis of the patterns of failure. Pancreatic cancer is characterized by early spread to peripancreatic tissues, perineural extension, and lymph node metastases. Fortner et al. (*11*) reported that 11 of 12 patients with primary tumors of 2.5 cm or less in diameter had peripancreatic soft tissue invasion microscopically. Lymphatic metastases of pancreatic cancer have been studied extensively by the Japanese (*12–16*). Lymph flows from the head of the pancreas to the anterior and posterior pancreaticoduodenal lymph nodes, the mesenteric artery nodes, the celiac trunk nodes, the hepatoduodenal ligament nodes, the para-aortic nodes, and the inter aorta-cava nodes. Routes from the body and tail of the pancreas lead to the celiac trunk nodes, splenic artery nodes, superior mesenteric artery nodes, para-aortic nodes, and nodes at the inferior border of the pancreas (Fig. 28.1). The overall incidence of metastases in pancreatic head carcinomas is of the order of 75%, and even in small tumors (≤2.5 cm), the incidence could be as high as 42% (*11*).

The reported incidence of nerve involvement either inside or outside of the pancreas is 53–90% (*15, 17–20*). Pathways of cancer spread along nerves from the pancreatic head to the regional nodes have been described (*21*); the plexus pancreaticus capitalis: (1) extends from the right celiac ganglion to the upper medial margin of the uncinate process of the pancreas, and the plexus pancreaticus capitalis, and (2) extends from the superior mesenteric artery to the medial margin of the uncinate process. Additional plexuses have been described around the superior mesenteric artery and hepatoduodenal ligament. More recently, a detailed anatomic study suggested a somewhat different route of perineural spread (*22*). Pancreatic head cancer spreads to the celiac plexus and ganglion along the posterior hepatic plexus; uncinate process cancer spreads to the superior mesenteric plexus along the inferior pancreaticoduodenal artery plexus; and cancers of the pancreatic body and tail spread to the splenic plexus, celiac plexus, and ganglion. It has been suggested that the perineurium represents a barrier for pancreatic cancer spread and that the cancer cells use the sites of blood vessel entry into the perineurium to invade nerves (*23*). Perineural involvement can be discontinuous, and is often related to the histologic grade of the tumor (*24*).

This pattern of spread has led many to advocate radical resections to locally eradicate pancreatic cancer. Recommendations have included removal of a wide margin, a complete plexus dissection and skeletonization around the superior mesenteric artery, common hepatic artery, and celiac axis. These wide retroperitoneal dissections have not been shown, to date, to improve survival.

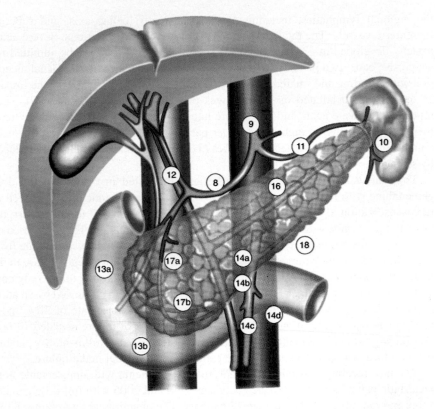

Fig. 28.1 Patterns of lymphatic spread of pancreatic cancer. Numbers indicate regional lymph node stations for pancreatic cancer metastasis. (Reproduced with permission from Gunderson LL, Tepper JA (eds.), Clinical radiation oncology. New York, Churchill Livingstone, 2006.)

For the same reasons, the primary tumor (or tumor bed), the duodenum, the draining lymph node basin, and the vascular trunks have been traditionally considered targets in the planning of external beam radiotherapy for pancreatic cancer (*25*). These large volumes can be treated safely (severe complication rate of <10%) to moderate doses (50–55 Gy) with concurrent 5-fluorouracil.

When gemcitabine was shown to be superior to 5-fluorouracil in patients with metastatic pancreatic cancer (*26*), a number of groups developed interest in combining it with radiation. Gemcitabine was shown to be a potent radiosensitizer of human tumor cells (*27, 28*) and these observations led to early clinical trials in lung and pancreatic cancer. It rapidly became clear that irradiating large volumes with concurrent gemcitabine will not be tolerated well because of the marked normal tissue toxicities.

Crane et al. (*29*) reported on 53 patients with locally advanced pancreatic cancer treated with gemcitabine (seven weekly cycles, 250–500 mg/m²) with concurrent radiotherapy. Patients were treated with a four-field technique with the beams equally weighted. The fields were designed to encompass the primary tumor and the regional lymphatics, including the porta hepatis, celiac axis, and superior mesenteric vessels. The total dose was 30–33 Gy in 10–11 fractions. Severe acute toxicity developed in 23% of patients, including 15% who had to be admitted for supportive care. Two patients (4%) developed severe late toxicity (duodenal ulceration with bleeding and small bowel obstruction). Additional evidence for the impact of the volume irradiated on toxicity was provided by Scalliet et al. (*30*). They reported six severe acute and four severe late complications (including three treatment-related deaths) in eight lung cancer patients treated with concurrent gemcitabine and radiation. In subsequent studies (*31, 32*) pulmonary toxicity was reduced by strictly limiting the target volume.

The University of Michigan group became interested in combining full-dose gemcitabine with radiation to simultaneously maximize systemic effects as well as radiosensitization. To reduce toxicity, the fields were designed to encompass the primary tumor only, without prophylactic lymph node irradiation. This was based on the thought that the majority of the benefit from radiation therapy would come from controlling the primary tumor and not from control of clinically occult disease in the nodes. In a phase I trial, 24–42 Gy in 15 fractions, delivered to the tumor only concurrently with gemcitabine (1,000 mg/m^2 on days 1, 8, and 15) followed by an additional cycle of gemcitabine, resulted in an objective response rate of 30% and a median survival of 11.6 months. Analysis of the pattern of failure revealed 14 failures (at any site) in 23 patients without metastatic disease at enrollment. Six patients suffered local progression and only one patient had a regional nodal failure.

We have recently expanded this analysis to all patients with unresectable non-metastatic pancreatic cancer treated between 1999 and 2005 with full-dose gemcitabine and radiotherapy. There were 77 patients. The planning target volume (PTV) was limited to the gross tumor volume (GTV) plus 1cm. The total dose was 24–42 Gy in 15 daily fractions. Pretreatment, treatment-planning, and follow-up CT scans were reviewed systematically for tumor size and evidence of local or systemic progression. In-field failure was defined as progression within the 80% isodose line. With a median follow-up time of 10.7 months (20.6 months in alive patients), local control was attained in 57 patients (74%) with a 1-year actuarial rate of 66%. Median time to progression was 7.4 months. The first site of progression was distant, local or combined in 30 patients (60% of failures), 15 (30%), and five (10%), respectively. Of the 15 patients who first progressed locally, 12 progressed in the GTV, two progressed in the GTV and with in-field lymph node metastases, and only one patient experienced a marginal peripancreatic lymph node failure.

We have also analyzed the toxicity associated with this regimen and its determinants. The medical records of 95 patients with unresectable pancreatic cancer treated with full-dose gemcitabine and radiation were reviewed and the following patient-and treatment-related variables were examined: race, age, gender, pre-existing microvascular disease, pretreatment abdominal surgery, biliary stent, GI or biliary bypass, pre-RT chemotherapy, total dose, PTV, volume receiving 20, 30, 35, and 40 Gy, the maximum dose to 1, 5, and 10 cm^3, and generalized equivalent uniform dose (gEUD) (*33, 34*) with $a = 6$ and $a = 10$. With a median follow-up time of 9.9 months (20.6 months in alive patients), 18 patients (19%)

developed severe toxicity: nine (9%) upper gastrointestinal bleeds, five (5%) diarrhea, four (4%) nausea/vomiting, one duodenal fistula, one radiation-induced colitis, one colon stricture, and one partial small bowel obstruction. There was a trend ($p = 0.13$) for larger PTVs to be associated with increased rates of any severe GI toxicity and for duodenal gEUD to be associated with severe duodenal toxicity. Patients with gEUD > 33 Gy (median; $a = 6$) and ≤33 had rates of 17% and 8%, respectively ($p = 0.09$). The rates of severe toxicity in women and men were 15% and 24% ($p = 0.017$). No other associations were found.

Thus, it appears that even when the PTV is limited to the GTV with a 1-cm margin, severe toxicity is related to volume, when radiation is combined with a potent radiosensitizer such a gemcitabine. It is also evident that such plans do not lead to marginal failures and exclusion of prophylactic lymph node irradiation in this setting does not compromise outcome. The potential advantage of a smaller PTV is better integration with more intensive systemic therapy and/or more intensive radiation dose-schedule. The latter is discussed at more length in the Intensity Modulated Radiotherapy (IMRT) section.

When PTVs are reduced, the risk of a geographic miss increases. In order for such a strategy to succeed, it is imperative that we know more about target motion and deformation. There is a paucity of data related to motion of the pancreas. Two small series have been published using implanted radio-opaque fiducial markers and fluoroscopy. The radiation oncology group at Stanford reported the results of one patient who had three 2-mm gold fiducial markers sutured into the tumor at the time of exploratory laparotomy as part of an aborted Whipple procedure. The patient was imaged fluoroscopically for one minute each in the anteroposterior (AP) and lateral directions to assess tumor motion during respiration. The maximal cranial-caudal (CC) movement was found to be 6 mm with breathing, and the lateral deviation 1 mm with aortic pulsation (35). The radiation oncology group at Massachusetts General Hospital reported a study of six patients who also underwent invasive marker placement and were observed fluoroscopically for 30 seconds each in the AP and lateral dimensions (36). The range of CC maximum motion was 6.5–18 mm, with an average of 4.4–12 mm. Movement in the AP dimension was much smaller, with a range of maximum values of 6.0–8.7 mm and a range of average values of 2.5–6.9 mm. While these small series provide important initial data regarding pancreatic movement, the use of fluoroscopy does not allow for analysis of pancreatic organ deformation and the relationship to adjacent organs.

In a more advanced study, Bussels et al. (37) recently reported their data using dynamic MRI to quantify pancreatic motion. They acquired one image every second for one minute in the axial and coronal planes. The pancreatic tumor was contoured on each image and the center of gravity on each frame was calculated. The movement over time of this center of gravity was analyzed in 12 patients. They found a larger degree of movement in the CC direction than reported by both the Stanford and Mass General groups, at 24 ± 16 mm.

We have recently reported preliminary data from our own study of breathing-related pancreas motion and deformation. We sought to characterize these changes in patients with unresectable pancreatic cancer and determine the dosimetric consequences of incorporating such data into Intensity IMRT planning. Six patients were imaged free breathing using noncontrast dynamic MRI on a 3T scanner. MR images were taken at a rate of three images/second, in a single plane (sagittal, coronal, and oblique), for 1 minute, using a 2D balanced fast field echo (BFFE) sequence. With the aid of an abdominal MRI radiologist, tumors were contoured, and the full extent of motion was determined in all six aspects of the target by relating it to a contour thought to represent the average end-exhale position. The observed motion was (range (mean)): superior 3–18 mm (8 mm), inferior 8–23 mm (16 mm), anterior 6–8 mm (7 mm), and posterior 2–8 mm (5 mm). There was no significant motion in the left to right direction.

Two IMRT plans were generated for each patient: one with no motion (assuming use of an Active Breathing Control (ABC) device), and another that incorporates individualized margins accounting for motion and deformation (assuming free breathing during treatment). GTV to CTV expansion was 5 mm in all patients. For each patient, two PTVs were then created: one with a 5-mm margin to account for setup uncertainty only (assuming use of ABC), the other also included the individualized extra margins for breathing. IMRT optimization was carried out using NEWOpt, our in-house optimization system that uses staged optimization and biological modeling in the objective function. The goals of optimization were to treat the GTV and also a surgical boost volume (SBV) encompassing 1 cm around the vasculature that was precluding resection. The optimization goals were prioritized to keep normal tissues in a clinically acceptable range (Table 28.1), increase the minimum target dose to 54 Gy, and then maximize gEUD in the PTV using a biological cost function, permitting target dose heterogeneity, with the highest dose localized to the SBV.

We found that PTV coverage was superior in plans that assume that motion has been eliminated. On average, the gEUD of the target PTV increased by 3 Gy (range 2–5Gy) for $a = -5$ and by 5 Gy (range 3–13 Gy) for $a = -15$. The gEUD of the SBV PTV increased even more: 4 Gy (range 1–12) for $a = -5$ and 5 Gy (range 1–13) for $a = -15$. These plans also delivered lower doses to normal tissues. For example, mean duodenal dose decreased on average by 3 Gy (range 2–5 Gy), and mean small-bowel dose decreased by 2 Gy (range 0–2 Gy) ($p = 0.002$ and $p = 0.005$, respectively).

Taken together, the available data suggest that motion and deformation of pancreatic tumors is substantial and varies considerably among patients. The use of ABC (or other methods to reduce breathing motion) is very important in pancreas IMRT or other plans that target the GTV with narrow margins. When patients are treated free-breathing, adequate expansions must be used to allow for target motion.

Table 28.1 Optimization goals for pancreatic cancer IMRT

Structure	Constraints
Kidney (L & R)	Max dose ≤20 Gy; not more than 10% of the volume can be between 18 and 20 Gy
Liver	Minimize NTCP
Stomach, Small intestine	Max dose ≤54 Gy; 2% of the volume can be between 50 and 54 Gy, 25% of the volume can be between 45 and 54 Gy
Spinal cord	Max dose ≤45 Gy
Duodenum	Max dose ≤60 Gy; not more than 33% of the volume can be between 45 and 60 Gy

3 Radiotherapy Dose

The radiation dose used currently in standard practice is grossly inadequate. Radiation doses of the order of 50–54 Gy are typically prescribed because of the low radiation tolerance of the surrounding small intestine, duodenum, stomach, kidneys, and spinal cord. To overcome these limitations and avoid dose to the organs at risk, some investigators combined preoperative external beam irradiation with intraoperative radiation or an interstitial radioactive implant (38–41). A more common approach has been to combine external-beam radiotherapy with a radiosensitizer (typically 5-fluorouracil), to preferentially enhance cytotoxic effects in the tumor.

Attempts to increase the physical radiation dose have resulted in severe complications. Ceha et al. (42) treated 44 patients with unresectable pancreatic carcinoma on a prospective phase II study at the Academic Medical Center in Amsterdam. Contrast-enhanced spiral CT scanning was used for 3D treatment planning. The gross tumor volume (GTV) consisted of the demonstrable extent of disease and included the primary tumor alone in 61% of patients or the primary tumor plus enlarged adjacent lymph nodes in 39% of patients. The planning target volume (PTV) was defined as the GTV plus a 1-cm margin in all directions but PTVs were not allowed to exceed 9 cm in any direction. This was an arbitrary choice in order to limit the treated volume to reduce toxicity. The total radiation dose was 70 Gy in the first 10 patients and 72 Gy in the subsequent 34 patients. Radiotherapy was delivered in 2 Gy fractions, 5 days a week. The maximal spinal cord dose was not allowed to exceed 46 Gy. One-third of one kidney was allowed to receive a dose exceeding 25 Gy provided that the contralateral kidney was not irradiated. The maximum allowed dose to the stomach was 50 Gy. Because of the proximity of the duodenum to the tumor, a maximum of 30% of its volume (the part directly adjacent to the pancreas) was allowed to exceed 50 Gy. Severe acute toxicity (grade 3 fatigue, nausea, upper gastrointestinal bleeding, and death of sepsis) was observed in five patients (11%). Late toxicity developed in 18% of patients. It included grade 3 upper gastrointestinal bleedings (7%), grade 4 stomach perforation (2%) and duodenal obstruction (2%), and three deaths of gastrointestinal bleeding (7%). Despite the excessive toxicity, the median overall survival time was an encouraging 10 months from the start of radiotherapy and the 1-year survival rate was 39%.

4 Radiotherapy Techniques

4.1 Three-dimensional Conformal Radiotherapy

Three-dimensional conformal radiotherapy (3DCRT) planning should be based on a helical CT obtained in the treatment position following administration of oral and double-phase intravenous contrast. The GTV is defined as the primary tumor (or tumor bed) plus any involved regional lymph nodes. The clinical treatment volume (CTV) may include the uninvolved regional lymph nodes. There are no standards that define the extent of the coverage of these lymph nodes. When treating with concurrent full-dose gemcitabine, the CTV includes the GTV with 0.5 cm margin, with no prophylactic irradiation of uninvolved nodes. The PTV encompasses the CTV with 1- to 2-cm margin to allow for set-up errors and target motion. When treating with concurrent full-dose gemcitabine, the CTV to PTV expansion has traditionally been 0.5 cm margin, although it is becoming apparent that such expansion is probably not sufficient. Multiple planar or non-coplanar beams should be used. Figures 28.2 and 28.3 demonstrate typical plans used at the University of Michigan in the postoperative setting and for the treatment of unresectable disease, respectively.

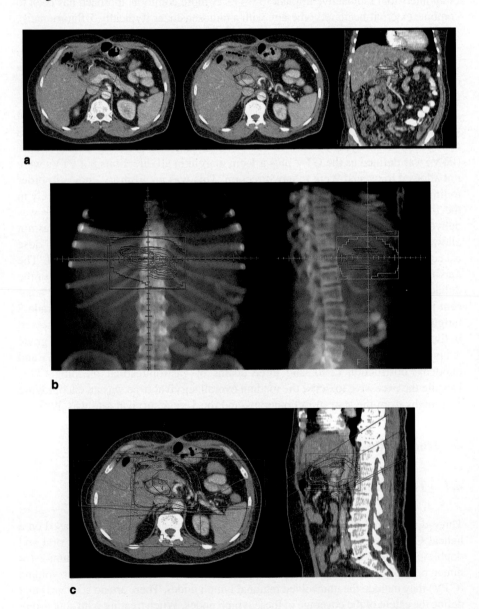

a

b

c

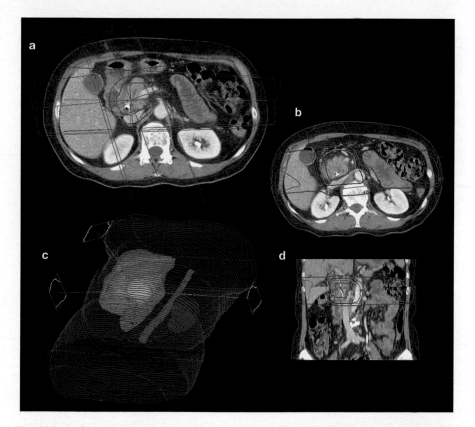

Fig. 28.3 Definitive radiotherapy plan for a patient with unresectable pancreatic cancer. The patient received concurrent full-dose gemcitabine. **A.** The GTV *(blue)* and PTV *(yellow)*. Beam arrangement is shown in **(A)**. **B.** Radiation was delivered through a left lateral and two right anterior oblique fields. Also shown are the spinal cord *(green)*, left kidney *(red)*, right kidney *(yellow)*, liver *(gray)*, and PTV *(pink)*. **C–D.** Dose distribution in an axial and coronal plane, respectively

4.2 Intensity Modulated Radiotherapy

Technological improvements over the past decade may now allow us to overcome the limitations described in the preceding. With the use of intensity modulated radiotherapy (IMRT), pancreatic tumors can be treated to higher radiation doses, whereas lower doses are delivered to OARs.

◄

Fig. 28.2 Postoperative radiation treatment plan. A. Tumor bed *(blue)*, portal (red), and celiac *(green)* lymph node regions, as well as a composite PTV *(pink)* in axial and coronal planes. The patient was treated with right and left lateral fields and an anterior inferosuperior oblique field. B. Beam-eye's view of the fields used. C. The resultant dose distribution

Landry et al. (*43*) evaluated the influence of IMRT with inverse treatment planning on the DVHs of normal tissue compared to 3DCRT in 10 patients with pancreatic cancer. The goal was to deliver 61.2 Gy to the GTV and 45 Gy to the CTV while maintaining critical normal tissues to below specified tolerances. They found IMRT plans to be more conformal than 3DCRT plans. The average dose delivered to one third of the small bowel was lower with the IMRT plan compared with 3DCRT. The dose delivered to one third of the small bowel was 30.2 Gy and 38.5 Gy with IMRT and 3DCRT plans, respectively ($p = 0.006$). The median volume of small bowel receiving >50 Gy or 60 Gy was reduced with IMRT. The median volume of small bowel >50 Gy was 19.2% and 31% for IMRT and 3DCRT, respectively. The median volume of small bowel exceeding 60 Gy was 12.5% and 19.8% for IMRT and 3DCRT, respectively. The normal-tissue complication probability model predicted a small bowel complication probability of 9.3% with IMRT compared to 24.4% with 3DCRT delivery of dose ($p = 0.021$).

There is very little clinical experience with the use of IMRT in pancreatic cancer. The Wayne State University group has reported on 15 patients (seven treated adjuvantly after curative resection and eight treated for unresectable disease) (*44*). IMRT was planed using the CORVUS system and delivered with a segmented multileaf collimator, using a 6 MV photon beam and ten intensity steps. Two target volumes were entered; target 1 consisted of the gross tumor volume (in unresectable cases) or the tumor bed (in post surgical cases) and target 2 consisted of the draining lymph nodes. Both targets were treated simultaneously in 25 daily fractions, 5 days a week. In the postoperative setting the total dose to target 1 was 45–54 Gy (median: 54 Gy). For unresectable disease the dose was 54–55 Gy (median: 54 Gy). The total dose to target 2 was 45 Gy in all patients. Patients were treated with one of two six-field beam arrangements that had been found to produce superior dose distributions in prior studies. Capecitabine was given at 1,600 mg/m^2/day in two divided doses, 5 days per week, concurrently with radiotherapy. In addition, most patients (73%) received gemcitabine-based chemotherapy. Systemic chemotherapy was given before, after, or both before and after chemo-radiotherapy in 47%, 7%, and 20% of patients, respectively. Treatment was tolerated well. Only one patient (7%) developed grade III toxicity: gastric ulceration that responded to medical management. Encouragingly, in the unresectable group, the 1-year actuarial survival rate was 69% and two patients (25%) converted to resectability.

At the University of Michigan, we have explored the potential of IMRT to escalate the dose to the target while respecting normal tissue tolerances. We hypothesized that by allowing greater heterogeneity across the PTV, we will be able to deposit substantially greater doses within the PTV. To drive the process of dose escalation in a biologically meaningful way, we elected to use the concept of gEUD. Originally introduced by Niemierko (*33*), gEUD is the biologically equivalent dose that, if given uniformly, would lead to the same level of tumor cell kill as the actual nonuniform dose distribution at hand. Subsequently, the concept was extended to normal tissues (*34*). Additional work showed that gEUD can be used for IMRT optimization (*45*). Comparing dose-volume–based and gEUD–based optimization of IMRT plans for prostate and head and neck cancer patients, Wu et al. (45) found that the latter allowed similar or better target coverage with a parallel reduction in dose to OAR.

We compared 3DCRT and IMRT treatment plans for 15 patients with locally advanced unresectable pancreatic cancer. GTV was defined as the imaged tumor on a pancreas protocol CT. PTV was defined as the GTV plus 1 cm expansion, as per planning guidelines in our previous institutional clinical trials. In addition, within the GTV, we defined the area of vascular involvement precluding surgical resection as the surgical boost volume (SBV). One of the level 2 goals (see the following) was to preferentially escalate the dose within this volume. The constraints for OAR in the IMRT plan are detailed in Table 28.1. A previously described (44), six-field non-coplanar beam arrangement with 5 mm IMRT beamlets was used (Fig. 28.4A).

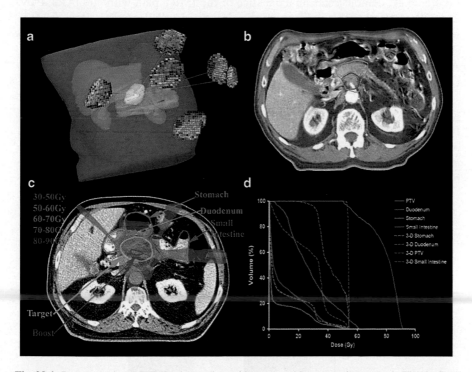

Fig. 28.4 Representative IMRT plan in a patient with unresectable pancreatic cancer. **A.** The six-field non-coplanar beam arrangement typically used, with their intensity maps. Also shown are the PTV *(pink)*, duodenum *(yellow)*, small intestine *(tan)*, stomach *(green)*, kidneys *(blue)*, and liver *(brown)*. **B.** The GTV *(pink)* and surgical boost volume *(red)*. **C.** Dose distribution and OAR and PTV. Note the high dose achievable in a large part of the PTV and the rapid falloff, meeting stringent constraints in OAR. **D.** Dose-volume histograms comparing IMRT *(solid lines)* and 3DCRT *(dashed lines)*. Note that IMRT results in substantial increases in dose to PTV and substantial decreases in dose to OAR

Optimization was performed using lexicographic ordering. The hierarchical planning goals are categorized into several levels of priority. The various priority level goals are optimized sequentially, one level of priority at a time, with the least important planning goals addressed last. By subdividing a large multicriteria problem into several somewhat smaller problems based on priority levels, the complex space of tradeoffs can be significantly simplified, greatly decreasing the need for iterative optimization trials before a solution that satisfies the goals of the protocol is found. In this study, the OAR dose goals were identified as the most important, therefore addressed at the first level. After the dose limits for the OARs were ensured, the next goal of escalating the PTV dose (maximize the minimum target dose, maximize the target gEUD, and keep maximum target dose <90Gy) was pursued at the second level. Finally, a general goal of dose reduction to all normal tissues was pursued at the last level.

An example IMRT plan is provided in Fig. 28.4. The beam arrangement is shown in Fig. 28.4A and target volume definitions are shown in Fig. 28.4B. Figure 28.4C demonstrates an axial slice of the IMRT plan with all OARs, PTV, and SBV defined with a color wash showing the dose distribution. A steep dose gradient exists in the overlap regions of OARs and PTV. In Fig. 28.4D, DVHs are shown comparing the 3DCRT and IMRT plans (dashed and solid lines, respectively). As can be seen, in the IMRT plan the PTV dose is higher and the mean dose in OARs is reduced.

Comparing the dose distributions in 15 patients, we found that the mean PTV gEUD achieved with IMRT was substantially higher. Figure 28.5A shows gEUD for two a values, -5 (66 ± 5 Gy versus 52 ± 11, $p < 0.005$) or -15 (59 ± 4 Gy versus 50 ± 13, $p < 0.005$). Simultaneous escalating the dose in the SBV resulted in an average gEUD in the vascular interface of 85 Gy, regardless of a value. At the same time, gEUD was significantly reduced in OARs. Figure 28.5B demonstrates the

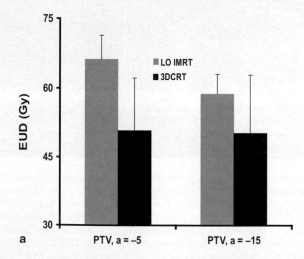

Fig. 28.5 (continued)

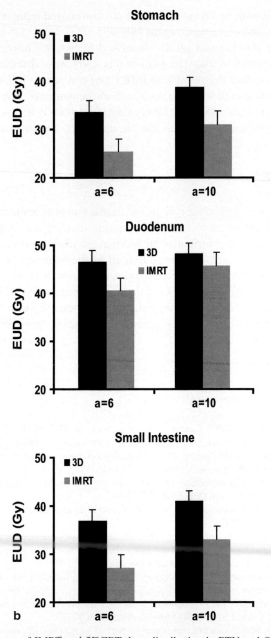

Fig. 28.5 Comparison of IMRT and 3DCRT dose distribution in PTV and OAR. **A.** IMRT can achieve substantial escalation of EUD in the PTV. The bars represent mean ± standard deviation in 15 pancreatic cancer cases (*a* = –5 represents a radiosensitive tumor and *a* = –15 represents a radioresistant tumor). **B.** IMRT can achieve reduced EUD in OAR. Bars represent mean doses ± standard deviation in 15 cases (*a* values of 6 and 10 have been used for normal tissues based on previous publications)

gEUD calculated with two *a* values (6 and *10*) considered representative of the tissue tolerance of gastrointestinal organs (*46–48*).

Based on the rational and results discussed herein, we have initiated a phase I radiation dose escalation trial. The goals of this study are to determine the maximum tolerated radiation dose delivered with IMRT and concurrent full-dose gemcitabine in patients with unresectable adenocarcinoma of the pancreas. The radiation dose to the PTV is escalated from 45 Gy in 1.8 Gy fractions to 60 Gy in 2.4 Gy fractions. The SBV is treated concurrently to doses that are up to 30% higher than the PTV doses.

5 Summary

Radiotherapy has an important role in the management of cancer of the pancreas, and with the advent of more effective systemic therapy, the importance of local control and its potential contribution to survival are likely to become more evident. Radiotherapy for this disease has been limited by the tolerance of normal tissues in the upper abdomen, but modern technologies may now allow us to overcome these limitations. Clinical implementation of the methodologies described in this chapter could result not only in improved palliation, but potentially in improvements in survival by delaying time to local progression and/or by improving resectability of borderline-resectable tumors.

References

1. Evans DB, Rich TA. 1997, Cancer of the pancreas. In: DeVita HS, Rosenberg SA (eds.) Cancer: principles and practice of oncology. Lippincott-Raven, Philadelphia. 1059–1060.
2. Haslam JB, Cavanaugh PJ, Stroup SL. 1973, Radiation therapy in the treatment of irresectable adenocarcinoma of the pancreas. Cancer 32(6):1341–1345.
3. Glimelius B, 1996, Chemotherapy improves survival and quality of life in advanced pancreatic and biliary cancer. Ann Oncol 7(6):593–600.
4. Palmer KR, 1994, Chemotherapy prolongs survival in inoperable pancreatic carcinoma. Br J Surg 81(6):882–885.
5. Gastrointestinal Tumor Study Group. Treatment of locally unresectable carcinoma of the pancreas: comparison of combined-modality therapy (chemotherapy plus radiotherapy) to chemotherapy alone. J Natl Cancer Inst 1988, 80(10):751–755.
6. Jain S, 2005, Carcinoma of the pancreas with portal vein involvement—our experience with a modified technique of resection. Hepatogastroenterology 52(65):1596–1600.
7. Geer RJ, Brennan MF. 1993, Prognostic indicators for survival after resection of pancreatic adenocarcinoma. Am J Surg 165(1):68–72; discussion 72–73.
8. Bold RJ, 1999, Major vascular resection as part of pancreaticoduodenectomy for cancer: radiologic, intraoperative, and pathologic analysis. J Gastrointest Surg 3(3):233–243.
9. Lygidakis NJ, 2004, Mono-bloc total spleno-pancreaticoduodenectomy for pancreatic head carcinoma with portal-mesenteric venous invasion. A prospective randomized study. Hepatogastroenterology 51(56):427–433.
10. Ammori JB, 2003, Surgical resection following radiation therapy with concurrent gemcitabine in patients with previously unresectable adenocarcinoma of the pancreas. J Gastrointest Surg 7(6):766–772.

11. Fortner JG, 1996, Tumor size is the primary prognosticator for pancreatic cancer after regional pancreatectomy. Ann Surg 223(2):147–153.
12. Kayahara M, 1992, Lymphatic flow in carcinoma of the head of the pancreas. Cancer 70(8):2061–2066.
13. Kayahara M, 1995, Surgical strategy for carcinoma of the pancreas head area based on clinico-pathologic analysis of nodal involvement and plexus invasion. Surgery 117(6):616–623.
14. Nagakawa T, 1993, The pattern of lymph node involvement in carcinoma of the head of the pancreas. A histologic study of the surgical findings in patients undergoing extensive nodal dissections. Int J Pancreatol 13(1):15–22.
15. Nagakawa T, 1993, A clinical study on lymphatic flow in carcinoma of the pancreatic head area—peripancreatic regional lymph node grouping. Hepatogastroenterology 40(5): 457–462.
16. Nakao A, 1997, Lymph node metastasis in carcinoma of the body and tail of the pancreas. Br J Surg 84(8):1090–1092.
17. Fortner JG, 1977, Regional pancreatectomy: en bloc pancreatic, portal vein and lymph node resection. Ann Surg 186(1):42–50.
18. Nagakawa T, 1993, Perineural invasion of carcinoma of the pancreas and biliary tract. Br J Surg 80(5):619–621.
19. Nakao A, 1996, Clinical significance of carcinoma invasion of the extrapancreatic nerve plexus in pancreatic cancer. Pancreas 12(4):357–361.
20. Takahashi T, 1997, Perineural invasion by ductal adenocarcinoma of the pancreas. J Surg Oncol 65(3):164–170.
21. Yoshioka H, Wakabayashi. T. 1958, Therapeutic neurotomy on head of pancreas for relief of pain due to chronic pancreatitis: a new technical procedure and its results. AMA Arch Surg 76(4):546–554.
22. Yi SQ, 2003, Innervation of the pancreas from the perspective of perineural invasion of pancreatic cancer. Pancreas 27(3):225–229.
23. Nagakawa T, 1992, A clinicopathologic study on neural invasion in cancer of the pancreatic head. Cancer 69(4):930–935.
24. Hirai I, 2002, Perineural invasion in pancreatic cancer. Pancreas 24(1):15–25.
25. Foo M, Gunderson L, Urrutia R. 2000, Pancreatic cancer. In: Gunderson L, Tepper JE (eds.) Clinical radiation oncology. Churchill Livingstone, Philadelphia, 700–702.
26. Burris HA 3rd,1997, Improvements in survival and clinical benefit with gemcitabine as first-line therapy for patients with advanced pancreatic cancer: a randomized trial. J Clin Oncol 15(6):2403–2413.
27. Shewach DS, 1994, Metabolism of 2',2'-difluoro-2'-deoxycytidine and radiation sensitization of human colon carcinoma cells. Cancer Res 54(12):3218–3223.
28. Lawrence TS, 1996, Radiosensitization of pancreatic cancer cells by 2',2'-difluoro-2'-deoxy-cytidine. Int J Radiat Oncol Biol Phys 34(4):867–872.
29. Crane CH, 2002, Is the therapeutic index better with gemcitabine-based chemoradiation than with 5-fluorouracil-based chemoradiation in locally advanced pancreatic cancer? Int J Radiat Oncol Biol Phys 52(5):1293–1302.
30. Scalliet PGC, Galdermans D, Meerbeek J, et al. GEMZAR (trade) (Gemcitabine) with thoracic radiotherapy—a phase II pilot study in chemonaive patients with advanced nonsmall cell lung cancer (NSCLC). Proc Am Soc Clin Oncol, 1998, 1923.
31. Groen HGA, van Putten J, van der Leest A, et al. Phase I study of gemcitabine (G) and high-dose thoracic radiation (RTf) in stage III non-small lung cancer (NSCLC). Proc Am Soc Clin Oncol 2000, 2123.
32. Vokes EE, 2002, Randomized phase II study of cisplatin with gemcitabine or paclitaxel or vinorelbine as induction chemotherapy followed by concomitant chemoradiotherapy for stage IIIB non-small-cell lung cancer: cancer and leukemia group B study 9431. J Clin Oncol 20(20):4191–4198.
33. Niemierko A. 1997, Reporting and analyzing dose distributions: a concept of equivalent uniform dose. Med Phys 24(1):103–110.

34. Niemierko A, 1999, A generalized concept of equivalent uniform dose (EUD) (Abstract). Med Phys 26:1100.
35. Murphy MJ, 2002, The effectiveness of breath-holding to stabilize lung and pancreas tumors during radiosurgery. Int J Radiat Oncol Biol Phys 53(2):475–482.
36. Gierga DP, 2004, Quantification of respiration-induced abdominal tumor motion and its impact on IMRT dose distributions. Int J Radiat Oncol Biol Phys 58(5):1584–1595.
37. Bussels B, 2003, Respiration-induced movement of the upper abdominal organs: a pitfall for the three-dimensional conformal radiation treatment of pancreatic cancer. Radiother Oncol 68(1):69–74.
38. Dobelbower RR Jr, 1986, 125I interstitial implant, precision high-dose external beam therapy, and 5-FU for unresectable adenocarcinoma of pancreas and extrahepatic biliary tree. Cancer 58(10):2185–2195.
39. Mohiuddin M, 1992, Long-term results of combined modality treatment with I-125 implantation for carcinoma of the pancreas. Int J Radiat Oncol Biol Phys 23(2):305–311.
40. Roldan GE, 1988, External beam versus intraoperative and external beam irradiation for locally advanced pancreatic cancer. Cancer 61(6):1110–1116.
41. Mohiuddin M, 1995, Combined intraoperative radiation and perioperative chemotherapy for unresectable cancers of the pancreas. J Clin Oncol 13(11):2764–2768.
42. Ceha HM, 2000, Feasibility and efficacy of high dose conformal radiotherapy for patients with locally advanced pancreatic carcinoma. Cancer 89(11):2222–2229.
43. Landry JC, 2002, Treatment of pancreatic cancer tumors with intensity-modulated radiation therapy (IMRT) using the volume at risk approach (VARA): employing dose-volume histogram (DVH) and normal tissue complication probability (NTCP) to evaluate small bowel toxicity. Med Dosim 27(2):121–129.
44. Ben-Josef E, 2004, Intensity-modulated radiotherapy (IMRT) and concurrent capecitabine for pancreatic cancer. Int J Radiat Oncol Biol Phys 59(2):454–459.
45. Wu Q, 2002, Optimization of intensity-modulated radiotherapy plans based on the equivalent uniform dose. Int J Radiat Oncol Biol Phys 52(1):224–235.
46. Schwarz M, 2004, Sensitivity of treatment plan optimisation for prostate cancer using the equivalent uniform dose (EUD) with respect to the rectal wall volume parameter. Radiother Oncol 73(2):209–218.
47. Rancati T, 2004, Fitting late rectal bleeding data using different NTCP models: results from an Italian multi-centric study (AIROPROS0101). Radiother Oncol 73(1):21–32.
48. Ghilezan M, 2004, Online image-guided intensity-modulated radiotherapy for prostate cancer: how much improvement can we expect? A theoretical assessment of clinical benefits and potential dose escalation by improving precision and accuracy of radiation delivery. Int J Radiat Oncol Biol Phys 60(5):1602–1610.

Chapter 29
The Evolution of Chemoradiation Strategies for Locally Advanced Pancreatic Cancer

A. William Blackstock and Stacy Wentworth

1 Introduction

In the United States, the incidence of pancreatic cancer has been on the rise since the 1930s and has seemed to level out since the 1970s. In 2008, it is projected that an estimated 37,680 new cases of pancreatic cancer will be diagnosed in the United States, resulting in approximately 34,290 deaths from the disease (*1*). Mortality rates closely follow incidence rates because of the poor prognosis of pancreatic cancer. In the United States, it is the fourth and the fifth most common cancer in men and women, respectively, and has the lowest 5-year survival rate of any cancer; generally <5% with little improvement in survival observed in the past 20 years (*1, 2*). Most patients who have pancreatic cancer succumb to metastatic disease, and current available treatments have had little impact on survival, indicating a lack of adequate systemic treatments. Surgery offers the only potential cure for pancreatic carcinoma, yet <20% of the patients present with tumors that are ultimately deemed resectable. Approximately two thirds of all pancreatic cancer patients have metastatic disease at the time of diagnosis, whereas the majority of the remaining patients have locally advanced unresectable disease. Cures for patients with locally advanced/unresectable pancreatic cancer are only anecdotal.

Patients with pancreatic cancer are staged according to the recently updated American Joint Committee on Cancer (AJCC) TNM staging system (*3*), in which disease stage is determined by the size of the primary tumor, its relationship to the celiac axis and the superior mesenteric artery (T), presence or absence of regional node involvement (N), and presence or absence of distant metastases (M). For general treatment purposes, pancreatic cancers are divided into categories that include resectable disease (T1–T3), locally advanced/unresectable disease (T4), and metastatic disease (M1). A locally advanced, unresectable pancreatic cancer is defined broadly as a tumor with evidence of extrapancreatic disease (extensive peripancreatic lymph node involvement and/or distant metastases), direct involvement of the celiac axis, superior mesenteric artery, inferior vena cava or aorta, or encasement or occlusion of the superior mesenteric vein–portal vein confluence (Fig. 29.1). Ultimately, determination of the pathologic AJCC stage and tumor resectability can only be established during laparotomy, when direct visualization and histologic

A.M. Lowy et al. (eds.) *Pancreatic Cancer.*
doi: 10.1007/978-0-387-69252-4, © Springer Science+Business Media, LLC 2008

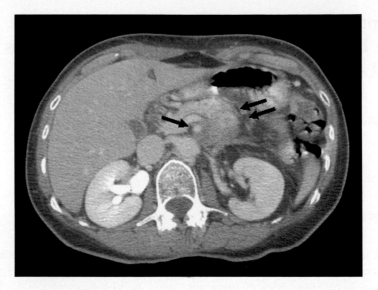

Fig. 29.1 Locally advanced pancreatic cancer: mass in the head of the pancreas *(double arrows)* surrounding the superior mesenteric artery *(arrow)*

confirmation is possible. For patients diagnosed with pancreatic cancer for which laparoscopic staging is not an option, physicians must rely on clinical evaluation and radiographic findings to base treatment decisions and estimate prognosis.

Therapeutic options for patients with locally advanced pancreatic cancer include radiation, chemotherapy, or radiation combined with chemotherapy. Trials incorporating newer targeted agents are currently underway and will be reviewed.

2   Radiation Delivery Strategies

Although external beam radiation therapy (EBRT) alone can result in palliation of pancreatic cancer related pain and obstructive symptoms (*4*), it does not provide optimal tumor control. Local failure exceeds 70% when conventional doses (40–60 Gy) of EBRT are used alone (*5*). Thus, techniques that increase the radiation dose to the tumor volume without increasing normal tissue toxicity have been investigated. Permanent Iodine-125 radioactive seed implantation and intraoperative electrons (IOERT) have been used as a dose-escalation technique in combination with chemotherapy and external beam radiation. IOERT allows for the direct visualization and delivery of radiation to the tumor, and allows sparing of the surrounding normal tissue. Data from single institution studies indicate that IOERT used at appropriate doses can be used safely and result in an improvement in local control when compared to conventional external beam techniques (*5–11*). In a study from Willett et al., 150 patients were treated with IOERT, external beam radiation, and chemotherapy. The 3- and 5-year survival for patients with locally advanced pancreatic cancer were reported to be 7% and 4%, respectively, with long-term survival demonstrated in eight patients who had small tumors. The authors conclude that IOERT may provide a benefit for selected patients with small, unresectable tumors (*12*).

Both Iodine-125 and Palladium-103 have been used for interstitial brachytherapy treatment for unresectable pancreatic cancer alone or in combination with external beam radiation ± 5-FU. Three small studies reported on patients with unresectable pancreatic cancer who were treated with iodine-125 implant (120–210 Gy), followed external beam radiation using standard fractionation plus 5-FU. Two of the three studies reported palliation of pain in approximately 60% of patients, and one study reported an 84% local control rate. Unfortunately, a number of treatment-related complications were reported, including gastrointestinal bleeding, fistula formation, gastric or small bowel obstruction, intra-abdominal abscess, and deep vein thrombosis/ pulmonary embolism (*13–17*).

Patients have also been treated with fast neutron particle beam therapy with or without conventional external beam radiation ± chemotherapy in attempt to improve local control (*18–20*). The only randomized study was performed by the RTOG, in which 49 patients were randomized to receive either 64 Gy standard radiation (photons) versus an equivalent dose of neutrons, or combined photons and neutrons. Although there was no significant difference in median survival or local control observed between the groups, there was an increase in moderate to life-threatening gastrointestinal or hepatic toxicity for patients receiving neutron therapy (*21*). In a related trial, 49 patients with locally advanced disease were randomized to either helium ion radiation therapy (60–70 Gy equivalent dose) or split-course standard beam radiation (60 Gy), with or without adjuvant 5-FU. Although the experimental arm showed a slight improvement in median survival, 7.8 months versus 6.5 months, respectively, the results did not warrant further investigation (*22*).

At present, more modern radiation technologies are being integrated into current treatment approaches in an attempt to improve the outcome for patients with locally advanced pancreatic cancer. Three-dimensional conformal radiotherapy, using CT-based treatment planning to optimize beam tumor targeting, beam orientation and weighting, and reduce the dose to surrounding normal tissues, is becoming more routine in the United States. Intensity-modulated radiation therapy (IMRT) is a newer technology that further refines this approach using inverse treatment planning that permits computerized optimization of a radiation treatment plan. This results in a computer-controlled, non-uniform radiation treatment, delivered in a precise, conformal manner, with further reductions in normal tissue irradiation. IMRT is currently being investigated in clinical trials for the treatment of a variety of intra-abdominal malignancies, including pancreatic cancer (*23–25*). Stereotactic radiotherapy (SRT) is another method of delivering radiation precisely to a targeted area of the body. It incorporates the use of a stereotactic body frame for immobilization and a linear accelerator that delivers a large single fraction, or hypofractionated external beam radiation therapy course, often in conjunction with IMRT. Two phase II trials have evaluated the use of SRT in patients with locally advanced pancreatic cancer. In one study, 16 patients received 45 Gy IMRT with concurrent 5-fluorouracil followed by a 25 Gy boost using SRT in a single fraction. Fifteen of these patients were free of local progression until death and only two patients experienced significant toxicity. The authors concluded that this approach provides excellent local control, is tolerable, but did not impact survival (26). In the second study, 22 patients were given 45 Gy delivered in three fractions over 5 to 10 days. Although standard radiographic evaluation proved difficult, 9% of patients were found to have partial response. The authors concluded that the treatment was associated with unacceptable toxicity and questionable benefit (27).

In summary, while improvements in the delivery of local radiation therapy are promising, the impact on outcome for patients with locally advanced pancreatic cancer is unclear.

3   Chemoradiation for Locally Advanced Unresectable Disease

3.1   Radiation Therapy with 5-Fluorouracil

An early study from the Mayo Clinic was the first to randomize unresectable gastrointestinal cancers to receive external beam radiation (35–40 Gy) with or without 5-fluorouracil (5-FU). The results from this 32-patient trial showed a significant improvement in median survival with the addition of 5-FU (10.4 months versus 6.3 months) (28). The results of this study led to a subsequent Gastrointestinal Tumor Study Group (GITSG) trial, which randomized patients to receive radiation with or without 5-FU. Specifically patients were randomized to one of three arms; high dose (60 Gy) radiation alone versus the same radiation with 5-FU chemotherapy versus moderate dose (40 Gy) radiation with 5-FU. Patients randomized to the concurrent chemoradiation arms also received several additional months of maintenance 5-FU. The median survival of both the high dose and moderate dose radiation groups receiving combined modality therapy exceeded that of the high dose radiation alone group, 9.2, 9.6, and 5.2 months, respectively (29). A second GITSG trial randomized 143 patients to receive either split-course radiation therapy (60 Gy) with concurrent and maintenance 5-FU, or 40 Gy with concurrent weekly doxorubicin, followed by maintenance 5-FU and doxorubicin. Although no survival difference was observed between the two groups, the observed toxicity for patients randomized to the doxorubicin-containing treatment arm was unacceptable (30).

The results of trials comparing chemotherapy alone with chemoradiation have also been reported. A GITSG trial reported in 1988 randomized 43 patients with locally advanced disease to receive either streptozotocin, mitomycin, and 5-flururacil (SMF) chemotherapy alone versus radiation (54 Gy) with concurrent bolus 5-FU followed by adjuvant SMF. The chemoradiation arm demonstrated a significant survival advantage over the chemotherapy alone arm at 1 year (41% versus 19%, respectively) (*31*). In contrast to the GITSG study, a trial from the Eastern Cooperative Oncology Group (ECOG) randomized 91 patients with locally advanced pancreatic cancer to either radiation (40 Gy) plus concurrent bolus 5-FU (600 mg/m^2 daily for 3 days during week 1 only) followed by weekly maintenance 5-FU, or 5-fluorouracil alone (600 mg/m^2 weekly). The investigators observed no significant difference in median survival between the groups (8.3 versus 8.2 months) (*32*). Significant methodologic flaws, including high rates of patient ineligibility, poor radiation technique, and the inclusion of gastric cancer patients, limit its impact on clinical practice.

As investigators began to understand the mechanism of radiosensitization by 5-FU, the protracted venous infusion (PVI-5-FU) dosing schedule gained popularity. PVI-5-FU allows for an increase in the cumulative drug dose without increased toxicity, and the protracted drug exposure potentially optimizes the 5-FU radiation sensitization. In addition, clinical trials that utilized concomitant PVI-5-FU and radiation in other gastrointestinal malignancies demonstrated potential advantages (*33*). A phase I trial from ECOG established the maximum-tolerated dose (MTD) of PVI-5-FU when delivered concurrently with conventional radiation for patients with locally advanced pancreatic cancer to be 250 mg/m^2/day. One-year progression-free, median, and 2-year survival were reported to be 40%, 11.9 months, and 18%, respectively (*34*). While Poen et al. in a retrospective study demonstrated PVI-5-FU chemoradiation resulted in less toxicity and greater chemotherapy and radiation dose intensity compared with bolus 5-FU, there have been no randomized trials comparing these two strategies (*35*). Concurrent radiation with PVI-5-FU has become an established approach and a common dosing schedule being investigated in combination with other novel agents.

In addition, the orally available 5-fluorouracil pro-drug, capecitabine, has been used in combination with radiation with or without the addition of other agents in the treatment of locally advanced pancreatic cancer, and appears to be comparable to PVI-5-FU (*36–38*). In studies from Ben-Josef et al. (*36*) and Saif et al. (*37*), the recommended capecitabine dose was 1,600 mg/m^2 given daily—5 days per week with radiation. Other investigators (*38*) utilize a daily dose of 1330 mg/m^2 given 7 days per week during radiation. To date, there have been no randomized trials comparing PVI-5-FU and radiation versus capecitabine and radiation in locally advanced pancreatic cancer patients.

In summary, treatments incorporating 5-FU–based chemotherapy and radiation have yielded the most consistent results and reflect the current standard of care for patients with locally advanced pancreatic cancer.

3.2   Radiation Therapy with Gemcitabine

The concept of combining gemcitabine with radiation for patient with locally advanced pancreatic cancer gained interest initially because of gemcitabine's demonstrated clinical benefit for patients with metastatic disease (*39*). Gemcitabine also has significant radiation sensitizing properties as demonstrated in in vitro and in vivo studies (*40–42*). As a result, the optimal use of gemcitabine delivered in concert with conventional radiation chemoradiation has been widely investigated.

The gemcitabine dose necessary to control occult disease in advanced pancreatic cancer as a single agent is in the range of 1,000 mg/m^2 per week (*41*), but is very schedule dependent. Although full-dose gemcitabine delivered in conjunction with conventional radiation therapy would hypothetically produce the best outcome, early trials using this strategy proved to be toxic (*42, 43*). Several phase I studies have been performed to determine the maximal tolerated dose (MTD) of concurrent gemcitabine and conventional radiation dose. Data from Blackstock et al. emphasizing the radiosensitizing effects of gemcitabine, evaluated a twice-weekly gemcitabine schedule. The MTD for twice-weekly gemcitabine was 40 mg/m^2 when delivered with conventional radiation fractionation and doses (*44*). Pipas et al. published a similar phase I study evaluating twice-weekly gemcitabine in which the MTD determined to be 50 mg/m^2 given twice weekly (*45*). Unfortunately, several subsequent phase II studies of twice-weekly gemcitabine proved disappointing (*46, 47*). An alternative approach was pursued by the University of Michigan, where full-dose gemcitabine was delivered at 1000 mg/m^2 on days 1, 8, and 15 of each 28-day cycle, with concurrent conformal radiotherapy, delivered in 15 fractions over 3 weeks. As reported by McGinn et al., the treated tumor volume was restricted to the gross tumor with a 1-cm margin. The radiation dose was escalated from 24 to 42 Gy (1.6 to 2.8 Gy daily fractions) and the recommended dose was 36 Gy (2.4 Gy daily) (*48*).

There have been several studies evaluating once-weekly gemcitabine with concurrent radiation with attenuated gemcitabine doses. Data from Crane et al. utilized a short-course radiation regimen (30–33 Gy delivered over 2 weeks) with gemcitabine doses ranging from 200 to 500 mg/m^2. Unfortunately, this regimen demonstrated significant side effects—24% acute severe treatment-related toxicity (*49*). A related experience published by Wolff et al. also used a radiation dose of 30 Gy (3-Gy fractions over 2 weeks) and concurrent weekly gemcitabine and found the MTD to be 350 mg/m^2, decreased from the starting dose of 400 mg/m^2 (*50*). These studies demonstrate the toxicities of combining short-course radiotherapy with gemcitabine and the moderate doses of gemcitabine that can be delivered. Additional studies have investigated using more conventional fractionated radiation therapy (45–50 Gy) with escalating doses of weekly gemcitabine. A study from Ikeda et al. established the MTD for concurrent weekly gemcitabine using this strategy to be 250 mg/m^2 (*51*). This led to a subsequent phase II study using this chemoradiation dosing schedule, followed by maintenance gemcitabine; the median survival was an encouraging 9.5 months (*52*). A similar experience has been reported by Epelbaum et al. The investigators utilized a 7-week gemcitabine induction therapy, followed by weekly gemcitabine delivered at a dose of 400 mg/m^2 (3 out of every 4 weeks) concurrent with conventional radiation. The results were encouraging as three of the 10 patients were able to undergo pancreatectomy, and only fibrosis was found at the time of surgery in one patient (*53*).

A retrospective review of 114 patients with locally advanced pancreatic cancer at MD Anderson compared the relative benefit of using 5-FU versus gemcitabine concurrently with radiotherapy. Sixty-one patients received continuous infusion 5-FU (200–300 mg/m^2/day) with radiation (30 Gy delivered in 10 fractions), and 53 patients received gemcitabine (250–300 mg/m^2) weekly over 7 weeks with the same radiation. There was no statistically significant improvement in median survival observed at short follow-up (11 months for gemcitabine and 9 months for 5-FU). There was significantly more toxicity encountered for the patients who received gemcitabine as compared with those receiving 5-FU (23% and 2%, respectively; $p = 0.0001$) (54). In an interesting phase III study reported by Li et al., gemcitabine-based chemoradiation was compared with 5-FU-based chemoradiation. Thirty-four patients were randomized to receive weekly concurrent gemcitabine (600 mg/m^2) versus concurrent bolus 5-FU for 3 consecutive days delivered every 2 weeks with radiotherapy followed by maintenance gemcitabine (all patients). The investigators observed a statistically significant improvement in median survival for the gemcitabine-based chemoradiation regimen (14.5 months) versus the 5-FU treated patients (6.7 months) (55).

3.3   Radiation with Chemotherapy Doublets

More recently, a number of investigators have attempted to add a second agent to standard 5-FU–based chemoradiation regimens. In a phase I ECOG trial, 5-FU delivered as a continuous infusion (7 days per week) and weekly gemcitabine was given in combination with conventional radiation therapy to a total dose of 59.4 Gy. Unfortunately, significant toxicity was observed and the trial was closed early. Five of seven patients enrolled suffered dose-limiting gastric or duodenal ulcers, thrombocytopenia, and Stevens-Johnson syndrome, leaving the authors to conclude this regimen was not feasible (56). A subsequent and similar phase I/II study was conducted in 32 patients, in which the continuous infusion 5-FU was given 5 days per week with weekly gemcitabine and external beam radiation (50.4 Gy). This slightly different regimen was tolerable at the MTD gemcitabine dose of 200 mg/m^2 (57). Discrepancies in toxicity between these two studies are thought to be related to the lower dose of radiation delivered, smaller radiation portals, and that the continuous infusion 5-FU was delivered 5 days per week, not 7 days per week. A subsequent 80-patient phase II CALGB study of this doublet (gemcitabine-5-FU) resulted in an encouraging median survival of over 12 months (H. Mamon, personal communication).

Several investigators have evaluated chemoradiation strategies incorporating the taxanes in this clinical setting. Similar to gemcitabine, paclitaxel has established radiation sensitizing properties and has systemic activity in pancreatic cancer. A phase I study reported by Safran et al. demonstrated the feasibility of combining weekly gemcitabine (75 mg/m^2) with paclitaxel (40 mg/m^2), and concurrent conventional radiotherapy (58). A subsequent RTOG (RTOG-9812) evaluated this strategy in a 109 patient phase II trial. The 1- and 2-year survival rates were 43% and 13%, respectively, and the median survival was 11.2 months. A 26% partial response rate, and 7% complete response rate were observed (59). The treatment regimen proved somewhat toxic, as four patients experienced grade IV toxicity and one died from treatment-related complications. Ashmalla et al. utilizing a hyperfractionated radiotherapy approach (63.8–1.1 Gy twice daily) determined the MTD for concurrent paclitaxel to be 60 mg/m^2 weekly. The investigators observed a complete response in two of the 17 evaluable patients in this limited phase I study (60). Viret et al. in a study escalating the dose of weekly docetaxel delivered with concurrent conventional radiation was not able to establish the MTD as the trial was halted at the 35 mg/m^2 dose level (61). While the investigators indicate this dose was well tolerated with concurrent radiation, 28% of the patients entered in to the study had to be hospitalized. Table 29.1 summarizes trials of concurrent chemoradiation strategies.

3.4 Radiation with Targeted Systemic Agents

Recently, the pathogenesis of pancreatic cancer has become better understood due to improved understanding of the molecular biology of the disease. As a result, a variety of specific targeted molecular and biologic therapies are currently under investigation. There is preclinical evidence that many of these approaches may provide synergistic or additive effects when combined with conventional chemotherapy and radiation. Crane et al. at MD Anderson recently completed a phase I trial establishing feasibility integrating the anti-VEGF antibody, bevacizumab, into current chemoradiation strategies (62). In this study, 48 patients with locally advanced, unresectable disease received 50.4 Gy of external beam radiation with concurrent capecitabine (final dose: 825 mg/m^2 bid, Monday–Friday) and escalating doses of bevacizumab. Bevacizumab was administered 2 weeks prior to radiotherapy, every 2 weeks concurrent with chemoradiotherapy, and then adjuvantly until disease progression. The overall response rate was 20% and the median survival was 11.6 months. Four patients underwent successful pancreaticoduodenectomy. The addition of bevacizumab did not increase the acute toxicity of chemoradiotherapy; however, bleeding and intestinal perforations were reported. The Radiation Therapy and Oncology Group (RTOG 0411) opened a phase II study based on these results that has recently closed; results are anticipated soon. The Eastern Cooperative Group (ECOG 2204) is also moving forward with an Intergroup study of adjuvant radiation plus bevacizumab and capecitabine in resected pancreatic cancer patients based upon the findings of this trial.

Table 29.1 Concurrent chemoradiation for locally advanced pancreatic cancer

Study	Phase	Number	RT (Gy)	CT	MS months	1-YS %	2-YS %
GITSG 1981	III	111	60 split	None	5.2	10	5
		117	40 split	5FU+maintenance	9.6	40	10
		25	60 split	5FU+maintenance	9.2	40	10
GITSG 1985	III	73	60 split	5FU	8.4		12
		70	60 split	DOXO	7.5		6
GITSG 1988	III	31	54	5FU-SMF	6.5	41	
		26	–	SMF	5.1	19	
ECOG 1985	III	47	40	5FU	5.1	32	6
		144	–	5FU	6.5	32	13
Li 2003	III	16	50.4–61.2	5FU	6.7	31	0
		18	50.4–61.2	GEM weekly 600 mg/m^2	14.5	56	15
Crane 2002	RS	61	30	FU-CI	9		
			–	200–300 mg/m^2	–		
			30	GEM weekly 250–300 mg/m^2	11		
CALGB 2003	II	38	50.4	GEM 40 mg/m^2 twice weekly then weekly × 5	8.2		5
Crane 2001	I/II	51	30–33	GEM weekly 200–500 mg/m^2 then weekly × 7	11		
Okusaka 2004	I	42	50.4	GEM weekly 250 mg/m^2	9.5	28	
McGinn 2001	I	37	24–42	GEM weekly 1,000 mg/m^2 3 times each 4 weeks	11.6		
			MTD 36 @ 2.4/day				
RTOG 2004	II	109	50.4	TXL weekly 50 mg/m^2	11.2	43	13
Mishra 2005	II	20	50.4	IND CPT+GEM	8.8	20	
				GEM 40 mg/m^2 twice weekly			

ADJ, Adjuvant; BID, twice daily; CAP, capecitabine; CISP, cisplatin; CPT, irinotecan; CT, chemotherapy; DOXO, doxorubicin; 5FU, 5-fluorouracil; GEM, gemcitabine; IMRT, intensity modulated radiation therapy; IND, induction (two cycles); MITO-C, mitomycin C; MS, median survival time; MTD, maximum tolerated dose; OR, overall response rate; RS, retrospective study; RT, radiation; SMF, streptozocin, mitomycin and 5-fluorouracil; TXL, paclitaxel; TXT, docetaxel; 1-YS, 1-year survival rate, 2-YS, 2-year survival rate.

Combinations of radiation, chemotherapy and cyclo-oxygenase2 (COX-2) inhibitors have also been explored. A Phase II study from MD Anderson combining EBRT/gemcitabine and the COX-2 inhibitor celecoxib demonstrated higher radiosensitivity but unacceptably high toxicity (63). Omitting radiation, Ferrari et al. found lower rates of toxicity with a median survival of 9.1 months and a 9% partial response rate (64). Additional studies combining celecoxib and 5-FU showed lower toxicity but no improvements in survival (65, 66). Results of combination therapy with gemcitabine, cisplatin and celecoxib have also been disappointing, with a median survival of <6 months.

Studies evaluating the inhibition of members of the ErbB family of epidermal growth factor receptors (EGFr) also appear to be promising. Epidermal growth factor (EGF) is known to stimulate DNA synthesis and rapid cell growth in pancreatic cancer cells. Overexpression of EGF receptors (EGFr) has been associated with a poorer prognosis in pancreatic cancer patients (67, 68). EGFr inhibitors thus have been investigated in order to block this molecule and thus arrest or prevent replication of malignant cells. Cetuximab, a humanized monoclonal antibody to EGFr, and trastuzumab, an antibody to ErbB2 have been combined with gemcitabine in patients with advanced pancreatic cancer (69, 70). Kormansky et al. recently reported the results of a phase I trial combining erlotinib and chemoradiation for patients with locally advanced pancreatic cancer (71). In this study, patients received twice-weekly gemcitabine, conventional radiation followed by maintenance erlotinib (150 mg daily). The MTD for erlotinib was 100 mg daily. Eight patients were treated using this regimen, seven of whom demonstrated stable disease, and one subsequently underwent resection. In a second phase I study, investigators combined erlotinib concurrent with weekly gemcitabine (75 mg/m^2), paclitaxel (40 mg/m^2), and standard radiation followed by maintenance erlotinib (150 mg daily). The MTD of erlotinib using this regimen was reported to be 50 mg daily. The median survival was an encouraging 15 months and 46% of patients demonstrated a partial response (72). Other dual EGFr and VEGF inhibitors show promise in preclinical models and provide an intriguing model for multiple pathway targets.

4   Conclusions

The treatment of patients with locally advanced pancreatic cancer remains a challenge. A number of trials are underway investigating the potential benefits of newer systemic agents delivered in combination with current chemoradiation techniques. It is possible that significant improvements in survival can be achieved by exploiting the molecular aberrations associated with pancreatic cancers; thus combining the expanding number of targeted agents with conventional chemotherapy and radiation in this clinical setting. Anti-angiogenic agents show promising results; however, they remain investigational at this time.

References

1. Jemal A, Siegel R, Ward E, 2008, Cancer statistics. CA Cancer J Clin 58(2):71–96.
2. Evans D, Abbrezzese J, Willett C. 2001, Cancer of the pancreas. Lippincott Williams & Wilkins, Philadelphia, .
3. American Joint Committee on Cancer Staging Manual. Exocrine pancreas, 6th ed. New York, Springer, 2002.
4. Minsky BD, Hilaris B, Fuks Z. 1988, The role of radiation therapy in the control of pain from pancreatic carcinoma. J Pain Symptom Manage 3(4):199–205.
5. Roldan GE, Gunderson LL, Nagorney DM, 1988, External beam versus intraoperative and external beam irradiation for locally advanced pancreatic cancer. Cancer 61(6): 1110–1116.
6. Shipley WU, Wood WC, Tepper JE, 1984, Intraoperative electron beam irradiation for patients with unresectable pancreatic carcinoma. Ann Surg 200(3):289–296.
7. Wood WC, Shipley WU, Gunderson LL, 1982, Intraoperative irradiation for unresectable pancreatic carcinoma. Cancer 49(6):1272–1275.
8. Tepper JE, Shipley WU, Warshaw AL, 1987, The role of misonidazole combined with intraoperative radiation therapy in the treatment of pancreatic carcinoma. J Clin Oncol 5(4):579–584.
9. Garton GR, Gunderson LL, Nagorney DM, 1993, High-dose preoperative external beam and intraoperative irradiation for locally advanced pancreatic cancer. Int J Radiat Oncol Biol Phys 27(5):1153–1157.
10. Sindelar WF, Kinsella TJ. 1999, Studies of intraoperative radiotherapy in carcinoma of the pancreas. Ann Oncol 10(Suppl 4):226–230.
11. Tepper JE, Noyes D, Krall JM, 1991, Intraoperative radiation therapy of pancreatic carcinoma; a report of RTOG-8505. Radiation Therapy Oncology Group. Int J Radiat Oncol Biol Phys 21(5):1145–1149.
12. Willett CG, Castillo CF, Del Shih HA, 2005, Long-term results of intraoperative electron beam irradiation (IOERT) for patients with unresectable pancreatic cancer. Ann Surg 241(2):295–299.
13. Shipley WU, Nardi GL, Cohen AM, 1980, Iodine-125 implant and external beam irradiation in patients with localized pancreatic carcinoma: a comparative study to surgical resection. Cancer 45(4):709–714.
14. Syed AM, Puthawala AA, Neblett DL. 1983, Interstitial iodine-125 implant in the management of unresectable pancreatic carcinoma. Cancer 52(5):808–813.
15. Dobelbower RR, Jr., Merrick HW, 3rd., Ahuja RK, 1986, 125I interstitial implant, precision high-dose external beam therapy, and 5-FU for unresectable adenocarcinoma of pancreas and extrahepatic biliary tree. Cancer 58(10):2185–2195.
16. Mohiuddin M, Cantor RJ, Biermann W, 1988, Combined modality treatment of localized unresectable adenocarcinoma of the pancreas. Int J Radiat Oncol Biol Phys 14(1):79–84.
17. Peretz T, Nori D, Hilaris B, 1989, Treatment of primary unresectable carcinoma of the pancreas with I-125 implantation. Int J Radiat Oncol Biol Phys 17(5):931–935.
18. Smith FP, Schein PS, Macdonald JS, 1981, Fast neutron irradiation for locally advanced pancreatic cancer. Int J Radiat Oncol Biol Phys 7(11):1527–1531.
19. Al-Abdulla AS, Hussey DH, Olson MH, 1981, Experience with fast neutron therapy for unresectable carcinoma of the pancreas. Int J Radiat Oncol Biol Phys 7(2):165–172.
20. Cohen L, Woodruff KH, Hendrickson FR, 1985, Response of pancreatic cancer to local irradiation with high-energy neutrons. Cancer 56(6):1235–1241.
21. Thomas FJ, Krall J, Hendrickson F, 1989, Evaluation of neutron irradiation of pancreatic cancer. Results of a randomized Radiation Therapy Oncology Group clinical trial. Am J Clin Oncol 12(4):283–289.
22. Linstadt D, Quivey JM, Castro JR, 1988, Comparison of helium-ion radiation therapy and split-course megavoltage irradiation for unresectable adenocarcinoma of the pancreas. Final

report of a Northern California Oncology Group randomized prospective clinical trial. Radiology 168(1):261–264.

23. Crane CH, Antolak JA, Rosen II, 2001, Phase I study of concomitant gemcitabine and IMRT for patients with unresectable adenocarcinoma of the pancreatic head. Int J Gastrointest Cancer 30(3):123–132.

24. Milano MT, Chmura SJ, Garofalo MC, 2004, Intensity-modulated radiotherapy in treatment of pancreatic and bile duct malignancies: toxicity and clinical outcome. Int J Radiat Oncol Biol Phys 59(2):445–453.

25. Landry JC, Yang GY, Ting JY, 2002, Treatment of pancreatic cancer tumors with intensity-modulated radiation therapy (IMRT) using the volume at risk approach (VARA): employing dose-volume histogram (DVH) and normal tissue complication probability (NTCP) to evaluate small bowel toxicity. Med Dosim 27(2):121–129.

26. Koong AC, Christofferson E, Le QT, 2005, Phase II study to assess the efficacy of conventionally fractionated radiotherapy followed by a stereotactic radiosurgery boost in patients with locally advanced pancreatic cancer. Int J Radiat Oncol Biol Phys 63(2):320–323.

27. Hoyer M, Roed H, Sengelov L, 2005, Phase-II study on stereotactic radiotherapy of locally advanced pancreatic carcinoma. Radiother Oncol 76(1):48–53.

28. Moertel CG, Childs DS, Jr., Reitemeier RJ, 1969, Combined 5-fluorouracil and supervoltage radiation therapy of locally unresectable gastrointestinal cancer. Lancet 2(7626):865–867.

29. Moertel CG, Frytak S, Hahn RG, 1981, Therapy of locally unresectable pancreatic carcinoma: a randomized comparison of high dose (6000 rads) radiation alone, moderate dose radiation (4000 rads + 5-fluorouracil), and high dose radiation + 5-fluorouracil: The Gastrointestinal Tumor Study Group. Cancer 48(8):1705–1710.

30. Radiation therapy combined with Adriamycin or 5-fluorouracil for the treatment of locally unresectable pancreatic carcinoma. Gastrointestinal Tumor Study Group. Cancer 1985, 56(11):2563–2568.

31. Gastrointestinal Tumor Study Group: Treatment of locally unresectable carcinoma of the pancreas: A comparison of combined modality therapy (chemotherapy plus radiotherapy) to chemotherapy alone. J Natl Cancer Inst 1988, 80:751–755.

32. Klassen DJ, MacIntyre JM, Catton GE, 1985, Treatment of locally unresectable cancer of the stomach and pancreas: a randomized comparison of 5-flurouracil alone with radiation plus concurrent and maintenance 5-fluorouracil—An Eastern Cooperative Oncology Group Study. J Clin Oncol 3(3):373–378.

33. O' Connell MJ, Martenson JA, Wieand HS, 1994, Improving adjuvant therapy for rectal cancer by combining protracted-infusion flurouracil with radiation therapy after curative surgery. N Engl J Med 331:502–507.

34. Whittington R, Neuberg D, Tester WJ, 1995, Protracted intravenous fluorouracil infusion with radiation therapy in the management of localized pancreaticobiliary carcinoma: a phase I Eastern Cooperative Oncology Group Trial. J Clin Oncol 13:227–232.

35. Poen JC, Collins HL, Niederhuber JE, 1998, Chemo-radiotherapy for localized pancreatic cancer: increased dose intensity and reduced acute toxicity with concomitant radiotherapy and protracted venous infusion 5-fluorouracil. Int J Radiat Oncol Biol Phys 40(1):93–99.

36. Ben-Josef E, Shields AF, Vaishampayan U, 2004, Intensity-modulated radiotherapy (IMRT) and concurrent capecitabine for pancreatic cancer. Int J Radiat Oncol Biol Phys 59:454–459.

37. Saif MW, Eloubeidi MA, Russo S, 2005, Phase I study of capecitabine with concomitant radiotherapy for patients with locally advanced pancreatic cancer: expression analysis of genes related to outcome. J Clin Oncol 23:8679–8687.

38. Schneider BJ, Ben-Josef E, McGinn CJ, 2005, Capecitabine and radiation therapy preceded and followed by combination chemotherapy in advanced pancreatic cancer. Int J Radiat Oncol Biol Phys 63:1325–1330.

39. Burris HA, 3rd., Moore MJ, Andersen J, 1997, Improvements in survival and clinical benefit with gemcitabine as first-line therapy for patients with advanced pancreas cancer: a randomized trial. J Clin Oncol 15:2403–2413.

40. Fields MT, Eisbruch A, Normolle D, 2000, Radiosensitization produced in vivo by once- vs. twice-weekly 2'2'-difluoro-2'-deoxycytidine (gemcitabine). Int J Radiat Oncol Biol Phys. 47(3):785–791 .
41. Lawrence TS, Chang EY, Hahn TM, 1996, Radiosensitization of pancreatic cancer cells by 2',2'-difluoro-2'-deoxycytidine. Int J Radiat Oncol Biol Phys 34:867–872.
42. Milas L, Fujii T, Hunter N, 1999, Enhancement of tumor radioresponse in vivo by gemcitabine. Cancer Res 59:107–114.
43. Poggi MM, Kroog GS, Russo A, 2002, Phase I study of weekly gemcitabine as a radiation sensitizer for unresectable pancreatic cancer. Int J Radiat Oncol Biol Phys 54:670–676.
44. Blackstock AW, Bernard SA, Richards F, 1999;Phase I trial of twice-weekly gemcitabine and concurrent radiation in patients with advanced pancreatic cancer. J Clin Oncol 17:2208–2212.
45. Pipas JM, Mitchell SE, Barth RJ, Jr., 2001, Phase I study of twice-weekly gemcitabine and concomitant external-beam radiotherapy in patients with adenocarcinoma of the pancreas. Int J Radiat Oncol Biol Phys 50(5):1317–1322.
46. Blackstock AW, Tepper JE, Niedwiecki D, 2003, Cancer and leukemia group B (CALGB) 89805: phase II chemoradiation trial using gemcitabine in patients with locoregional adenocarcinoma of the pancreas. Int J Gastrointest Cancer 34:107–116.
47. Mishra G, Butler J, Ho C, 2005, Phase II trial of induction gemcitabine/CPT-11 followed by a twice-weekly infusion of gemcitabine and concurrent external beam radiation for the treatment of locally advanced pancreatic cancer. Am J Clin Oncol 28:345–350.
48. McGinn CJ, Zalupski MM, Shureiqi I, 2001, Phase I trial of radiation dose escalation with concurrent weekly full-dose gemcitabine in patients with advanced pancreatic cancer. J Clin Oncol 19:4202–428.
49. Crane CH, Janjan NA, Evans DB, 2001, Toxicity and efficacy of concurrent gemcitabine and radiotherapy for locally advanced pancreatic cancer. Int J Pancreatol 29(1):9–18.
50. Wolff RA, Evans DB, Gravel DM, 2001, Phase I trial of gemcitabine combined with radiation for the treatment of locally advanced pancreatic adenocarcinoma. Clin Cancer Res 7(8):2246–2253.
51. Ikeda M, Okada S, Tokuuye K, 2002, A phase I trial of weekly gemcitabine and concurrent radiotherapy in patients with locally advanced pancreatic cancer. Br J Cancer 86(10):1551–1554.
52. Okusaka T, Ito Y, Ueno H, 2004, Phase II study of radiotherapy combined with gemcitabine for locally advanced pancreatic cancer. Br J Cancer 91(4):673–677.
53. Epelbaum R, Rosenblatt E, Nasrallah S, 2002, Phase II study of gemcitabine combined with radiation therapy in patients with localized, unresectable pancreatic cancer. J Surg Oncol 81(3):138–143.
54. Crane CH, Abbruzzese JL, Evans DB, 2002, Is the therapeutic index better with gemcitabine-based chemoradiation than with 5-fluorouracil-based chemoradiation in locally advanced pancreatic cancer? Int J Radiat Oncol Biol Phys 52(5):1293–1302.
55. Li CP, Chao Y, Chi KH, 2003, Concurrent chemoradiotherapy treatment of locally advanced pancreatic cancer: gemcitabine versus 5-fluorouracil, a randomized controlled study. Int J Radiat Oncol Biol Phys 57(1):98–104.
56. Talamonti MS, Catalano PJ, Vaughn DJ, 2000, Eastern Cooperative Oncology Group Phase I trial of protracted venous infusion fluorouracil plus weekly gemcitabine with concurrent radiation therapy in patients with locally advanced pancreas cancer: a regimen with unexpected early toxicity. J Clin Oncol 18(19):3384–3389.
57. Willett CG, Czito BG, Bendell JC, 2005, Locally advanced pancreatic cancer. J Clin Oncol 23:4538–4544.
58. Safran H, Dipetrillo T, Iannitti D, 2002, Gemcitabine, paclitaxel, and radiation for locally advanced pancreatic cancer: a Phase I trial. Int J Radiat Oncol Biol Phys 54(1):137–141.
59. Rich T, Harris J, Abrams R, 2004, Phase II study of external irradiation and weekly paclitaxel for nonmetastatic, unresectable pancreatic cancer: RTOG-98-12. Am J Clin Oncol 27(1):51–56.

60. Ashamalla H, Zaki B, Mokhtar B, 2003, Hyperfractionated radiotherapy and paclitaxel for locally advanced/unresectable pancreatic cancer. Int J Radiat Oncol Biol Phys 55(3):679–687.

61. Viret F, Ychou M, Goncalves A, 2003, Docetaxel and radiotherapy and pancreatic cancer. Pancreas 27(3):214–219.

62. Crane CH, Ellis LM, Abbruzzese JL, 2006, Phase I trial evaluating the safety of bevacizumab with concurrent radiotherapy and capecitabine in locally advanced pancreatic cancer. J Clin Oncol 24(7):1145–1115.

63. Crane CH, Mason K, Janjan NA, 2003, Initial experience combining cyclooxygenase-2 inhibition with chemoradiation for locally advanced pancreatic cancer. American J Clin Oncol 26(4):S81–S84.

64. Ferrari V, Valcamonico F, Amoroso V, 2006, Gemcitabine plus celecoxib (GECO) in advanced pancreatic cancer: a phase II trial. Cancer Chemother Pharmacol 57(2):185–190.

65. Rayes BF, El Zalupski MM, Shields 2005, A phase II study of celecoxib, gemcitabine, and cisplatin in advanced pancreatic cancer. Invest New Drugs 23(6):583–590.

66. Milella M, Gelibter A, Cosimo S, Di 2004, Pilot study of celecoxib and infusional 5-fluorouracil as second-line treatment for advanced pancreatic carcinoma. Cancer 101(1):133–138.

67. Xiong HQ, Abbruzzese JL. 2002, Epidermal growth factor receptor-targeted therapy for pancreatic cancer. Semin Oncol 29(5 Suppl 14):31–37.

68. Dong M, Nio Y, Guo KJ, 1998, Epidermal growth factor and its receptor as prognostic indicators in Chinese patients with pancreatic cancer. Anticancer Res 18(6B):4613–4619.

69. Xiong HQ, Rosenberg A, LoBuglio A, 2004, Cetuximab, a monoclonal antibody targeting the epidermal growth factor receptor, in combination with gemcitabine for advanced pancreatic cancer: a multicenter phase II Trial. J Clin Oncol 22(13):2610–2616.

70. Safran H, Iannitti D, Ramanathan R . 2004, Herceptin and gemcitabine for metastic pancreatic cancers that overexpress HER-2/neu. Cancer Invest 22:706–712.

71. Moore MJ, Goldstein D, Hamm J et al. Erlotinib improves survival when added to gemcitabine in patients with advanced pancreatic cancer: A phase III trial of the national Cancer Institute of Canada Clinical Trials Group (NCIC-CTG). Paper presented at: 2005 Gastrointestinal Cancers Symposium: Current status and future directions for prevention and management; January 27–29; Holly wood, FL. Abstract 77. Available at: http://www.asco.org.

72. Kortmanksy JS, O'Reilly EM, Minksy BD, 2005; A phase I trial of erlotinib, gemcitabine and radiation for patients with locally advanced, unresectable pancreatic cancer. J Clin Oncol 23(Suppl):334s (abstract 4107).

Chapter 30
Optimum Cytotoxic Therapy for Advanced Pancreatic Cancer

Sameer P. Desai and Mark M. Zalupski

1 Introduction

The effectiveness of treatment for pancreatic cancer is limited by the combination of early metastases and de novo resistance to cytotoxic therapies, rendering most patients candidates for palliative systemic therapy. Despite more than four decades of study, the benefit of systemic therapy is limited to a minority of patients and the impact on survival is marginal. In the pre-gemcitabine era, 5-fluorouracil (5FU) was commonly used, either alone or as a component of combination therapy. Based on low response rates, toxicity, and minimal impact on survival, some even questioned the use of cytotoxic treatment. However, following initial studies, gemcitabine quickly became a standard treatment for pancreatic cancer based on the combination of tolerability and symptom control. While acknowledging an overall improvement with gemcitabine, there clearly remains a need for more effective therapies. Increasingly, phase I and II studies have been performed in this disease, investigating dose and schedule questions of gemcitabine delivery and/or the addition of one or more drugs to gemcitabine. Reports from many of these trials describe improved efficacy or increased tolerance. Confirmatory phase III studies, however, have generally defined these apparent gains as either modest or nonexistent. The rapid introduction of a wide array of targeted agents into the clinic is leading to a new generation of studies, bringing hope to the many patients suffering from this difficult disease.

Interpretation of clinical studies in pancreatic cancer is challenging. With improvements in imaging modalities, patients are diagnosed earlier and there has been an increase in the percentage of patients correctly identified as advanced disease, paradoxically with a smaller volume of metastatic disease. In the past, patients were often planned for therapy as locally advanced or metastatic, with many of the former receiving radiation therapy. Most recent trials enroll both clinical groups as advanced disease. Nevertheless, outcomes to therapy are clearly related to stage and volume of disease and the proportion of patients in any trial with metastatic disease will influence survival. A primary measure of efficacy in oncologic clinical trials has been tumor response rate, a difficult measure in non-metastatic pancreatic cancer due to the desmoplastic stroma of the primary tumor and the difficulty of identifying

A.M. Lowy et al. (eds.) *Pancreatic Cancer*.
doi: 10.1007/978-0-387-69252-4, © Springer Science+Business Media, LLC 2008

pre- and post-treatment extent of disease. The carbohydrate tumor associated antigen CA 19-9 has been considered as a measure of response, but its utility is lessened by fluctuations in its value due to biliary obstruction and cholangitis, as well as by a fraction of patients who do not have any elevation at baseline.

The goals of therapy in pancreatic cancer include symptom control and improved survival. Recent phase III trials emphasized overall survival as the primary endpoint. As data have accumulated, phase III trials have increased in size to identify disappointingly small improvements in survival as statistically significant. Additionally, as options for treatment increase, second-line therapy may have an impact on a survival endpoint, as has been demonstrated in colorectal cancer. Quality of life (QOL) measures support the use of treatment as compared to supportive care only in advanced disease but are difficult to interpret in phase II and III trials due to subjectivity, therapy related toxicities and patient attrition. Clinical benefit response (CBR), a measure of performance status (PS), pain intensity and control, and weight, have been employed in pancreatic cancer trials but its use requires initial symptoms and a somewhat subjective assessment of PS and pain control. Progression-free survival often parallels QOL and CBR but is subject to the inherent difficulties in objectively defining progression and the intervals at which disease is evaluated.

Percutaneous and endoscopic treatment of biliary and gastric outlet obstruction has effectively palliated many patients with advanced pancreatic cancer and has permitted subsequent use of systemic therapy. Clinical research has expanded and clinical trials and accrual in this disease have increased dramatically. Following is a review of past and recent clinical trials of systemic therapy in advanced pancreatic cancer with an emphasis on those studies that have impacted on clinical practice, defined standard treatment and serve as a platform for future work in this disease.

2   Fluoropyrimidine Therapy

Activity of 5FU in pancreatic cancer was reported as far back as 1960 (*1*). Results of those early studies of bolus 5FU were highly variable and interpretation likely compromised by lack of standardized reporting criteria (*2*). More recent phase II studies evaluating bolus 5FU with leucovorin (5FU/LV) have generally reported low response rates and moderate gastrointestinal toxicity. In one such study, 42 patients with pancreatic cancer were treated on a weekly schedule (5FU 600 mg/m², LV 500 mg/m²) with 3 (7%) partial responses observed (*3*). Diarrhea requiring hydration occurred in 21% of patients, and there was one treatment-related death. In retrospect, the dose of 5FU was higher than what is generally used currently. A second study used daily bolus 5FU (370 mg/m²) for 5 consecutive days with continuous infusion of LV (500 mg/m²/day) for 6 days, monthly. In 20 evaluable patients, objective response was not seen (*4*). Toxicity was moderate, including seven patients hospitalized for mucositis, diarrhea, and myelosuppression. More recently, 5FU has been evaluated using infusional schedules of administration. In one study, a 24-hour infusion of 5FU (2,600 mg/m^2) with LV was given weekly to 33 patients. Partial response was seen in three (9%) and grade III/IV toxicities were less frequent than with bolus administration (diarrhea 8%, vomiting 5%, and hand-foot syndrome 14%) (5). The oral fluoropyrimidine pro-drug capecitabine, demonstrated tolerance and activity in a study of 42 patients with advanced pancreatic cancer. Using a total daily dose of 2,500 mg/m^2 for 14 days every 3 weeks, partial responses were seen in three (7%) patients and CBR in 25%, and median survival approached 6 months (6). Grade III/IV toxicities included hand-foot syndrome 17%, nausea 10%, and diarrhea 17%, with no treatment-related deaths. These and other data suggest that in pancreatic cancer, infusional 5FU is better tolerated, may have improved efficacy, and is likely to be easier to combine with other myelosuppressive agents than bolus or intermittent administration of 5FU.

Combination chemotherapy in the pre-gemcitabine era most often utilized 5FU as a component of treatment. The two most widely evaluated regimens combined 5FU and mitomycin C with either doxorubicin (FAM) or streptozotocin (SMF). Although both regimens showed encouraging results in early studies, when evaluated in phase III studies, response rates and survival were disappointing. The Gastrointestinal Tumor Study Group (GITSG) compared the two regimens in 133 patients with advanced pancreatic cancer and reported response rates of 13% for FAM and 15% for SMF (7). The Cancer and Acute Leukemia Group B (CALGB) studied these regimens in 196 patients with advanced pancreatic cancer and found response rates of 14% for FAM and 4% for SMF (8). Both reports described moderate toxicity without an apparent commensurate benefit. A small randomized study of 40 patients using 5FU, cyclophosphamide, methotrexate, vincristine, and mitomycin C found a survival advantage for chemotherapy when compared with best supportive care (median survival 44 weeks versus 9 weeks) (9). However, when this regimen was compared in a randomized study involving 187 patients to 5FU alone or 5FU, doxorubicin and cisplatin, there was no survival advantage to any of the regimens and median survival of the entire group was 4.5 months (10).

Although the value of chemotherapy in advanced pancreatic cancer in the pre-gemcitabine era has been debated, it was noted that some patients achieved an improvement in the quality of their lives, particularly a marked reduction in pain (2). This led to studies probing not only quantity, but also QOL. Using the EORTC-QLC-C30 instrument, QOL was evaluated in a study of 90 patients with advanced pancreatic or biliary cancer randomized to chemotherapy or best supportive care. This study found improved QOL and quality adjusted survival time for patients randomized to chemotherapy (11). A general acceptance of the importance of improvements in QOL led to the development of composite parameters to quantify these benefits. Clinical benefit response (CBR) arose as a surrogate marker of clinical efficacy in pancreatic cancer evaluating for changes in performance status, weight, pain intensity, and analgesic consumption (12). Studies that utilized CBR as the primary endpoint in patients with pancreatic cancer ultimately led to the approval of gemcitabine in this disease.

3   Single-Agent Gemcitabine

Gemcitabine is a fluorine substituted deoxycytidine analog. Gemcitabine functions as an antimetabolite, arresting cells at the G1/S interphase. Gemcitabine requires facilitated uptake into the cell by a nucleoside transport system, and following uptake, must be phosphorylated for cytotoxicity. The diphosphate metabolite inhibits ribonucleotide reductase, leading to depletion of triphosphated nucleotides necessary for DNA synthesis. Gemcitabine-triphosphate is incorporated into DNA, interfering with DNA chain elongation and leading to cell death. Although gemcitabine is a very schedule-dependent drug, nearly all studies in pancreatic cancer have used a simple 30-minute IV infusion until recently, when a fixed dose rate infusion schedule of gemcitabine (10 $mg/m^2/minute$) was investigated. Resistance to gemcitabine is seen when cells are deficient or inefficient in nucleoside transport of the drug into the cell or in the setting of increased intracellular concentrations of ribonucleotide reductase.

Gemcitabine has a broad spectrum of cytotoxic activity in a variety of nonhematologic tumors. Two initial phase II investigations in pancreatic cancer motivated further study, which ultimately led to FDA approval of gemcitabine for this disease. These initial trials involved previously untreated patients and used a regimen of gemcitabine 800-1,250 mg/m^2 over 30 minutes weekly for 3 of 4 weeks. In the first study, five of 35 evaluable patients (14%) had a partial response and an additional 14 patients had stable disease for a disease control rate of 54% (13). The median duration of response was 13 weeks and median survival in all patients was 5.6 months. In the second study, two of 32 evaluable patients (6%) had a partial response and disease control was seen in 25% with median survival of 6.3 months (14). Toxicity was mild in both studies. A phase II study in previously treated patients used gemcitabine 1,000 mg/m^2 weekly for 7 weeks, followed by a week of rest, then weekly infusions for 3 of every 4 weeks (15). This study used Clinical Benefit Response (CBR) as its primary endpoint, defining responders as those who obtained and sustained for at least 4 weeks improvements in pain intensity, daily analgesic consumption, and/or performance status. Seventeen of 63 treated patients (27%) obtained CBR for a median duration of 3.5 months. Median survival in this previously treated population was 3.9 months and therapy was well tolerated.

The pivotal phase III study randomized 126 patients with advanced, symptomatic pancreatic cancer to either weekly gemcitabine 1,000 mg/m^2 over 30 minutes or weekly bolus 5FU 600 mg/m^2 using CBR as the primary endpoint (16). The study found CBR more commonly in the gemcitabine-treated patients (23.8% versus 4.8%, $p = 0.002$). Gemcitabine treatment also led to a statistically improved median survival (5.6 versus 4.4 months) and 1-year survival (18% versus 2%) as compared with 5FU. Tumor response was infrequent in both arms (5.4% gemcitabine versus 0% 5FU). Toxicity with gemcitabine was mild, with the most common toxicity being uncomplicated grade III/IV neutropenia in 26% of the patients.

Additional experience with gemcitabine in advanced pancreatic cancer was reported from a compassionate use Investigational New Drug (IND) treatment protocol in which a total of 3,023 patients with unresectable or metastatic pancreatic cancer, with at most one previous chemotherapy regimen, were treated (*17*). Disease-related symptom improvement was prospectively determined using analgesic requirement, pain intensity, performance status, and weight gain, with 18.4% of patients cumulatively experiencing benefit after the fourth cycle. Tumor response information was available at the time of reporting in 982 patients, with 14 patients (1.4%) having complete response and 104 patients (10.6%) achieving a partial response, for an overall response rate of 12%. Survival data were either available or censored at the time of reporting in 2,380 patients, with median survival of 4.8 months and 1-year survival rate of 15%. Expectedly, patients with a better baseline performance status and/or those who were chemotherapy naïve lived longer. Gemcitabine was remarkably well tolerated in this population of advanced pancreatic cancer, with only a 4.6% discontinuation rate due to adverse events.

4   Pharmacologic Manipulation of Gemcitabine

The very modest clinical benefit for gemcitabine in advanced cancer prompted the investigation into possibilities of increasing the active phosphate concentrations within tumor cells. Both a higher dose over a standard infusion time of 30 minutes and longer infusion times have been evaluated. A phase II study reported on 43 previously untreated patients with metastatic pancreatic cancer using 2,200 mg/m^2 of gemcitabine every 14 days. In this study one complete and eight partial responses were seen, for an overall response rate of 21%. Eighteen additional patients had stable disease for a disease control rate of 63%. Median time to progression (TTP), median survival, and 1-year survival were 5.3 months, 8.8 months, and 26%, respectively (*18*). Toxicity was mild, predominantly myelosuppression.

Preclinical data supported a pharmacokinetic means of dose intensification of gemcitabine by lengthening the infusion time to 10 mg/m^2/minute, known as fixed dose rate (FDR) infusion. The basis for this strategy of administration was to overcome the saturability of deoxycytidine kinase, the rate-limiting step in gemcitabine intracellular phosphorylation. Investigators compared these two means of gemcitabine intensification by randomizing 92 patients to receive gemcitabine 2,200 mg/m^2 over 30 minutes (standard arm) or gemcitabine 1,500 mg/m^2 over 150 minutes (FDR), weekly for 3 of every 4 weeks (*19*). In 49 patients receiving high-dose gemcitabine, median survival and 1-year survival rate were 5.0 months and 9%, respectively, considerably poorer than in the previous study. In the 43 patients treated in the FDR arm, improved median survival of 8.0 months ($p = 0.013$) and a 1-year survival rate of 29% ($p = 0.014$) was noted. Toxicity, predominantly grade III/IV neutropenia and thrombocytopenia was significantly higher in the FDR arm. An Italian group used FDR gemcitabine 1,000 mg/m^2 over 100 minutes in 40 patients with advanced pancreas and biliary cancer and found response and stable disease in six (15%) and 20 (50%) patients. The median survival and 1-year survival were 9.2 months and 25.8%, respectively, and treatment was well tolerated (*20*). Despite these encouraging results with FDR infusion of gemcitabine, a recent

Eastern Cooperative Oncology Group (ECOG) phase III study randomized 833 patients with advanced pancreatic cancer (88% metastatic) to one of three arms. The study compared gemcitabine 1,000 mg/m^2 weekly over 30 minutes (standard) to FDR gemcitabine using 1,500 mg/m^2 over 150 minutes weekly for 3 of every 4 weeks. In a preliminary report (*21*), median overall survival was 4.96 months for standard gemcitabine and 6.01 months for FDR gemcitabine, respectively. The hazard ratio comparing these two arms was 1.21 and reached borderline statistical significance only.

5 Gemcitabine-Based Combination Cytotoxic Therapies

Although gemcitabine as a single agent in advanced pancreatic cancer has utility, enthusiasm has been muted considering the limited benefit it provides over either fluoropyrimidines or no therapy. Evaluations of combination therapies incorporating gemcitabine as the primary component have logically followed.

5.1 Gemcitabine-Fluoropyrimidine Doublets

Fluoropyrimidines have been investigated in doublet regimens using bolus 5FU, infusional 5FU, and the oral pro-drug capecitabine.

A phase II study evaluated gemcitabine 1,000 mg/m^2 followed by bolus 5FU 600 mg/m^2 weekly for 3 of 4 weeks in 36 eligible patients with metastatic pancreatic cancer. Partial response was seen in five patients (14%), and median survival of 4.4 months and 1-year survival rate of 8.6% was reported. Grade III/IV toxicity consisted predominantly of myelosuppression, with one treatment-related death from sepsis (*22*). A second phase II study used the same regimen adding leucovorin 20 mg/m^2 as a 30-minute infusion simultaneously with the gemcitabine in 29 patients with either unresectable or metastatic pancreatic cancer. Overall response rate was 21% and median and 1-year survival were an encouraging 8.4 months and 36%, respectively (*23*). A subsequent phase III study conducted by ECOG randomized 327 patients with advanced pancreatic cancer (90% metastatic) to either gemcitabine alone 1,000 mg/m^2 or gemcitabine followed by bolus 5FU 600 mg/m^2, weekly for 3 of every 4 weeks. There was a statistically significant improvement favoring the combination in progression-free survival (2.2 months versus 3.4 months, $p = 0.022$) and a trend toward improved median survival (5.4 months to 6.7 months, $p = 0.09$) without substantive differences in toxicities (*24*). Despite an improvement in progression-free survival, similar toxicity profile and a trend toward improved overall survival, the study was considered negative due to lack of a statistically different overall survival. Using a different schedule of gemcitabine and 5FU, a recent phase II study treated 42 patients with locally advanced ($n = 11$) or metastatic ($n = 31$) pancreatic cancer. Patients received gemcitabine 1,000 mg/m^2 on day 1 and leucovorin 100 mg/m^2 and bolus 5FU 400 mg/m^2 days 1-3 repeated every 2 weeks. There were two complete and 11 partial responses, for an overall response rate of 31%. Median TTP and overall survival were 9.75 months and 13.1 months in a well-tolerated regimen (25).

Several phase II studies have combined gemcitabine with infusional 5FU with or without modulators in various schedules. One study treated 38 patients with locally advanced ($n = 7$) or metastatic ($n = 31$) pancreatic cancer with gemcitabine 1,000 mg/m^2 followed by leucovorin 200 mg/m^2 and 5FU 750 mg/m^2 administered as a 24-hour continuous infusion weekly for 4 of every 6 weeks. There were two partial responses (5%), median survival was 9.3 months and 1-year survival was 32% (26). Another study evaluated 46 patients treated with gemcitabine 1,400 mg/m^2 and 5FU 3,000 mg/m^2 as a continuous infusion over 48 hours weekly for 3 of every 4 weeks. Response rate, median survival and 1-year survival were 7%, 5.2 months, and 25%, respectively. Grade III/IV toxicity included neutropenia 45%, mucositis 7.5%, and hyperbilirubinemia 10.5% (27). A bimonthly regimen was evaluated in 56 patients with either unresectable ($n = 12$) or metastatic ($n = 45$) pancreatic cancer. Treatment consisted of leucovorin 400 mg/m^2 in 2 hours followed by 5FU 1,000 mg/m^2 over 22 hours and then gemcitabine 800–1,250 mg/m^2 given in a FDR infusion of 10 mg/m^2/minute. Objective response rate was 19% and median survival was 7.2 months. Toxicity was mild but complete alopecia was seen in 36% (28).

Protracted venous infusions (PVI) of 5FU have been combined with gemcitabine including a study that evaluated 25 patients, most of whom (92%) had metastatic disease. Patients received gemcitabine 1,000 mg/m^2 weekly for 3 of every 4 weeks along with PVI 5FU 200 mg/m^2/day. Partial response was seen in five patients (20%) and median survival was 6.2 months, 1-year survival was 20% in this well-tolerated regimen (29). Another study randomized 94 patients with advanced pancreatic cancer to gemcitabine 1,000 mg/m^2 weekly for 7 weeks followed by a 2-week rest, then weekly for 3 of every 4 weeks or the same in combination with PVI 5FU 200 mg/m^2/day for 6 weeks followed by 2 weeks of rest and then for 3 of every 4 weeks. Toxicities were mild in both arms with no treatment-related deaths. There was no benefit seen in terms of response rate, progression-free, or overall survival to the addition of PVI 5FU (30). A recent study evaluated the use of gemcitabine combined with intra-arterial 5FU in 24 patients with locally advanced ($n = 3$) or metastatic ($n = 21$) pancreatic cancer. Gemcitabine was given at 1,000 mg weekly for 3 of every 4 weeks IV and 5FU 250 mg/day was given as a continuous arterial infusion on days 1-5 every week. The intra-arterial catheter was placed to allow the distribution of 5FU to include the pancreas tumor and liver after occlusion of the gastric and pancreaticoduodenal arteries. Grade III/IV neutropenia was seen in 30%, gastroduodenal ulceration occurred in four patients and cholangitis in five patients. Partial response was seen in five patients (21%), median survival and 1-year survival rate were an encouraging 14 months and 51%, respectively (31). The logistics of intra-arterial delivery of 5FU may limit the application of this approach.

The development of oral fluoropyrimidines has led to the incorporation of these agents into combination regimens. Capecitabine is an oral pro-drug that is preferentially activated to 5FU in tumor tissue. The combination of gemcitabine 1,000 mg/m^2 on days 1, 8 and capecitabine 650 mg/m^2 BID days 1-14 every 21 days was evaluated in 53 patients with locally advanced ($n = 8$) or metastatic ($n = 45$) pancreatic cancer. The response rate, median survival, and 1-year survival were 19%, 8 months, and 35%, respectively. Toxicity was mild, although grade III/IV neutropenia was seen in 34% and febrile neutropenia in 4% (*32*). This combination regimen was compared with standard gemcitabine in a phase III study conducted by the Central European Cooperative Oncology Group. In a preliminary abstract (*33*), a trend toward improved survival was noted with the combination (8.4 months versus 7.3 months, *p* = 0.314). Additionally, another European phase III study involving 533 patients (70% with metastasis) was recently presented comparing standard gemcitabine 1,000 mg/m^2 weekly for 3 of 4 weeks to a combination of gemcitabine with capecitabine 830 mg/m^2 BID days 1-21 every 28 days. At the time of an interim analysis in May 2005, there was a significantly improved overall survival for the combination with hazard ratio 0.80 (95% CI: 0.65-0.98; *p* = 0.026); median survival was 7.4 months for the combination and 6.0 months for gemcitabine alone (*34*).

In the studies discussed in the preceding, especially the phase II studies, the proportion of patients treated with nonmetastatic disease has considerable influence on progression-free and overall survival, making comparisons across studies or evaluation of schedule and dose modifications of either drug difficult. The ECOG and the two capecitabine phase III trials suggest incremental improvement in survival with a gemcitabine and fluoropyrimidine doublet. It seems likely that the combination of gemcitabine and a fluoropyrimidine does provide additional benefit as compared with gemcitabine alone, without undue toxicity. The optimal use of the fluoropyrimidine, likely infusional 5FU, or capecitabine requires additional study, and this combination has not yet been embraced as a standard of care.

5.2   Gemcitabine-Platinum Doublets

Gemcitabine has been combined with cisplatin in phase II studies. In one study, 42 patients with locally advanced ($n = 4$) or metastatic ($n = 38$) pancreatic cancer received gemcitabine 1,000 mg/m^2 on days 1, 8, 15, and cisplatin 50 mg/m^2 on days 1, 15 repeated every 28 days. There was one complete response and 10 partial responses for an overall response rate of 26%. Median and 1-year survival was 7.1 months and 19%. Grade III/IV myelosuppression was common with neutropenia in 64%, thrombocytopenia in 62%, and anemia in 48%. However, there was only one patient with febrile neutropenia and no treatment-related deaths (*35*). Another study treated 45 patients with locally advanced ($n = 6$) or metastatic ($n = 39$) pancreatic cancer with gemcitabine 1,000 mg/m^2 and cisplatin 35 mg/m^2, both given weekly for 2 of every 3 weeks. There was one complete and four partial responses for an overall response rate of 9%. Median TTP and overall survival was 3.6 months and 5.6 months. Toxicity was mild, including grade III/IV neutropenia and thrombocytopenia in 6% and 10%, respectively (*36*). More recently, cisplatin has

Select phase II trials of gemcitabine + fluorouracil

Treatment[a,b] gemcitabine 1,000 mg +	Ref	n	% M$_1$ disease	Response rate	Median Survival	1-Year survival	Comments
5FU 600 mg wkly	22	36	100%	14%	4.4 mos	9%	Subsequent ph III trial (ref 24)
LV 20 mg 5FU 600 mg wkly	23	29	–	21%	8.4 mos	36%	–
LV 100 mg 5FU 400 mg d 1-3 every 14 d	25	42	74%	31%	13.1 mos	–	Tx well tolerated
LV 200 mg 5FU 750 mg for 24 h wkly × 4 every 6 wks	26	38	82%	5%	9.3 mos	32%	Median TTP 7.1 mos
Gem 1,400 mg 5FU 3,000 mg for 48 h wkly	27	46	–	7%	5.2 mos	25%	~Grade 3 neutropenia in 45%
LV 400 mg 5FU 1,000 mg 24 h	28	56	–	19%	7.2 mos	–	Gem by FDR
5FU 200 mg LDCI for 3/4 wks	29	25	92%	20%	6.2 mos	20%	
5FU 200 mg LDCI for 3/4 wks	30	45	67%	11%	6.9 mos	20%	Tx well tolerated
Capecitabine 650 mg BID d 1-14 every 3 wks	32	53	85%	19%	8.0 mos	35%	Subsequent ph III trial (ref 33)

[a] Gemcitabine 1,000 mg/m^2 over 30 minutes unless otherwise stated.
[b] All mg doses /m^2. FDR, fixed dose rate infusion; LDCI, low-dose continuous infusion; LV, leucovorin; M$_1$, metastatic disease; TTP, time to progression.

been combined with FDR gemcitabine. In 51 patients with metastatic pancreatic cancer, gemcitabine 1,000 mg/m^2 over 100 minutes and cisplatin 20 mg/m^2 were given on days 1, 8 every 3 weeks. The majority of patients (62.7%) required adjustment to an every-other-week schedule due to myelosuppression. Objective response rate, median survival, and estimated 1-year survival were 19%, 7.1 months and 29%, respectively. Toxicity was primarily hematologic with grade III/IV neutropenia in 53% and thrombocytopenia in 16%, but no episodes of febrile neutropenia or treatment-related deaths (37).

A small phase III study was performed comparing gemcitabine 1,000 mg/m^2 alone given weekly for 7 weeks followed by a 2-week rest, then weekly for 3 of 4 weeks to the same regimen with cisplatin 25 mg/m^2 given weekly for 3 of every 4 weeks. The study involved 107 patients with unresectable ($n = 45$) or metastatic ($n = 62$) pancreatic cancer. There was a statistically significant improvement in response rate with the combination (9.2% versus 26.4%, $p = 0.02$) but only a trend toward improved survival (4.6 versus 6.9 months, $p = 0.43$). Nonsignificant differences in toxicity favoring gemcitabine alone included grade III/IV neutropenia (9%

versus 18%) and alopecia (2 versus 12%), and the difference in asthenia reached significance (9 versus 24%) (*38*). Another phase III study compared gemcitabine alone given weekly for 3 of every 4 weeks with gemcitabine 1,000 mg/m^2 plus cisplatin 50 mg/m^2 days 1, 15 repeated every 28 days in 195 patients (72.9% metastatic disease). In a preliminary report, progression-free survival was significantly improved from 2.8 months to 5.4 months ($p < 0.01$) with the combination, and median survival was improved from 6.0 months to 8.3 months ($p = 0.12$). Apart from nausea and vomiting, toxicity was similar between the arms (*39*).

The benefits of cisplatin and gemcitabine inspired evaluation of newer platinum derivatives that are better tolerated. Gemcitabine 800 mg/m^2 days 1, 8 was combined with carboplatin AUC 4 day 8 repeated every 3 weeks in a multicenter phase II study. In 47 evaluable patients with unresectable ($n = 11$) or metastatic ($n = 36$) pancreatic cancer, response rate, median survival and 1-year survival were 17%, 7.4 months, and 28%, respectively. Toxicity was mild with no treatment-related deaths (*40*). Another novel platinum derivative, oxaliplatin, has known activity in a variety of gastrointestinal malignancies. The combination of gemcitabine 1,000 mg/m^2 days 1, 8 and oxaliplatin 100 mg/m^2 day 1 every 3 weeks was studied in 46 patients with metastatic pancreatic cancer. One complete response and four partial responses were seen for an overall response rate of 11%. The median TTP and overall survival were 4.5 months and 6.2 months. Grade III/IV toxicity included neutropenia 51%, thrombocytopenia 24%, nausea 9%, and dehydration 11%. There were three patients with febrile neutropenia and one patient who died from hemolytic uremic syndrome (*41*). Another study used FDR gemcitabine 1,000 mg/m^2 over 100 minutes day 1 and oxaliplatin 100 mg/m^2 over 2 hours on day 2 every 2 weeks in 64 patients with locally advanced ($n = 30$) or metastatic ($n = 34$) pancreatic cancer. Twelve of the 30 patients with locally advanced disease received chemoradiotherapy after six cycles of the combination. Response rate, median survival, and 1-year survival in the 34 patients with metastatic disease were 30%, 8.7 months, and 26%, respectively. In the entire group, these same measures were 31%, 9.2 months, and 36%, respectively. Myelosuppression was much less common, and other grade III/IV toxicity included nausea or vomiting 14% and neuropathy 11%. There was one patient with febrile neutropenia and no treatment-related deaths (*42*).

This latter study prompted a phase III study using the same regimen combining oxaliplatin with FDR gemcitabine versus gemcitabine alone in 313 eligible patients (70% metastatic disease). The combination was found to be superior in terms of response rate (26.8% versus 17.3%, $p = 0.04$), progression-free survival (5.8 versus 3.7 months, $p = 0.04$) and clinical benefit (38.2% versus 26.9%, $p = 0.03$). There was a trend toward improved overall survival (9.0 months versus 7.1 months, $p = 0.13$), which did not meet statistical significance. Statistical differences in grade III/IV toxicity that favored the single agent included thrombocytopenia, vomiting, and neuropathy (*43*). This oxaliplatin with FDR gemcitabine regimen was included in the recent ECOG 3-arm phase III study described earlier. In a preliminary report, the median survival for the standard arm and gemcitabine-oxaliplatin arm were 4.96 months and 6.47 months, respectively, with a hazard ratio of 1.22, a difference not achieving statistical significance (*21*).

Although the results of the gemcitabine-platinum combinations in individual phase III trials have been negative for overall survival, a recent meta-analysis was presented combining results of four phase III trials using gemcitabine-cisplatin or gemcitabine-oxaliplatin versus gemcitabine alone. The overall survival in the combined analysis was significantly improved, favoring the platinum combination (6.7 versus 8.3 months, $p = 0.031$) (44). It seems clear that there is benefit to the combination of gemcitabine with a platinum agent compared with gemcitabine alone, but the benefit remains modest and is most clearly seen in younger and better-performing patients. The decision to use such combination chemotherapy in a palliative setting needs to be weighed against the increased toxicity and time commitments of that treatment.

5.3   Other Gemcitabine-Cytoxic Combinations

Camptothecin derivatives have activity in pancreatic cancer and have also been evaluated in combination with gemcitabine. The combination of irinotecan and gemcitabine was studied in 60 patients with locally advanced ($n = 9$) or metastatic ($n = 51$) pancreatic cancer using a 3-week schedule with gemcitabine 1,000 mg/m2 over 60 minutes on days 1, 8 and irinotecan 300 mg/m^2 on day 8. There was one

Select phase II trials of gemcitabine + a platinum compound

Treatment [a,b] gemcitabine 1,000 mg +	Ref	n	% M$_1$ disease	Response rate	Median survival	1-Year survival	Comments
Cisplatin 50 mg d 1,15 every 4 wks	35	42	90%	26%	7.1 mos	19%	≥ Grade 3 ANC 64% Plts 62%
Cisplatin 35 mg d 1, 8 every 3 wks	36	45	87%	9%	5.6 mos	–	≥ Grade 3 ANC 6% Plts 10%
Cisplatin 20 mg d 1, 8 every 3 wks	37	51	100%	19%	7.1 mos	29%	Gem by FDR
Carboplatin AUC 4 d 8 every 3 wks	40	47	77%	17%	7.4 mos	28%	Gem 800 mg d 1, 8
Oxaliplatin 100 mg d 1 every 3 wks	41	46	100%	11%	6.2 mos	18%c	≥ Grade 3 ANC 51% Plts 24%
Oxaliplatin 100 mg d 2, 16 every 4 wks	42	34	100%	30%	8.7 mos	26%	Gem d 1,15 By FDR

[a] Gemcitabine 1,000 mg/m^2 over 30 minutes unless otherwise stated.
[b] All mg doses/m^2.
[c] Estimated from Kaplan-Meier survival curve. ANC, neutropenia; FDR, fixed dose rate infusion; M$_1$, metastatic disease; plts, thrombocytopenia.

complete response and 14 partial responses, for an overall response rate of 25%. Median TTP and overall survival were 7 months, and 1-year survival was 22.7%. Neutropenia grade III/IV occurred in 45%, with 10 patients developing febrile neutropenia, nine were hospitalized and two died. Other grade III/IV toxicities included thrombocytopenia 15%, diarrhea 8%, and asthenia 15% (45). In another phase II study, 45 patients were treated with gemcitabine 1,000 mg/m^2 over 30 minutes followed by irinotecan 100 mg/m^2 on days 1, 8 of a 21-day cycle. Response rate was 20%, and median survival and 1-year survival were 5.7 months and 27%, respectively. Treatment was well tolerated with no febrile neutropenia or grade IV diarrhea, although one patient died from dehydration and renal failure (46). This latter schedule was compared with gemcitabine alone in 342 patients with advanced pancreatic cancer, 80% of whom had metastatic disease. Although there was an improved response rate with the combination, neither TTP nor median survival was improved. Grade III/IV diarrhea and febrile neutropenia was seen more often in the combination arm (47). The novel synthetic camptothecin derivative DX-8951F (Exatecan) in combination with gemcitabine versus gemcitabine alone was studied in 349 patients with locally advanced ($n = 75$) or metastatic ($n = 274$) disease. In a preliminary report, no difference was seen in TTP or median survival and only a trend toward improved clinical benefit was observed (48).

Taxanes as single agents are not particularly active in pancreatic cancer, but gemcitabine and docetaxel have been evaluated in a number of phase II studies using a variety of doses and schedules. In one study, 38 evaluable patients with locally advanced ($n = 9$) or metastatic ($n = 29$) pancreatic cancer were treated with gemcitabine 750 mg/m^2 and docetaxel 35 mg/m^2 weekly for 3 of 4 weeks. Response rate, median survival and 1-year survival were 27%, 7 months, and 19.3%, respectively. Grade III/IV neutropenia was seen in 37% of patients and there were four deaths within the first 30 days, one of which was attributed to therapy (49). In another study, 32 patients with locally advanced ($n = 10$) or metastatic ($n = 22$) pancreatic cancer were treated with docetaxel 75 mg/m^2, followed by gemcitabine 2,000 mg/m^2 every 2 weeks. Two complete and two partial responses were seen, for an overall response rate of 12.5%. Median survival was only 4.7 months and toxicity included grade III/IV neutropenia in 47%, grade 3 neuropathy in 16%, and two deaths while on therapy (50). Thirty-four patients (unresectable 10, metastatic 24) were treated with two different dose/schedules of this combination. The first 18 patients received gemcitabine 800 mg/m^2 days 1, 8, 15, and docetaxel 75 mg/m^2 day 1 every 28 days. Due to a high incidence of myelosuppression, treatment was altered to gemcitabine 1,000 mg/m^2 and docetaxel 40 mg/m^2, both agents given days 1, 8 every 3 weeks. In 33 evaluable patients, response rate, median survival, and 1-year survival were 30%, 10.5 months, and 41%. Grade III neutropenia was seen in 30% and one death was attributed to pulmonary toxicity (51). Recently the EORTC randomized 89 evaluable patients with locally advanced ($n = 15$) or metastatic ($n = 74$) pancreatic cancer to either 21 day cycles of gemcitabine 800 mg/m^2 days 1, 8 and docetaxel 85 mg/m^2 day 8 or docetaxel 75 mg/m^2 and cisplatin 75 mg/m^2 both on day 1 only. In the gemcitabine and docetaxel arm, response rate, median survival, and 1-year survival were 19%, 7.4 months, and 30%, respectively.

In the docetaxel and cisplatin arm, respective results were 23.5%, 7.1 months, and 16%. Toxicity in the gemcitabine containing arm included grade III/IV neutropenia in 47% with 9% febrile neutropenia and two deaths, one of which was attributed to treatment. In the cisplatin-containing arm, grade III/IV toxicity neutropenia was seen in 55% with febrile neutropenia in 16% and no deaths (52).

Additional cytotoxic agents have been evaluated in combination with gemcitabine. Epirubicin 20 mg/m^2 followed by gemcitabine 1,000 mg/m^2 weekly for 3 of 4 weeks was given to 44 patients with locally advanced ($n = 10$) or metastatic ($n = 34$) pancreatic cancer. Response rate, median survival, and 1-year survival were 25%, 10.9 months, and 23%. Toxicity including myelosuppression was mild with no hospitalizations or deaths (53). The multitargeted antifolate pemetrexed was evaluated in combination with gemcitabine in a phase III study versus gemcitabine alone in 536 patients (90% metastatic). There was no benefit to the combination in terms of TTP or survival and toxicity was significantly increased, predominantly myelosuppression (54). The thymidylate synthetase inhibitor raltitrexed was evaluated in combination with gemcitabine. A Belgian multicenter study treated 33 patients with locally advanced (n = 5) or metastatic ($n = 28$) pancreatic cancer with gemcitabine 1,000 mg/m^2 days 1, 8 and raltitrexed 3,000 mg/m^2 day 1 repeated every 3 weeks. Response rate, median survival and 1-year survival were 30%, 4.7 months, and 21%, respectively. Toxicity included 42% grade III/IV neutropenia

Select phase II trials of gemcitabine + docetaxel

Treatment[a,b] gemcitabine 1,000 mg +	Ref	n	% M$_1$ disease	Response rate	Median survival	1-Year survival	Comments
Docetaxel 35 mg d 1,8, 15 every 4 wks	49	38	76%	27%	7.0 mos	19%	Gem 750 mg
Gem 2000 mg + Docetaxel 75 mg every 2 wks	50	32	69%	12%	4.7 mos	18%[c]	50% pts experienced grade 4 tox
Docetaxel 75 mg every 4 wks modified to 40 mg every 3 wks	51	33	71%	30%	10.5 mos	41%	Modified secondary to toxicity
Docetaxel 85 mg d 8, every 3 wks	52	47	82%	19%	7.4 mos	30%	Gem 800 mg d 1, 8
Capecitabine 1.5–2 g d1-14, Docetaxel 30 mg d 4, 11 each 21 d	59	23	100%	39%	–	–	Gem 750 mg FDR d 4,11 "GTX"

[a] Gemcitabine 1,000 mg/m^2 over 30 minutes unless otherwise stated.
[b] All mg doses /m^2.
[c] Estimated from Kaplan-Meier survival curve. FDR, fixed dose rate infusion.

with one febrile neutropenia and one death (55). Another study treated 27 patients with locally advanced ($n = 11$) or metastatic ($n = 16$) pancreatic cancer with gemcitabine 800 mg/m^2 days 1, 8 and raltitrexed 3,500 mg/m^2 day 1 every 3 weeks. Response rate was only 4%, median survival 5.5 months, and 1-year survival 11%. Neutropenia was seen in 18% and hospitalization for diarrhea occurred in four patients (56).

Combinations of three or more cytoxic drugs have been evaluated in the first line setting using gemcitabine as a backbone. The combination of gemcitabine, cisplatin and infusional 5FU was investigated in two phase II studies. One study treated 47 patients with locally advanced ($n = 16$) or metastatic ($n = 31$) disease with gemcitabine 1,000 mg/m^2 days 1, 8, 15; cisplatin 50 mg/m^2 days 1, 15; and PVI 5FU 175 mg/m^2/day days 1-15 repeated every 28 days. Response rate, median survival, and 1-year survival were 26%, 8.6 months, and 36%, respectively. Toxicity included grade III/IV neutropenia in 60%, thrombocytopenia in 42%, and mucositis in 22%. There were 13 hospitalizations and two deaths related to treatment (57). Another study treated 34 patients (six unresectable and 28 metastatic) with gemcitabine 1,000 mg/m^2 weekly on weeks 1, 2, 5, 6; cisplatin 20 mg/m^2 weekly for 6 weeks; and PVI 5FU 200 mg/m^2/day days 1-42, repeated every 8 weeks. Responses were seen in 19% and median and 1-year survival was 9 months and 26%. Toxicity was milder and included grade III/IV neutropenia in 24% and grade III/IV thrombocytopenia in 22% (58). Recently reported in preliminary abstract form was a study involving 23 patients with metastatic pancreatic cancer treated with capecitabine 1,500 mg/m^2 days 1-14, and gemcitabine 750 mg/m^2 over 75 minutes and docetaxel 30 mg/m^2 days 4, 11. Using CT scanning, response rate in metastatic sites was 39%, including 17% complete responses. Toxicity included one patient with lung toxicity and another patient with grade IV mucositis and sepsis (59). Based on a phase II study, another group randomized 99 patients with locally advanced ($n = 29$) or metastatic ($n = 70$) pancreatic cancer to either gemcitabine alone ($n = 47$) or the combination of gemcitabine 600 mg/m^2 days 1, 8; cisplatin 40 mg/m^2 day 1, epirubicin 40 mg/m^2 day 1 and PVI 5FU 200 mg/m^2 days 1-28 repeated every 4 weeks (PEFG, $n = 52$). Response rate (38.5% versus 8.5%) and 1-year survival (38.5% versus 21.4%) favored the PEFG group as compared with gemcitabine alone. Toxicity with the combination included grade III/IV neutropenia (43%) and thrombocytopenia (30%) and three hospitalizations (60).

In summary, the combination of gemcitabine with one more cytoxic agent(s) seems to increase response rate, median survival, and the fraction of patients alive at 1 year in advanced pancreatic cancer. These advantages come at the expense of greater toxicity and an increased burden of therapy. An individual phase III trial has not yet been published that describes a statistically significant survival advantage to a cytotoxic combination; therefore, one has not emerged as a standard replacing single-agent gemcitabine. However, data do support the use of gemcitabine and cis- or oxaliplatin, especially in younger patients with good performance status, as well as the gemcitabine and capecitabine combination. These incremental improvements provided by combination therapy may not be sufficient to have a major impact in metastatic disease, but may afford an advantage over single-agent gemcitabine in the adjuvant, neoadjuvant, or locally advanced disease setting.

5.4   Gemcitabine with Novel Agents

The recent introduction of numerous targeted agents has led to studies combining these agents with gemcitabine in patients with pancreatic cancer. Initial studies evaluated gemcitabine and the farnesyl transferase inhibitor tipifarnib, as well as gemcitabine and the matrix metalloproteinase inhibitor marimastat. Both agents were subsequently evaluated in large, phase III, placebo-controlled studies comparing the combination with gemcitabine and placebo. Neither study demonstrated an improvement in outcome with the combination (61, 62). Despite these results, enthusiasm for novel targeted molecules in pancreatic cancer was renewed by a recent report of a prolongation of survival in patients treated with the combination of gemcitabine and erlotinib.

Erlotinib is an oral tyrosine kinase inhibitor (TKI) of the epidermal growth factor receptor (EGFR). Following a phase IB study demonstrating tolerance of the combination (63) a large phase III trial comparing gemcitabine and erlotinib with gemcitabine and placebo was conducted. This study randomized 569 patients and reported an improved median survival (6.2 months versus 5.9 months, $p = 0.038$), 1-year survival (23% versus 17%), and progression-free survival (hazard ratio, 0.77; $p = 0.004$) with the gemcitabine-erlotinib combination (64). In the fall of 2005, the FDA approved the use of this combination in patients with advanced pancreatic cancer based on these data.

Phase II and III studies have evaluated monoclonal antibodies in combination with gemcitabine. Cetuximab, an EGFR-directed monoclonal antibody, was combined with gemcitabine in 41 patients (35 metastatic) with evidence of EGFR staining of their tumor. Response rate, median survival, and 1-year survival were 12%, 7.1 months, and 32%, respectively (65). Although these results were promising, a follow-up phase III trial by the Southwest Oncology Group comparing gemcitabine with or without cetuximab was recently presented as a negative study (66). The monoclonal antibody trastuzumab, directed against another EGFR family member HER-2/neu, was evaluated in combination with gemcitabine in 34 patients with metastatic pancreatic cancer and 2+/3+ HER2/neu overexpression by immunohistochemistry. Response rate, median survival, and 1-year survival were 6%, 7 months, and 19%, respectively (67). The recombinant humanized anti-vascular endothelial growth factor (VEGF) monoclonal antibody bevacizumab was investigated in combination with gemcitabine in 52 patients with metastatic pancreatic cancer. Response rate, median survival, and 1-year survival were 21%, 8.8 months, and 29% (68). Unfortunately, a follow-up phase III trial by the Eastern Cooperative Oncology Group comparing gemcitabine with or without bevacizumab was recently reported as showing no advantage to the combination (69).

    Additional novel agents have been combined with gemcitabine without clear
indication of enhanced efficacy. The oligonucleotide anti-sense inhibitor of H-ras,
ISIS-2503, was given by continuous infusion combined with gemcitabine to 48
patients with either locally advanced ($n = 5$) or metastatic ($n = 43$) pancreatic cancer. Response rate, median survival, and 6-month survival were 10%, 6.6 months,
and 58%. Grade III/IV neutropenia was seen in 56% and thrombocytopenia in 40%
(70). The proteosome inhibitor bortezomib was combined with gemcitabine in a
randomized study. In 42 evaluable patients with metastatic disease receiving the
combination treatment, response rate, 6-month survival, and median survival were
10%, 41%, and 4.8 months without unanticipated toxicity (71). The selective cyclo-
oxygenase-2 (COX-2) inhibitor celecoxib has been combined with chemotherapy
in pancreatic cancer. In one study, 42 patients (16 locally advanced, 26 metastatic)
were treated with celecoxib and gemcitabine. Response rate was 9% and median
survival was 9.1 months with generally mild toxicity (72). A second study evaluated celecoxib with FDR gemcitabine and cisplatin in 22 patients with metastatic
disease. Response rate was 14%, median survival 5.8 months, and 1-year survival
13% and increased hematologic toxicity was observed (73).

6   Non-gemcitabine Treatments

Following approval of gemcitabine for treatment of pancreatic cancer, there had been
a paucity of investigation and/or development of successful non-gemcitabine-containing
regimens in this disease. With the recognition of the limits of gemcitabine-based
therapies, more attention and study of alternatives to gemcitabine are likely to be
forthcoming, with some selected approaches described in the following.

    The FOLFOX-6 combination has been evaluated as a first-line treatment in
advanced pancreatic cancer. In one phase II study of 30 patients (22 with metastatic
disease) a response rate of 27.6% was reported (74). Median time to progression
and survival were 4.0 and 7.5 months, respectively. Toxicity was mild.

    The Southwest Oncology Group recently reported a phase II combination
chemotherapy trial in pancreatic cancer without gemcitabine that is of some interest
(75). Based on preclinical rationale, mitomycin (10 mg/m^2 day 1 every 6 weeks)
and dipyridamole (75 mg orally three times daily) were added to weekly leucovorin
(30 mg/m^2) and infusional 5FU (200 mg/m^2/day for 4 weeks) in 50 patients with
locally advanced pancreatic cancer. Dipyridamole was intended to modulate 5FU
by inhibiting nucleotide transport and sustaining the depleted intracellular triphosphate nucleotide concentrations induced by 5FU. Survival probability at 1 year in
this group of patients was 54%. In the 47 patients evaluable for response, objective
response rate was 26% and two complete responses were seen.

    Ixabepilone, a non-taxane tubulin-binding agent, has been evaluated in untreated
patients with advanced pancreatic cancer in a phase II study by the Southwest
Oncology Group (76). Sixty patients with metastatic disease received ixabepilone
40 mg/m^2 every 21 days. The estimated 6-month survival was 60%, median survival

Select phase II trials of non-gemcitabine therapies

Treatment[a]	Ref	n	% M$_1$ disease	Response rate	Median survival	1-Year survival	Comments
Capecitabine 2,500 mg d–1-14 every 3 wks	6	42	–	7%	6.0 mos	–	CBR in 24%
Docetaxel 75 mg +Cisplatin 75 mg d–1 every 3 wks	52	47	84%	23%	7.4 mos	16%	febrile neutropenia in 16%
Oxaliplatin 100 mg d 1 5FU 400 mg, LV 400 mg d 1, 5FU 3,000 mg by 46 h inf every 2 wks	74	30	73%	28%	7.5 mos	18%	Folfox-6 regimen
Ixabepilone 40 mg every 3 wks	76	60	100%	9%	7.2 mos	25%[b]	Initial dose 50 mg decreased due to neurotoxicity

[a] All mg doses/m^2.
[b] Estimated from Kaplan-Meier survival curve. CBR, clinical benefit response.

was 7.2 months, and time to treatment failure was 2.3 months. The confirmed response rate was 9%. Based on these encouraging results, further development of ixabepilone in pancreatic cancer is ongoing.

7   Second-Line Cytotoxic Therapy

Currently there is no standard second line chemotherapy for advanced pancreatic cancer. A randomized trial presented in preliminary form compared a combination of weekly 5FU 2,000 mg/m^2 over 24 hours and leucovorin 200 mg/m^2 with oxaliplatin 85 mg/m^2 day 8, 22 given for 4 consecutive weeks, repeated every 42 days to best supportive care (BSC) in patients with gemcitabine refractory pancreatic cancer. After 46 of a planned 165 patients were enrolled, the BSC arm was closed. Despite the small number of patients, a survival benefit was seen favoring treatment (40 weeks versus 34 weeks, $p = 0.03$) (77). A phase II study in 30 patients with advanced pancreatic cancer that were gemcitabine refractory used the same three agents (oxaliplatin 50 mg/m^2, 5FU 500 mg/m^2, and leucovorin 50 mg/m^2) given weekly by bolus injection until progression was reported. Median duration of disease control and overall survival were 22 and 25 weeks, respectively. Eight patients developed febrile neutropenia with no treatment-related deaths (78). Oxaliplatin has also been studied alone or in combination with other agents in previously treated patients. One study treated 18 patients with locally advanced ($n = 5$) or metastatic ($n = 13$) pancreatic cancer refractory to gemcitabine with oxaliplatin 130 mg/m^2 every 21 days. Clinical benefit was seen in 28% and median survival was 3.5 months in this generally well tolerated regimen (*79*). In another study, 30 patients with metastatic pancreatic cancer refractory to gemcitabine based chemotherapy were treated with oxaliplatin 60 mg/m^2 days 1, 15, and irinotecan 60 mg/m^2 days 1, 8, 15, every 4 weeks. Response rate, clinical benefit and overall survival were 10%, 20%, and 5.9 months, respectively, and treatment was well tolerated (*80*). The combination of FDR gemcitabine and oxaliplatin in gemcitabine refractory patients was studied in 31 evaluable patients and showed a response rate of 22.6% and median survival of 6 months (*81*). Raltitrexed 3,000 mg/m^2 every 3 weeks has been studied in combination with irinotecan or oxaliplatin in previously treated patients with advanced pancreatic cancer. With irinotecan 200 mg/m^2 and raltitrexed every 3 weeks, response rate, clinical benefit, and median survival were 16%, 29%, and 6.5 months. Treatment was generally well tolerated with grade III/IV neutropenia in 21% (*82*). With oxaliplatin 130 mg/m^2 and raltitrexed every 3 weeks, response rate was 24% and median survival was 5.2 months and treatment was well tolerated (*83*).

8 Summary

Despite scores of phase II and many phase III studies (Table 30.1) trying to improve upon the modest benefits of, and supplant single-agent gemcitabine, there is no one regimen that emerges as the preferred choice for all patients with advanced pancreatic cancer. The median survival in single institution studies occasionally reaches double digit figures when reported in months, but randomized multicenter studies have generally shown median survivals between 6 and 9 months for combination therapy. Survival benefits have now been described in preliminary reports with gemcitabine-erlotinib as well as gemcitabine-capecitabine. However, enthusiasm has been tempered by the modest increments in survival (0.5–1.5 months) and significant costs of these agents. There is an expectation that the newer generation of targeted agents, some of which have multiple targets, may provide more favorable results. It is also likely that combinations of two or more cytotoxics and/or targeted agents may be required for best outcomes. The approach of individualizing therapy for the patient by determining the molecular abnormalities within their cancer is on the horizon.

At the present time, patients with advanced pancreatic cancer first need to decide whether they are interested in therapy directed at the cancer, given the relatively modest benefits of treatment. Those that are symptomatic should understand the potential for clinical benefit with treatment. Acceptable approaches to palliative therapy include single-agent gemcitabine, infused over 30 minutes, weekly. Fixed dose rate gemcitabine, gemcitabine-capecitabine, gemcitabine-platinum, and gemcitabine-erlotinib combinations are all reasonable alternatives for patients, especially those with good performance status, and a desire for more aggressive therapy. When available, clinical trial participation should be offered and encouraged. Only when disease control in response to therapy is expected and lasting, can that

Table 30.1 Randomized trials comparing gemcitabine alone vs. gemcitabine + agent in advanced pancreatic cancer

Agent	Reference	Number	Prog-free survival in months	Median survival in months
Bolus 5FU	24	327	2.2 vs 3.4; $p = 0.02$	5.4 vs 6.7; $p = 0.09$
Capecitabine	33	319		7.3 vs 8.4; $p = 0.31$
Capecitabine	34	533		6.0 vs 7.4; $p = 0.026$
Cisplatin	38	107	1.9 vs 4.7; $p = 0.48$	4.7 vs 7.0; $p = 0.48$
Cisplatin	39	195	2.8 vs 5.4; $p < 0.01$	6.0 vs 8.3; $p = 0.12$
Oxaliplatin	43	313	3.7 vs 5.8; $p = 0.04$	7.1 vs 9.0; $p = 0.13$
Irinotecan	47	342	3.0 vs 3.5; $p = 0.35$	6.6 vs 6.3; $p = 0.79$
Pemetrexed	54	536	3.3 vs 3.9; $p = 0.11$	6.3 vs 6.2; $p = 0.85$
Tipifarnib	61	688	3.6 vs 3.7; $p = 0.72$	6.1 vs 6.4; $p = 0.75$
Marimastat	62	239	3.2 vs 3.1; $p = 0.68$	5.5 vs 5.5; $p = 0.95$
Erlotinib	64	569	3.5 vs 3.7; $p = 0.004$	5.9 vs 6.2; $p = 0.038$
Cetuximab	66	766	3.0 vs 3.5; $p = 0.058$	5.9 vs 6.4; $p = 0.14$
Bevacizumab	69	602	4.7 vs 4.9; $p = 0.99$	6.1 vs 5.8; $p = 0.78$

treatment be considered optimal. Increased understanding of the biology of pancreatic cancer, the mechanisms of resistance to systemic treatment and identification and development of new agents will lead to discovery of optimal systemic therapy for pancreatic cancer.

References

1. Cornell GN, Cahow CE, et al. Clinical experience with 5-fluorouracil (NSC-19893) in the treatment of malignant disease. Cancer Chemother Rep 1960, 9:23–30.
2. Ahlgren JD. 1996, Chemotherapy for pancreatic carcinoma. Cancer 1960, 78(3 Suppl):654–663.
3. DeCaprio JA, Mayer RJ, 1991, Fluorouracil and high-dose leucovorin in previously untreated patients with advanced adenocarcinoma of the pancreas: results of a phase II trial. J Clin Oncol 9(12):2128–2133.
4. Crown J, Casper ES, 1991, Lack of efficacy of high-dose leucovorin and fluorouracil in patients with advanced pancreatic adenocarcinoma. J Clin Oncol 9(9):1682–1686.

5. Rijswijk RE, Van Jeziorski K, 2004, Weekly high-dose 5-fluorouracil and folinic acid in metastatic pancreatic carcinoma: a phase II study of the EORTC GastroIntestinal Tract Cancer Cooperative Group. Eur J Cancer 40(14):2077–2081 .
6. Cartwright TH, Cohn A, 2002, Phase II study of oral capecitabine in patients with advanced or metastatic pancreatic cancer. J Clin Oncol 20(1):160–164.
7. GITSG. Phase II studies of drug combinations in advanced pancreatic carcinoma: fluorouracil plus doxorubicin plus mitomycin C and two regimens of streptozotocin plus mitomycin C plus fluorouracil. The Gastrointestinal Tumor Study Group. J Clin Oncol 1986, 4(12):1794–1798.
8. Oster MW, Gray R, 1986, Chemotherapy for advanced pancreatic cancer. A comparison of 5-fluorouracil, Adriamycin, and mitomycin (FAM) with 5-fluorouracil, streptozotocin, and mitomycin (FSM). Cancer 57(1):29–33.
9. Mallinson CN, Rake MO, 1980, Chemotherapy in pancreatic cancer:results of a controlled, prospective, randomised, multicentre trial. Br Med J 281(6255):1589–1591.
10. Cullinan S, Moertel GC, 1990, A phase III trial on the therapy of advanced pancreatic carcinoma. Evaluations of the Mallinson regimen and combined 5-fluorouracil, doxorubicin, and cisplatin. Cancer 65:(10)2207–2212.
11. Glimelius B, Hoffman K, 1996, Chemotherapy improves survival and quality of life in advanced pancreatic and biliary cancer. Ann Oncol 7(6):593–600.
12. Heinemann V. 2001, Gemcitabine: progress in the treatment of pancreatic cancer. Oncology 60(1):8–18.
13. Casper ES, Green MR, 1994, Phase II trial of gemcitabine (2,2Î-difluorodeoxycytidine) in patients with adenocarcinoma of the pancreas. Invest New Drugs 12(1):29–34.
14. Carmichael J, Fink U, 1996, Phase II study of gemcitabine in patients with advanced pancreatic cancer. Br J Cancer 73(1):101–105.
15. Rothenberg ML, Moore MJ, 1996, A phase II trial of gemcitabine in patients with 5-FU-refractory pancreatic cancer. Ann Oncol 7(4):347–353.
16. Burris HA 3rd., Moore MJ, 1997, Improvements in survival and clinical benefit with gemcitabine as first-line therapy for patients with advanced pancreatic cancer: a randomized trial. J Clin Oncol 15(6):2403–2413.
17. Storniolo AM, Enas NH, 1999, An investigational new drug treatment program for patients with gemcitabine: results for over 3000 patients with pancreatic carcinoma. Cancer 85(6):1261–1268.
18. Ulrich-Pur H, Kornek GV, 2000, A phase II trial of biweekly high dose gemcitabine for patients with metastatic pancreatic adenocarcinoma. Cancer 88(11):2505–2511.
19. Tempero M, Plunkett W, 2003, Randomized phase II comparison of dose-intense gemcitabine: thirty-minute infusion and fixed dose rate infusion in patients with pancreatic adenocarcinoma. J Clin Oncol 21(18):3402–3408.
20. Gelibter A, Malaguti P, 2005, Fixed dose-rate gemcitabine infusion as first-line treatment for advanced-stage carcinoma of the pancreas and biliary tree. Cancer 104(6):1237–1245.
21. Poplin E, Levy DE, 2006, Phase III trial of gemcitabine (30-minute infusion) versus gemcitabine (fixed-dose-rate infusion[FDR]) versus gemcitabine + oxaliplatin (GEMOX) in patients with advanced pancreatic cancer (E6201). J Clin Oncol 24(18S):LBA4004.
22. Berlin JD, Adak S, 2000, A phase II study of gemcitabine and 5-fluorouracil in metastatic pancreatic cancer: an Eastern Cooperative Oncology Group Study (E3296). Oncology 58(3):215–218.
23. Marantz A, Jovtis S, 2001, Phase II study of gemcitabine, 5-fluorouracil, and leucovorin in patients with pancreatic cancer. Semin Oncol 28(3 Suppl 10):44–49.
24. Berlin JD, Catalano P, 2002, Phase III study of gemcitabine in combination with fluorouracil versus gemcitabine alone in patients with advanced pancreatic carcinoma: Eastern Cooperative Oncology Group Trial E2297. J Clin Oncol 20(15):3270–3275.
25. Correale P, Messinese S, 2003, A novel biweekly pancreatic cancer treatment schedule with gemcitabine, 5-fluorouracil and folinic acid. Br J Cancer 89(2):239–242.
26. Oettle H, Arning M, 2000, A phase II trial of gemcitabine in combination with 5-fluorouracil (24-hour) and folinic acid in patients with chemonaive advanced pancreatic cancer. Ann Oncol 11(10):1267–1272.

27. Santasusana JM, Garcia Lopez JL, 2005, A phase II trial of gemcitabine and weekly high-dose 5-fluorouracil in a 48-hour continuous-infusion schedule in patients with advanced pancreatic carcinoma. A study of the Spanish Cooperative Group for Gastrointestinal Tumour Therapy (TTD). Clin Transl Oncol 7(11):493–498.
28. Andre T, Noirclerc M, 2004, Phase II study of leucovorin, 5-fluorouracil and gemcitabine for locally advanced and metastatic pancreatic cancer (FOLFUGEM 2). Gastroenterol Clin Biol 28(8–9):645–650.
29. Rauch DP, Maurer CA, 2001, Activity of gemcitabine and continuous infusion fluorouracil in advanced pancreatic cancer. Oncology 60(1):43–48.
30. Costanzo F, Di Carlini P, 2005, Gemcitabine with or without continuous infusion 5-FU in advanced pancreatic cancer: a randomised phase II trial of the Italian oncology group for clinical research (GOIRC). Br J Cancer 93(2):185–189.
31. Takamori H, Kanemitsu K, 2005, 5-Fluorouracil intra-arterial infusion combined with systemic gemcitabine for unresectable pancreatic cancer. Pancreas 30(3):223–226.
32. Stathopoulos GP, Syrigos K, 2004, Front-line treatment of inoperable or metastatic pancreatic cancer with gemcitabine and capecitabine: an intergroup, multicenter, phase II study. Ann Oncol 15(2):224–229.
33. Herrmann R, Bodoky G, 2005, Gemcitabine (G) plus Capecitabine (C) versus G alone in locally advanced or metastatic pancreatic cancer. A randomized phase III study of the Swiss Group for Clinical Cancer Research (SAKK) and the Central European Cooperative Oncology Group (CECOG). J Clin Oncol, 23(16S):4010.
34. Cunningham D, Chau I, 2005, PS11 Best of ECCO 13 Phase III randomised comparison of gemcitabine (GEM) versus gemcitabine plus capecitabine (GEM-CAP) in patients with advanced pancreatic cancer. Eur J Cancer Suppl 3(4):12.
35. Philip PA, Zalupski MM, 2001, Phase II study of gemcitabine and cisplatin in the treatment of patients with advanced pancreatic carcinoma. Cancer 92(3):569–577.
36. Cascinu S, Labianca R, 2003, Weekly gemcitabine and cisplatin chemotherapy: a well-tolerated but ineffective chemotherapeutic regimen in advanced pancreatic cancer patients. A report from the Italian Group for the Study of Digestive Tract Cancer (GISCAD). Ann Oncol 14(2):205–208.
37. Ko AH, Dito E, 2006, Phase II study of fixed dose rate gemcitabine with cisplatin for metastatic adenocarcinoma of the pancreas. J Clin Oncol 24(3):379–385.
38. Colucci G, Giuliani F, 2002, Gemcitabine alone or with cisplatin for the treatment of patients with locally advanced and/or metastatic pancreatic carcinoma: a prospective, randomized phase III study of the Gruppo Oncologia dell'Italia Meridionale. Cancer 94(4):902–910.
39. Heinemann V, Quietzsch D, 2003, A phase III trial comparing gemcitabine plus cisplatin versus gemcitabine alone in advanced pancreatic carcinoma. Proc Amer Soc Clin Oncol 22:1003.
40. Xiros N, Papacostas P, 2005, Carboplatin plus gemcitabine in patients with inoperable or metastatic pancreatic cancer: a phase II multicenter study by the Hellenic Cooperative Oncology Group. Ann Oncol 16(5):773–779.
41. Alberts SR, Townley PM, 2003, Gemcitabine and oxaliplatin for metastatic pancreatic adenocarcinoma: a North Central Cancer Treatment Group phase II study. Ann Oncol 14(4):580–585.
42. Louvet C, Andre T, 2002, Gemcitabine combined with oxaliplatin in advanced pancreatic adenocarcinoma: final results of a GERCOR multicenter phase II study. J Clin Oncol 20(6):1512–1518.
43. Louvet C, Labianca R, 2005, Gemcitabine in combination with oxaliplatin compared with gemcitabine alone in locally advanced or metastatic pancreatic cancer: results of a GERCOR and GISCAD phase III trial. J Clin Oncol 23(15):3509–3516.
44. Louvet C, Hincke A, 2006, Increased survival using platinum analog combined with gemcitabine as compared to gemcitabine single agent in advanced pancreatic cancer (APC): pooled analysis of two randomised trials, the GERCOR/GISCAD Intergroup Study and a German Multicenter Study. J Clin Oncol 24(18S):4003.
45. Stathopoulos GP, Rigatos SK, 2003, Treatment of pancreatic cancer with a combination of irinotecan (CPT-11) and gemcitabine: a multicenter phase II study by the Greek Cooperative Group for Pancreatic Cancer. Ann Oncol 14(3):388–394.

46. Rocha Lima CM, Savarese D, 2002, Irinotecan plus gemcitabine induces both radiographic and CA 19-9 tumor marker responses in patients with previously untreated advanced pancreatic cancer. J Clin Oncol 20(5):1182–1191.
47. Rocha Lima CM, Green MR, 2004, Irinotecan plus gemcitabine results in no survival advantage compared with gemcitabine monotherapy in patients with locally advanced or metastatic pancreatic cancer despite increased tumor response rate. J Clin Oncol 22(18):3776–3783.
48. Cheverton P, Friess H, 2004, Phase III results of exatecan (DX-8951f) versus gemcitabine (Gem) in chemotherapy-naïve patients with advanced pancreatic cancer (APC). J Clin Oncol 22(14S):4005.
49. Schneider BP, Ganjoo KN, 2003, Phase II study of gemcitabine plus docetaxel in advanced pancreatic cancer: a Hoosier Oncology Group study. Oncology 65(3):218–223.
50. Shepard RC, Levy DE, 2004, Phase II study of gemcitabine in combination with docetaxel in patients with advanced pancreatic carcinoma (E1298). A trial of the eastern cooperative oncology group. Oncology 66(4):303–309.
51. Jacobs AD, Otero H, 2004, Gemcitabine combined with docetaxel for the treatment of unresectable pancreatic carcinoma. Cancer Invest 22(4):505–514.
52. Lutz MP, Cutsem EV, 2005, Docetaxel plus gemcitabine or docetaxel plus cisplatin in advanced pancreatic carcinoma: randomized phase II study 40984 of the European Organisation for Research and Treatment of Cancer Gastrointestinal Group. J Clin Oncol 23(36):9250–9256.
53. Neri B, Cini G, 2002, Weekly gemcitabine plus Epirubicin as effective chemotherapy for advanced pancreatic cancer: a multicenter phase II study. Br J Cancer 87(5):497–501.
54. Oettle H, Richards D, 2005, A phase III trial of pemetrexed plus gemcitabine versus gemcitabine in patients with unresectable or metastatic pancreatic cancer. Ann Oncol 16(10):1639–1645.
55. Laethem JL, Van Maele P, Van, 2004, Raltitrexed plus gemcitabine (TOMGEM) in advanced pancreatic cancer. Results of a Belgian multicentre phase II study. Oncology 67(5–6):338–343.
56. Arends JJ, Sleeboom HP, 2005, A phase II study of raltitrexed and gemcitabine in patients with advanced pancreatic carcinoma. Br J Cancer 92(3):445–448.
57. El-Rayes BF, Zalupski MM, 2003, Phase II study of gemcitabine, cisplatin, and infusional fluorouracil in advanced pancreatic cancer. J Clin Oncol 21(15):2920–2925.
58. Novarino A, Chiappino I, 2004, Phase II study of cisplatin, gemcitabine and 5-fluorouracil in advanced pancreatic cancer. Ann Oncol 15(3):474–477.
59. Fine RL, Fogelman DR, 2006, Gemcitabine, docetaxel, and capecitabine (GTX) in the treatment of metastatic pancreatic cancer (PC): a prospective phase II study. J Clin Oncol 24(18S):14024.
60. Reni M, Cordio S, 2005, Gemcitabine versus cisplatin, epirubicin, fluorouracil, and gemcitabine in advanced pancreatic cancer: a randomised controlled multicentre phase III trial. Lancet Oncol 6(6):369–376.
61. Cutsem E, Van Velde H, van de, 2004, Phase III trial of gemcitabine plus tipifarnib compared with gemcitabine plus placebo in advanced pancreatic cancer. J Clin Oncol 22(8): 1430–1438.
62. Bramhall SR, Schulz J, 2002, A double-blind placebo-controlled, randomised study comparing gemcitabine and marimastat with gemcitabine and placebo as first line therapy in patients with advanced pancreatic cancer. Br J Cancer 87(2):161–167.
63. Porterfield BW, Dragovich T, 2004, Erlotinib + gemcitabine in patients with unresectable pancreatic carcinoma: results from a phase IB trial. J Clin Oncol 22(14S):4110.
64. Moore MJ, Goldstein D, 2007, Erlotinib plus gemcitabine compared with gemcitabine alone in patients with advanced pancreatic cancer: a phase III trial of the National Cancer Institute of Canada Clinical Trials Group. J Clin Oncol 25(15):1960–1966.
65. Xiong HQ, Rosenberg A, 2004, Cetuximab, a monoclonal antibody targeting the epidermal growth factor receptor, in combination with gemcitabine for advanced pancreatic cancer: a multicenter phase II Trial. J Clin Oncol 22(13):2610–2616.

66. Philip PA, Benedetti J, 2007, Phase III study of gemcitabine [G] plus cetuximab [C] versus gemcitabine in patients [pts] with locally advanced or metastatic pancreatic adenocarcinoma [PC]: SWOG S0205 study. J Clin Oncol 25(18S):LBA4509.
67. Safran H, Iannitti D, 2004, Herceptin and gemcitabine for metastatic pancreatic cancers that overexpress HER-2/neu. Cancer Invest 22(5):706–712.
68. Kindler HL, Friberg G, 2005, Phase II trial of bevacizumab plus gemcitabine in patients with advanced pancreatic cancer. J Clin Oncol 23(31):8033–8040.
69. Kindler HL, Niedzwiecki D, 2007, A double-blind, placebo-controlled, randomized phase III trial of gemcitabine (G) plus bevacizumab (B) versus gemcitabine plus placebo (P) in patients (pts) with advanced pancreatic cancer (PC): a preliminary analysis of Cancer and Leukemia Group B (CALGB). J Clin Oncol 25(18S):4508.
70. Alberts SR, Schroeder M, 2004, Gemcitabine and ISIS-2503 for patients with locally advanced or metastatic pancreatic adenocarcinoma: a North Central Cancer Treatment Group phase II trial. J Clin Oncol 22(24):4944–4950.
71. Alberts SR, Foster NR, 2005, PS-341 and gemcitabine in patients with metastatic pancreatic adenocarcinoma: a North Central Cancer Treatment Group (NCCTG) randomized phase II study. Ann Oncol 16(10):1654–1661.
72. Ferrari V, Valcamonico F, 2006, Gemcitabine plus celecoxib (GECO) in advanced pancreatic cancer: a phase II trial. Cancer Chemother Pharmacol 57(2):185–190.
73. El-Rayes BF, Zalupski MM, 2005, A phase II study of celecoxib, gemcitabine, and cisplatin in advanced pancreatic cancer. Invest New Drugs 23(6):583–590.
74. Ghosn M, Farhat F, 2007, FOLFOX-6 combination as the first-line treatment of locally advanced and/or metastatic pancreatic cancer. Am J Clin Oncol 30(1):15–20.
75. Isacoff WH, Bendetti JK, 2007, Phase II trial of infusional fluorouracil, leucovorin, mitomycin, and dipyridamole in locally advanced unresectable pancreatic adenocarcinoma: SWOG S9700. J Clin Oncol 25(13):1665–1669.
76. Whitehead RP, McCoy S, 2006, A phase II trial of epothilone B analogue BMS-247550 (NSC #710428) ixabepilone, in patients with advanced pancreatic cancer: a Southwest Oncology Group study. Invest New Drugs 24:515–520.
77. Oettle H, Pelzer U, 2005, Oxaliplatin/folinic acid/5-fluorouracil [24h] (OFF) plus best supportive care versus best supportive care alone (BSC) in second-line therapy of gemcitabine-refractory advanced pancreatic cancer (CONKO 003). J Clin Oncol 23(16S):4031.
78. Tsavaris N, Kosmas C, 2005, Second-line treatment with oxaliplatin, leucovorin and 5-fluorouracil in gemcitabine-pretreated advanced pancreatic cancer: a phase II study. Invest New Drugs 23(4):369–375.
79. Androulakis N, Syrigos K, 2005, Oxaliplatin for pretreated patients with advanced or metastatic pancreatic cancer: a multicenter phase II study. Cancer Invest 23(1):9–12.
80. Cantore M., Rabbi C, 2004, Combined irinotecan and oxaliplatin in patients with advanced pre-treated pancreatic cancer. Oncology 67(2):93–97.
81. Demols A, Peeters M, 2006, Gemcitabine and oxaliplatin (GEMOX) in gemcitabine refractory advanced pancreatic adenocarcinoma: a phase II study. Br J Cancer 94(4):481–485.
82. Ulrich-Pur H, Raderer M, 2003, Irinotecan plus raltitrexed versus raltitrexed alone in patients with gemcitabine-pretreated advanced pancreatic adenocarcinoma. Br J Cancer 88(8):1180–1184.
83. Reni M, Pasetto L, 2006, Raltitrexed-eloxatin salvage chemotherapy in gemcitabine-resistant metastatic pancreatic cancer. Br J Cancer 94(6):785–791.

Chapter 31
Adjuvant Chemoradiation for Pancreatic Cancer: Past, Present and Future

Michael C. Garofalo and William F. Regine

1 Introduction

Adjuvant chemoradiation began to be investigated for pancreatic cancer over three decades ago. During the intervening years we have achieved a better understanding of the molecular and genetic basis of pancreatic cancer; however the survival of patients treated with the best modern therapies has changed very little. According to data from the American Cancer Society, the 5-year survival for pancreatic cancer patients remains a dismal 5%, up from a historical 3% three decades ago (*1*). In 2007, an estimated 37,170 newly diagnosed cases of pancreatic cancer in the United States will be nearly equaled by an estimated 33,170 pancreatic cancer deaths (*1*). This underscores the continued need to develop novel multimodality treatment approaches to this disease. Surgery remains the cornerstone to any hope for long-term survival, however only approximately 10–20% of newly diagnosed patients present with non-metastatic and potentially resectable disease (*2*). Pancreatic cancer is considered uniformly fatal in patients unable to undergo a resection. With respect to the minority of patients with resectable disease, cooperative groups both in the United States (US) and Europe have conducted randomized clinical trials in recent decades that have sought to define the potential benefit of adjuvant chemotherapy or adjuvant chemoradiotherapy versus surgery alone for patients with resectable disease. The results of these trials have been conflicting and as a consequence, no current standard exists with respect to adjuvant therapy. Gemcitabine appears to be the most promising agent based on recent phase III trials and may provide a foundation on which to build future trial designs (*3, 4*). Refinements in delivery techniques for continuous-course modern radiation therapy (RT) as well as promising targeted therapies may also improve upon historical outcomes when added to a gemcitabine backbone. The ideal time sequence of combined adjuvant therapies is also an area of active deliberation. Though there is no current standard for adjuvant therapy in pancreatic cancer, continued investigations into combinations of chemotherapy, radiation therapy, and biologic therapy are warranted. This chapter reviews the historical trials that have defined the potential benefits for adjuvant chemoradiation and examine ongoing and future trial concepts for adjuvant chemoradiation.

A.M. Lowy et al. (eds.) *Pancreatic Cancer.*
doi: 10.1007/978-0-387-69252-4, © Springer Science+Business Media, LLC 2008

2 Rationale for Adjuvant Therapy in Pancreatic Cancer

For the select few who present with resectable nonmetastatic disease, surgery is vital toward a curative-intent treatment approach. Unfortunately, even after pathologically complete (R0) resections, most patients eventually fail and ultimately die of disease progression (5, 6). It has been estimated that up to approximately 75% of patients with recurrent disease have a component of local-regional failure following surgery, and that approximately 25% of patients have local only failures. The high rate of both locoregional and distant disease recurrence in pancreatic cancer following surgery provides a strong rationale for developing novel combinations of adjuvant therapies toward improved clinical outcomes for these patients (5, 7–12). The retroperitoneal location of the pancreas and its proximity to major vascular structures make resections with widely negative margins challenging, which often results in close or microscopically positive surgical margins. Residual microscopic locoregional disease can be eradicated by adjuvant chemoradiation. Considering other gastrointestinal malignancies, the locoregional control benefits conveyed by adjuvant chemoradiation have been proven in phase III trials to translate into improved overall survival (13, 14). The historical "split-course" adjuvant chemoradiation trials performed by the Gastrointestinal Tumor Study Group (GITSG) and European Organization for Research and Treatment of Cancer (EORTC) groups suggested a benefit to adjuvant chemoradiation in pancreatic cancer patients whereas the recent ESPAC-1 trial conducted by the European Study Group for Pancreatic Cancer (ESPAC) suggested a detriment to adjuvant radiation therapy (15–21). These important historical trials and the recently reported results of the Radiation Therapy Oncology Group (RTOG) 97-04 trial provide the foundation on which future adjuvant chemoradiation trials will be built (4).

3 Historical "Split-Course" Chemoradiation Trials

Investigations into the potential benefit of adjuvant chemoradiation for patients with resected pancreatic cancers were borne out of the positive results of chemoradiation in patients with locally advanced, inoperable pancreatic cancers (22, 23). The benefits of combining 5-fluorouracil (5-FU) with radiation therapy in the locally advanced population prompted the GITSG to initiate the first prospective phase III randomized trial designed to evaluate the potential benefit of adjuvant chemoradiation in patients with resected disease. Two European phase III trials, the EORTC trial and the ESPAC-1 trial, followed the GITSG trial and the conflicting results of these trials have set the stage for the ongoing controversy surrounding adjuvant therapy in pancreatic cancer. These three trials have in common "split-course" radiation therapy delivery and 5-FU. Modern trial designs have moved away from split-course radiation therapy delivery to continuous-course and have incorporated the more active agent gemcitabine (4).

3.1   GITSG Trial (1974–1982)

The GITSG trial randomized patients with pancreatic adenocarcinoma who were felt to have undergone potentially curative (R0) resections with negative margins to chemoradiation versus observation. Therapy involved a split-course of 40 Gy of external beam radiation therapy (EBRT) delivered over a period of 6 weeks with a 2-week break after the first 20 Gy. EBRT was delivered in daily 2Gy fractions, and chemotherapy consisted of 5-FU (500 mg/m^2 IV bolus) given on days 1–3 of weeks 1 and 5, followed by weekly infusions of maintenance 5-FU for 2 years or until disease progression. Although terminated early due to slow patient accrual and an increasing difference in survival between the arms, analysis of 43 patients enrolled revealed a statistically significant doubling in median survival and modest improvement in 5-year survival for patients receiving adjuvant split-course chemoradiation. Twenty-one patients randomized to adjuvant split-course chemoradiation had a median survival of 21 months, 2-year survival of 43%, and 5-year survival of 19% compared to 11 months, 18%, and 5%, respectively, for the observation group ($p = 0.03$). There were no life-threatening complications or deaths attributable to therapy (15, 16). Only two of the 51 treated patients (4%) in the GITSG study developed possible late treatment-related complications. Criticisms of this trial included poor patient accrual (limited power), lack of RT quality assurance, and the fact that over one third of the patients in the treatment arm did not complete maintenance therapy as intended. In reaction to small patient numbers, the GITSG sought to confirm the results of the randomized trial with an additional cohort of 32 patients that were assigned the identical adjuvant chemoradiotherapy treatment. This non-randomized cohort of patients achieved outcomes similar to those in the randomized trial, with median, 2-year and 5-year survivals of 18 months, 46% and 17%, respectively (17). These additional results further substantiated the benefit seen with adjuvant chemoradiation and led to the adoption of adjuvant chemoradiation as the standard of care in the United States.

3.2   EORTC Trial (1987–1995)

In the second randomized, multicenter trial to evaluate the potential benefit of adjuvant chemoradiation, the EORTC randomized resected patients to chemoradiation or observation. This trial was similar to the GITSG design, save for the following four major differences: (1) nonpancreatic periampullary adenocarcinomas were included in the study, (2) no maintenance chemotherapy was included in the treatment arm, (3) patients with positive surgical margins were allowed in the study without stratification, and (4) chemotherapy consisted of continuous infusion 5-FU (25 mg/kg) instead of bolus 5-FU. Of 207 patients eligible for analysis, 103 were randomized to observation and 104 to a split-course chemoradiotherapy regimen similar to that used in the GITSG study. When compared with patients randomly assigned to observation, the patients assigned to adjuvant chemoradiation had no significant improvement in median survival, 2-year survival, or 5-year survival (*18*). The median overall survival was 24.5 months and the 2-year survival was 51% for the treatment arm, compared with 19 months and 41% for the observation group, respectively ($p = 0.208$). Similar to the GITSG trial, adjuvant treatment was well tolerated with no grade IV or V toxicities and only seven patients developing grade III toxicities.

Criticisms of the EORTC trial included: (1) the inclusion of patients with positive margins without stratification, (2) the lack of RT quality assurance, (3) inclusion of nonpancreatic periampullary cancers that are well known to have a better prognosis, and (4) statistical design. To address the criticism of the inclusion of the periampullary cancers, the authors reported a subanalysis including only the patients with pancreatic head cancers ($n = 114$). The median survival for patients with pancreatic head cancers treated with adjuvant chemoradiotherapy (versus observation) was 17.1 months (versus 12.6 months), 2-year survival rates were 37% (versus 23%), and 5-year survival rates were 20% (versus 10%) in favor of adjuvant chemoradiotherapy. Statistical significance was not reached ($p = 0.099$); however, the power to detect a statistical significance was diluted for this unplanned subanalyses. The authors concluded from these results that the chemoradiation regimen used in the study could not be recommended as standard adjuvant treatment for pancreatic cancer. Statistical reanalysis of the EORTC data using a one-sided log-rank test demonstrates that the 14% survival difference is statistically significant ($p = 0.049$) (*19*). The differences in interpretation of the EORTC trial have contributed to the continuing controversy over the potential benefits of adjuvant chemoradiation.

3.3 ESPAC-1 Trial (1994–2000)

The European Study Group for Pancreatic Cancer (ESPAC) conducted the prospective multicenter ESPAC-1 trial in Europe between 1994 and 2000. This trial included patients with resected adenocarcinomas of the pancreas (irrespective of margin status) and sought to establish the benefit of adjuvant chemotherapy or chemoradiotherapy when compared with observation. The trial design was highly complex and has led to difficulty and controversy in interpreting the study findings. A total of 541 patients were randomized to one of three arms: (1) chemotherapy versus no chemotherapy, (2) chemoradiation versus no chemoradiation, or (3) a 2 × 2 factorial design of observation versus chemotherapy versus chemoradiation with maintenance chemotherapy. An early intent-to-treat analysis of this trial with a median follow-up of 10 months was reported by Neoptolemos et al. and suggested no benefit to chemoradiation (compared with no chemoradiation) and a benefit to chemotherapy (compared with no chemotherapy) with pooled data from all three arms (*20*).

The mature results of ESPAC-1 were reported in 2004, and the analysis was restricted to patients in the third arm of the trial (2 × 2 factorial design) (*21*). In this analysis, patients underwent double randomization according to a 2 × 2 factorial design resulting in a total of four groups assigned to observation, chemotherapy, chemoradiation, or chemoradiation and further chemotherapy. Radiation therapy employed in this trial mirrored the split-course paradigm used in both the GITSG and EORTC trials, in that patients received 10 daily 2 Gy fractions over 2 weeks, followed by another course after a 2-week break. Chemotherapy given as part of concomitant chemoradiotherapy consisted of 5-FU IV bolus doses (500 mg/m^2) given on days 1–3 of each course, identical to the GITSG study. Chemotherapy utilized in the chemotherapy alone arm (or as maintenance after concomitant chemoradiotherapy) was administered using the Mayo Clinic regimen (a 5-day schedule of 5-FU at 425 mg/m^2/day and folinic acid at 20 mg/m^2/day repeated every four weeks) for a total of 6 cycles. After a median follow up of 47 months, the estimated 5-year survival of patients randomized to chemoradiotherapy versus no chemoradiotherapy was 10% versus 20% (p = 0.05). The patients who received chemotherapy had a significantly higher 5-year survival when compared with those who did not receive chemotherapy (21% versus 8%, p = 0.009). Detailed results of this complex trial can be found in Table 31.1 in context with the results of the other phase III cooperative group adjuvant chemoradiation trials.

The authors of this trial concluded that the use of adjuvant chemotherapy resulted in a significant improvement in overall survival and that postoperative chemoradiation worsened survival because it delayed the administration of chemotherapy. The controversial results of this trial resulted in several letters to the editor addressing the problems with the design and conduct of this study (24–27).

Table 31.1 Results of randomized multicenter phase III trials evaluating adjuvant chemoradiotherapy

Study Group	n	Treatment Schema	Overall survival (actuarial) 2y	5y	Median survival
GITSG (16)	21	5-FU + RT	43%	19%	21.0 mo †
	22	(control)	19%	5%	10.9 mo
Klinkenbijl et al (18)	60	5-FU + RT	37%	20%	17.1 mo §
(EORTC)	54	(control)	23%	10%	12.6 mo
Neoptolemos et al (21)	145	CRT	29%	10%	15.8 mo
(ESPAC–1)	144	no CRT	41%	20%	17.8 mo †
	147	C	40%	21%	20.1 mo †
	142	no C	30%	8%	15.5 mo
Regine et al (4)	187	5-FU + CRT + 5-FU	NR	22% (3yOS)	16.9 mo
RTOG 97–04	201	G + CRT + G	NR	31% (3yOS)	20.5 mo †,*

5-FU = 5-fluorouracil
C = chemotherapy (5-FU)
CRT = chemoradiotherapy (5-FU + RT)
G = gemcitabine
mo = month
NR = not reported
RT = radiation therapy
† = statistically significant
§ = statistically significant on reanalysis
* = pancreatic head cancers only

Table 31.2 Results of randomized multicenter phase III trials in the gemcitabine era

Study Group	n	Treatment Schema	Overall survival (actuarial)		Median survival
			3y	5y	
Regine et al (4)	187	5-FU + CRT + 5-FU	22%	NR	16.9 mo
RTOG 97–04	201	G + CRT + G	31%	NR	20.5 mo †,*
Oettle et al (3)	177	(control)	21%	12%	20.2 mo
(CONKO-001)	179	GEM	34%	23%	20.6 mo †,*

5-FU = 5-fluorouracil
CRT = chemoradiotherapy (5-FU + RT)
G = gemcitabine
mo = month
NR = not reported
† = statistically significant
* = pancreatic head cancers only
§ = trend toward improved overall survival, p=0.06

Examples of such criticism include lack of centralized quality assurance of radiation therapy dose and fields. Per protocol, patients were intended to receive a total of 40 Gy. However, only 75% of patients received this dose. Some patients received less than this target dose, whereas others received up to 60 Gy. In addition, the 2×2 factorial design allowed for "background therapy" (chemoradiotherapy or chemotherapy), which can directly influence compliance with future randomized treatments and thus potentially influence results. Irrespective of the criticisms of this trial, it should be noted that the controversial results of ESPAC-1 stand alone with respect to the conclusion that adjuvant chemoradiation worsens survival. Both the GITSG and EORTC trials suggested benefits, not detriments. The reasons for the inferior radiation results in ESPAC-1 are unclear, and the fact that the median overall survival (15.5 months) for patients receiving surgery alone were much better than that seen in the GITSG (10.9 months) or EORTC (12.6 months) trials is also unexplained. Thus, the unique results of ESPAC-1 need further validation before any conclusions can be drawn regarding the role of chemotherapy or chemoradiation in the adjuvant setting.

Nevertheless, the authors concluded from this trial that adjuvant chemotherapy (without radiation) should be considered standard adjuvant therapy. Consequently, the design of the subsequent ESPAC-2 and ESPAC-3 studies has focused on adjuvant chemotherapy only paradigms. The currently accruing ESPAC-3(v2) trial is a large three-arm phase III study comparing the chemotherapy regimen used in ESPAC-1 (bolus 5-FU and folinic acid) versus gemcitabine versus observation following resection (28). The results of this study will be important for two principal reasons: (1) it will help to validate the results of CONKO-001 (discussed later in this chapter) demonstrating an advantage to adjuvant gemcitabine versus observation, and (2) it will establish the potential benefit of adjuvant gemcitabine versus the historically utilized 5-FU.

4   Modern "Continuous-Course" Chemoradiation Trials

Modern adjuvant chemoradiation trials incorporate continuous-course daily fractionated radiation therapy to higher doses and the most active chemotherapeutic
agent in pancreatic cancer, gemcitabine. Single-agent gemcitabine has been
established as the standard treatment for advanced pancreatic cancer based on a
randomized study demonstrating a very modest survival advantage over 5-FU
(29). Therefore, the RTOG sought to evaluate the potential benefit of adding
gemcitabine to adjuvant 5-FU based chemoradiotherapy. RTOG 97-04 is the first
and only phase III adjuvant trial to evaluate gemcitabine-based chemoradiation
and also the first to incorporate modern, continuous-course radiation therapy
delivery. The results demonstrate an advantage to gemcitabine-based adjuvant chemoradiation and will serve as a framework for future trial design within the US
cooperative group.

4.1   RTOG 97-04 (1998–2002)

RTOG 97-04 represents the most recent randomized cooperative group trial evaluating adjuvant chemoradiotherapy, the final results of which were recently reported
in JAMA (4). This intergroup trial was conducted by several US cooperative groups,
including the Radiation Therapy Oncology Group (RTOG), the Eastern Cooperative
Oncology Group (ECOG), and the Southwest Oncology Group (SWOG). Considering
the criticisms that weaken the conflicting results of the "historical" phase III trials,
the RTOG mandated that all radiation treatment fields and diagnostic studies (imaging films, reports, and operative notes) be centrally reviewed and approved prior to
the start of therapy. All patients enrolled in the study had histologically proven adenocarcinoma of the pancreas. Patients of pathologic stages T1-4, N0-1, M0 were eligible
for randomization following a gross total resection and were stratified according to
surgical margins (positive versus negative versus unknown), tumor diameter (<3 cm
versus ≥3 cm) and nodal status (involved versus uninvolved). Protocol therapy was
required to begin 3–8 weeks after surgical resection.

Patients were randomized to one of two "sandwich" treatment arms: (1) 5-FU,
followed by 5-FU based chemoradiotherapy, followed by further 5-FU, or (2)
gemcitabine, followed by 5-FU based chemoradiotherapy, followed by further
gemcitabine. The chemoradiotherapy component of the treatment was the same in
both arms and consisted of continuous-course fractionated radiation therapy to a
total dose of 50.4 Gy (in 1.8 Gy daily fractions) combined with concomitant 5-FU
(250 mg/m^2/day) delivered by continuous infusion throughout the 5½ weeks of RT.
RT fields included the tumor bed (as defined by preoperative CT imaging) and
regional lymph nodes (pancreatic, celiac, mesenteric, para-aortic, duodenal, and
hepatic portal). At least 4-MV photons and a minimum three- to four-field approach
was utilized. Following an initial dose of 45 Gy, a final 5.4 Gy was delivered to a
"boost" field of the tumor bed as defined by the preoperative tumor volume. The

chemotherapy (3 weeks up front and 3 months out back) consisted of either: (1) gemcitabine (1,000 mg/m^2), or (2) 5-FU (250 mg/m^2/day).

Of 538 enrolled patients, 451 were found to be eligible for analysis. Failure to send serum for CA-19-9 analysis was the most common reason for patient ineligibility. Of the 451 patients analyzed, 230 were randomly assigned to the 5-FU based regimen and 221 were assigned to the gemcitabine. Demographics were similar between the two patient groups, save for T stage. Patients randomized to the gemcitabine-based arm had a higher percentage of patients with T3/4 disease than patients in the 5-FU based arm (81 versus 70%, $p = 0.013$). The majority (86%) of tumors were of the pancreatic head. Over half of the patients had microscopically positive or unknown surgical margins. Based on an analysis of 388 eligible patients with pancreatic head tumors, a statistically significant overall survival advantage was seen for patients treated with gemcitabine-based therapy. The median survival and 3-year overall survival for patients treated with gemcitabine-based chemoradiotherapy was 20.5 months and 31% versus 16.9 months and 22% for the 5-FU based arm Gemcitabine-based treatment was found to be statistically improved over 5-FU-based treatment for patients with pancreatic head tumors after adjusting for protocol-specified stratification variables on multivariate analysis (HR of 0.80; 95% CI, 0.63–1.00; p=0.05). Overall survival of patients with pancreatic head tumors was a primary endpoint of this study, not an unplanned subanalysis. No significant difference in survival was found when patients with body/tail tumors were included in the analysis.

With prospective RT quality assurance on RTOG 97-04, only 5% of patients treated on protocol were found to have an unacceptable protocol variance. Abrams et al. have reported the impact of RT quality assurance and compliance on survival in RTOG 97-04 in abstract form at the annual meeting of the American Society for Therapeutic Radiology and Oncology in 2006 (30). While grade III/IV hematologic toxicity was greater in the gemcitabine-based arm (58%) compared with the 5-FU arm (9%), there were no differences in febrile neutropenia or infection between the two groups, and approximately 90% of patients were able to complete therapy as per study design. Based on these results, the authors concluded that gemcitabine was superior to 5-FU when added to chemoradiation, and that future adjuvant chemoradiotherapy trials should build upon a gemcitabine-based chemoradiotherapy backbone.

4.2   The Gemcitabine Era (RTOG 97-04 and CONKO-001)

The preliminary results of RTOG 97-04 were made available shortly before the mature results of the Charité Onkologie (CONKO)-001 trial were reported. These two trials are the only reported phase III multicenter trials evaluating the potential benefit of gemcitabine in the adjuvant setting of pancreatic cancer. The CONKO-001 trial was not a trial testing adjuvant chemoradiotherapy, but rather a phase III multicenter trial that randomized patients with resected pancreatic cancers to either observation or adjuvant gemcitabine. Radiation therapy was excluded from the design in keeping with the conclusions from the prior phase III European studies in the adjuvant setting. Unlike ESPAC-1, the experimental design of CONKO-001 was simple and patients with a history of prior chemotherapy or radiotherapy were excluded from the study. Patients were required to have a gross total resection (R0 or R1) and were stratified for resection, nodal involvement and T stage. The primary endpoint of CONKO-001 was disease free survival (DFS) and was powered to demonstrate an improvement in median DFS of at least 6 months. The treatment arm included a total of six cycles of gemcitabine on days 1, 8, and 15 of a 4-week cycle. Based on an analysis of 354 eligible patients (179 in the gemcitabine arm and 175 in the observation arm), with a median follow-up of 53 months, the investigators found a significant increase in median disease free survival for patients assigned to the gemcitabine arm (13.4 months versus 6.9 months, $p < 0.001$) (3). There was a trend toward improved median overall survival for patients treated with gemcitabine versus those in the observation arm (22.1 months versus 20.2 months, $p = 0.061$).

The RTOG 97-04 and CONKO-001 trials represent the modern phase III evaluation of gemcitabine-based treatment in the adjuvant setting. Unfortunately, the results of RTOG 97-04 cannot be directly compared with the CONKO-001 results because of fundamental differences in treatment design and patient characteristics. CONKO-001 had more favorable patients than RTOG 97-04, with 83% of patients undergoing R0 resections (versus 40%) and all patients having a postoperative CA19-9 ≤90 (versus no upper limit). Pertinent to the differences in patient selection for these two trials, Berger et al. have reported an analysis of the prognostic significance of postoperative CA19-9 level as a predictor for overall survival following chemoradiation (31). For purposes of comparison with the CONKO-001 trial outcome, further analysis of the subset of patients enrolled on RTOG 9704 with postoperative CA19-9 levels ≤90 (identical to all CONKO-001 patients enrolled) versus those with postoperative CA19-9 levels >90 demonstrated a significant difference in survival following gemcitabine-based chemoradiation favoring those with lower postoperative CA19-9 levels (22.8 months versus 9.6 months median survival, $p < 0.0001$). The median and 3-year overall survival for patients with pancreatic head tumors treated with gemcitabine based chemoradiation with good quality assurance for RT treatment delivery and a postoperative CA 19-9 of ≤90 was 25.2 months and 46%, respectively (32). Although it is hazardous to compare outcomes across two separate randomized trials, this is the best that we can do at this time in terms of trying to define the benefit of chemoradiation versus chemotherapy alone as adjuvant treatment for pancreatic cancer in the gemcitabine era. If delivered with good quality assurance, radiation therapy combined with gemcitabine appears to enhance the median survival for patients with adenocarcinomas of the pancreatic head when compared with gemcitabine alone. Given that several analyses have demonstrated the strong prognostic value of factors such as postoperative CA19-9, surgical margin status, and quality assurance of radiation delivery— the only way to truly answer the question of whether chemoradiation is better than chemotherapy alone as adjuvant therapy is to design a randomized trial that incorporates these prognostic factors and good quality assurance into the design so that treatment groups are fairly balanced.

At present, what we can conclude is that the CONKO-001 trial suggested a 2-month trend toward improved overall survival with gemcitabine alone, and the results of RTOG 97-04 demonstrate a 4-month trend toward improved overall survival when gemcitabine was added to radiation therapy in patients with pancreatic head cancers. Taking together the strong trends in the above two trials favoring gemcitabine and the known benefits of gemcitabine over 5-FU or observation in the metastatic disease setting, future investigations should focus on building trials around a gemcitabine backbone.

5   Current and Future Adjuvant Chemoradiation Trials

Current and future adjuvant chemoradiotherapy trials will thematically help to refine the following: (1) the ideal timing of radiation therapy when combined with gemcitabine, (2) delivery of radiation therapy with better precision and consequent reductions in toxicity, (3) the potential benefits of adding active biologic agents to a gemcitabine/RT backbone, (4) prognostic factors that help to define which subgroups of patients are most likely to benefit from adjuvant chemoradiation, and (5) establish whether adjuvant chemoradiation improves upon adjuvant chemotherapy alone in a balanced patient population. Considering improving upon radiation therapy delivery, intraoperative radiation therapy (IORT) has been utilized at specialized centers since its inception in 1983 at the National Cancer Institute (33). Investigations into the potential survival benefit of IORT have been inconclusive given that the number of patients in these reports is limited and not well balanced with respect to eligibility criteria, radiation dose, or the use of other adjuvant therapy (34–39). Given that the majority of these studies are institutional and retrospective in nature and the fact that IORT continues to be available only at a select few centers, it is impractical to incorporate IORT as part of a national cooperative group trial. A more widely available modern radiation therapy delivery technique known as intensity modulated radiation therapy (IMRT) can reduce the radiation dose to nearby normal tissues and thus result in potential reductions in toxicity during chemoradiation and/or allow for safer dose escalation of radiation therapy. Several studies have suggested that inverse planned IMRT can reduce the side effects associated with chemoradiotherapy; therefore, it is likely to be investigated in future trials as a potential improvement in radiation therapy treatment technique (40–42).

To address the question of whether chemoradiation is more effective than chemotherapy in the gemcitabine era, the EORTC recently conducting a European phase II/III trial comparing adjuvant gemcitabine-based chemoradiation versus gemcitabine alone in patients with resected pancreatic cancer. Patients received either two cycles of gemcitabine and then gemcitabine-based chemoradiation or four cycles of gemcitabine alone (43). This study has recently closed to accrual and the results are anticipated with great interest. At present the RTOG is considering design concepts for the follow-up American trial to 97-04. This trial has yet to be finalized but is likely to take the form of several cycles of gemcitabine and a targeted biologic agent followed by randomization of patients who have not developed distant metastatic disease to further chemotherapy and a targeted biologic versus chemoradiation followed by further chemotherapy and a targeted biologic. Conceptually, this trial would: (1) allow for self-selection of patients destined to develop distant metastases early (i.e., during their initial chemotherapy prior to randomization) who are unlikely to benefit from chemoradiation, (2) investigate the added benefit of a biologic such as erlotinib to gemcitabine in the adjuvant setting, and (3) incorporate inverse-planned intensity modulated radiation therapy in the patients randomized to chemoradiation, which will result in reduced potential for radiation-related toxicity. Stratification by prognostic factors and good prospective radiation therapy quality assurance will continue to be essential to effective trial design. At present, there is no definite standard with respect to adjuvant therapy in pancreatic cancer. Given the relatively poor outcomes of patients, a clinical trial should be considered the preferred treatment. The optimal combination and sequence of adjuvant therapies has yet to be established and continues to be the subject of ongoing and future clinical trials.

References

1. Jemal A, Siegel R, Ward E, et al. 2007 Cancer statistics, CA Cancer J Clin 2007. 57, 43–66,2007.
2. Warshaw AL, Fernandex del-Castillo C, 1992, Pancreatic adenocarcinoma. N Engl J Med 326(7):455–465.
3. Oettle H, Post S, Neuhaus P, 2007, Adjuvant chemotherapy with gemcitabine versus observation in patients undergoing curative-intent resection of pancreatic cancer. JAMA 297:267–277.
4. Regine WF, Winter KA, Abrams RA, 2008, Fluorouracil vs gemcitabine chemotherapy before and after fluorouracil-based chemoradiation following resection of pancreatic adenocarcinoma: a randomized controlled trial. JAMA 299(9):1019–1026.
5. Griffin JF, Smalley SR, Jewell W, 1990, Patterns of failure after curative resection of pancreatic carcinoma. Cancer 66:56–61.
6. Foo ML, Gunderson LL, Nagorney DM, 1993, Patterns of failure in grossly resected pancreatic ductal adenocarcinoma treated with adjuvant irradiation ± 5 fluorouracil. Int J Radiat Oncol Biol Phys 26:483–489.
7. Tepper J, Nardi G, Suit H. 1973, Carcinoma of the pancreas: review of MGH experience from 1963 to 1973. Analysis of surgical failure and implications for radiation therapy. Cancer 37(3):1519–1524.
8. Whittington R, Bryer MP, Haller DG, 1991, Adjuvant therapy of resected adenocarcinoma of the pancreas. Int J Radiat Oncol Biol Phys 21(5):1137–1143.
9. Hishinuma S, Ogata Y, Tomikawa M, 2006, Patterns of recurrence after curative resection of pancreatic cancer, based on autopsy findings. J Gastrointest Surg 10(4):511–518.
10. Sperti C, Pasquali C, Piccoli A, 1997, Recurrence after resection for ductal adenocarcinoma of the pancreas. World J Surg 21(2):195–200.
11. Kayahara M, Nagakawa T, Ueno K, 1993, An evaluation of radical resection for pancreatic cancer based on the mode of recurrence as determined by autopsy and diagnostic imaging. Cancer 72(7):2118–2123.
12. Griffin JF, Smalley SR, Jewell W, 1990, Patterns of failure after curative resection of pancreatic carcinoma. Cancer 66(1):56–61.
13. Macdonald JS, Smalley SR, Benedetti J, 2001, Chemoradiotherapy after surgery compared with surgery alone for adenocarcinoma of the stomach or gastroesophageal junction. N Engl J Med 345:725–230.

14. Krook JE, Moertel CG, Gunderson LL, 1991, Effective surgical adjuvant therapy for high-risk rectal carcinoma. N Engl J Med 324:709–715.
15. Kalser MH, Ellenberg SS. 1985, Pancreatic cancer. Adjuvant combined radiation and chemotherapy following curative resection. Arch Surg 120:899–903.
16. Douglass HO, Strablein DM. 1990, Ten year follow-up of first generation surgical adjuvant studies of the Gastrointestinal Tumor Study Group. In: Salmon SE (ed.) Adjuvant therapy of cancer, vol 4. WB Saunders, Philadelphia, 405–415.
17. Gastrointestinal Tumor Study Group. Further evidence of effective adjuvant combined radiation and chemotherapy following curative resection of pancreatic cancer. Cancer 1987, 59:2006–2010.
18. Klinkenbijl JH, Jeekel J, Sahmoud T, 1999, Adjuvant radiotherapy and 5-fluorouracil after curative resection of cancer of the pancreas and periampullary region: a phase III trial of the EORTC gastrointestinal tract cancer cooperative group. Ann Surg 230(6):776–782.
19. Garofalo MC, Regine WR, Tan MT. 2006, On statistical reanalysis, the EORTC trial is a positive trial for adjuvant chemoradiation in pancreatic cancer. Ann Surg 244(2):332–333.
20. Neoptolemos JP, Dunn JA, Stocken DD, 2001, Adjuvant chemoradiotherapy and chemotherapy in respectable pancreatic cancer: a randomized controlled trial. Lancet 358:1576–1585.
21. Neoptolemos JP, Stocken DD, Friess F, 2004, A randomized trial of chemoradiotherapy and chemotherapy after resection of pancreatic cancer. N Engl J Med 350(12):1200–1210.
22. Moertel CG, Childs DS JrReitemeier RJ, 1969, Combined 5-fluorouracil and supervoltage radiation therapy of locally unresectable gastrointestinal cancer. Lancet 2:865–867.
23. Hasalam JB, Cavenaugh PJ, Stroup SL. 1973, Radiation therapy in the treatment of irresectable adenocarcinoma of the pancreas. Cancer 32:1341–1345.
24. Choti MA. 2004, Adjuvant therapy for pancreatic cancer—the debate continues. N Engl J Med 350(12):1249–1251.
25. Morris SL, Beasley M, Leslie M. 2004, Chemotherapy for pancreatic cancer. N Engl J Med 350(26):2713 [letter to the editor].
26. Crane CH, Ben-Josef E, Small W. 2004, Chemotherapy for pancreatic cancer. N Engl J Med 350(26):2713–2714 [letter to the editor].
27. Bydder S, Spry N. 2004, Chemotherapy for pancreatic cancer. N Engl J Med 350(26):2714 [letter to the editor].
28. ESPAC-3(v2): Phase III adjuvant trial in pancreatic cancer comparing 5FU and D-L-folinic acid versus gemcitabine. (Accessed 11/15/07 at http://pfsearch.ukcrn.org.uk/StudyDetail. aspx?TopicID=&StudyID=669).
29. Burris HA 3rdMoore MJ, Andersen J, 1997, Improvements in survival and clinical benefit with gemcitabine as first-line therapy for patients with advanced pancreas cancer: a randomized trial. J Clin Oncol 15(6):2403–2413.
30. Abrams RA, Winter KA, Regine WF, 2006, Radiotherapy quality assurance review and survival. Proceedings of ASTRO, Int J Radiat Oncol Biol Phys 66(3):S22.
31. Berger AC, Winter K, Hoffman J, et al. Post-resection CA 19-9 predicts overall survival (OS) in patients treated with adjuvant chemoradiation: A secondary endpoint of RTOG 9704. J Clin Oncol 2007, 25(18S):Abstract 4522.
32. Regine WF, Garcia M, Berger AC, 2007, Post-resectional CA 19-9 values <90 are associated with significantly worse survival in patients with pancreatic carcinoma treated with adjuvant therapy on RTOG 9704—implications for current and future trials. Int J Radiat Oncol Biol Phys 69(3):S78; Abstract 137.
33. Sindelar WF, Kinsella T, Tepper J, 1983, Experimental and clinical studies with intraoperative radiotherapy. Surg Gynecol Obstet 157:205–219.
34. Zerbi A, Fossati V, Parolini D, 1994, Intraoperative radiation therapy adjuvant to resection in the treatment of pancreatic cancer. Cancer 73:2930–2935.
35. Kokubo M, Nishimura Y, Shibamoto Y, 2000, Analysis of the clinical benefit of intraoperative radiotherapy in patients undergoing macroscopically curative resection for pancreatic cancer. Int J Radiat Oncol Biol Phys 48:1081–1087.

36. Sunamura M, Kobari M, Lozonschi L, 1998, Intraoperative radiotherapy for pancreatic adenocarcinoma. J Hepatobiliary Pancreat Surg 5:151–156.
37. Coquard R, Ayzac L, Gilly FN, 1997, Intraoperative radiotherapy in resected pancreatic cancer: feasibility and results. Radiother Oncol 44(3):271–275.
38. Farrell TJ, Barbot DJ, Rosato FE. 1997, Pancreatic resection combined with intraoperative radiation therapy for pancreatic cancer. Ann Surg 226(1):66–69.
39. Reni M, Panucci MG, Ferreri AJ, 2001, Effect on local control and survival of electron beam intraoperative irradiation for resectable pancreatic adenocarcinoma. Int J Radiat Oncol Biol Phys 50:651–658.
40. Landry JC, Yang GY, Ting JY, 2002, Treatment of pancreatic cancer tumors with intensity-modulated radiation therapy (IMRT) using the volume at risk approach (VARA): employing dose-volume histogram (DVH) and normal tissue complication probability (NTCP) to evaluate small bowel toxicity. Med Dosim 27(2):121–129.
41. Bai YR, Wu GH, Guo WJ, 2003, Intensity modulated radiation therapy and chemotherapy for locally advanced pancreatic cancer: results of feasibility study. World J Gastroenterol 9(11):2561–2564.
42. Milano MT, Chmura SJ, Garofalo MC, 2004, Intensity modulated radiation therapy (IMRT) in the treatment of pancreatic and bile duct malignancies: toxicity and outcome. Int J Radiat Oncol Biol Phys 59(2):445–453.
43. EORTC-40013 (NCT00064207). Phase II/III randomized study of gemcitabine followed by chemoradiotherapy with gemcitabine versus gemcitabine alone after prior curative resection in patients with pancreatic head adenocarcinoma. (Accessed 11/15/07 at http://www.cancer.gov/clinicaltrials/EORTC-40013).

Chapter 32
Neoadjuvant Treatment for Resectable and Locally Advanced Pancreatic Cancer

Rebecca P. Petersen, Johanna C. Bendell, Brian G. Czito, and Douglas S. Tyler

1 Rationale for Neoadjuvant Therapy in Resectable Disease

Pancreatic carcinoma is the fourth leading cause of cancer death in the United States, resulting in over 30,000 deaths per year. The overall prognosis is poor, with a 5-year survival rate of 4% for all stages (*1*). Although it is debatable if this disease can be cured through surgical resection, only a minority of patients (15–20%) present with potentially resectable disease that warrants an attempt at surgery. Even with advances in operative techniques and perioperative care, prognosis remains suboptimal for patients undergoing complete resection, as the 5-year survival is <20% (*2*). Efforts to improve on outcomes with radical surgery have focused on combined strategies of adjuvant and neoadjuvant chemotherapy alone or in conjunction with radiation therapy.

In an attempt to improve upon the efficacy of adjuvant chemoradiation therapy, interest in neoadjuvant treatment approaches has increased. Approximately one third of patients who undergo resection do not receive planned postoperative therapy due to complications of surgery or delayed recovery (*3, 4*). In contrast, all patients who are resected following neoadjuvant therapy have received the potential benefit of multimodality therapy and there appears to be a significantly lower rate of major complications post-pancreaticoduodenectomy, such as pancreatic leaks (*5*). Other theoretical advantages include improved delivery of chemotherapy and radiosensitizing oxygen to tissues whose blood supply has not been disrupted by surgery, as well as the avoidance of irradiation to fixed loops of bowel postoperatively.

Neoadjuvant therapy may also potentially downsize or improve resectability of tumors, such as those with celiac or superior mesenteric artery involvement; however, current evidence suggests low conversion resectability rates following "neoadjuvant" therapy for patients with locally advanced disease. In a study from New England Deaconess Hospital, 16 patients with locally advanced unresectable pancreatic cancer were treated neoadjuvantly with 5-FU chemotherapy and 45 Gy of EBRT and infusional 5-FU. Of these 16 patients, only two (13%) were able to undergo resection (*6*). Similarly, investigators from Duke University reported that only two (8%) of 25 patients with locally advanced pancreatic cancer treated with

A.M. Lowy et al. (eds.) *Pancreatic Cancer*.
doi: 10.1007/978-0-387-69252-4, © Springer Science+Business Media, LLC 2008

45 Gy of EBRT and 5-FU (with or without cisplatin or mitomycin C) subsequently underwent complete resection with negative margins (*7*). A prospective study of 87 patients with locally advanced pancreatic cancer from Memorial Sloan-Kettering Cancer Center treated with combined modality therapy found that only three patients achieved a complete response. These patients were taken for resection, two were found to still have locally advanced disease, and one was resected with negative margins only to recur and die 18 months later (*8*). In addition, an estimated 20% of patients have occult metastatic disease at time of initial diagnosis that will become apparent during administration of the neoadjuvant regimen. Recognition of these patients leads to improved selection of patients for surgery, as patients with occult but aggressive tumor biology are spared the potential morbidity, potential mortality, and costs associated with surgery (*9, 10*).

Although there are clear theoretical benefits to the neoadjuvant treatment approach to pancreatic cancer, it is important to recognize that not all patients are appropriate candidates. Exclusion criteria include severe comorbid conditions, lack of a tissue diagnosis, or requirement of immediate surgical management of biliary obstruction. As a consequence, neoadjuvant chemotherapy should be considered as one of several approaches to treating pancreatic cancer. This chapter reviews screening and appropriate selection of patients for neoadjuvant therapy and describes the various combinations of treatment strategies and the evidence supporting their use.

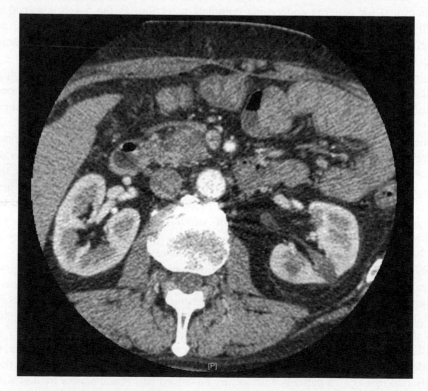

Fig. 32.1 Resectable pancreatic cancer

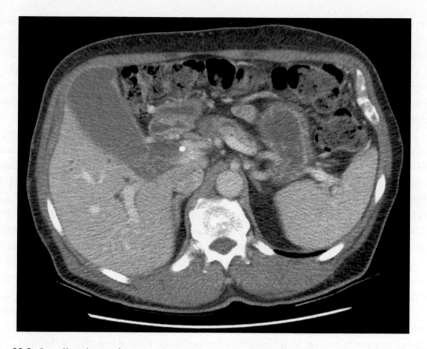

Fig. 32.2 Locally advanced pancreatic cancer involving the celiac artery

1.1 Diagnostic Algorithm to Assess Eligibility for Neoadjuvant Therapy

All patients suspected of having pancreatic carcinoma should undergo standard pre-treatment evaluation that includes thorough physical examination, thin-section, contrast-enhanced, multiphase spiral computed tomography (CT) of the abdomen, and chest radiography. Eligibility for a neoadjuvant approach to treatment requires that the tumor is nonmetastatic on initial radiographic imaging studies. Although the definition of resectable pancreatic cancer varies among operators, standard nomenclature exists to characterize the extent of the tumor among potentially eligible patients. (see Figure 32.1) Locally advanced disease is typically defined by arterial abutment/encasement or venous occlusion on radiographic imaging studies (see Figure 32.2). Patients with enlarged lymph nodes are also frequently included in the locally advanced group. Potentially resectable disease is defined as having no arterial or significant venous involvement. Patients having venous involvement but no evidence of venous occlusion are also generally considered potentially resectable.

Following radiographic characterization of the tumor, the next step in determining whether a patient is eligible for neoadjuvant therapy is the need to establish a tissue diagnosis of malignancy, which is necessary for any patient to be treated with chemotherapy and/or radiation therapy. In patients presenting with painless, obstructive jaundice, frequently the initial approach to diagnosis is endoscopic retrograde cholangiopancreatography (ERCP) during which time common bile duct brushings can be obtained and a biliary stent placed to relieve symptomatic pruritus. Unfortunately, endoscopic brushings only result in a conclusive diagnosis in 20% of pancreatic cancer patients; thus, ERCP is not routinely performed at our initial diagnostic procedure for patients not requiring biliary decompression. However, obstructed patients who undergo neoadjuvant therapy require biliary decompression by ERCP stent placement prior to initiation of treatment.

For patients without a clinical indication for ERCP or with negative endoscopic brushings, the tissue diagnosis is typically established by endoscopic ultrasound (EUS)-guided fine-needle aspirate (FNA) or by CT or ultrasound imaging–guided FNA. In a randomized controlled trial comparing EUS-guided FNA with CT or ultrasound guided FNA (11), the sensitivity of detecting pancreatic malignancy was not statistically significant, based upon a relatively small sample size. If the initial FNA is nondiagnostic then a repeat procedure is recommended, and it is not unreasonable to use an alternative imaging modality to perform the FNA. If a tissue diagnosis is unable to be obtained after two attempts, then consideration should be given to surgical exploration. Interestingly, there has been concern of increased risk of developing peritoneal carcinomatosis in patients undergoing biopsy via a percutaneous approach, potentially related to tumoral seeding (12). However, as the procedures for diagnosis depend on experience, use of a specific approach may vary among centers based on availability and experience with a specific technique.

2 Neoadjuvant Chemoradiation Regimens and Supporting Evidence

Principles for the combined use of chemotherapy and radiation therapy in neoadjuvant regimens are based on studies of both adjuvant therapies for pancreatic cancer and therapies for locally advanced pancreatic cancer. Although a randomized controlled trial conducted in United States has demonstrated increased survival from the use of adjuvant chemoradiation therapy, European studies have found that chemotherapy was effective, but radiation was found to be ineffective and possibly harmful (3, 4, 14–17). All of these studies have been criticized in their design and methods, although a discussion of this is beyond the scope of this chapter. The treatment of locally advanced pancreatic cancer is also somewhat controversial, with some randomized trials suggesting benefit of chemoradiation in this setting and one showing no benefit (14–17). As most neoadjuvant studies have been conducted in the United States, the majority of these have incorporated radiation therapy in the neoadjuvant therapy regimen (Tables 32.1 and 32.2). Among the varying regimens, the dose of radiation has ranged between 30 and 60 Gy based on practice patterns at individual institutions. Several chemotherapeutic agents have been evaluated in neoadjuvant regimens both as monotherapies and in combination. Specific agents include 5-fluorouracil (5-FU), doxorubicin, streptozocin, mitomycin C, cisplatin, gemcitabine, paclitaxel, capecitabine, and docetaxel. Studies have typically identified populations based on the radiographic

Table 32.1 Selected studies of neoadjuvant therapy for locally advanced pancreatic cancer

Study	Design	Total n	Neoadjuvant therapy	Resected n	Median survival (months)
GITSG 1981 (14)	Randomized multicenter	169 (arm 1) 25 (arm 2)	RT (40–60 Gy) 5-FU RT alone (60 Gy)	NA	10[c] 5.3[c]
GITSG 1985 (15)	Randomized multicenter	73 (arm 1) 70 (arm 2)	RT (60 Gy) 5-FU RT (40 Gy) Doxorubicin	NA	8.5[c] 7.6[c]
ECOG 1985 (17)	Randomized multicenter	47 (arm 1) 44 (arm 2)	RT 5-FU 5-FU	NA	8.3[c]
GITSG 1988 (16)	Randomized multicenter	22 (arm1) 21 (arm 2)	RT(54 GY)/5- FU→ SMF SMF alone	NA	9.7[c] 7.4[c]
Jessup et al. 1993 (18)	Single center prospective	16	RT (45 Gy) 5-FU	NR	9.6[a]
Kamthan et al. 1997 (19)	Single center prospective	35	RT (54 Gy) 5-FU Cisplatin Streptozocin	5	15[a] 31[b] 11[c]
Wanebo et al. 2000 (20)	Single center prospective	14	RT (45 Gy) 5-FU Cisplatin	9	9[a] 19[b]
Snady et al. 2000 (21)	Single center prospective	68	RT (54 Gy) 5-FU Streptozocin Cisplatin	20	23.6[a] 32.3[b] 21.2[c]
Ammori et al. 2003 (22)	Single center prospective	67	RT (50 Gy) Gemcitabine ± Cisplatin	9	11.9[a] 17.6[b]
Aristu et al. 2003 (23)	Single center prospective	47	RT (45 Gy) 5FU Cisplatin ± Paclitaxel or Gemcitabine or Docetaxel	9	11[a] 23[b] 10[c]
White et al. 2004 (24)	Single center prospective	88	RT (45 Gy) 5-FU Cisplatin Mitomycin C	18	23 [b]
Joensuu et al. 2004 (25)	Single center prospective	28	RT (50 Gy) Gemcitabine	20	25[a] 25[b] 14[c]
Pipas et al. 2005 (26)	Single center prospective	24	RT (50.4 Gy) Gemcitabine Docetaxel	13	14[a]

[a] All patients, resectable and unresectable.
[b] Resectable patients.
[c] Unresectable patients.
5-FU, Fluorouracil; NA, surgery not attempted; NR, not reported; RT, radiation therapy; SMF, streptozocin, mitomycin C, fluorouracil.

Table 32.2 Selected studies of neoadjuvant therapy for potentially resectable pancreatic cancer

Study	Design	Total n	Neoadjuvant therapy	RR	Resected n	Median survival (months)
Yueng et al. 1993 (28)	Single center prospective	26	RT (50.4 Gy) 5-FU Mito-mycin C	23%	12	12[b]
Staley et al. 1996 (32)	Single center prospective	39	RT (30, 50.4 Gy) 5-FU IORT	NR	33	19[b]
Spitz et al. 1997 (27)	Single center prospective	91	RT (30, 50.4 Gy) 5-FU	NR	41	19.2[b] 7.2[c]
Hoffman et al. 1998 (29)	Multicenter prospective	53	RT (50.4 Gy) 5-FU Mito-mycin C	15%	24	9.7[a] 15.7[b]
Pisters et al. 1998 (33)	Single center prospective	35	RT (30 Gy) 5-FU IORT	66%	20	25[b]
Pisters et al. 2002 (34)	Single center prospective	37	RT (30 Gy) Paclitaxel IORT	11%	20	12[a] 19[b] 10[c]
Wolff et al. 2002 (35)	Single center prospective	86	RT (30 Gy) Gemcitabine	58%	63	36[b]
White et al. 2004 (24)	Single center prospective	96	RT (45 Gy) 5-FU Cisplatin Mitomycin C	NR	53	23 [b]
Moutardier et al. 2004 (30)	Single center prospective	61	RT (30 Gy) 5-FU Cisplatin RT	NR	40	13[a] 26.6[b] 8.6[c]
Meszoely et al. 2004 (36)	Single center prospective	63	Gemcitabine	NR	41	20[b] 9[c]
Mornex et al. 2005 (31)	Single center prospective	41	RT (50 Gy) 5-FU Cisplatin	10%	26	11.5[a] 12.5[b] 8.1[c]
Talamonti et al. 2006 (37)	Multicenter prospective	20	RT (36 Gy) Gemcitabine	15%	17	26[b]

[a] All patients, resectable and unresectable.
[b] Resectable patients.
[c] Unresectable patients.
5-FU, Fluorouracil; IORT, intraoperative radiation therapy; NR, not reported; RR, response rate (partial + complete); RT, radiation therapy.

characteristics of the primary tumor with regard to its potential for surgical resection, and most are single center studies describing the median survivals and response rates of the various regimens. As targeted agents have shown some promise in the treatment of metastatic disease, studies using these agents in the neoadjuvant and locally advanced setting have also begun.

2.1   Therapy for Locally Advanced Pancreatic Cancer

Five randomized trials have evaluated the use of chemoradiation therapy for patients with locally advanced, unresectable pancreatic cancer. The Mayo Clinic performed a randomized trial in the 1960s in which 64 patients with locally unresectable, nonmetastatic pancreatic adenocarcinoma received radiation (35–40 Gy) with 5-FU versus radiation with a placebo. A significant survival advantage was seen for patients receiving radiation with 5-FU versus radiation alone (10.4 months versus 6.3 months) (13). The Gastrointestinal Tumor Study Group (GITSG) followed with a similar trial of 194 patients with confirmed unresectable and nonmetastatic pancreatic cancer who were randomized to one of three arms: (1) radiation alone (60 Gy), (2) radiation (40 Gy) plus 5-FU, or (3) radiation (60Gy) plus 5-FU. The radiation alone arm was closed early as a result of an inferior survival rate. The 1-year survival rate in the two combined modality therapy arms was 36% and 38%, respectively, versus 11% for the radiation alone arm (14).

The second GITSG trial of this series randomized 157 locally advanced pancreatic cancer patients to radiation/5-FU or radiation/5-FU plus doxorubicin. A significant increase in treatment related toxicity was seen in the doxorubicin arm. However, no survival difference was observed between the two groups (median survival 37 versus 33 weeks) (15). A follow-up GITSG trial compared chemotherapy alone to chemoradiation, again in surgically confirmed unresectable tumors. Forty-three patients were randomized to receive combination streptozocin, mitomycin-C, and 5-FU (SMF) chemotherapy or 54 Gy of radiation with 5-FU chemotherapy followed by adjuvant SMF chemotherapy. The chemoradiation arm demonstrated a significant survival advantage over the chemotherapy alone arm (1-year survival 41% versus 19%) (16).

In contrast, the Eastern Cooperative Oncology Group (ECOG) reported no benefit to chemoradiation versus chemotherapy only. In this study, patients with unresectable, nonmetastatic pancreatic or gastric adenocarcinoma were randomized to receive either 5-FU chemotherapy alone or radiation (40 Gy) with 5-FU. Patients with locally recurrent disease as well as patients undergoing surgery with residual disease were eligible for this trial. In the 91 analyzable pancreatic patients, no survival difference was observed between the two groups (median survival 8.2 versus 8.3 months) (17).

Unlike the randomized trials conducted in locally advanced pancreatic cancer patients in whom surgery was never attempted, subsequent studies began to investigate the role of "neoadjuvant" therapy in this patient population. The intention was that some of these patients may be eligible for resection following therapy. Initially, the majority of these studies were small, prospective observational studies conducted at single institutions (18–26).

Early studies of neoadjuvant therapy in this patient population evaluated 5-FU in conjunction with radiation therapy, which was incorporated into most neoadjuvant regimens until recent studies with gemcitabine. Subsequent regimens have incorporated cisplatin as a component of a combined chemotherapy regimen. In a single center observational study of 35 patients receiving 5-FU, streptozocin, cisplatin, and radiation, a 43% overall response rate was noted in all patients. In addition, a median survival of 31 months was realized for the five (14%) patients who became eligible for resection following neoadjuvant therapy (19). A similar observational study of 68 patients using the same regimen showed a 32% overall response rate and a median survival of 32 months for the 20 (29%) patients who became eligible for surgery and subsequently underwent resection following combined chemoradiation therapy (n = 20) (21). In contrast, patients not eligible for surgery following chemoradiation therapy had a 21-month median survival. Another report describing the combination of cisplatin, 5-FU, and radiation in 14 patients reported an overall response rate of 64% with a median survival of 19 months among patients who became eligible for surgery following therapy (20). A report describing the addition of mitomycin C to this regimen in 58 patients showed a 58% response rate with a median survival of 23 months following combined chemoradiation therapy (24). Based on these studies, 5-FU has been the agent most frequently utilized in conjunction with radiation in the neoadjuvant setting.

More recently, gemcitabine has been studied in this patient population as both a monotherapy with radiation treatment and in combination with other chemotherapeutic agents. Among patients treated with gemcitabine monotherapy with 50 Gy of radiation, median survival of 25 months for resected patients has been reported (25). Other studies have combined gemcitabine with docetaxel, paclitaxel or cisplatin with radiation, but survival has not been as impressive (22, 23, 26). Unfortunately, in the absence of a randomized controlled trial of these various regimens, it remains unclear which chemotherapeutic agents alone or in combination with radiation therapy result in optimal survival. To date, the majority of neoadjuvant studies in this population are uncontrolled, single center experiences with small sample sizes.

2.2 Neoadjuvant Chemotherapy or Chemoradiotherapy for Potentially Resectable Pancreatic Cancer

Studies of neoadjuvant chemoradiation among patients with potentially resectable pancreatic cancer have also evaluated similar combinations of therapies. In a study of 91 patients receiving 5-FU alone with radiation (30 or 50.4 Gy), median survival was 19.2 months among resected patients (27). Other studies evaluating the combination of 5-FU and mitomycin C have found median survivals ranging from 12 to 15.7 months among resected patients (28, 29). Studies of patients treated with 5-FU and cisplatin have found variation in survival rates with one series of 61 patients experiencing a median survival of 26.6 months (30), whereas another series of 41 patients described a median survival of 12.5 months (31).

Other studies have evaluated the use of intraoperative radiation therapy (IORT) in conjunction with standard radiation therapy with varying combinations of chemotherapeutic agents. Patients treated with the combination of IORT with external beam irradiation and 5-FU were found to have a median survival ranging from 19 to 25 months (32–34). IROT was also evaluated in combination with external beam irradiation and paclitaxel, resulting in a 19-month median survival (34).

Three series of monotherapy with gemcitabine in addition to radiation therapy have also been published (35–37). In the first, a 58% response rate was found, with a median survival of 36 months for resected patients (35). Two subsequent studies found lower response rates of 15% or less with median survivals ranging from 20 to 26 months (36, 37). A study conducted at the Fox Chase Cancer Center consisted of 63 potentially resectable patients who were treated with preoperative gemcitabine-based chemoradiation therapy. Of these 63 patients, 31 underwent preoperative chemoradiation therapy followed by surgery and then by adjuvant chemotherapy alone. Eight patients underwent preoperative chemoradiation therapy followed by surgery without adjuvant chemotherapy, and 21 patients were found not to be appropriate surgical candidates following preoperative chemoradiation therapy either at the time of postinduction staging or at surgical exploration. The median survival for patients undergoing induction chemoradiation therapy who subsequently underwent resection was 20 months (n = 41) (36). The most recent phase II trial reported by Talamonti et al. consisted of 20 patients with resectable pancreatic cancer who received three cycles of gemcitabine, with radiation during their second cycle. Nineteen patients (95%) completed the planned regimen and 17 patients (85%) underwent resection. Of the 17 patients undergoing resection, 16 (94%) had negative margins. The median survival for patients undergoing resection was 26 months (37).

2.2.1 Duke Experience with Neoadjuvant Chemoradiation Therapy

In 1994, Duke University Medical Center began offering neoadjuvant chemoradiation therapy to all patients with biopsy-proven, localized pancreatic adenocarcinoma as determined by radiographic imaging. The neoadjuvant chemoradiation regimen has varied over the past 12 years, but has predominantly been 5-FU based. One-hundred eighty-four patients with either locally advanced or resectable disease have undergone such therapy. Of 96 potentially resectable patients receiving neoadjuvant therapy, >70% underwent surgical exploration, and 55% (53 patients) were resected. This resectability rate is consistent with previous studies, ranging from 45 to 57% (7, 27, 29). In a separate cohort of 88 locally advanced patients undergoing "neoadjuvant" chemoradiation therapy, 53% underwent surgical exploration, and 18% (16 patients) were resected. In the locally advanced patients eligible for surgical resection following neoadjuvant therapy (n = 16), all had arterial abutment on CT scan as opposed to arterial encasement. These and other data suggest that a small but significant number of patients who originally present with locally advanced disease as assessed by radiographic imaging may be converted to potentially resectable disease following neoadjuvant chemoradiation therapy. Patients who underwent neoadjuvant therapy followed by a complete resection (n=67) had a 5-year survival of 28% with an overall median survival of 23 months

(*24*). Treatment-related morbidity, specifically complications related to endoscopic stenting for biliary decompression, occurred in 34% of patients, with 15% requiring hospitalization. One death was related to cholangitis, which occurred during chemoradiation therapy.

In addition to evaluating the various chemoradiation therapy regimens by comparing overall median survival rates, it may be more appropriate to integrate more immediate surrogate markers of prognosis into clinical trials and management in this very select population of resected pancreatic cancer patients. A recent study conducted at Duke by White et al. investigated the significance of histologic responses to neoadjuvant chemoradiation therapy. The study consisted of 70 patients receiving neoadjuvant chemoradiation therapy followed by surgery whose specimens were reviewed by an independent pathologist for evidence of tumor necrosis, tumor fibrosis, residual tumor load, and tumor differentiation. The authors identified tumor necrosis, large tumor residual load, and poor differentiation to be significant, independent predicators of poor prognosis (*38*). This study suggests that histologic responses to neoadjuvant chemoradiation therapy may serve as a useful surrogate marker for treatment efficacy, notably, as we begin to identify innovative molecular targets that may be used in conjunction with standard chemotherapy and radiation in hopes of improving ultimate outcomes.

3   Future Directions

The addition of targeted therapies may potentially offer new hope and a variety of novel treatment strategies for patients with pancreatic cancer. The ability to potentially predict outcome based upon pathologic response to neoadjuvant treatment (*9*) suggests that the neoadjuvant setting may be the ideal one to develop novel approaches and define the role of targeted approaches to therapy. Several studies are currently underway to investigate the use of antiangiogenic agents, tyrosine kinase inhibitors, proteasome inhibitors, and other molecular targets; however, these agents have been studied most extensively in the metastatic setting.

Initial efforts to antagonize vascular endothelial growth factor (VEGF) in patients with pancreatic cancer evaluated the efficacy of gemcitabine in combination with the antiangiogenic agent, bevacizumab, in patients with unresectable pancreatic cancer (*39*). The response rate was found to be 27% versus 5.6% when compared with historical controls treated with gemcitabine alone, and the 1-year survival rate was 53%. Subsequently, a phase II trial of the combination of gemcitabine and bevacizumab found a response rate of 21% with a median progression-free survival of 5.4 months and median overall survival of 8.8 months. In addition, studies have suggested that anti-VEGF therapy potentially enhances not only the delivery of chemotherapies by eliminating inefficient tumor neovasculature, but also reduces tumor interstitial pressure and enhances the effectiveness of radiation therapy. However, the most recent CALBG randomized trial (CALGB 80303) comparing the combination of gemcitabine and bevacizumab with gemcitabine alone did not find a meaningful clinical response (*40*). Currently, the Radiation Therapy Oncology Group (RTOG 0417) is undertaking a phase II study combining bevacizumab and capecitabine.

The only targeted agent to date that has shown a statistically significant survival benefit in the metastatic setting compared to chemotherapy alone is erlotinib, an anti-EGFR tyrosine kinase inhibitor. Although the survival benefit was statistically significant with a increase in 1-year survival from 17% to 24%,in addition the median progression- free survival and overall survival benefits for the gemcitabine plus erlotinib arm versus gemcitabine alone was also significant (3.75 versus 3.55 months, $p = 0.003$ and 6.37 versus 5.91 months, $p = 0.025$, respectively). In patients with locally advanced pancreatic cancer, a phase I study of erlotinib, gemcitabine, and radiation therapy for patients has found a maximal tolerated dose of erlotinib 100 mg daily, gemcitabine 40 mg/m^2 biweekly, and radiation therapy (50.4 Gy) (*41*). Additional studies have also been conducted to evaluate the combination of erlotinib, gemcitabine, paclitaxel, and radiation therapy.

Cetuximab, another EGFR inhibitor, has been evaluated in combination with gemcitabine in a phase II study in the patients with metastatic disease. Overall, the response rate was 12%, with a median progression-free survival of 3.8 months and median overall survival of 7.1 months (*42*). In addition, two small trials comparing cetuximab in combination with gemcitabine and radiation therapy for localized pancreatic cancer have demonstrated that cetuximab can be given at full dose with chemotherapy and radiation therapy without significantly increased toxicity (*43, 44*). Currently, a phase III randomized study of gemcitabine plus cetuximab versus gemcitabine (SWOG S0205) has completed enrollment and follow-up is ongoing.

4   Summary and Conclusions

Although neoadjuvant therapy remains investigational for patients with resectable pancreatic cancer, it is becoming a more accepted approach for patients with locally advanced disease. Potential advantages of neoadjuvant therapy include improved delivery of therapy prior to surgery, fewer postoperative complications than with more traditional adjuvant therapy, and improved respectability of the tumor. Although most neoadjuvant regimens have included radiation therapy, there is no clear consensus regarding the dose. In addition, equivocal results have been found from studies of varying chemotherapies and combination regimens and all studies have significant methodologic limitations. Analysis of histologic response to neoadjuvant therapy at Duke University Medical Center has suggested that some features may predict clinical outcomes. Currently research is ongoing to identify key molecular markers to better understand tumor biology and classify tumors. Ultimately, this approach may lead to targeted therapies based on individual tumor characteristics.

References

1. Jemal A, Siegel R, Ward E, Cancer statistics, 2006. CA Cancer J Clin 2006, 56:106.
2. Sohn TA, Yeo CJ, Cameron JL, 2000, Resected adenocarcinoma of the pancreas—616 patients: results, outcomes, and prognostic indicators. J Gastrointest Surg 4:567–579 .
3. Klinkenbijl JH, Jeekel J, Sahmoud T, 1999, Adjuvant radiotherapy and 5 fluorouracil after curative resection of cancer of the pancreas and periampullary region: phase III trial of the EORTC gastrointestinal tract cancer cooperative group. Ann Surg 230:776–782.
4. Yeo CJ, Abrams RA, Grochow LB, 1997, Pancreaticoduodenectomy for pancreatic adenocarcinoma: postoperative adjuvant chemoradiation improves survival. A prospective, single-institution experience. Ann Surg 225:621–633.
5. Cheng T, Sheth K, White RR, 2006, Effect of Neoadjuvant Chemoradiation on Operative Mortality and Morbidity for Pancreaticoduodenectomy. Ann Surg Oncol 13:66–74.
6. Willett CG, Warshaw AL. Intraoperative electron beam irradiation in pancreatic cancer. Frontiers in Bioscience, 1998.
7. White R, Hurwitz H, Lee C, 2001, Neoadjuvant chemoradiation for localized adenocarcinoma of the pancreas. Ann Surg Oncol 8:758–765.
8. Kim HJ, Czischke K, Brennan MF, 2002, Does neoadjuvant chemoradiation downstage locally advanced pancreatic cancer? J Gastrointest Surg. 6(5):763–769.
9. White RR, Kattan MW, Haney JC, 2006, Evaluation of preoperative therapy for pancreatic cancer using a prognostic nomogram. Ann Surg Oncol 13:1485–1492.
10. Evans DB, Abbruzzese JL, Willett CG. 2001, Cancer of the pancreas. In: DeVita VT Jr Hellman S, Rosenberg SA (eds.) Cancer: principles and practice of oncology, 6 th ed. Lippincott, Philadelphia, 1138th ed..
11. Horwhat JD, Paulson EK, McGrath K, 2006, A randomized comparison of EUS-guided FNA versus CT or US-guided FNA for the evaluation of pancreatic mass lesions. Gastroint Endosc 63:966–975.
12. Micames C, Jowell P, White R, 2003, Lower frequency of peritoneal carcinomatosis in patients with pancreatic cancer diagnosed by EUS-guided FNA vs percutaneous FNA. Gastrointest Endosc 58:690–695.
13. Moertel CG, Childs DS Jr, Reitemeier RJ, Colby My Jr, Holbrook MA, 1969, Combined 5-fluorouracil and supervoltage radiation therapy of locally unresectable gastrointestinal cancer. Lancet 2(7626): 865–867.
14. Moertel CG, Frytak S, Hahn RG, 1981, Therapy of locally unresectable pancreatic carcinoma: a randomized comparison of high dose (6000 rads) radiation alone, moderate dose radiation (4000 rads + 5-fluorouracil), and high dose radiation + 5-fluorouracil: The Gastrointestinal Tumor Study Group. Cancer 48:1705–1710.
15. Radiation therapy combined with Adriamycin or 5-fluorouracil for the treatment of locally unresectable pancreatic carcinoma. Gastrointestinal Tumor Study Group. Cancer 1985, 56:2563–2568.
16. Treatment of locally unresectable carcinoma of the pancreas: comparison of combined-modality therapy (chemotherapy plus radiotherapy) to chemotherapy alone. Gastrointestinal Tumor Study Group. J Natl Cancer Inst 1988, 80:751–755.
17. Klaassen DJ, MacIntyre JM, Catton GE, 1985, Treatment of locally unresectable cancer of the stomach and pancreas: a randomized comparison of 5-fluorouracil alone with radiation plus concurrent and maintenance 5-fluorouracil—an Eastern Cooperative Oncology Group study. J Clin Oncol 3:373–378.
18. Jessup JM, Steele G JrMayer RJ, 1993, Neoadjuvant therapy for unresectable pancreatic adenocarcinoma. Arch Surg 128:559.
19. Kamthan AG, Morris JC, Dalton J, 1997, Combined modality therapy for stage II and stage III pancreatic carcinoma. J Clin Oncol 15:2920–2927.
20. Wanebo HJ, Glicksman AS, Vezeridis MP, 2000, Preoperative chemotherapy, radiotherapy, and surgical resection of locally advanced pancreatic cancer. Arch Surg 135:81–87.

21. Snady H, Bruckner H, Cooperman A, 2000, Survival advantage of combined chemoradio-therapy compared with resection as the initial treatment of patients with regional pancreatic carcinoma. An outcomes trial. Cancer 89:314–327.
22. Ammori JB, Colletti LM, Zalupski MM, 2003, Surgical resection following radiation therapy with concurrent gemcitabine in patients with previously unresectable adenocarcinoma of the pancreas. J Gastrointest Surg 7(6):766–772.
23. Aristu J, Canon R, Pardo F, 2003, Surgical resection after preoperative chemoradiotherapy benefits selected patients with unresectable pancreatic cancer. Am J Clin Oncol 26:30–36.
24. White RR, Tyler DS. 2004, Neoadjuvant therapy for pancreatic cancer: the Duke experience. Surg Oncol Clin North Am 13:675–684.
25. Joensuu TK, Kiviluoto T, Kärkkäinen P, 2004, Phase I-II trial of twice-weekly gemcitabine and concomitant irradiation in patients undergoing pancreaticoduodenectomy with extended lymphadenectomy for locally advanced pancreatic cancer. Rad Oncol 60:444–452.
26. Pipas MJ, Barth RK, Zaki B, 2005, Docetaxel/gemcitabine followed by gemcitabine and external beam radiotherapy in patients with pancreatic adenocarcinoma. Ann Surg Oncol 12:995–1004.
27. Spitz FR, Abbruzzese JL, Lee JE, 1997, Preoperative and postoperative chemoradiation strate-gies in patients treated with pancreaticoduodenectomy for adenocarcinoma of the pancreas. J Clin Oncol 15(3):928–937.
28. Yeung RS, Weese JL, Hoffman JP, 1993, Neoadjuvant chemoradiation in pancreatic and duo-denal carcinoma. A Phase II Study. Cancer 72:2124–2133.
29. Hoffman JP, Lipsitz S, Pisansky T, 1998, Phase II trial of preoperative radiation therapy and chemotherapy for patients with localized, resectable adenocarcinoma of the pancreas: an Eastern Cooperative Oncology Group Study. J Clin Oncol 16:317–312.
30. Moutardier V, Magnin V, Turrini O, 2004, Assessment of pathologic response after preopera-tive chemoradiotherapy and surgery in pancreatic adenocarcinoma. Int J Radiat Oncol Biol Phys 60:437.
31. Mornex F, Girard N, Delpero JR, 2005, Radiochemotherapy in the management of pancreatic cancer—part I: neoadjuvant treatment. Semin Radiat Oncol 15:226–234.
32. Staley CA, Lee JE, Cleary KA, 1996, Preoperative chemoradiation, pancreaticoduodenec-tomy, and intraoperative radiation therapy for adenocarcinoma of the pancreatic head. Am J Surg 171:118.
33. Pisters PW, Abbruzzese JL, Janjan NA, 1998, Rapid-fractionation preoperative chemoradia-tion, pancreaticoduodenectomy, and intraoperative radiation therapy for resectable pancreatic adenocarcinoma. J Clin Oncol 16:3843.
34. Pisters PW, Wolff RA, Janjan NA, 2002, Preoperative paclitaxel and concurrent rapid-frac-tionation radiation for resectable pancreatic adenocarcinoma: toxicities, histologic response rates, and event-free outcome. J Clin Oncol 20:2537.
35. Wolff RA, Evans DB, Crane CH, 2002, Initial results of preoperative gemcitabine-based chemora-diation for resectable pancreatic adenocarcinoma (abstract). Proc Am Soc Clin Oncol 21:130a.
36. Meszoely IM, Wang H, Hoffman JP. 2004, Preoperative chemoradiation therapy for adenocar-cinoma of the pancreas: The Fox Chase Cancer Center experience, 1986–2003. Surg Oncol Clin North Am 13(4):685–696.
37. Talamonti MS, Small W, Mulcahy MF, 2006, A multi-institutional Phase II trial of preopera-tive full-dose gemcitabine and concurrent radiation for patients with potentially resectable pancreatic carcinoma. Ann Surg Oncol 13:150–158.
38. White R, Xie B, Gotfried M, 2005, Prognostic significance of histologic response to preopera-tive chemoradiation of periampullary malignancies. Ann Surg Oncol 12:214–221.
39. Kindler HL, Friberg G, Singh DA, 2005, Phase II trial of bevacizumab plus gemcitabine in patients with advanced pancreatic cancer. J Clin Oncol 31:8033–8040.
40. Kindler HL, Friberg G, Singh DA, 2005, Phase II trial of bevacizumab plus gemcitabine in patients with advanced pancreatic cancer. J Clin Oncol 1(23):8033–8040.
41. Kortmansky S, O'Reilly EM, Minsky BD, 2005, A phase I trial of erlotinib, gemcitabine and radiation for patients with locally advanced, unresectable pancreatic cancer. J Clin Oncol 23:4107.

42. Xiong HQ, Rosenberg A, LoBuglio A. 2004, Cetuximab, a monoclonal antibody targeting the epidermal growth factor receptor, in combination with gemcitabine for advanced pancreatic cancer: a multicenter phase II trial. J Clin Oncol 22:2610–2616.
43. Pipas JM, Zaki B, Suriawinata AA, et al. Cetuximab, intensity-modulated radiotherapy (IMRT), and twice-weekly gemcitabine for pancreatic adenocarcinoma. Proc Am Soc Clin Oncol 2006 (abstract 14056).
44. Krempien RC, Munter MW, Timke C, et al. Phase II study evaluating trimodal therapy with cetuximab intensity modulated radiotherapy (IMRT) and gemcitabine for patients with locally advanced pancreatic cancer (ISRCTN56652283). Proc Am Soc Clin Oncol, 2006 (abstract 4100).

Section VII
Emerging Targeted Therapies

Chapter 33
An Overview of Clinical Trials of Targeted Therapies in Pancreatic Cancer

Bassel El-Rayes

1 Introduction

Pancreatic cancer is the fourth leading cause of cancer mortality in the United States (1). Over 75% of patients with pancreatic cancer have locally advanced or metastatic disease at diagnosis (2). The median survival of patients with metastatic and locally advanced pancreatic cancer is 3–6 months and 8–10 months, respectively. The only potentially curative treatment is surgical resection. Patients who undergo a potentially curative resection have a median survival of 14–20 months and <20% are long-term survivors because of the development of metastatic disease. Therefore, improvement in the outcome of patients with pancreatic cancer is dependent on the development of more effective systemic therapies.

Gemcitabine is considered the standard chemotherapy in advanced pancreatic cancer. The response rate, median survival and 1-year survival in patients with advanced pancreatic cancer treated with gemcitabine in the pivotal trial were 5.4%, 5.6 months, and 18%, respectively (3). Combination chemotherapy did not demonstrate any significant survival advantage in randomized trials as compared with single-agent gemcitabine (4, 5). In the adjuvant setting, gemcitabine has been shown to be superior to observation (6) or 5-fluorouracil (7). Therefore, the impact of cytotoxic chemotherapy in pancreatic cancer has been at best modest. Nevertheless, most of the new drug development using targeted agents has been based on a gemcitabine platform.

Fundamental processes associated with carcinogenesis include molecular aberrations involving cell cycle control, signal transduction, apoptosis, angiogenesis, and invasion. The identification of agents that target these abnormalities offers an opportunity for the development of effective and selective systemic treatments for pancreatic cancer. Unfortunately, recently conducted clinical trials evaluating the role of novel targeted therapies in pancreatic cancer have demonstrated somewhat disappointing results (Table 33.1). This chapter reviews the clinical studies that have been undertaken in patients with pancreatic cancer using targeted agents.

A.M. Lowy et al. (eds.) *Pancreatic Cancer*.
doi: 10.1007/978-0-387-69252-4, © Springer Science+Business Media, LLC 2008

Table 33.1 Summary of completed trials of targeted agents in pancreatic cancer

Targeted agent	Target	Phase	Regimen	Results
Marimastat	MMPI[a]	III	Marimastat vs Gemcitabine	No significant difference
		III	Marimastat/gemcitabine vs Gemcitabine	No significant difference
Bay 12-9566	MMPI	III	Bay 12-9566 vs Gemcitabine	OS in favor of gemcitabine
Celecoxib	COX-2[b]	II	Gemcitabine	Response rate 17%
		II	Gemcitabine/cisplatin	6-Month survival 46%
Bortezomib	Proteasome	II	Single-agent Gemcitabine	Median survival 2.5 months Median survival 4.8 months
Bevacizumab	VEGF[c]	II	Gemcitabine	Median survival 8.8 months
		III	Bevacizumab/gemcitabine vs Gemcitabine	No significant difference
Tipifarnib	FTI[d]	III	Tipifarnib/gemcitabine vs gemcitabine	No significant difference
ISIS-2503	Ras	II	Gemcitabine	Median survival 6.6 months
Erlotinib	EGFR[d]	III	Erlotinib/gemcitabine vs gemcitabine	Significant improvement in survival in favor of erlotinib gemcitabine
Cetuximab	EGFR	III	Cetuximab/gemcitabine vs gemcitabine	No significant difference

[a] Matrix metalloproteinase inhibitors.
[b] Cyclo-oxygenase-2.
[c] Vascular endothelial growth factor.
[d] Epidermal growth factor receptor.

2   Matrix Metalloproteinase Inhibitors

The matrix metalloproteinases (MMP) are a family of zinc-containing endoproteinases that degrade collagen and proteoglycans (8). Degradation of the extracellular matrix is an essential step in angiogenesis, invasion, and metastasis. MMPs are overexpressed in a variety of human malignancies, including pancreatic cancer. A correlation between tumor aggressiveness and MMP expression has been reported in pancreatic cancer (9). In preclinical animal models, MMP inhibitors were found to decrease cancer implantation and improve survival (10, 11). Consequently, MMPs were considered a rationale target for new drug development in pancreatic cancer.

Marimastat was evaluated in two randomized clinical trials. In the first study, 414 patients with previously untreated metastatic pancreatic cancer were randomized to receive three different dose levels of the drug versus a control arm of standard dose and schedule of gemcitabine alone (12). There was no significant difference between marimastat at the highest dose level (25 mg twice daily) and gemcitabine (1,000 mg/m^2) with respect to median survival

(125 versus 167 days). Progression-free survival was significantly better in the gemcitabine arm. The lower doses of marimastat (5, 10 mg) resulted in a median and 1-year survival, which were inferior to gemcitabine. In the second trial, 239 patients were randomized to receive gemcitabine plus marimastat (10 mg) versus gemcitabine alone (*13*). No significant difference was observed with respect to survival (primary endpoint), time to treatment failure, or objective response rate.

A second MMP inhibitor was also tested in advanced pancreatic cancer. BAY 12-9566 is a specific inhibitor of MMP-2, MMP-3, MMP-9, and MMP-13 (*14*). Two hundred seventy-seven patients with advanced pancreatic cancer were randomized to receive BAY 12-9566 or gemcitabine. The primary endpoint of the trial was overall survival. The trial was terminated early due to a significant difference in survival in favor of gemcitabine (6.59 versus 3.74 months, $p < 0.01$). Failure of MMP inhibitors to show any anticancer effects in advanced pancreatic cancer has dampened any interest in their further development in this disease.

3 Cyclo-oxygenase-2 Inhibitors

The cyclo-oxygenase (COX) enzyme catalyzes a key step in the synthesis of prostaglandins that play a critical role in inflammation, angiogenesis, and regulation of cell cycle and apoptosis (*15*). Two isoforms of the COX enzyme were identified in human tissues. COX-1 is constitutively expressed in most tissues, whereas COX-2 is inducible by certain physiologic and pathologic stimuli (*16*). COX-2 over-expression by immunohistochemistry is observed in 57–67% of pancreatic adenocarcinoma (*17*). Furthermore, COX-2 expression is absent in the nonmalignant surrounding pancreatic tissue. COX-2 inhibitors such as sulindac (*16*), celecoxib (*16, 17*), or SN-398 (*18*) inhibit growth of pancreatic cell lines. Celecoxib sensitized human pancreatic cancer cell lines to the proapoptotic effects of gemcitabine (*19, 20*).

Two phase II trials evaluated celecoxib in combination with chemotherapy in advanced pancreatic cancer. In the first trial, celecoxib at a dose of 400 mg twice daily was administered in combination with gemcitabine and cisplatin (21). The primary endpoint was survival at 6 months. Twenty-two patients with metastatic pancreatic cancer were enrolled. The median and 6-month survival rates were 5.8 months and 46%, respectively. In the second trial, Smith et al. reported on 20 patients treated with gemcitabine and celecoxib (*22*). The observed response rate was 17% and no unexpected toxicities were observed. The results of both trials do not demonstrate an apparent improvement in the clinical activity of gemcitabine when combined with celecoxib. With the failure of celecoxib to impart an anticancer benefit in other cancers such as colorectal cancer, further development of this or other COX-2 blocking agents has been halted.

4 Proteasome Inhibitors

The regulation of cell signaling pathways is dependent on the activation and subsequent degradation of key regulatory proteins (*23*). The proteasomes are involved in the degradation of proteins and as such regulate cell cycle and apoptosis. The pro-apoptotic effects of proteasome inhibition are largely due to inhibition of the NF-κB signaling pathway (*24, 25*). NF-κB is a transcriptional factor that may be activated in response to stressful stimuli that include cytotoxic or radiation therapy and is constitutively activated in approximately 70% of pancreatic cancer (*26*). The activation of NF-κB and its translocation to the nucleus results in transcription of genes involved in proliferation, angiogenesis, and survival.

Bortezomib is a selective proteasome inhibitor. In preclinical models, bortezomib-induced apoptosis and sensitized pancreatic cancer cell lines to the effects of cytotoxic agents (*27, 28*). Based on the preclinical observation and the novel mechanism of action, the North Central Cancer Treatment Group (NCCTG) conducted a randomized phase II trial evaluating bortezomib as a single agent or in combination with gemcitabine in patients with metastatic pancreatic cancer (*29*). In the 42 patients who were treated with bortezomib, no objective responses were observed and the median survival was 2.5 months. In the 39 patients treated with gemcitabine and bortezomib, the response rate and median survival were 10% and 4.8 months, respectively. The results of the combination were comparable to the activity of single-agent gemcitabine and therefore did not support further development of bortezomib in pancreatic cancer. Nevertheless, the concept of developing other strategies to target NF-κB remains very attractive.

5 Angiogenesis Inhibitors

Tumor progression is dependent on the proliferation of endothelial cells that is largely achieved through activation of receptors on these cells by angiogenic growth factors secreted by the tumor cells. The new blood vessels within tumor deposits have increased permeability, resulting in dysregulated circulation that raises the intratumoral interstitial pressure and impedes the efficient delivery of cytotoxic molecules to target cells (*30*). Vascular Endothelial Growth Factor (VEGF) is the growth factor central to tumor angiogenesis (*31*). VEGF expression is dysregulated in pancreatic cancer (*32*) as a result of a number of molecular and physiologic aberrations, including but not limited to oncogene activation and tumor hypoxia (*33*). In pancreatic cancer, high tumoral expression of VEGF is also associated with poor prognosis (*34*). Elevated serum VEGF is correlated with poor survival after surgical resection (*34–36*). Inhibition of the VEGF pathway sensitizes pancreatic cancer cell lines to the cytotoxic effects of gemcitabine (*37*).

Major strategies aimed at targeting the VEGF signaling pathway include VEGF receptor tyrosine kinase inhibitors, anti-VEGF monoclonal antibodies, and binding VEGF to soluble VEGF receptors (VEGF trap). Bevacizumab is a recombinant anti-VEGF monoclonal antibody with relatively broad spectrum activity in advanced colorectal, breast, and non-small cell lung cancers. Bevacizumab in combination with gemcitabine was evaluated in advanced pancreatic cancer (38). A total of 52 patients with advanced pancreatic cancer were enrolled on the initial phase II study. The response and estimated 1-year survival rates were 21% and 29%, respectively. Based on this trial, a prospective randomized phase III trial comparing bevacizumab and gemcitabine with gemcitabine plus placebo was completed (39). The primary endpoint was overall survival. A total of 602 patients were enrolled on the trial. No significant difference was observed between the two arms with respect to median survival (5.8 months on combination versus 6.1 months on gemcitabine plus placebo and 1-year survival (18% versus 20%).

6   Ras Inhibitors

The *ras* proto-oncogene family includes *H-ras,* K-rasA, K-rasB, and *N-ras* (40). Ras lies at the center of signaling cascades of several proliferation promoting growth factors, such as the epidermal growth factor receptor (EGFR) pathway (40). Activation of ras results in downstream signaling through the PI-3 kinase/Akt and raf/MAPK pathways promoting cellular proliferation and survival (41). Activating mutations involving K-ras gene are present in 75–90% of pancreatic cancer (42). Activation of K-ras protein requires post-translational modification by farnesyl transferase (43). In pancreatic cancer cell lines, H-ras promotes growth in response to transforming growth factor (TGF-α) (44). Therefore, it is thought that the ras family that is commonly dysregulated in pancreatic cancer may play a central role in tumor growth and present a rational target for drug development.

Two agents targeting the ras signaling pathway were evaluated in pancreatic cancer patients. Tipifarnib is a farnesyl transferase inhibitor (FTI) that inhibited growth of human pancreatic cancer cells in xenograft models (45). Van Cutsem et al. conducted a randomized phase III trial of tipifarnib and gemcitabine versus gemcitabine in patients with advanced pancreatic cancer (46). Six hundred eighty-eight patients were enrolled on the trial. No significant differences were observed with respect to median survival (primary endpoint) or 1-year survival. ISIS-2503, an H-ras antisense molecule was evaluated in combination with gemcitabine in patients with advanced pancreatic cancer (47). Forty-eight patients were enrolled. The response, median, and 6-month survival rates were 10%, 6.6 months, and 57%, respectively. It was concluded that the addition of ISIS-2503 to gemcitabine did not improve survival of patients with pancreatic cancer. The results of these early studies in pancreatic cancer with a goal to target ras signaling pathway were disappointing given the high frequency of *ras* mutations. The choice of agents and/or the redundant signaling pathways may be major factors in the failure of those agents in the clinic.

7 Epidermal Growth Factor Receptor Inhibitors

Ligand activation of the epidermal growth factor receptor (EGFR) by EGF or
TGF-α results in receptor dimerization and activation of the tyrosine kinase
domain (48). The EGFR transmits cellular signals through at least two different pathways: MAP kinase and PI3-Kinase/Akt (49). Activation of the EGFR
signaling induces growth, chemoresistance and invasiveness of pancreatic
tumors (50, 51). The two strategies targeting the EGFR currently in clinical
trials are receptor tyrosine kinase inhibitors and anti-EGFR monoclonal
antibodies.

Erlotinib (OSI-774) is an oral receptor kinase inhibitor. In a phase III trial,
569 patients with locally advanced or metastatic pancreatic cancer were randomized to gemcitabine plus placebo or gemcitabine and erlotinib (52). Erlotinib
was administered at a dose of 100 mg in 515 patients and 150 mg in 47 patients.
The primary endpoint was survival with secondary endpoints of progression-
free survival, response rate, and improvement in the quality of life. The median
survival favored the erlotinib arm with a hazard ratio of 0.82 (95% CI; 0.67–
0.97, $p = 0.034$). Fifty-eight percent (58%) of the patients survived 6 months or
longer on the erlotinib arm. The 12-month survival was 24% and 17% for the
erlotinib and gemcitabine arms, respectively. In multivariate analysis significant
predictors for survival were treatment with erlotinib, favorable performance
status, locally advanced disease, and normal serum albumin concentration. The
progression-free status was also improved in the erlotinib arm (3.75 versus 3.55
months) with a hazard ratio of 0.76 ($p = 0.03$). A higher incidence of rash (71%
versus 29%), diarrhea (51% versus 36%), infection (41% versus 31%), and stomatitis (23% versus 14%) were observed in the erlotinib arm. No significant
difference in grade III or IV toxicities was observed between the two arms.
A nonsignificant increase in the incidence of infection, interstitial lung disease,
and mild hepatic toxicity were observed in the erlotinib arm. No correlation was
found between EGFR expression by immunohistochemistry and clinical benefit
from erlotinib. Based on the results of this trial, erlotinib in combination with
gemcitabine was approved for pancreatic cancer in the United States and subsequently the European Union.

Cetuximab is a chimeric anti-EGFR monoclonal antibody that inhibits EGFR-
dependent proliferation and survival of human pancreatic cancer cells in vitro (53),
and in an orthotropic nude mouse model of pancreatic cancer. These effects were
potentiated by the coadministration of gemcitabine. A phase II trial of gemcitabine
plus cetuximab in patients with advanced pancreatic cancer ($n = 41$) showed a
1-year survival rate of 31.7% and median survival duration of 7.1 months (54).
Based on the favorable results of this trial, the South Western Oncology Group
(SWOG) conducted a randomized phase III trial comparing gemcitabine to gemcitabine and cetuximab (55). The primary endpoint of the trial was survival. The total
number of patients accrued was 766. No significant difference was observed with
respect to survival, progression-free survival, or time to treatment failure. Therefore,

the addition of cetuximab to gemcitabine, although well tolerated, did not improve the overall survival.

8   Targeted Drugs Currently in Clinical Trials

Table 33.2 summarizes the targeted agents currently in development in pancreatic cancer.

Table 33.2   Selected targeted agents currently in clinical trials in pancreatic cancer

Targeted agent	Target	Disease stage	Regimen
Isoflavone	Akt/ NF-κB	III/IV (1st line)	Gemcitabine, erlotinib
Curcumin	NF-κB/ EGFR/HIF	III/IV (1st line)	Gemcitabine
Flavopiridol	Cyclin-dependent kinase	III (1st line) III/IV (2nd line)	Radiation Docetaxel
Depsipeptide	Histone deacetylase	III/IV (1st line)	Gemcitabine
Bortezomib	Proteasome	III/IV (1st line)	Carboplatin
AZD0430	Src	III/IV (1st line)	Gemcitabine
Lapatinib	Pan-erb tyrosine kinase	III/IV (1st line)	Gemcitabine Oxaliplatin, Gemcitabine
Cetuximab	EGFR	III/IV (1st line)	Ixabepilone
Gefitinib	EGFR tyrosine kinase	III/IV (2nd line)	Docetaxel
Enzastaurln	PKC-β	III/IV (1st line)	Gemcitabine, enzastaurin
Bevacizumab	VEGF	III/IV (1st line) III/IV (2nd line)	Cetuximab ± gemcitabine Gemcitabine/cisplatin Erlotinib/gemcitabine/ Capecitabine Gemcitabine/ Capecitabine Gemcitabine/ Erlotinib or cetuximab Docetaxel Erlotinib
		III (1st line) Adjuvant	FOLFOX/radiation Gemcitabine
PTK787/ ZK222584	VEGFR tyrosine kinase	III/IV (1st line)	Gemcitabine
Sunitinib	VEGFR/PDGFR/cKIT	III/IV (2nd line)	
Sorafinib	VEGFR/PDGFR/Raf	III/IV (1st line)	Gemcitabine
AG013736	VEGFR/PDGFR	III/IV (1st line)	Gemcitabine
Volociximab	Integrin α5β1	III/IV (1st line)	Gemcitabine
GV1001	Telomerase peptide vaccine	III/IV (1st line)	Gemcitabine
Ipilimumab	Cytotoxic T-lymphocyte (CTLA4)	III/IV (1st line)	
Mistletoe	Immune modulation	III/IV (1st line)	Gemcitabine
TNFerade gene therapy	TNF	III	5FU and radiation

[a] HIF, Hypoxia-induced factor; EGFR, epidermal growth factor receptor; PDGF, platelet-derived growth factor; PKC, protein kinase C; VEGF, vascular endothelial growth factor.

8.1 EGFR HER Signaling

The clinical benefit from targeting the EGFR pathway in pancreatic cancer has been at best modest. Three approaches for targeting this pathway are still being explored in clinical trials. The first approach is to use a pan-erb tyrosine kinase inhibitor (lapatinib) in combination with gemcitabine-based chemotherapy. The rationale is that the EGFR can heterodimerize with other members of the erb family of receptors. Therefore, inhibition of the receptor tyrosine kinase of the EGFR may not be sufficient for the inhibition of the EGFR signaling. The second approach is evaluating the effects of combining EGFR blockade with cytotoxic agents other than gemcitabine such as docetaxel or ixabepilone. The third approach is to evaluate combination therapy of targeted agents. The rationale is that pancreatic cancer cells have multiple gene abnormalities that contribute to tumor growth, metastasis, and chemoresistance. The targeting of one pathway such as EGFR may be in sufficient to alter the natural history of the disease. Ongoing trials are evaluating combining EGFR inhibitors with VEGF inhibitors (bevacizumab), or Akt/NF-kB inhibitors (isoflavone).

8.2 Vascular Endothelial Growth Factor Signaling

Trials are evaluating the effects of combining bevacizumab with either gemcitabine-based combination chemotherapy regimens (cisplatin or capecitabine) or with non-gemcitabine regimens (FOLOFOX/radiation or docetaxel). Other anti-angiogenic agents are being evaluated in pancreatic cancer and those include: VEGFR tyrosine kinase inhibitors (PTK787/ZK222584, sunitinib, sorafenib, AG013736), VEGF trap, PKC-beta inhibitors (enzastaurin), or anti-integrin $\alpha5\beta1$ (volociximab).

Other n Novel targets that are being evaluated in pancreatic cancer include the src pathway inhibitors (AZD0430), proteasome inhibitors (Bortezomib), cyclin-dependent kinase inhibitors (flavopiridol), or histone deacetylases (depsipeptide). Immune mediated targeted therapies currently in clinical trials include vaccines (GV1001), monoclonal antibodies (ipilimumab), or nonspecific immune modulators (mistletoe). Gene therapy approach is also currently in clinical trials in locally advanced pancreatic cancer.

9 Conclusion

Targeted agents represent a rational choice for drug development in pancreatic cancer. The studies conducted until now have failed to show a major impact for targeted agents in pancreatic cancer. The challenge for future trials will be the incorporation of new trial designs that can better evaluate the activity of targeted agents.

References

1. Jemal A, Siegel R, Ward E, et al. Cancer statistics, 2007. Cancer 2007, 57:43–66.
2. El-Rayes BF, Philip PA. A review of systemic therapy for advanced pancreatic cancer. Clin Adv Hematol Oncol 2003, 1:430–434.
3. Burris HA 3rd Moore MJ, Andersen J, et al. Improvements in survival and clinical benefit with gemcitabine as first-line therapy for patients with advanced pancreatic cancer: a randomized trial. J Clin Oncol 1997, 15:2403–2413.
4. Rocha Lima CM, Green MR, Rotche R, et al. Irinotecan plus gemcitabine results in no survival advantage compared with gemcitabine monotherapy in patients with locally advanced or metastatic pancreatic cancer despite increased tumor response rate. J Clin Oncol 2004, 22:3776–3783.
5. Louvet C, Labianca R, Hammel P, et al. 2005, Gemcitabine in combination with oxaliplatin compared with gemcitabine alone in locally advanced or metastatic pancreatic cancer: results of a GERCOR and GISCAD phase III trial. J Clin Oncol 23:3509–3516.
6. Oettle H, Post S, Neuhaus P, et al. 2007, Adjuvant chemotherapy with gemcitabine vs observation in patients undergoing curative-intent resection of pancreatic cancer: a randomized controlled trial. JAMA 297:267–277.
7. Regine W, Winter W, Abrams R. RTOG 9704 a phase III study of adjuvant pre and post chemoradiation 5-FU vs. gemcitabine for resected pancreatic cancer. ASCO 2006.
8. Koshiba T, Hosotani R, Wada M, et al. 1998, Involvement of matrix metalloproteinase-2 activity in invasion and metastasis of pancreatic carcinoma. Cancer 82:642–650.
9. Bramhall SR. 1997, The matrix metalloproteinases and their inhibitors in pancreatic cancer. From molecular science to a clinical application. Int J Pancreatol 21:1–12.
10. Watson SA, Morris TM, Robinson G, et al. 1995, Inhibition of organ invasion by the matrix metalloproteinase inhibitor batimastat (BB-94) in two human colon carcinoma metastasis models. Cancer Res 55:3629–3633.
11. Chirivi RG, Garofalo A, Crimmin MJ, et al. 1994, Inhibition of the metastatic spread and growth of B16-BL6 murine melanoma by a synthetic matrix metalloproteinase inhibitor. Int J Cancer 58:460–464.
12. Bramhall SR, Rosemurgy A, Brown PD, et al. 2001, Marimastat as first-line therapy for patients with unresectable pancreatic cancer: a randomized trial. J Clin Oncol 19:3447–3455.
13. Bramhall SR, Schulz J, Nemunaitis J, et al. 2002, A double-blind placebo-controlled, randomised study comparing gemcitabine and marimastat with gemcitabine and placebo as first line therapy in patients with advanced pancreatic cancer. Br J Cancer 87:161–167.
14. Moore MJ, Hamm J, Dancey J, et al. 2003, Comparison of gemcitabine versus the matrix metalloproteinase inhibitor BAY 12-9566 in patients with advanced or metastatic adenocarcinoma of the pancreas: a phase III trial of the National Cancer Institute of Canada Clinical Trials Group. J Clin Oncol 21:3296–3302.
15. Williams CS, Mann M, DuBois RN. 1999, The role of cyclooxygenases in inflammation, cancer, and development. Oncogene 18:7908–7916.
16. Molina MA, Sitja-Arnau M, Lemoine MG, et al. 1999, Increased cyclooxygenase-2 expression in human pancreatic carcinomas and cell lines: growth inhibition by nonsteroidal anti-inflammatory drugs. Cancer Res 59:4356–4362.
17. Merati K, Said Siadaty M, Andea A, et al. 2001, Expression of inflammatory modulator COX-2 in pancreatic ductal adenocarcinoma and its relationship to pathologic and clinical parameters. Amer J Clin Oncol 24:447–452.
18. Yip-Schneider MT, Barnard DS, Billings SD, et al. 2000, Cyclooxygenase-2 expression in human pancreatic adenocarcinomas. Carcinogenesis 21:139–146.
19. Li M, Wu X, Xu XC. 2001, Induction of apoptosis in colon cancer cells by cyclooxygenase-2 inhibitor NS398 through a cytochrome c-dependent pathway. Clin Cancer Res 7:1010–1016.
20. El-Rayes BF, Ali S, Sarkar FH, et al. 2004, Cyclooxygenase-2-dependent and -independent effects of celecoxib in pancreatic cancer cell lines. Mol Cancer Ther 3:1421–1426.

21. El-Rayes BF, Zalupski MM, Shields AF, et al. 2005, A phase II study of celecoxib, gemcitabine, and cisplatin in advanced pancreatic cancer. Invest New Drugs 23:583–590.
22. Smith E, Burris H, Loehrer P, et al. Preliminary report of a phase II trial of gemcitabine combined with celecoxib for advanced pancreatic cancer. ASCO 2003.
23. Adams J, Kauffman M. 2004, Development of the proteasome inhibitor Velcade (Bortezomib). Cancer Invest 22:304–311.
24. Teicher BA, Ara G, Herbst R, et al. 1999, The proteasome inhibitor PS-341 in cancer therapy. Clin Cancer Res 5:2638–2645.
25. Adams J, Palombella VJ, Sausville EA, et al. 1999, Proteasome inhibitors: a novel class of potent and effective antitumor agents. Cancer Res 59:2615–2622.
26. Wang W, Abbruzzese JL, Evans DB, et al. 1999, The nuclear factor-kappa B RelA transcription factor is constitutively activated in human pancreatic adenocarcinoma cells. Clin Cancer Res 5:119–127.
27. Chandler NM, Canete JJ, Callery MP, 2004, Increased expression of NF-kappa B subunits in human pancreatic cancer cells. J Surg Res 118:9–14.
28. Bold RJ, Virudachalam S, McConkey DJ, 2001, Chemosensitization of pancreatic cancer by inhibition of the 26S proteasome. J Surg Res 100:11–17.
29. Nawrocki ST, Bruns CJ, Harbison MT, et al. 2002, Effects of the proteasome inhibitor PS-341 on apoptosis and angiogenesis in orthotopic human pancreatic tumor xenografts. Mol Cancer Ther 1:1243–1253.
30. Alberts SR, Foster NR, Morton RF, et al. 2005, PS-341 and gemcitabine in patients with metastatic pancreatic adenocarcinoma: a North Central Cancer Treatment Group (NCCTG) randomized phase II study. Ann Oncol 16:1654–1661.
31. Korc M. 2003, Pathways for aberrant angiogenesis in pancreatic cancer. Mol Cancer 2:8.
32. Bergers G, Benjamin LE. 2003, Tumorigenesis and the angiogenic switch. Nat Rev 3:401–410.
33. Cherrington JM, Strawn LM, Shawver LK. 2000, New paradigms for the treatment of cancer: the role of anti-angiogenesis agents. Adv Cancer Res 79:1–38.
34. Ikeda N, Adachi M, Taki T, et al. 1999, Prognostic significance of angiogenesis in human pancreatic cancer. Br J Cancer 9:1553–1563.
35. Luo J, Guo P, Matsuda K, et al. 2001, Pancreatic cancer cell-derived vascular endothelial growth factor is biologically active in vitro and enhances tumorigenicity in vivo. Int J Cancer 92:361–369.
36. Knoll MR, Rudnitzki D, Sturm J, et al. 2001, Correlation of postoperative survival and angiogenic growth factors in pancreatic carcinoma. Hepato-gastroenterology 48:1162–1165.
37. Bruns CJ, Shrader M, Harbison MT, et al. 2002, Effect of the vascular endothelial growth factor receptor-2 antibody DC101 plus gemcitabine on growth, metastasis and angiogenesis of human pancreatic cancer growing orthotopically in nude mice. Int J Cancer 102:101–108.
38. Kindler HL, Friberg G, Singh DA, et al. 2005, Phase II trial of bevacizumab plus gemcitabine in patients with advanced pancreatic cancer. J Clin Oncol 23:8033–8040.
39. Kindler H, Niedzwiecki D, Hollis D, et al. A double-blind, placebo-controlled, randomized phase III trial of gemcitabine (G) plus bevacizumab (B) versus gemcitabine plus placebo (P) in patients (pts) with advanced pancreatic cancer (PC): A preliminary analysis of Cancer and Leukemia Group B (CALGB). ASCO 2007.
40. Rebollo A, Martinez AC, 1999, Ras proteins: recent advances and new functions. Blood 94:2971–2980.
41. Bollag G, McCormick F, 1991, Regulators and effectors of ras proteins. Annu Rev Cell Biol 7:601–632.
42. Bos JL. 1989, ras oncogenes in human cancer: a review. Cancer Res 49:4682–4689.
43. Leonard DM. 1997, Ras farnesyltransferase: a new therapeutic target. J Med Chem 40:2971–2990.
44. Seufferlein T, Van Lint J, Liptay S, et al. 1999, Transforming growth factor alpha activates Ha-Ras in human pancreatic cancer cells with Ki-ras mutations. Gastroenterology 116:1441–1452.
45. End DW, Smets G, Todd AV, et al. 2001, Characterization of the antitumor effects of the selective farnesyl protein transferase inhibitor R115777 in vivo and in vitro. Cancer Res 61:131–137.

46. Van Cutsem E, van de Velde H, Karasek P, et al. 2004, Phase III trial of gemcitabine plus tipi-farnib compared with gemcitabine plus placebo in advanced pancreatic cancer. J Clin Oncol 22:1430–1438.
47. Alberts SR, Schroeder M, Erlichman C, et al. 2004, Gemcitabine and ISIS-2503 for patients with locally advanced or metastatic pancreatic adenocarcinoma: a North Central Cancer Treatment Group phase II trial. J Clin Oncol 22:4944–4950.
48. El-Rayes BF, LoRusso PM, 2004, Targeting the epidermal growth factor receptor. Br J Cancer 91:418–424.
49. Perugini RA, McDade TP, Vittimberga FJ Jr, et al. 2000, Pancreatic cancer cell proliferation is phosphatidylinositol 3-kinase dependent. J Surg Res 90:39–44.
50. Wagner M, Cao T, Lopez ME, et al. 1996, Expression of a truncated EGF receptor is associated with inhibition of pancreatic cancer cell growth and enhanced sensitivity to cisplatinum. Int J Cancer 68:782–787.
51. Yamanaka Y, Friess H, Kobrin MS, et al. 1993, Coexpression of epidermal growth factor receptor and ligands in human pancreatic cancer is associated with enhanced tumor aggressiveness. Anticancer Res 13:565–569.
52. Moore MJ, Goldstein D, Hamm J, et al. 2007, Erlotinib plus gemcitabine compared with gemcitabine alone in patients with advanced pancreatic cancer: a phase III trial of the National Cancer Institute of Canada Clinical Trials Group. J Clin Oncol 25:1960–1966.
53. Bruns CJ, Harbison MT, Davis DW, et al. 2000, Epidermal growth factor receptor blockade with C225 plus gemcitabine results in regression of human pancreatic carcinoma growing orthotopically in nude mice by antiangiogenic mechanisms. Clin Cancer Res 6:1936–1948.
54. Xiong HQ, Rosenberg A, LoBuglio A, et al. 2004, Cetuximab, a monoclonal antibody targeting the epidermal growth factor receptor, in combination with gemcitabine for advanced pancreatic cancer: a multicenter phase II Trial. J Clin Oncol 22:2610–2616.
55. Philip PAJ, Fenoglio-Preiser C, Zalupski M, et al. Phase III study of gemcitabine [G] plus cetuximab [C] versus gemcitabine in patients [pts] with locally advanced or metastatic pancreatic adenocarcinoma [PC]: SWOG S0205 study. ASCO 2007.

Chapter 34
Utility of Animal Models in Pancreatic Cancer Research

Asfar S. Azmi, Mussop Mohammad, Ahmed O. Kaseb, Fazlul H. Sarkar, and Ramzi M. Mohammad

1 Introduction

The vast majority of human pancreatic cancers (~95%) are classified as ductal adenocarcinomas (1, 2), whereas acinar cell carcinomas and other histologic types are much less common. The cell origin of ductal adenocarcinomas is still under debate (3). Some studies have suggested that it arises from metaplasia (transdifferentiation) of acinar cells or even endocrine (islet) cells to ductal cells leading to ductal adenocarcinoma (3, 4) Although this has been based on cell lines and animal models, observations on human carcinomas, however, imply a different scenario. Hyperplastic and dysplastic epithelial lesions of the pancreatic ducts have been identified frequently in association with ductal adenocarcinomas (5), and these are now referred to as pancreatic intraepithelial neoplasia (PanINs) (6, 7). The evidence thus suggests that ductal adenocarcinomas may simply be originating from ductal cells, although it cannot be ruled out that ductal metaplasia of other cell types, especially acinar cells or centro-acinar cells (trans-differentiation or formation of ductular structures) could also be involved in the development of ductal adenocarcinoma under different situations, including genetic or epigenetic processes. Moreover, recent studies by Guerra et al. provided strong evidence for a role for pancreatic tissue damage and pancreatitis in the etiology of pancreatic ductal adenocarcinoma (PDAC) (9).

It is certain that the etiology of PDACs is fairly complex and poorly understood. This chapter provides an overview of the histologic and molecular complexities of pancreatic neoplasia as they apply to and correlate with different animal models, with a focus on transgenic mice and mice bearing human pancreatic tumor cells as xenografts, and their potential utility for developing preventive and/or therapeutic strategies.

2 Toward Developing Pancreatic Cancer Animal Models

There is an obvious need for the development of animal models to study pancreatic cancer biology as it relates to what is seen in the clinic. This could be further justified based on the fact that pancreatic cancer is usually diagnosed at an advanced stage and,

A.M. Lowy et al. (eds.) *Pancreatic Cancer*.
doi: 10.1007/978-0-387-69252-4, © Springer Science+Business Media, LLC 2008

as such, the processes of PDAC in humans are poorly understood. Furthermore, more challenges lie in the unique characteristics of the human pancreas. Among these factors are the high levels of nucleases and proteinases in the pancreatic tissue, in addition to the anatomic location of the pancreas, which explain the difficulty in obtaining sufficient tissue for pathologic analysis. Hence, drug dose, route of administration, and frequency of dosing that are essential components of drug development can only be assessed through preclinical efficacy models rather than in humans. The development of PDAC in animal models is simply dependent on the successful targeting of proliferating ductal epithelial cells, which has been an ongoing challenge, although xenograft models do not pose such challenges and, as such, xenograft models are useful for assessing antitumor activity of new and novel drugs.

3 Genes Involved in Differentiation and Development That Are Potential Targets for Drug Development

Prior to the development of transgenic or knock-out animals for PDAC, one must understand the normal developmental process of the pancreas. The pancreas first arises in the human embryo as dorsal and ventral buds of endoderm off the foregut/midgut at Carnegie Stage 12 (dorsal pancreas) and Carnegie Stage 13–14 (ventral pancreas), which corresponds to days 26–32. Subsequently, they fuse by 6 weeks (Carnegie Stage 17), following the rotation of the duodenum and stomach after ducts and acini become evident, such that the dorsal and ventral buds fuse to form a single pancreatic rudiment connected by ducts to the midgut (*10*) (Fig. 34.1). Dissection of the signaling pathways and genes encoding critical proteins in this embryologic process have been proposed as key targets in the gene-based development of new pharmaceuticals, which control signals on cellular

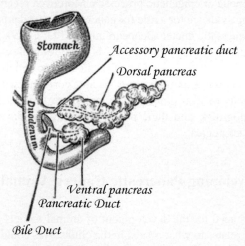

Fig. 34.1 Human pancreas

proliferation and differentiation in the adult pancreas (*11–14*). The key genes so far identified include notch, nestin (*15*), K-ras (*16, 17*), transforming growth factor (TGF)-α, and Hedgehog (*18, 19*). Endocrine cells are present at the earliest stages of pancreatic development but subsequently migrate from the exocrine epithelium to form separate islets. Notably, signals from adjacent embryonic structures are crucial for ultimate pancreatic development. Explant studies have demonstrated that the development of the early pancreatic endoderm requires secreted factors from the notochord.

The key role of the notochord in pancreatic development involves inhibition of Sonic Hedgehog (Shh) in the pancreatic endoderm, possibly through the secretion of fibroblast growth factor 2 (FGF2) and activin-betaB (*20*). The pancreatic endoderm lacks the Shh expression and, accordingly, inhibition of Shh has been reported to be sufficient for pancreatic gene expression. Differentiation of exocrine and endocrine portions of the pancreas necessitates mesenchymal signaling (*21*). Hence, gene knock-out experiments in mice have contributed (although not significantly) to our understanding of the genetic changes and transcription factors associated with pancreatic embryogenesis and to some extent carcinogenesis, leading to the development of PDAC.

4   Genetic Mutations in Pancreatic Carcinoma

Genetic alterations and over-expression of certain genes such as K-ras mutation, inactivation of the p53, p16, and DPC4 genes (*22*) and frequent chromosomal loss of the 17 (*23*) are characteristics of pancreatic cancer (Table 34.1; Fig. 34.2). This chapter briefly reviews those in the following paragraphs as they relate to the development of animal models.

Table 34.1 Genes frequently altered in pancreatic tumors

Gene/locus	Chromosomal location	Common alteration	Frequency of alteration	Refs
K-ras (K-ras2)	12p12.1	Point mutation codon 12,13, or 67	74–100%	24, 76, 77
Her2/neu (ERBB2)	17q21	Overexpression	66–69%	25
p16INK4a (CDKN2A)	9p21.3	Missense and homozygous deletions	25–98%	78, 79
p19ARF	9p21.3		30–82%	78
p15INK4b (CDKN2B)	9p21.3	Homozygous deletions		1
P53	17p13			80
DPC4/Smad4	18q21.1	Homozygous deletion, point mutation, LOH	~48–50%	22, 23, 29
Palladin (PNCA1)	4q32–34	Mutation, RNA over-expression	Unknown	81, 82
Rb1	13q14.1– 13q14.2	point mutation	50%	83
CDKN1A or P21 waf	6p21.2	Missense and homozygous deletions	Unknown	28, 84

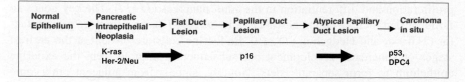

Fig. 34.2 Mutations in genes at different stages of pancreatic cancer progression

4.1 K-ras

Mutations of the K-ras gene occur in >90% of pancreatic carcinomas. No other human tumor comes close in mutational frequency that is observed in PDAC. The Ras pathway is important in the transmission of growth-promoting signals from the cell surface receptors, toward the nucleus, where these signals affect the production and regulation of other key proteins. It is interesting that although most mutations in genes are expected to cause their inactivation, with the Ras genes the opposite happens— they become more active in signaling. Ras mutations involve only certain amino acids, those that interfere with the GTPase activity. In pancreatic cancer, mutations are essentially seen only at the twelfth position (codon or amino acid 12), with rare exceptions seen at codon 13. Most mutations in pancreatic cancer change a glycine at codon 12 to a valine or aspartate (*24*). The mutation to serine is quite unusual in pancreatic cancer, a peculiar finding since it is a common mutation in other tumor types, which have K-ras mutations. K-ras mutation has been a potential target for the development of transgenic model, which is described later in this chapter.

4.2 Her-2/Neu

The HER-2/neu gene appears to be over-expressed in approximately 70% of invasive PDAC (*25*). In noninvasive lesions, over-expression of HER-2/neu is an early event, encountered in 82% of PanIN-1A lesions. An interesting finding is that the expression of HER-2/neu appears to decrease from PanIN-3 (100%) to invasive carcinoma (70%) (*26*), and as such, the relevance of this finding is not clear. Moreover, there is no report toward the development of animal models using HER-2/neu, although this has been documented for other cancers.

4.3 p53

Mutation of the p53 is the most common somatic alteration in human cancers. The p53 protein plays a central role in modulating cellular responses to cytotoxic stresses by contributing to both cell cycle arrest and programmed cell death. Loss of p53 function may lead to increased cell survival, genetic instability, and inappropriate cell growth (*27*). This tumor suppressor gene is inactivated in 50–75% of infiltrating pancreatic adenocarcinoma, being rare in chronic pancreatitis (*28*), and as such has been used for the development of animal models as described later.

4.4 DPC4/Smad4

A possible "pancreas specific" recessive oncogene is DPC4 (deleted in pancreatic adenocarcinoma 4) or Smad4, which is located on chromosome 18q (*22, 29*). DPC4 is inactivated in approximately half of pancreatic tumors, usually by mutations or allelic deletion. It has been shown that mice null for DPC4 (Smad4), the polyp adenomas progress into malignant and invasive adenocarcinomas without additional mutations (*30*). This indicates that mutations in DPC4 (SMAD4) play a significant role in the malignant progression of pancreatic tumors. Targeting this gene for the development of transgenic animal models has been limited.

4.5 p16INK4A

Approximately 80% of pancreatic adenocarcinomas feature loss of p16 function by mutations, homozygous deletions, or hypermethylation (*31–33*). P16INK4A has been suggested to be a negative prognostic marker in resected pancreatic cancer (*34*). The p16 along with p53 and Rb are believed to be key players in the regulation of cell cycle at the G1/S level. Because of its role in human pancreas cancer, p16 deletion has been used for the development of knock-out animals toward the development of PDAC.

4.6 p19ARF

p19ARF (alternate reading frame) gene mutations, which are found in 30–80% of pancreatic cancers. The p19ARF function is critical for maintaining the appropriate function of p53 in cells much like p16INK4a function is critical for appropriate pRb function. Numerous workers have established that disruptions of p16INK4A and the p19ARF-p53 circuit play critical and cooperative roles in PDAC progression, with specific tumor suppressor genotypes provocatively influencing the tumor biological phenotypes and genomic profiles of the resultant tumors (*35, 36*). Therefore, numerous attempts have been made for the development of knock-out animals by knocking out p19ARF alone, p16INK4a, p53 alone, or their combinations, as discussed later. However, debate is still continuing regarding targeting these gene knock-outs in specific cell types that may relate to the development of PDAC in humans.

5 Cells of Origin of Pancreatic Cancer

As indicated, the determination of the cellular origin of pancreatic cancer is very important in the development of tumor models to study human pancreas cancer and its treatment. The human pancreas is composed of endocrine and exocrine portions. The epithelial cells of both parts have a common embryologic origin, the gut endoderm (*37*). The exocrine part is composed of acinar secretory cells, connected to large ducts that drain into the duodenum. Acinar cells account for the most predominant pancreatic cells, and secrete nucleases, proteases, lipases, and amylases. Cells lining the pancreatic ducts secrete bicarbonate and mucous. The endocrine pancreas can be subdivided into four distinct types according to their secretory products, which include insulin, glucagon, somatostatin, and pancreatic polypeptide.

The cell origin of PDAC is still under debate (*9*). Some studies have suggested that it arises from metaplasia (transdifferentiation) of acinar cells or even endocrine (islet) cells to ductal cells leading to ductal adenocarcinoma (*3, 4*) (Fig. 34.3). Although this has been the impression based on cell lines and animal models, observations from human pancreatic cancers do not fully support this hypothesis, which could be partly due to lack of true understanding about the processes of carcinogenesis of PDAC in humans. Hyperplastic and dysplastic epithelial lesions of the pancreatic ducts are frequently identified in association with ductal adeno-carcinomas (*5*); these are currently classified as pancreatic intraepithelial neoplasia (PanINs) (*6*). Observations from human pancreatic cancer suggest that PDAC may simply arise from ductal cells. However, it cannot be ruled out that ductal metapla-sia of other cell types, especially acinar cells, may be involved in the development of ductal adenocarcinoma under different conditions. Other studies have suggested that regardless of the specific cellular origin, pancreatic PDAC most likely arises from the clonal expansion of cells that acquire a growth advantage through

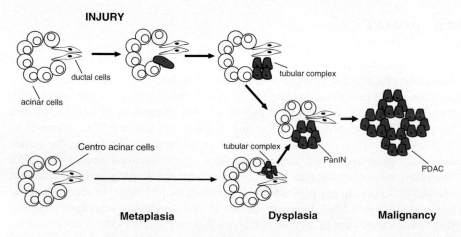

Fig. 34.3 Plausible cellular origin of pancreatic cancer

oncogene activation and tumor suppressor gene inactivation. Examples include K-ras mutations and deletions or mutations in p53, p16INK4a, p19ARF, and DPC4 (22, 38, 39). The following paragraphs summarize many attempts toward development of animal models for PDAC, although the cell of origin for the development of PDAC in humans is still under intense debate.

6   Rodent Models of Mouse, Rat, and Syrian Hamster

The laboratory mouse model is one of the most well-studied animal model systems for understanding the processes of carcinogenesis as well as its use for testing the therapeutic efficacy of newly developed drugs, because of its small size, lower cost, ease of breeding, short life span of about 1–2 years as well as molecular and pathological similarities to humans. The murine and rodent models for cancer investigation have progressed through several phases of complexity, which include use of chemical or viral carcinogens, xenograft tumors derived from pancreatic cancer cell lines or explants, and several variations of genetically engineered mice. Each approach has its advantages and disadvantages. It is important to choose the most appropriate model to address a particular question that is relevant to the development of human PDAC.

Carcinogen induce pancreas cancer have been studied for several decades; for example, Azaserine exposure in rats resulted in predominantly acinar rather than ductal carcinomas in one study (40). In contrast, pancreatic ductal adenocarcinomas induced in the Syrian golden hamster (SGH) by nitroso-bis(2-oxopropyl) amine was found to share many similarities with the human disease, including mutations of the K-ras oncogene (41). In addition, several other studies have confirmed that SGH PDAC share a molecular identity with the human disease through the high prevalence of K-ras mutations (42–45). These mutations were also similar in their G to A transition, localization in the second position of codon 12, and additional p53 mutations (46). However, this model of pancreatic cancer was compromised by the development of concomitant malignancies in the liver and lung (47). Siveke and Schmid (48) established a mouse model of metastatic pancreatic cancer in which K-ras and p53 were shown to enhance together with chromosome instability leading to metastasis. Deletion of both alleles of DPC4/Smad4 in the pancreatic cells of mice has no effect on pancreatic development physiologically. However, when combined with K-ras gene activation, DPC4/Smad4 deficiency led to rapid progression to activated K-ras-initiated neoplasm (35).

Several attempts have been made to develop a rat model that expresses the pathologic features of human PDAC. In one study, surgical methods to position chemical carcinogens in the proximity to proliferating ductal cells resulted in the preferential development of ductal adenocarcinomas (49). The study demonstrated that PD mutations of the K-ras gene occur in >90% of pancreatic carcinomas. No other human tumor comes close in mutational frequency that is observed in PDAC. K-ras mutation has been a potential target for the development of transgenic model, which is described later.

PDAC can easily be induced in the rat with dimethylbenz(a)anthracine (DMBA) implantation. The development of hyperplastic, atypical, and dysplastic changes preceding and accompanying pancreatic carcinomas suggested that this model is likely to be useful for studying early stages of pancreatic carcinogenesis. The chemical carcinogen–induced model systems have been extensively used for genetic and preclinical studies, including identification of oncogenes, tumor suppressor genes, the mapping of tumor susceptibility traits, and to check the effect of chemopreventive agents of different classes. However, such model systems have certain disadvantages and limitations. These include a restricted subset of tumor types and grades with incomplete penetrance and latency, and as such the role of carcinogenesis in the development of human PDAC is not clear. Such limitations prompted the development of newer technologies to provide mouse cancer models that reflect more accurately the common forms of human cancer, which allows better investigation opportunities of tumor genetics and gene environment interactions as discussed later.

7 Xenograft Models

Xenograft by definition means the surgical graft of tissue or cells from one species to an unlike species. Currently, the most commonly used preclinical animal models are tumor xenografts in immunodeficient mice. This type of model system can be subdivided into two different subtypes: (a) subcutaneous model in which the tumor graft/cells are implanted into the animal subcutaneously (Fig. 34.4); and (b) orthotopic model in which the graft is injected into an appropriate organ (Fig. 34.5). The subcutaneous xenograft still remains the standard for drug screening in pharmaceutical industries. These models are simple to grow and can be studied easily as the tumor growth on the mouse flank, which can be measured by a simple caliper, but the tumor environment is not ideal for the organ of interest. On the other hand, the orthotopic xenograft model is more advanced and the microenvironment is similar to what actually happens in human PDAC, although the measurement of the tumor growth is harder due to the deep-seated location of tumors in organs such as pancreas, even though newer and more sophisticated imaging tools are being developed for accurate measurement of tumors grown in the orthotopic site. In theory the tumors that arise from orthotopic implant closely resemble human tumors because the nearby blood vessel system and other supporting tissue better mirror the tumors microenvironment. Currently the orthotopic model is used to study a wide array of different cancer types, which include models for acute lymphoblastic leukemia (ALL), acute and myelogenous leukemia (AML), bladder cancer, bone and connective tissue, brain, breast, cervix, colon, head and neck, lung, ovarian, pancreas, prostate, renal, skin, stomach, and uterine cancer.

Although most human malignant tumors grow well as a xenograft in nude or SCID mice in the subcutaneous site, they seldom metastasize despite their malignant characteristics (*50, 51*). Therefore, an attempt to mimic the pattern of local growth of pancreatic cancer in the pancreatic organ, a human pancreatic tumor cell

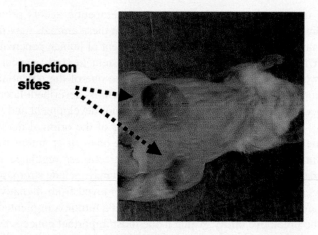

Fig. 34.4 Subcutaneous model of human pancreatic cancer established as a xenograft in SCID mouse

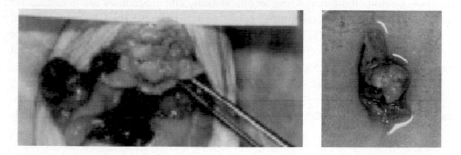

Fig. 34.5 Orthotopic model for human pancreatic cancer. The pancreas of SCID mouse is shown with large tumor during dissection *(left panel)*. The pancreas was surgically removed from the mouse, notice the nodularity of the pancreas due to tumor metastases *(right panel)*

line was injected (implanted) in the pancreas of nude mice and was found to produce local and distant dissemination with a 100% take rate and 50% metastatic behavior in nude mice (*52*). The orthotopic model of human pancreatic cancer in the SCID mouse, however, was not documented prior to our studies. We have shown that pancreatic cancer cells or tissues from human PDAC could be implanted in the pancreas of SCID mice, resulting in the development of PDAC in mice (*53*). Moreover, our laboratory has successfully investigated the subcutaneous implantation of human primary pancreatic tissue in SCID mice to evaluate the efficacy of chemotherapy. In addition, the cultured pancreatic tumor cell line HPAC, implanted in both a subcutaneous site and the pancreas, was used to study the antitumor effect of chemotherapeutic drugs, as well as gene-based therapy (*54*) (Fig. 34.6A,B). Our results strongly suggest that the subcutaneous as well as orthotopic model in SCID mice can be used to elucidate the efficacy of therapeutic agents prior to human phase II studies, and the study result obtained from these animals may facilitate the discovery of novel agents for the successful treatment of human pancreatic cancer.

Xenograft models give a reasonably good system to study cancer mutations. Among the well studied mutations, K-ras has been one of the potential targets for the development of the transgenic model, which is described later. Although xenograft mice models are very useful to study tumor development and progression, they may still not completely mimic the behavior of the original malignant cells. This phenomenon could be best explained on the basis of an interaction between tumor and surrounding host tissues (55). Tumor cells are regulated by different modes of signaling from a variety of sources, which may include stroma, endothelial, and immune cells. Therefore, when a tumor is removed from its native site these interactions are interrupted. The same is true when a tumor is implanted into a new host. Thus, the predictive utility, which is the most important concept in preclinical models, is not preserved in the most commonly used models. This highlights the urgent need for the development of a more reliable model that will emulate human PDAC. It is relatively easy to identify disadvantages of orthotopic transplantation, the most obvious limitation being technical skill. The procedures are generally far more difficult and time consuming, hence more expensive than for conventional subcutaneous (sc) models. Endpoints for determining the effects of therapy are more complex than the normal tumor measurement in sc models and ensuring that animal suffering is kept to a minimum, although essential, can be difficult.

As imaging studies are developed and improved and become more widely available, the endpoint becomes less of a problem and animal use can be reduced as the ability to follow the effects of therapy sequentially in individual animals

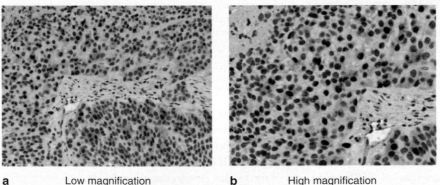

a   Low magnification   b   High magnification

Fig. 34.6 Human pancreatic tumor cells (stained with antibody to NF-kB) growing in an orthotopic model of pancreatic cancer establish in nude mice. In these unpublished photographs, sections are stained with antibody to NF-kB. The tumors are established by orthotopic transplantation of BxPC3 in nude mice. These stained sections demonstrate that the high expression of NF-kB typically seen in human tumors is maintained in the orthotopic graft. NF-kB activation has been shown to inhibit apoptosis in response to chemotherapeutic agents and ionizing radiation in cancer cells

becomes possible. The availability of new xenograft animal models for human pancreatic cancer provides an important tool for evaluating new agents, combinations, or concepts in a preclinical in vivo setting. Compared with clinical trials in humans, an investigation utilizing preclinical xenografts models is faster, less expensive, and does not involve heterogeneity of tumors that is inherent in human cancers. The development of a mouse strain deficient in both humoral and cellular immunity (SCID) has opened new avenues of research in numerous fields such as oncology, hematology, and immunology and, such, SCID mice could be utilized for the transplantation of fresh human cancer tissue or established cell lines. These are usually transient models developed for specific short-term research questions. Pancreatic cancer xenografts are often used for drug trials to determine the efficacy of new anticancer agents, natural products as well as standard chemotherapeutic drugs. These models test the effect of drugs directly on human-derived cell lines or tissues isolated from patient's tumor, which are then injected subcutaneously in several sites in SCID mice (see Fig. 34.2).

In the orthotopic model, human pancreatic cancer cells are implanted directly into the pancreas of the SCID mouse (53, 56, 57). These are the most commonly used models, but they have certain limitations. For example, not all human pancreatic cancer cells will grow in these animals for still unknown reasons. In addition, pancreatic cancer cells may retain certain molecular and histologic features of the adjacent normal cells, which may preclude the tested drug from selectively destroying the cancer cells without affecting the normal cells. Another reason to use the xenograft models is that the cancer in mice does not actually develop via a chronic pathologic process, i.e., the mice are in a more favorable health condition than patients with pancreas cancer; thus, they can better tolerate the treatment. In chemical-induced models of carcinogenesis in which tumors develop spontaneously, the chemical carcinogens are used at high doses for extended periods; therefore, death from systemic toxicity is a major concern and, as such, the relevance of a given carcinogen may not truly represent the human situation for PDAC. The overall toxic effects likely influence the actual metabolism of the tested drugs, in addition to compromising the health of the animal. Furthermore, chemical-induced carcinogenesis can be a long-term process, which makes it difficult to determine when the treatment can be started.

8   Genetically Engineered Mouse Models of Pancreatic Cancer

Genetically engineered models are the most advanced animal models of human cancers. Currently there are a number of such models that accurately mimic the pathophysiologic and molecular aspects of human malignancies. Tumors in humans develop through the accumulation of multiple genetic mutations that predispose to increased cell survival, growth, and dissemination of tumors. Therefore, the most compelling concept in preclinical testing is manipulation of the model to induce mutations that closely mimic the state of human tumors. As such, notch gene knock-in and knock-out strategies have been used successfully.

Genetically engineered mouse (GEM) models provide an in situ tumor development in an immunocompetent animal setting. They provide a promising preclinical model and have the potential to advance our understanding of the pathobiology of pancreatic tumors and our ability to develop novel tests for the early detection and new treatment modalities for pancreatic cancer. Some of the commonly used genetically engineered animal models that recapitulate human solid cancers are discussed in the following.

8.1 Transgenic Model

Mutant animals, especially mice that express oncogenes or dominant suppressive tumor suppressor genes in a nonphysiologic manner, attributing to ectopic enhancer and promoter elements, are commonly termed transgenic genetically engineered mice (58). A classical transgenic mouse is generated by pronuclear injection of cDNA constructs that contain promoter elements designed to restrict tissue tropism. This model carries most of the features of translocated or amplified proto-oncogenes. Such mice have been extremely informative in establishing and verifying the basic tenets of cancer biology and also in laying the groundwork for the development of more advanced genetically engineered models. The advantages of the transgenic mice model include the ability to reversibly regulate target gene expression with exogenous ligands such as doxycycline or interferon (59). This model system also takes advantage of the tetracycline operon. Further increasing its utility, the transgenic model has been engineered so that tetracycline, or its noncytotoxic analog doxycycline, can either promote or inhibit transcription as determined by tissue specific expression of tetracycline-regulated transcription factors. This model has been used to identify the feasibility of treating different cancers with therapeutics that target crucial oncogene, such as H-Ras, K-ras, Myc, Bcr-abl, and ErbB2/Neu (HER-2/neu) in the maintenance of melanoma (60), lung adenocarcinoma (61), AML, T-cell lymphoma (62), B-cell leukemia, and breast cancer (63), respectively. One drawback of this system is that it is difficult to influence the control necessary to induce oncogenes at physiologic levels, an important factor considering the fact that many oncogenes cause toxic effects, including senescence or apoptosis, when over-expressed in vivo.

In transgenic models, particular concern should be considered regarding the homozygous or heterozygous status of transgene carriers. These animals are frequently bred by mating a heterozygous male with a heterozygous female to increase the frequency of transgenic pups. This breeding procedure produces a mixture of homozygous and heterozygous pups. Southern blot analysis with radioactive probes is the most common method to distinguish homozygous from heterozygous pups. Because the mice bearing two alleles of one transgene may show different sensitivity to the agent to be tested, compared with those bearing only one allele, animals bred this way cannot be used for accurate testing of drug efficacy. As mentioned, pancreatic cancer can be induced by chemical carcinogens administered to the animals (*18*). For example, in the hamster, pancreatic cancer can be induced by N-nitroso-*bis*-(2-oxopropyl) amine (BOP) (*64, 65*). The tumors are ductal phenotypes with obvious fibrosis, progress rapidly with strong invasive potential, and tumor cells metastasize to the liver. Moreover, the hamster tumors also show high frequency of K-ras mutations, as seen in human pancreatic cancer. Interestingly, pancreatic cancer induced by the same chemical in mice or rats is usually acinar cell carcinoma and seldom demonstrates K-ras mutations. Thus, it is apparent that the K-ras mutation alone is not adequate to induce the full carcinogenic effect; other genes are involved. Results from other studies indicate K-ras mutation with deficiency of the p16-Ink4a, p19Arf, or p53 tumor suppressor gene, led to ductal adenocarcinomas that showed propensity to metastasize to the liver (*1*). However, it takes only one round of the breeding procedure to segregate the transgenic alleles; the second round of breeding needs to start from heterozygous breeders again, which limits the usefulness of such animal models for therapeutic purposes.

8.2   Endogenous Genetically Engineered Mice

This is a variation of the traditional transgenic mice model and consists of mutant mice that lose the expression of tumor suppressor genes from their native promoters (*58*). Pancreatic cancer has up till now received much less attention for its treatment or usage in drug-targeted development, although it is one of the leading causes of cancer deaths with incidences even higher than prostate cancer. A number of transgenic mouse models have been established, but none is perfect for drug discovery studies involving pancreatic cancers. Drug discovery studies require large numbers of animals that are of the same gender and age because it is now well recognized that the gender and age of animals influences drug metabolism. Thus, it is believed that using a single transgene model represents the best way to convene the requirement. Unfortunately, no single-transgene animal model has been established thus far that can consistently mimic PDAC. The MT100 line of *tgfα* transgenic mice has been one of the most promising models to study the prevention of pancreatic cancer. In this model female mice yield ductal proliferation with 100% penetrance at several months of age. However, in future studies efforts should be targeted toward identification of gene promoters or enhancers that are specific for ductal cells of the pancreas or even acinar cells. Efforts are needed to make these cells highly active in vivo, yielding large numbers of cells, such that a model can be utilized in testing potential molecules for discovery of new drugs. Table 34.2 gives a brief description of the available animal model systems for pancreatic cancer, highlighting their advantages as well as disadvantages. The following paragraphs also summarize additional transgenic animals that are available for therapeutic studies, indicating their advantages and disadvantages.

An international workshop, sponsored by The National Cancer Institute and the University of Pennsylvania, was held in 2004 with two main goals: (1) describing the histopathology of pancreatic exocrine neoplasia in existing genetically engineered mouse models, and (2) developing a standard nomenclature for these lesions (7). The main goal was to standardize the process of reporting pancreatic pathologic changes in genetically engineered mouse models and facilitate comparisons among these models and with that of human pancreas cancer. It is important to note that genetically engineered mice differ significantly from humans, and that mouse tumors that are histologically similar to human tumors may be genetically or biologically different.

The workshop proposed a two-phase approach to evaluate mouse models of pancreatic neoplasia. First, every affected compartment in general was described. Second, the specific pathologic changes to establish a defined diagnosis were

Table 34.2 Advantages and disadvantages of different animal models

Tumor model	Advantages	Disadvantages	Ideal for
Subcutaneous implantation	Use of human tumor cells in an in vivo system, Simple to initiate, tumor volume measurement is easy	Microenvironment differs from that of the pancreas	Assay for tumorigenicity
Orthotopic transplantation	Use of human tumor cells in an in vivo system, More closely replicates tumor microenvironment	More technically complex to initiate, Difficult to measure tumor size.	Studies of therapeutics, imaging of metastatic disease
Transgenic animal model (RCAS-TVA models)	Allows for study of single gene effects in a variety of cell types	Although quite close but still not an accurate replication of human pancreatic cancer histology	Characterization of single gene effects
Conditional K-ras mouse models	Accurately recapitulates histology, signaling pathways seen in early stages of pancreatic cancer	Cancers less genetically complex than in humans, Time consuming and expensive to maintain	Studies of chemoprevention, diagnostics, ras pathway, Ability to study effects of additional mutational events added to K-ras
Immortalized pancreatic duct cells	Retain characteristics of untransformed pancreatic duct cells	Might not represent cell of origin of pancreatic duct cancer, More difficult to maintain and manipulate in culture	Studies of single gene effects, signaling pathways, Perhaps best control for cell culture studies using pancreatic cancer cellcancer cell lines

described. This resulted in the identification of several pathologic differences between these models and human PDAC. Among these differences in ductal adenocarcinomas was that it tends in humans to be moderately or poorly differentiated, whereas in mice it is more frequently anaplastic. In addition, multi-lineage differentiation, including acinar differentiation, and multi-focality, were found to be more associated with genetically engineered mice. Moreover, pancreatic intraepithelial neoplasia in humans occurs in normal pancreatic parenchyma and is intensely desmoplastic, whereas in mice it develops in the setting of metaplasia with less frequency of desmoplasia. Research into identification of changes between genetically engineered tumors and those of human origin remains an evolving field at the present time.

9 Genetic Intervention Strategies for Preclinical Mouse Modeling

Both *Knock-out alleles,* in which a gene is deleted, and *targeted mutant alleles,* which harbor subtle mutations in the endogenous locus, are useful for modeling hereditary tumor syndromes that result from the loss of one copy of a tumor-suppressor gene (e.g., hereditary retinoblastoma) (*66*), or the subtle mutation of an oncogene or tumor-suppressor gene (e.g., familial gastrointestinal stromal tumors; GIST) (*67*). However, they may result in embryonic lethality, and hence are not ideally suited for modeling spontaneous cancers. Therefore, *conditional alleles* have been developed to allow controlled deletion, reactivation, or mutation of endogenous genes. This can be achieved through the incorporation of bacterial recombinase systems, such as Cre/lox (*68*). These enzymes catalyze either the excision or inversion of sequences flanked by associated recognition sites, depending on the relative orientation of the sites. Another model is the *conditional recombination alleles* that incorporate drug-sensitive elements (e.g., tamoxifen analogue) (*69*). This is especially useful in settings in which the genes in the target tissue/organ used for spatial restriction are expressed early in development, potentially hitting primitive cells unrelated to the origin of the targeted tumor type.

10 Evaluating Preclinical Models of Cancer

Mouse models of cancer can be used as an investigational research tool to study tumor biology, discover new therapies, and develop clinical assays. Successful candidate models for preclinical research should meet certain criteria because the principal role of these models is to substitute for human subjects in early research. Among these criteria is the ability of the system to undergo genetic manipulations that accurately reflect the known genetic mutations in patients with pancreatic cancer. This must include the maintenance of similarity in the genetics of both the targeted cells and nontargeted cells. This involves producing controlled mutations in endogenous genes in targeted cells, meanwhile leaving an effectively wild-type genotype in the nontargeted cells. These limitations in genetic manipulations should alert researchers to any subsequent phenotypic deviations.

In addition, the histology of the tumor model should be as similar as possible to that of human tumors. Moreover, pathophysiologic conditions associated with the presence of the tumor in the host, such as cachexia, should also be studied and established. Another step in animal model validation is to compare the tumor phenotype at a molecular level, including but not limited to, gene expression assessment. A very innovative approach involves administering drugs with predictable human effects to potential animal candidates. It is proposed that the experiment should be done even when such therapy is ineffective in humans, which in turn will provide an idea about the similarity between the animal model and PDAC in humans (70).

However, further considerations must be given to the histologic complexities that are observed both in human PDAC as well as different animal models. Several chemical- or transgene-induced animal models of pancreatic carcinogenesis are available. The morphologic traits of pancreatic lesions from most transgenic models have been reviewed by a bevy of pathologists in a workshop in 2004, as indicated earlier (8) and further summarized in a recent review article (6). However, only few of these transgenic models have really been studied in a systematic manner; thus, the morphologic details related to age, gender, genetic background, and hetero-/homozygous status are inadequate, suggesting that further advance research is needed in this area along with more sophisticated ultrastructural data. Human PDAC exhibits changes in a variety of genetic markers (71). In order to understand the complexities of histologic findings in human PDACs and the similarities in the animal counterpart, one must also appreciate the molecular complexities of pancreatic cancers. As such, more work is needed both in the human PDAC as well as in transgenic animal models so that therapeutic trials using animal models could emulate or predict what could happen in a human clinical trial, which is highly expensive.

11 Tumor Imaging in Mouse Models of Cancer

With spontaneous mouse models, it is often unclear which animals have developed tumors. For example, KPC mice survive between 2 and 10 months before developing PDAC. Therefore, choosing a time point at which to study the animals might result in treating numerous mice that do not harbor a tumor. Identifying an effective and noninvasive method to detect early PDAC is an optimal strategy. Almost all of the imaging techniques that are used in humans (e.g., MRI, CT, endoscopic ultrasonography, FDG-PET) have been adapted for use in small animals. In addition, techniques based on imaging genetically engineered alleles are also available, e.g., optical imaging that detects fluorescence. In short, much sophistication is still needed for animal imaging by reducing cost and ease of operational techniques, all of which will collectively advance our research for optimal uses of animal models for assessing and validating the therapeutic efficacy of novel and needed drugs that can be successfully used for the treatment of human PDAC with better survival.

12 Preclinical Studies of Novel Compounds Developed Specifically for the Treatment of Pancreatic Cancer

One of the signaling pathways generating interest in pancreatic cancer is the hedgehog pathway, which has led to the use of the small molecule inhibitor (SMI) purmorphamine for therapeutic purposes (72–75). Serum or plasma specimens could also be analyzed for the disposition of drugs and their metabolites that can also be used as surrogates for tumor exposure and tumoral concentrations of these drugs. Mouse models can also provide critical information in regard to the tissue level of the drug, despite differences in drug disposition between human and mouse models. The pharmacodynamic effect on target tissues can also be done in this context as well, through immunohistochemical and expression profiling techniques. Thus, collection of pharmacodynamic and pharmacokinetic data will aid in determining the maximum tolerated dose for mice that could be related to target effect of a given drug.

13 Example of Practical Aspects in Tumor Model Maintenance and Treatment

Currently, human pancreatic tumors are maintained in a mouse strain exhibiting severe combined immune deficiency (SCID) mice, and are transplanted into naïve groups of SCID mice for therapy trials, although transgenic animal models appear to be the future for such trials. In SCID animals all mice should weigh over 19 g at the start of therapy, and body weight for individual mice within each experiment should not vary by more than 5 g. The mice are kept in sterile conditions and supplied with sterile food and water. The food should be soft, easy to eat with a high fat content, and easily available. To initiate a study, animals are pooled and each implanted bilaterally with 30–60 mg tumor fragments injected subcutaneously by a 12-gauge trocar.

The tumor-implanted mice are again pooled before random distribution to the separate treatment and control groups. In order to check the effect of early treatment in slow-growing tumors, drug therapy is started 1–3 days after tumor implantation when the number of cancer cells is relatively small (10^7–10^8 cells). In contrast, in rapidly growing tumors (e.g., HPAC and KCI-MOH1) (54, 56) treatment should start on the day after implantation. Subcutaneous tumors should be measured three times weekly using a microcaliper. Mice are sacrificed when their tumors reach an estimated 1,500–2,000 mg to avoid animal discomfort.

14 Assessment of Antitumor Activity of an Agent

The following quantitative endpoints are frequently used to assess antitumor activity
of the subcutaneous model as described in the preceding.

14.1 Tumor Growth Delay (T-C Value) Analysis

In tumor growth delay analysis, T is the median time (in days) required for the
treatment group tumors to reach an estimated 750 mg and C is the median time (in
days) in which the tumors in the control group reach this estimated weight. For
tumor growth delay calculations (T-C), tumors need to be measured frequently,
especially if the tumor is considered as rapidly growing tumor. Some tumors have
a doubling time (Td) of 24 or 48 hours. Such tumors need to be measured at least
three times per week. Measurements of the control group need to be obtained as
soon as the tumors can be detected (100–150 mg).

14.2 Tumor Growth Inhibition (T/C Value) Analysis

For the T/C value, the median tumor mass in each group is determined at the time
when the control group's median tumor mass is ~750 mg. A T/C value ≤0.42% is
considered to represent significant antitumor activity and <10% is considered a
high antitumor activity, as determined by the National Cancer Institute-Drug
Evaluation Branch of the Division of Cancer Treatment. The T/C percent value is
a surrogate for antitumor efficacy of a tested drug. This size range of tumor burden
was chosen for it represents tumors in exponential growth phase. Calculation performed
during this growth phase is ideal, for as the tumor grows, the tumor-doubling time
will become longer and the true efficacy of a targeted drug cannot be accurately
determined. One reason for the increased doubling time is that tumors destroy their
own blood supply, thus limiting their oxygen and nutrient supply, and hence slowing
growth. In order to get reliable exponential tumor doubling time, early measurements
of subcutaneous tumors in the control group are needed. The Td is essential to
calculate the Log10 tumor cell kill. As for slow growing tumors, when their
doubling time is >60 hours, twice a week measurements are enough.

14.3 Tumor Cell Kill (Total) Analysis

The $\log_{10}$ cell kill can be calculated from the following equation:

$$\text{Log}_{10} \text{ cell kill (total)} = (T-C)/(3.32)\,(Td)$$

where, $T - C$ = tumor growth delay (in days), Td = tumor volume doubling time (in days), and 3.32 is a constant value. Td can be calculated using a log-linear growth plot of estimated tumor size from the untreated-group measured during exponential growth phase (200–1,000 mg).

14.4 Log_{10} Cell Kill (net) = $(T - C)$ – (treatment duration)/ (3.32) (Td)

The net Log_{10} cell kill for the treatment duration (in days) can be determined by using the above equation, the value of the log_{10} cell kill (total) is usually higher compared with the log_{10} cell kill (net). This is due to the subtraction of treatment days from tumor growth delay. It is important that the same person on a given experiment performs these measurements, since different people have different way of measuring subcutaneous tumors using the same caliper.

14.5 Percent Increase in Host Life Span for Orthotopic Models

In orthotopic models, in which one cannot measure the tumor diameters using calipers, percent increased life span (%ILS) is usually used as endpoint for assessing antitumor activity of an agent. %ILS can be calculated as follows: (%ILS) = 100 (MDD (median day of death of the treated tumor-bearing mice) – (MDD of the tumor-bearing control mice)/MDD of the tumor bearing control mice. It is worth noting that body weight loss of $\geq 20\%$ in treated animals is used to indicate an excessively toxic dose in most single-course trials.

15 Summary

The development of xenograft models enabled rapid and facile in vivo assessment of tumor tissue and cell lines in immunocompromised mice. Indeed patient-specific models have recently been proposed as a means to prospectively personalize treatment regimens. Gene knock-out and gene alterations in mice will not only provide insights into neoplastic mechanisms, but could also be used for personalized and targeted therapy. Human pancreatic tumor xenografts (orthotopic or subcutaneous) will still be useful for drug discovery and development based on the sophisticated mechanistic understanding of the genetic makeup of tumor cells as well as molecular targeting for therapy. On the other hand, the transgenic mouse models of pancreatic cancer that utilize conditional knock-in of the K-ras oncogene have already provided strong evidence supporting that PanIN lesions are the precursor lesions to invasive PDAC. This further suggests that the presence of a previously unrecognized cell population that expresses transcription factors could be critically important, not only in pancreatic development and lineage specification, but also on elucidating the cell of origin for PDAC for further refinement of the model for therapeutic trials. Overall, pancreatic cancer recovery remains rare because of the genetic complexity and resultant biologic aggressiveness of the disease. The recent advancement of tools for pancreatic cancer investigation outlined herein suggest the promise of more rapid progress toward understanding the crucial events in pancreatic carcinogenesis, and the methods to detect and target them successfully in order to have an impact in the lives of patients diagnosed with this devastating disease and the lives of their families and friends.

Acknowledgments The authors would like to thank Dr. Goustin for helping to prepare this chapter. The National Cancer Center Institute, NIH grant R01CA109389 (RM Mohammad) and Leukemia and Lymphoma Society grant 8028-07 (RM Mohammad) are acknowledged.

References

1. Hezel AF, Kimmelman AC, Stanger BZ, et al. 2006, Genetics and biology of pancreatic ductal adenocarcinoma. Genes Dev 20:1218–1249.
2. Tuveson DA, Hingorani SR. 2005, Ductal pancreatic cancer in humans and mice. Cold Spring Harbor Symp Quant Biol 70:65–72.
3. Pour PM, Standop J, Batra SK. 2002, Are islet cells the gatekeepers of the pancreas? Pancreatology 2:440–448.
4. Schmid RM. 2002, Acinar-to-ductal metaplasia in pancreatic cancer development. J Clin Invest 109:1403–1404.
5. Andea A, Sarkar F, Adsay VN. 2003, Clinicopathological correlates of pancreatic intraepithelial neoplasia: a comparative analysis of 82 cases with and 152 cases without pancreatic ductal adenocarcinoma. Mod Pathol 16:996–1006.
6. Hruban RH, Adsay NV, Albores-Saavedra J, et al. 2001, Pancreatic intraepithelial neoplasia: a new nomenclature and classification system for pancreatic duct lesions. Am J Surg Pathol 25:579–586.
7. Hruban RH, Adsay NV, Albores-Saavedra J, et al. 2006a, Pathology of genetically engineered mouse models of pancreatic exocrine cancer: consensus report and recommendations. Cancer Res 66:95–106.
8. Hruban RH, Rustgi AK, Brentnall TA, et al. 2006b, Pancreatic cancer in mice and man: the Penn Workshop 2004. Cancer Res 2006b, 66:14–17.
9. Guerra C, Schuhmacher AJ, Canamero M, et al. 2007, Chronic pancreatitis is essential for induction of pancreatic ductal adenocarcinoma by K-Ras oncogenes in adult mice. Cancer Cell 11:291–302.
10. Park HW, Chae YM, Shin TS. 1992, Morphogenic development of the pancreas in the staged human embryo. Yonsei Med J 33:104–108.
11. Kawakami Y, Raya A, Raya RM, et al. 2005, Retinoic acid signalling links left-right asymmetric patterning and bilaterally symmetric somatogenesis in the zebrafish embryo. Nature 435:165–171.
12. Leach SD. 2995, Epithelial differentiation in pancreatic development and neoplasia: new niches for nestin and Notch. J Clin Gastroenterol 39:S78–82.
13. Miyamoto Y, Maitra A, Ghosh B, et al. 2003, Notch mediates TGF alpha-induced changes in epithelial differentiation during pancreatic tumorigenesis. Cancer Cell 3:565–576.

14. Murtaugh LC, Stanger BZ, Kwan KM, et al. 2003, Notch signaling controls multiple steps of pancreatic differentiation. Proc Natl Acad Sci U S A 100:14920–14925.
15. Means AL, Meszoely IM, Suzuki K, et al. 2005, Pancreatic epithelial plasticity mediated by acinar cell transdifferentiation and generation of nestin-positive intermediates. Development (Cambridge, England) 132:3767–3776.
16. Hingorani SR, Petricoin EF, Maitra A, et al. 2003, Preinvasive and invasive ductal pancreatic cancer and its early detection in the mouse. Cancer Cell 4:437–450.
17. Tuveson DA, Shaw AT, Willis NA, et al. 2004, Endogenous oncogenic K-ras (G12D) stimulates proliferation and widespread neoplastic and developmental defects. Cancer Cell 5:375–387.
18. Leach SD. 2004, Mouse models of pancreatic cancer: the fur is finally flying! Cancer Cell 5:7–11.
19. Pasca di Magliano M, Sekine S, Ermilov A, et al. 2006, Hedgehog/Ras interactions regulate early stages of pancreatic cancer. Genes Dev 20:3161–3173.
20. Kim SK, Hebrok M, Melton DA. 1997, Notochord to endoderm signaling is required for pancreas development. Development (Cambridge, England) 124:4243–4252.
21. Scharfmann R. 2000, Control of early development of the pancreas in rodents and humans: implications of signals from the mesenchyme. Diabetologia 43:1083–1092.
22. Hahn SA, Schutte M, Hoque AT, et al. 1996, DPC4, a candidate tumor suppressor gene at human chromosome 18q21.1. Science 271:350–353.
23. Hoglund M, Gorunova L, Jonson T, et al. 1998, Cytogenetic and FISH analyses of pancreatic carcinoma reveal breaks in 18q11 with consistent loss of 18q12-qter and frequent gain of 18p. Br J Cancer 77:1893–1899.
24. Dammann R, Schagdarsurengin U, Liu L, et al. 2003, Frequent RASSF1A promoter hypermethylation and K-ras mutations in pancreatic carcinoma. Oncogene 22:3806–3812.
25. Dugan MC, Dergham ST, Kucway R, et al. 1997, HER-2/neu expression in pancreatic adenocarcinoma: relation to tumor differentiation and survival. Pancreas 14:229–236.
26. Day JD, Diguiseppe JA, Yeo C. 1996, Immunohistochemical evaluation of Her–2/neu expression in pancreatic adenocarcinoma and pancreatic intraepithelial neoplasia. Human Pathol 27:119–124.
27 Kirsch DG, Kastan MB. 1998, Tumor suppressor p53: implication for tumor development and prognosis. J Clin Oncol 16:3158–3168.
28. Dergham ST, Dugan MC, Joshi US, et al. 1997a, The clinical significance of p21(WAF1/CIP-1) and p53 expression in pancreatic adenocarcinoma. Cancer 80:372–381.
29. Jonson T. Gorunova L, Dawiskiba S, et al. 1999, Molecular analyses of the 15q and 18q SMAD genes in pancreatic cancer. Genes Chromosomes Cancer 24:62–71.
30. Takaku K, Oshima M, Miyoshi H, et al. 1998, Intestinal tumorigenesis in compound mutant mice of both Dpc4 (Smad4) and Apc genes. Cell 92:645–656.
31. Caldas C, Hahn SA, Da Costa LT, et al. 1994, Frequent somatic mutations and homozygous deletions of the p16 (MTS1) gene in pancreatic adenocarcinoma. Nat Genet 8:27–32.
32. Schutte M, Hruban RH, Geradts J, et al. 1997, Abrogation of the Rb/p16 tumor–suppressive pathway in virtually all pancreatic carcinomas. Cancer Res 57:3126–3130.
33. Ueki T, Toyota M, Sohn T, et al. 2000, Hypermethylation of multiple genes in pancreatic adenocarcinoma. Cancer Res 60:1835–1839.
34. Gerdes B, Ramaswamy A, Ziegler A, et al. 2002, P16[INK4a] is a prognostic marker in resected ductal pancreatic cancer: An Analysis of p16[INK4a], p53, MDM2, an Rb. Ann Surg 235:51–59.
35. Bardeesy N, Aguirre AJ, Chu GC, et al. 2006, Both p16. Ink4a and the p19[Arf]-p53 pathway constrain progression of pancreatic adenocarcinoma in the mouseProc Natl Acad Sci U S A 103:5947–5952.
36. Bardeesy N, Cheng KH, Berger JH, et al. 2006, Smad4 is dispensable for normal pancreas development yet critical in progression and tumor biology of pancreas cancer. Genes Dev 20:3130–3146.
37. Slack JM. 1995, Developmental biology of the pancreas. Development 121:1569–1580.
38. Almoguera C, Shibata D, Forrester K, et al. 1988, Most human carcinomas of the exocrine pancreas contain mutant c-K-ras genes. Cell 53:549–554.

39. Berrozpe G, Schaeffer J, Peinado MA, et al. 1994, Comparative analysis of mutations in the p53 and K-ras genes in pancreatic cancer. Int J Cancer 58:185–191.
40. Lilja HS, Hyde E, Longnecker DS, et al. 1977, DNA damage and repair in rat tissues following administration of azaserine. Cancer Res 37:3925–3931.
41. Pour P, Mohr U, Cardesa A, et al. 1975, Pancreatic neoplasms in an animal model: morphological, biological, and comparative studies. Cancer 36:379–389.
42. Cerny WL, Mangold KA, Scarpelli DG. 1992, K-ras mutation is an early event in pancreatic duct carcinogenesis in the Syrian golden hamster. Cancer Res 52:4507–4513.
43. Fujii H, Egami H, Chaney W, et al. 1990, Pancreatic ductal adenocarcinomas induced in Syrian hamsters by N-nitrosobis(2-oxopropyl)amine contain a c-Ki-ras oncogene with a point-mutated codon 12. Mol Carcinogen 3:296–301.
44. Sugio K, Gazdar AF, Albores-Saavedra J, et al. 1996, High yields of K-ras mutations in intraductal papillary mucinous tumors and invasive adenocarcinomas induced by N-nitroso(2-hydroxypropyl)(2-oxopropyl)amine in the pancreas of female Syrian hamsters. Carcinogenesis 17:303–309.
45. van Kranen HJ, Vermeulen E, Schoren L, et al. 1991, Activation of c-K-ras is frequent in pancreatic carcinomas of Syrian hamsters, but is absent in pancreatic tumors of rats. Carcinogenesis 12:1477–1482.
46. Clapper ML, Wood M, Leahy K, et al. 1995, Chemopreventive activity of Oltipraz against N-nitrosobis(2-oxopropyl)amine (BOP)-induced ductal pancreatic carcinoma development and effects on survival of Syrian golden hamsters. Carcinogenesis 16:2159–2165.
47. Zalatnai A, Schally AV. 1990, Hepatic lesions in Syrian golden hamsters with pancreatic carcinoma induced by N-nitrosobis(2-oxopropyl)amine (BOP). Acta Morphologica Hungarica 38:119–130.
48. Siveke JT, Schmid RM. 2005, Chromosomal instability in mouse metastatic pancreatic cancer —it's K-ras and Tp53 after all. Cancer Cell 7:405–407.
49. Rivera JA, Graeme-Cook F, Werner J, et al. 1997, A rat model of pancreatic ductal adenocarcinoma: targeting chemical carcinogens. Surgery 122:82–90.
50. Fogh J, Orfeo T, Tiso J, et al. 1980, Twenty three new human tumor cell lines established in nude mice. Exp Cell Biol 48:229–239.
51. Sordat BC, Ueyama Y, Fogh J, et al. 1982, Metastasis of tumor xenografts in the nude mouse. In: Fogh J, Giovanella BC (eds.) The nude mouse in experimental and clinical research. vol 2, Academic Press, New York, 95–143.
52. Reyes G, Villanueva S, Garcia C, et al. 1996, Orthotopic xenografts of human pancreatic carcinomas aquire genetic abbrations during dissemination of nude mice. Cancer Res 56: 5713–5719.
53. Mohammad RM, Al-Katib A, Pettit GR, et al. 1998a, An orthotopic model of human pancreatic cancer in severe combined immunodeficient mice: potential application for preclinical studies. Clin Cancer Res 4:887–894.
54. Mohammad RM, Dugan MC, Mohamed AN, et al. 1998b, Establishment of a human pancreatic tumor xenograft model: potential application for preclinical evaluation of novel therapeutic agents. Pancreas 16:19–25.
55. Hanahan D, Weinberg RA. 200, The hallmarks of cancer. Cell 100:57–70.
56. Mohammad RM, Li Y, Mohamed AN, et al. 1999, Clonal preservation of human pancreatic cell line derived from primary pancreatic adenocarcinoma. Pancreas 19:353–361.
57. Shono M, Sato N, Mizumoto K, et al. 2001, Stepwise progression of centrosome defects associated with local tumor growth and metastatic process of human pancreatic carcinoma cells transplanted orthotopically into nude mice. Lab Invest J Tech Meth Pathol 81:945–952.
58. Tuveson DA, Jacks T. 2002, Technologically advanced cancer modeling in mice. Curr Opin Genet Dev 12:105–110.
59. Kuhn R, Schwenk F, Aguet M, et al. 1995, Inducible gene targeting in mice. Science 269:1427–1429.
60. Chin L, Tam A, Pomerantz J, et al. 1999, Essential role of oncogenic ras in tumor maintenance. Nature 400:468–472.

61. Fisher GH, Wellen SL, Klimstra D, et al. 2001, Induction and apoptotic regression of lung adenocarcinomas by regulation of a K-Ras transgene in the presence and absence of tumor suppressor genes. Genes Dev 15:3249–3262.
62. Felsher DW, Bishop JM. 1999, Reversible tumorigenesis by MYC in hematopoietic lineages. Mol Cell 4:199–207.
63. Moody SE, Sarkisian CJ, Hahn KT. 2002, Conditional activation of Neu in mammary epithelium of transgenic mice results in reversible pulmonary metastasis. Cancer Cell 2:451–461.
64. Kokkinakis DM, Scarpelli DG, Rao MS, 1983, Metabolism of pancreatic carcinogens N-nitroso-2,6-dimethylmorpholine and N-nitrosobis(2-oxopropyl)amine by microsomes and cytosol of hamster pancreas and liver. Cancer Res 43:5761–5767.
65. Kokkinakis DM, Wieboldt R, Hollenberg PF, et al. 1987, Structural relationships of pancreatic nitrosamine carcinogens. Carcinogenesis 8:81–90.
66. Clarke AR, Maandag ER, van Roon M, et al. 1992, Requirement for a functional Rb-1 gene in murine development. Nature 359:328–330.
67. Cristofano A, Di Pesce B, Cordon-Cardo C, et al. 1998, Pten is essential for embryonic development and tumour suppression. Nat Genet 19:348–355.
68. Orban PC, Chui D, Marth JD. 1992, Tissue- and site-specific DNA recombination in transgenic mice. Proc Natl Acad Sci U S A 89:6861–6865.
69. Indra AK, Warot X, Brocard J, et al. 1999, Temporally-controlled site-specific mutagenesis in the basal layer of the epidermis: comparison of the recombinase activity of the tamoxifen–inducible Cre–ER(T) and Cre–ER(T2) recombinases. Nucleic Acids Res 27:4324–4327.
70. Olive KP, Tuveson DA. 2006, The use of targeted mouse models for preclinical testing of novel cancer therapeutics. Clin Cancer Res 12:5277–5287.
71. Maitra A, Kern SE, Hruban RH. 2006, Molecular pathogenesis of pancreatic cancer. Best Pract Res Clin Gastroenterol 20:211–226.
72. Briscoe J. 2006, Agonizing hedgehog. Nat Chem Biol 2:10–11.
73. Riobo NA, Saucy B, Dilizio C, et al. 2006, Activation of heterotrimeric G proteins by Smoothened. Proc Natl Acad Sci U S A 103:12607–12612.
74. Sinha S, Chen JK. 2006, Purmorphamine activates the Hedgehog pathway by targeting Smoothened. Nature Chem Biol 2:29–30.
75. Weitzman JB. 2002, Agonizing hedgehog. J Biol 1:7.
76. Dergham ST, Dugan MC, Kucway R, 1997b, Prevalence and clinical significance of combined K-ras mutation and p53 aberration in pancreatic adenocarcinoma. Int J Pancreatol 21:127–143.
77. Luttges J, Schlehe B, Menke MA, et al. 1999, The K-ras mutation pattern in pancreatic ductal adenocarcinoma usually is identical to that in associated normal, hyperplastic, and metaplastic ductal epithelium. Cancer 85:1703–1710.
78. Attri J, Srinivasan R, Majumdar S, et al. 2005, Alterations of tumor suppressor gene p16INK4a in pancreatic ductal carcinoma. BMC Gastroenterol 5:22.
79. Huang L, Goodrow TL, Zhang SY, et al. 1996, Deletion and mutation analyses of the P16/MTS-1 tumor suppressor gene in human ductal pancreatic cancer reveals a higher frequency of abnormalities in tumor-derived cell lines than in primary ductal adenocarcinomas. Cancer Res 56:1137–1141.
80. Li Y, Bhuiyan M, Vaitkevicius VK, et al. 1998, Molecular analysis of the p53 gene in pancreatic adenocarcinoma. Diagn Mol Pathol 7:4–9.
81. Brentnall TA, Bronner MP, Byrd DR, et al. 1999, Early diagnosis and treatment of pancreatic dysplasia in patients with a family history of pancreatic cancer. Ann Int Med 131:247–255.
82. Pogue-Geile KL, Chen R, Bronner MP, et al. 2006, Palladin mutation causes familial pancreatic cancer and suggests a new cancer mechanism. PLoS Med 3:e516.
83. Yamano M, Fujii H, Takagaki T, et al. 2000, Genetic progression and divergence in pancreatic carcinoma. Am J Pathol 156:2123–2133.
84. Ruggeri BA, Huang L, Berger D, et al. 1997, Molecular pathology of primary and metastatic ductal pancreatic lesions: analyses of mutations and expression of the p53, mdm-2, and p21/WAF-1 genes in sporadic and familial lesions. Cancer 79:700–716.

Chapter 35
K-ras Inhibitors and Pancreatic Cancer

Steven R. Alberts

1 Introduction

The ras family includes a group of five guanosine triphosphate-binding proteins (H-ras, K-ras, M-ras, N-ras, and R-ras). In mammals ras-proto-oncogenes encode for four related and highly conserved proteins, H-ras, N-ras, K-ras 4A, and K-ras 4B (1). Ras proteins serve as important components of signaling pathways involved in a variety of cellular functions, including cell cycle control, cell adhesion, endocytosis, exocytosis, and apoptosis. In order for these proteins to perform their functions they need to bind guanosine triphosphate (GTP) (2). Guanosine triphosphate creates a conformational change allowing ras to attach more tightly to its intended target. Hydrolysis of GTP to guanosine diphosphate (GDP) inactivates ras. The ability of ras to exchange GDP for GTP is under the control of guanine nucleotide exchange factors (GEFs). The GEFs are activated by growth factors or cytokines and promote the release of GDP and therefore the binding of GTP. GTPase-activating proteins (GAPs) return ras to its inactive state.

Although a variety of genetic modifications have been identified in pancreatic carcinoma, mutations of K-ras are by far the most commonly occurring mutation. Mutations are seen in >85% of pancreatic ductal carcinomas (3). The development of mutations in K-ras appear early in the development of pancreatic cancer, having been observed in precursor lesions within the pancreatic duct (4). The mutations in K-ras in pancreatic cancer are also unique in that it typically involves codon 12, but may also rarely involve codons 13 or 61 (5, 6). These mutations in K-ras make it resistant to GAP and as a result lead to constitutive activation of downstream pathways, resulting in altered regulation of cellular proliferation. In preclinical studies, using the pancreatic cancer cell lines Panc-1 and MiaPaca-2, blocking activated K-ras resulted in increased apoptosis and loss of other malignant features supporting a pivotal role for K-ras in the development and maintenance the malignant phenotype.

Based on the frequency and apparent critical role of K-ras in pancreatic cancer several approaches have been developed to block activated K-ras. This includes both farnesyl transferase inhibitors and antisense oligonucleotides.

A.M. Lowy et al. (eds.) *Pancreatic Cancer.*
doi: 10.1007/978-0-387-69252-4, © Springer Science+Business Media, LLC 2008

2   Farnesyltransferase Inhibitors

In order for ras proteins to properly associate to the cell membrane they must undergo prenylation (7). This process involves the addition of a farnesyl isoprenoid to ras by the enzyme farnesyltransferase (FTase) and is a critical step in the post-translational modification of ras. The use of farnesyltransferase inhibitors (FTIs) inhibited cell growth in 70% of cancer cell lines tested in one previously reported preclinical study. This effect was independent of ras mutation status, with both mutated and wild-type ras showing a response to the FTIs (8). The use of FTIs appears to result in a gradual cell cycle block with eventual cell cycle arrest consistent with the progressive depletion of activated ras (9).

The FTIs can be divided into three categories of agents based on their mechanism of action. These categories include competitive inhibitors of farnesyl pyrophosphate (FPP), competitive inhibitors of CAAX, and analogs that have both of these properties (10). FPP is an enzyme involved in catalyzing protein prenylation by serving as the isoprenoid donor. The terminal amino acid sequence CAAX (C = cytosine, A = any aliphatic amino acid, X = serine or methionine) serves as the site of farnesylation and is present in all members of the ras family. For any of these inhibitors to appropriately exert their antineoplastic activity they must be given in a way that provides continuous exposure to the drug and thereby blocks the ongoing process of ras-related signal transduction.

The CAAX inhibitor SCH66336 is an orally bioavailable agent that has been assessed in a series of phase I and II trials. In vitro it is a potent inhibitor of cell lines with K-ras mutations, other ras mutations, and wild-type ras (11). Phase I trials in patients with non-hematologic cancers have been performed. In a trial of a 7-day administration every 3 weeks gastrointestinal toxicity (nausea, vomiting, and diarrhea) and fatigue were dose limiting (12). This trial also showed evidence of inhibition of farnesylation in buccal cells from patients treated in the trial. In two other trials of continuous daily administration similar toxicity was noted together with reversible myelosuppression and neurocortical toxicity (13, 14). In a subsequent phase I trial SCH66336 was combined with gemcitabine and showed gastrointestinal toxicity and moderate myelosuppression as the most common toxicities (15). Although no phase II or III trials with SCH66336 have been reported for pancreatic cancer, preclinical assessment with xenografts have shown activity with this tumor type (11).

Another CAAX inhibitor, R115777, has been evaluated in a clinical trial for pancreatic cancer. Whereas SCH66336 is a tricyclic drug derived from an anti-histamine lead compound, R115777 is a quinoline that was originally developed as an anti-fungal agent (16). Initial evidence of activity was noted in preclinical studies including pancreatic cancer xenografts (17). In subsequent phase I trials a variety of dosing schedules have been evaluated, including twice daily for 5 days every 2 weeks, twice daily for 21 days every 4 weeks, and continuous dosing (18–21). Early evidence of activity in pancreatic cancer was noted in these trials. The dose limiting toxicities were similar to those noted for SCH66336. A subsequent phase

I trial established a schedule for gemcitabine and R115777 (22). Evidence of activity in pancreatic cancer was also noted in this trial.

In a phase II trial of patients with previously untreated metastatic pancreatic cancer, R115777 was given as a twice daily dose of 300 mg for 21 days every 4 weeks. Twenty patients were accrued to this trial. No objective responses were seen. The median survival time was 19.7 weeks. Only a partial inhibition of farnesylation was observed in peripheral blood mononuclear cells obtained from patients enrolled in this trial (23). In a separate phase II trial of R115777 using the same dosing schedule, 58 patients with previously untreated either locally advanced or metastatic pancreatic cancer enrolled (24). In 53 evaluable patients from this trial a median survival of 2.6 months was reported.

While the phase II trials were underway a phase III trial of gemcitabine and R115777 was also undertaken. Using a randomized, double-blind, placebo-controlled design patients with previously untreated locally advanced, unresectable or meta-static pancreatic cancer were randomized to either gemcitabine and placebo or gemcitabine and R115777 (25). The R115777 was given at a dose of 200 mg twice a day continuously. The gemcitabine was given at a dose of 1,000 mg/m^2 over 30 minutes weekly for 7 weeks followed by a 1-week break for the first cycle and then weekly for 3 weeks followed by a 1-week break for subsequent cycles. A total of 688 patients were enrolled from 126 sites in 14 countries. Of these patients, 341 received gemcitabine and R115777 and 347 received gemcitabine and placebo. Median overall survival was the primary endpoint, with those receiving R115777 living 193 days versus 182 days for those receiving placebo ($p = 0.75$). No mean-ingful difference was seen in other endpoints including progression-free survival, response rate, or time-to-performance status deterioration.

Other FTIs are being evaluated for cancer in general. This includes L-778,123, a drug that blocks both FTase and geranylgernanyltransferase I (26). A combination of L-778,123 and radiation was recently evaluated in a phase I trial for patients with locally advanced pancreatic cancer (27). Although the combination was reasonably well tolerated, only limited efficacy was noted.

At this point the role of FTIs in the treatment of pancreatic cancer remains uncertain. The initial trials, including a phase III trial, do not show meaningful clinical results. Further work will be needed to determine if FTIs in combination with other targeted therapy may be of benefit.

3   Ras-Directed Antisense Therapy for Pancreatic Cancer

As the molecular changes leading to the development and progression of cancer have become more clearly understood a greater focus on molecular or targeted therapy has developed, with a large variety of approaches currently under evalua-tion. One potential approach of interest focuses on the use of oligonucleotides to interfere with the expression of RNA (28). Specifically, antisense oligonucleotides have been created that are able to bind to a complimentary target RNA and inhibits

its expression, thereby limiting the synthesis of proteins believed to be important in the development and progression of cancer. In general, this approach has led to a reduction of protein overexpression, but not complete elimination of protein synthesis (*29*). In this manner normal physiologic expression is preserved, thereby limiting potentially therapy-related toxicities. Other potential approaches with oligonucleotides have used the oligonucleotides as decoy binding sites (*30*). Support for this approach comes from both preclinical studies as well as the recognition of naturally occurring antisense RNAs that serve to regulate gene expression (*31*).

Early development of antisense oligonucleotides began in the late 1970s with the creation of an oligonucleotide sequence complementary to a portion of the Rous sarcoma virus that effectively blocked viral replication in fibroblasts (*32, 33*). Over the next two decades a large amount of preclinical data was generated on the use of this approach in many different settings. Based on a review of this work and its potential importance, the use of antisense oligonucleotides and their role in post-transcriptional gene silencing was recognized as the breakthrough of the year by *Science* in 2002 (*34*). In particular, the results of research in this field were recognized for the surprising ability of small RNA molecules to control DNA expression by shutting down genes or altering their levels of expression. The application of this technology to a number of medical fields is currently being investigated. However, only one antisense-based therapy has received full approval by the Food and Drug Administration (FDA). Fomivirsen (Vitravene™) was developed to target the major immediate-early gene of cytomegalovirus (CMV) as a means of treating CMV-induced retinitis in patients with acquired immunodeficiency syndrome (*35*).

A variety of the antisense oligonucleotides developed that have potential applicability in pancreatic cancer, including several directed at ras. Given the high frequency of K-ras mutation, particularly in one codon, therapeutic approaches that are very specific may be of greater benefit. Although an antisense oligonucleotide against K-ras has been developed (*36–38*), no antisense oligonucleotides directed specifically against K-ras have entered clinical trials for pancreatic cancer. However, an antisense oligonucleotide directed against H-ras has been evaluated in a phase II trial, based on in part on the preclinical observation that H-ras modulates mutated K-ras. The H-ras antisense inhibitor ISIS 2503 (phosphorothioate 29-oligodeoxyribonucleotide) is 20 nucleotides long and is designed to hybridize to a sequence in the initiation translation region of the human H-ras mRNA (*39*). Once hybridized to its target ISIS 2503 renders the hybridized mRNA amenable to degradation by RNaseH. Initial preclinical evaluation of ISIS 2503 showed activity inhibiting proliferation of cultured T24 bladder cells (*40*). Subsequent evaluation of ISIS 2503 in xenograft models showed activity against Mia-PaCa-2, a tumor known to possess K-ras mutations (*41*).

Following the establishment of appropriate schedules of administration for ISIS 2,503 as a single agent in phase I trials (*41, 42*), a phase I trial of ISIS 2503 combined with gemcitabine was performed (*43*). This trial established a schedule of gemcitabine 1,000 mg/m^2 on days 1 and 8 and ISIS 2503 6 mg/kg/day as a 14-day continuous infusion starting on day 1. Although neutropenia and thrombocytopenia were frequently encountered with this combination, no dose-limiting toxicity was incurred in this trial. Building on this phase I trial, a phase II trial of ISIS 2503 with gemcitabine for patients with locally advanced or metastatic pancreatic cancer was undertaken (*44*). A total of 48 patients were enrolled, of which 43 had metastatic disease. The median overall survival was 6.7 months, with one patient having a complete response and four patients having partial responses. These measures of outcomes were similar to those expected from gemcitabine alone indicating that ISIS 2503 provided no additional benefit.

4 Conclusion

Mutations in ras, particularly K-ras, are an early and apparent critical step in the development of pancreatic cancer. Therapeutic approaches directed at ras, with either FTIs or antisense oligonucleotides, have not made a meaningful change in patient outcomes. The reason for the lack of benefit remains unclear, although it is likely that other molecular changes may be able to overcome selective attempts to block overexpression of ras. Further work is needed to determine the potential role of ras-directed agents in combination with other targeted therapies for a cancer in which little progress has been made.

Reference

1. Lowy DR, Williamson BM. 1993, Function and regulation of ras. Annu Rev Biochem 62:851–891.
2. Wittinghofer A, Scheffzek K, Ahmadian MR. 1997, The interaction of Ras with GTPase-activating proteins. FEBS Letts 410:63–67.
3. Rozenblum E, Schutte M, Goggins M, 1997, Tumor-suppressive pathways in pancreatic carcinoma. Cancer Res 57:1731–1734.
4. Moskaluk CA, Hruban RH, Kern SE. 1997, p16 and K-ras gene mutations in the intraductal precursors of human pancreatic adenocarcinoma. Cancer Res 57:2140–2143.
5. Sakorafas GH. 1999, Pancreatic cancer. In: Kurzrock R, Talpaz M (eds.) Molecular biology in cancer medicine, 2nd ed. London, Martin Dunitz Ltd, 393–409.
6. Bos JL. 1989, ras oncogenes in human cancer: a review. Cancer Res 49:4682–4689.
7. Kato K, Cox AD, Hisaka MM, et al.1992, Isoprenoid addition to Ras protein is the critical modification for its membrane association and transforming activity. Proc Natl Acad Sci USA 89:6403–6407.
8. Sepp-Lorenzino L, Ma Z, Rands E, et al. 1995, A peptidomimetic inhibitor of farnesyl:protein transferase blocks the anchorage-dependent and -independent growth of human tumor cell lines. Cancer Res 55:5302–5309.
9. Moasser MM, Sepp-Lorenzino L, Kohl NE, et al. 1998, Farnesyl transferase inhibitors cause enhanced mitotic sensitivity to taxol and epothilones. Proc Natl Acad Sci U S A 95:1369–1374.
10. Crul M, Klerk GJ, de Beijnen JH, et al. 2001, Ras biochemistry and farnesyl transferase inhibitors: a literature survey. Anti-Cancer Drugs 12:163–184.
11. Liu M, Bryant MS, Chen J, et al. 1998, Antitumor activity of SCH 66336, an orally bioavailable tricyclic inhibitor of farnesyl protein transferase, in human tumor xenograft models and wap-ras transgenic mice. Cancer Res 58:4947–4956.

12. Adjei AA, Erlichman C, Davis JN, et al. 2000, A phase I trial of the farnesyl transferase inhibitor SCH66336: Evidence for biological and clinical activity. Cancer Res 60:1871–1877.
13. Awada A, Eskens F, Piccart M, et al. 2002, Phase I and pharmacological study of the oral farnesyltransferase inhibitor SCH 66336 given once daily to patients with advanced solid tumours. Eur J Cancer 38:2272–2278.
14. Eskens F, Awada A, Cutler DL, et al. 2001, Phase I and pharmacokinetic study of the oral farnesyl transferase inhibitor SCH 66336 given twice daily to patients with advanced solid tumors. J Clin Oncol 19:1167–1175.
15. Hurwitz H, Amado R, Prager D, et al. 2000, Phase I trial of the farnesyl transferase inhibitor SCH66336 plus gemcitabine in advanced cancers (abstract 717). Proc Am Soc Clin Oncol, 185a.
16. Venet M, End D, Angibaud P. et al. 2003, Farnesyl protein transferase inhibitor ZARNESTRA R115777—history of a discovery. Curr Top Med Chem 3:1095–1102.
17. End DW, Smets G, Todd AV, et al. 2001, Characterization of the antitumor effects of the selective farnesyl protein transferase inhibitor R115777 in vivo and in vitro. Cancer Res 61:131–137.
18. Crul M, Klerk GJ, de Swart M, et al. 2002, Phase I clinical and pharmacologic study of chronic oral administration of the farnesyl protein transferase inhibitor R115777 in advanced cancer. J Clin Oncol 20:2726–2735.
19. Lara PN, Jr., Law LY, Wright JJ, et al. 2005, Intermittent dosing of the farnesyl transferase inhibitor tipifarnib (R115777) in advanced malignant solid tumors: a phase I California Cancer Consortium Trial. Anti-Cancer Drugs 16:317–321.
20. Zujewski J, Horak ID, Bol CJ, et al. 2000, Phase I and pharmacokinetic study of farnesyl protein transferase inhibitor R115777 in advanced cancer. J Clin Oncol 18:927–941.
21. Punt CJ, van Maanen L, Bol CJ, et al. 2001, Phase I and pharmacokinetic study of the orally administered farnesyl transferase inhibitor R115777 in patients with advanced solid tumors. Anti-Cancer Drugs 12:193–197.
22. Patnaik A, Eckhardt SG, Izbicka E, et al. 2003, A phase I, pharmacokinetic, and biological study of the farnesyltransferase inhibitor tipifarnib in combination with gemcitabine in patients with advanced malignancies. Clin Cancer Res 9:4761–4771.
23. Cohen SJ, Ho L, Ranganathan S, et al. 2003, Phase II and pharmacodynamic study of the farnesyltransferase inhibitor R115777 as initial therapy in patients with metastatic pancreatic adenocarcinoma. J Clin Oncol 21:1301–1306.
24. Macdonald JS, McCoy S, Whitehead RP, et al. 2005, A phase II study of farnesyl transferase inhibitor R115777 in pancreatic cancer: a Southwest oncology group (SWOG 9924) study. Invest New Drugs 23:485–487.
25. Van Cutsem E, van de Velde H, Karasek P, et al. 2004, Phase III trial of gemcitabine plus tipifarnib compared with gemcitabine plus placebo in advanced pancreatic cancer. J Clin Oncol 22:1430–1438.
26. Lobell RB, Liu D, Buser CA, et al. 2002, Preclinical and clinical pharmacodynamic assessment of L-778,123, a dual inhibitor of farnesyl:protein transferase and geranylgeranyl:protein transferase type-I. Mol Cancer Ther 1:747–758.
27. Martin NE, Brunner TB, Kiel KD, et al. 2004, A phase I trial of the dual farnesyltransferase and geranylgeranyltransferase inhibitor L-778,123 and radiotherapy for locally advanced pancreatic cancer. Clin Cancer Res 10:5447–5454.
28. Wacheck V, Zangemeister-Wittke U. 2006, Antisense molecules for targeted cancer therapy. Crit Rev Oncol Hematol 59:65–73.
29. Phillips MI. 2005, Antisense therapuetics: a promise waiting to be fulfilled. In: Phillips MI (ed.) Antisense therapeutics, 2nd ed. Totowa, Humana Press NJ, 3–10.
30. Makeyev AV, Eastmond DL, Liebhaber SA. 2002, Targeting a KH-domain protein with RNA decoys. RNA 8:1160–1173.
31. Mizuno T, Chou MY, Inouye M. 1984, A unique mechanism regulating gene expression: Translational inhibition by a complementary RNA transcript (micRNA). Proc Natl Acad Sci USA 81:1966–1970.

32. Stephenson ML, Zamecnik PC. 1978, Inhibition of Rous sarcoma viral RNA translation by a specific oligodeoxyribonucleotide. Proc Natl Acad Sci U S A 75:285–288.
33. Zamecnik PC, Stephenson ML. 1978, Inhibition of Rous sarcoma virus replication and cell transformation by a specific oligodeoxynucleotide. Proc Natl Acad Sci U S A 75:280–284.
34. Couzin J. 2002, Small RNAs make big splash. Science 298:2296–2297.
35. Boyer DS, Cowen SJ, Danis RP, et al.2002, Randomized dose-comparison studies of intravitreous fomivirsen for treatment of cytomegalovirus retinitis that has reactivated or is persistently active despite other therapies in patients with AIDS. Am J Ophthalmol 133:475–483.
36. Nakada Y, Saito S, Ohzawa K, et al.2001, Antisense oligonucleotides specific to mutated K-ras genes inhibit invasiveness of human pancreatic cancer cell lines. Pancreatology 1:314–319.
37. Kita K, Saito S, Morioka CY, et al. 1999, Growth inhibition of human pancreatic cancer cell lines by anti-sense oligonucleotides specific to mutated K-ras genes. Int J Cancer 80:553–558.
38. Ohnami S, Matsumoto N, Nakano M, et al. 1999, Identification of genes showing differential expression in antisense K-ras-transduced pancreatic cancer cells with suppressed tumorigenicity. Cancer Res 59:5565–5571.
39. Cowsert LM. 1997, In vitro and in vivo activity of antisense inhibitors of ras: potential for clinical development. Anti-Cancer Drug Design 12:359–371.
40. Chen G, Oh S, Monia BP, et al. 1996, Antisense oligonucleotides demonstrate a dominant role of c-Ki-RAS proteins in regulating the proliferation of diploid human fibroblasts. J Biol Chem 271:28259–28265.
41. Cunningham CC, Holmlund JT, Geary RS, et al. 2001, A Phase I trial of H-ras antisense oligonucleotide ISIS 2503 administered as a continuous intravenous infusion in patients with advanced carcinoma. Cancer 92:1265–1271.
42. Gordon GS, Sandler AB, Holmlund JT, et al. 1999, A phase I trial of ISIS 2503, an antisense inhibitor of H-ras, administered by a 24-hour (hr) weekly infusion in patients (pts) with advanced cancer (abstract 604). J Clin Oncol 18:157a.
43. Adjei AA, Dy GK, Erlichman C, et al. 2003, A phase I trial of ISIS 2503, an antisense inhibitor of H-ras, in combination with gemcitabine in patients with advanced cancer. Clin Cancer Res 9:115–123.
44. Alberts SR, Schroeder M, Erlichman C, et al. 2004, Gemcitabine and ISIS-2503 for patients with locally advanced or metastatic pancreatic adenocarcinoma: a North Central Cancer Treatment Group phase II trial. J Clin Oncol 22:4944–4950.

Chapter 36
HER Family of Receptors as Treatment Targets in Pancreatic Cancer

Bhaumik B. Patel and Adhip P. N. Majumdar

1 Molecular Biology of Pancreas Cancer

Genetic mutation is the hallmark of the development and progression of cancer. The most commonly found mutations in pancreatic cancer are K-ras, CDKN2A (9p), p53 (17q), and smad4 (18q) (1). Smoking, which has been linked to the K-ras mutation, is the most common mutation in pancreatic cancer, with >70% of all pancreatic cancers harboring codon 12 mutations (2). Pancreatic cancer, like colon adenocarcinoma, is believed to follow a genetic progression model with a progressively increasing number of mutations being acquired in a seemingly temporal sequence with morphologic progression from a normal ductal cell to low-grade PanIN to high-grade PanIN, leading to frank invasive adenocarcinoma (Fig. 36.1) (1). K-ras and CDKN2A appear to occur early in the process of carcinogenesis, leading to increased proliferation and shortening of telomere length. Shortened telomere length promotes genetic instability (1). P53 and BRCA2 mutations appear in the later stages, such as high-grade PanIN and invasive cancer (1). These mutations cause an impaired DNA damage checkpoint and promote development of aneuploid tumors (see Fig. 36.1).

K-ras mutation is an early and almost universal finding in pancreatic cancer. Besides activation of various downstream pathways, which include but are not limited to mitogen activated protein kinase (MAPK) and phosphatidylinositol 3-kinase (PI3K), it also establishes autocrine HER family signaling in pancreatic cancer (1). This is evidenced by increased co-expression of various ligands and the signal transduction pathways induced by the member(s) of the HER family (1). Transforming growth factor-α (TGF-α), EGF, and EGFR are over-expressed by 15-, 10-, and threefold compared with that in normal pancreatic tissue in the same tumor. This strongly suggests the existence of an autocrine activation loop involving EGFR in pancreatic cancer (3).

A.M. Lowy et al. (eds.) *Pancreatic Cancer*.
doi: 10.1007/978-0-387-69252-4, © Springer Science + Business Media, LLC 2008

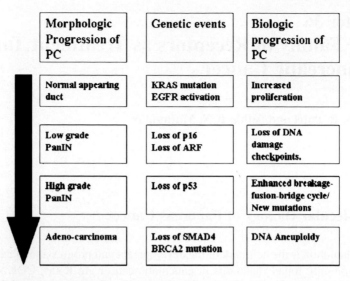

Fig. 36.1 Schematic representation of progression of pancreatic cancer from precancerous PanIN lesions to invasive carcinoma and associated molecular genetic changes associated with each stage of progression. (From Yarden Y, Ullrich A. Growth factor receptor tyrosine kinases. Ann Rev Biochem 1987, 57:443–487.)

2 HER Signaling Pathways

Accumulating evidence suggests that members of the receptor tyrosine kinase family, specifically epidermal growth factor receptor (EGFR/HER-1) and its family members are frequently implicated in experimental models of epithelial cell neoplasia as well as human cancers (4–8). The HER-1 receptor family represents a pleiotropic cell surface signaling system. The four transmembrane receptors (EGFR/HER-1, HER-2, HER-3, and HER-4) that comprise this family interact with members of the HER family of ligands to transform extracellular signals to net cell function (9, 10). There is increasing evidence to support the concept that the malignant behavior of some tumors is sustained by deregulated activation of one or more of these growth factor receptors. Such deregulation could result from either structural alterations of the receptor itself (11, 12), leading to the establishment of an autocrine loop whereby the cells produce growth factors that stimulate their own growth (13, 14) or the loss of growth factor receptor suppressor function.

All members of the HER family are cell surface allosteric enzymes consisting of a single transmembrane domain that separates the extracellular ligand binding domain from the intracellular kinase domain (Fig. 36.2). Under normal physiologic conditions, activation of HER receptors is regulated by the specific spatial and temporal expression of their ligands that are members of EGF family of growth factors (13). Ligand binding initiates homo/heterodimerization of the receptors, leading to auto and transtyrosine phosphorylation of the receptors (16). Tyrosine

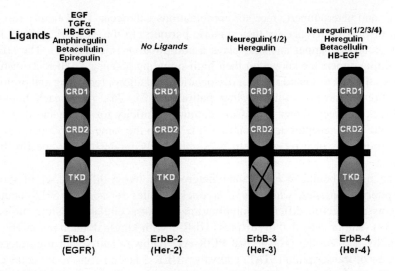

Fig. 36.2 Schematic representation of the four ErbB family members and their respective ligands. CRD, cystine rich domain; EGF, epidermal growth factor; HB-GF, heparin binding-EGF; TGF-α, transforming growth factor α;TKD, tyrosine kinase domain. There are no known ligands for ErbB-2 and the tyrosine kinase domain is non-functional in ErbB-3, as marked with a cross.

phosphorylation/activation of HER-1 kinase domain leads to recruitment of different proteins, initiating a downstream signaling cascade. The receptor tyrosine kinase signaling may be terminated by the endocytosis of the receptor-ligand complex (*17*). The downstream signaling by HER receptors results in transcriptional regulation of various genes, including proto-oncogenes such as jun, fos, and myc, in addition to some zinc-finger-containing transcription factors (*18*).

Signaling by Erb-B receptors is quite diversified and finely tuned at two levels of regulation. These include the specific binding of the ligand to their cognate receptor(s) and the ability of each receptor to form homo/heterodimers. The peptide ligands are produced as transmembrane precursors and their ectodomains are processed by proteolysis, which leads to shedding/secretion of the soluble form of growth factors (*19*). There are several HER-specific ligands, all sharing an EGF-like motif of 45–55 amino acids, including six cysteine residues that interact covalently to form three loops. Depending on the binding specificity conferred by this region, the ligands may be categorized into three groups (see Fig. 36.2). The first group includes epidermal growth factor (EGF), amphiregulin, and transforming growth factor-α (TGF-α), which bind specifically to HER-1. The second group includes betacellulin (BTC), heparin-binding EGF (HB-EGF), and epiregulin, which exhibits dual specificity for HER-1 and HER-4 (*20*). The third group includes neuregulins (Neu, also called Neu differentiation factors or Heregulins). This group is further divided into two subgroups depending on their ability to bind to HER-3 and HER-4, or only HER-4 (*21, 22*). The second level of regulation depends on the homo/heterodimerizing partners. Although, a total of nine possible homo- and heterodimeric receptor combinations can occur, HER family receptors often display preference for their dimeric partners. In this network, HER-2 is the most preferred partner and thus plays a coordinating role (23, 24). The HER-2-containing dimers are known for their high signaling potency, as HER-2 drastically reduces the rate of ligand receptor dissociation and allows for strong and prolonged activation of downstream signaling pathways (25, 26). Also, each homo/heterodimer has been shown to possess unique specificity for the ligand that would stimulate HER receptor activation (27-32). Within the same heterodimer, the signaling properties of a receptor can be significantly modulated by specific ligand binding.

The ligand-bound receptor homo/heterodimer has a different set of tyrosine phosphorylation sites, which serve as docking sites for specific SH2-containing proteins and recruit different combinations of intracellular signaling molecules (33, 34). Tumor cells that overexpress HER-1 with kinase domain mutations preferentially activate the pro-survival PI3K-Akt pathway and signal transducer and activator of transcription (STAT) pathways. HER-1 has no consensus sequence for the p85 adaptor subunit of PI3K; it couples to this pathway via GAB1. GAB1 in turn binds the growth factor receptor-bound protein 2 (GRB2), which docks at the phosphorylated tyrosine of the kinase domain of the activated HER-1. Similarly, there is no evidence for direct binding of STAT to the HER-1. However, it is proposed that this coupling is mediated via tyrosine 1068 and 1086 of HER-1 kinase domain (35). HER-2 couples to the mitogen-activated protein kinase (MAPK) pathway through GRB2, SHC, downstream of kinase-related (DOK-R) (36) and CRK. Phospholipase Cγ (PLCγ) binding has recently been implicated in transducing signals by HER-1 (37). Although HER-3 is able to bind neuregulins (NRGs), it has impaired kinase activity owing to substitutions in crucial residues in the tyrosine-kinase domain. Therefore, HER-3 gets phosphorylated and functions as a signaling entity only when it heterodimerizes with another HER receptor (38), HER-2 being the preferred partner. HER-3 contains six docking sites for the p85 adaptor subunit of PI3K (39) and couples very efficiently to this pathway (34).

3   Significance of HER Family Receptors in Pancreatic Cancer

Many studies have demonstrated that activation of HER-1 pathway that causes suppression of apoptotic signals and promotion of pro-survival signals lead to increased neo-angiogenesis and tumor invasion and ultimately metastasis in pancreatic cancer (40–43). Various EGF family ligands and receptors are over-expressed in pancreatic cancer (44, 45). EGF ligands such as EGF, TGF-α, amphiregulin, and HB-EGF, which are over-expressed in pancreatic cancer, are involved in autocrine activation of HER. Over-expression of HER-1, which is seen in >70% of pancreatic cancer, is associated with increased tumor size, advanced clinical stage at presentation, and poor survival (46, 47). High HER-1 expression as determined by immunohistochemistry (IHC) in the primary tumor is associated with poor differentiation and hepatic metastasis. Mutations involving EGFR tyrosine kinase domain is seen in only 3–4% of patients and is not the major mechanism of EGFR activation in pancreatic cancer (*48*). Over-expression resulting from amplification is seen in approximately 20% of poor prognosis breast cancer patients, whose tumors are particularly sensitive to anti-HER-2 antibody-based therapy (*49*). However, over-expression of HER-2 is less commonly observed in pancreatic cancer. HER-2 is over-expressed in only 17–25% of patients. In about 11–33% of the cases, over-expression of HER-2 is the result of gene amplification (*50*). Coexpression of HER-1 and HER-2 is seen in about 25% of patients, suggesting that HER-2 might be an important cooperating member of HER-1 in pancreatic cancer. HER-3 overexpression is seen in about 47% of pancreatic cancer, but it is not found to be either amplified or mutated (*51*). HER-3 overexpression, like HER-1 overexpression, is also associated with advanced clinical stage and poor prognosis (*51*). However, prognosis related to HER-4 over-expression in pancreatic cancer is controversial. HER-4 expression is not associated with poor survival and its role in tumor aggression is also not clear (*52*).

4 Targeting HER-1 and -2 with Small Molecule Tyrosine Kinase Inhibitors

The preponderance of EGFR and HER-2 in a wide variety of solid tumors has prompted extensive drug development efforts to design pharmacologic inhibitors of HER-1 and -2. Indeed, several small molecule inhibitors of HER-1 (quinazoline- or pyrimidine-based) have been developed to interrupt the intracellular signaling cascade of EGFR induced by ligand binding of the receptor (*53*). Small molecule inhibitors of HER-1 (Table 36.2), gefitinib (Iressa™, AstraZeneca Pharmaceuticals), and erlotinib (Tarceva™, OSI Pharmaceuticals) as well as dual HER-1 and -2 inhibitor lapatinib (Tykerb™, Glaxo-SmithKline) have been progressed to large-scale randomized clinical trials. It has recently been demonstrated that gefitinib and erlotinib are effective mainly in a subgroup of non-small cell lung cancer patients who have specific mutations in the EGFR gene (*54, 55*).

Since EGFR and its ligands play a very crucial role in the pathogenesis in pancreatic cancer and their overexpression promotes tumor growth and metastasis, it is reasonable to speculate that inhibition of EGFR pathway may improve survival in metastatic pancreatic cancer.

In preclinical studies using pancreatic xenograft model of two different pancreatic cell lines, one expressing high HER-1 with moderate HER-2 and the other with moderate HER-1 and high HER-2 levels, erlotinib either alone or in combination with gemcitabine caused a significant inhibition of tyrosine phosphorylation of HER-1 (*56*). This was translated into twofold induction of apoptosis only in the high HER-1 expressing cell line. There was no effect on PKB activation with erlotinib alone or a combination of gemcitabine and erlotinib (*56*). Another HER-1 tyrosine kinase inhibitor gefitinib also inhibited HER-1 activation and proliferation as well as invasiveness of pancreatic cancer cells in vitro (*57*). A phase I study of gemcitabine and erlotinib showed that the combination was tolerable with no excess toxicity when erlotinib was added to gemcitabine. There were 12 patients with pancreatic cancer in this study (*58*). Of 12 patients, one had partial response, three had a minor response, and six had stable disease (*58*). The high disease control rate (70%) observed with this combination prompted a phase III trial comparing gemcitabine and placebo with gemcitabine plus erlotinib in patients with locally advanced and metastatic pancreatic cancer (*59*). Five hundred sixty-nine patients were randomized to receive a standard dose of gemcitabine with or without erlotinib at 100 mg/day dose (a small Canadian cohort of 48 patients was treated with 150 mg/day dose) (*59*). The combination of erlotinib with gemcitabine was well tolerated except for increased grade I or II rash, diarrhea, and stomatitis (*59*). Of note, 2.1% of patients on the treatment arm developed interstitial lung disease compared with 0.4% in the control group. The study met the primary objective of improvement in overall survival. Gemcitabine and erlotinib combination resulted in a statistically significant improvement in median survival (6.4 months versus 5.9 months, $p = 0.025$) and 1-year survival rate (25% versus 17%) compared with placebo-treated control (*59*). Although there was no increase in partial response, gemcitabine and erlotinib combination resulted in a better disease control rate (58% versus 49%) compared with the controls (*59*). This led to FDA approval of the combination therapy of gemcitabine and erlotinib as a first-line treatment of locally advanced and metastatic pancreatic cancer. HER-1 tyrosine kinase inhibitors have also been looked at in combination with chemotherapy in patients who progressed on gemcitabine-based therapy (*60-62*). In a phase II trial, 30 patients who failed gemcitabine therapy were treated with capecitabine 1,000 mg/m^2 twice a day (14 out of a 21-day cycle) and erlotinib 150 mg/m^2/day (*60*). All patients had an ECOG performance status of 0 or 1. The regimen was well tolerated, with the exception of grade III diarrhea (14%), rash (14%), and hand-foot syndrome (11%). The regimen was active, with 11% partial responses and 57% stable disease, resulting in 68% disease control (*60*). Gefitinib was also investigated as a second-line therapy of metastatic pancreatic cancer in combination with docetaxel. However, in a phase II trial, the combination was poorly tolerated with a significant neutropenic infection when docetaxel was given at a dose of 75 mg/m^2, which led to reduction of the docetaxel dose to 60 mg/m^2 (*61*). Two separate phase II trials of docetaxel and erlotinib combination failed to show significant activity, with best response measured as stable disease (*61, 62*).

Although treatment with inhibitors of HER-1 showed signs of success in some patients, failure in others could partly be due to co-expression of multiple members of the EGFR family, which may lead to an enhanced transforming potential and worsened prognosis (*63, 64*). Most solid tumors, including those in the pancreas, express more than one member of the EGFR family (*53, 65*). Therefore, identification of inhibitor(s) targeting multiple members of the EGFR family is likely to provide a therapeutic benefit to a broad patient population. A number of small molecule inhibitors, such as canertinib dihydrochloride (Pfizer) and Tykerb®

(Glaxo-SmithKline) targeting tyrosine kinase activity of HER-1 and other member(s) of its family have been developed (*66, 67*). Baerman et al. (*68*) demonstrated that lapatinib inhibits basal as well as EGF and heregulin-induced activation of HER-1, -2, and -3. It also causes inhibition of AKT phosphorylation, but not MAPK 42/44. This translates into inhibition of anchorage-dependent as well as independent growth of pancreatic cancer cells (*68*). These encouraging in vitro results led to a phase I clinical trial of lapatinib in combination with: (*1*) gemcitabine and (*2*) gemcitabine and oxaliplatin (GEMOX) in patients with advanced adenocarcinoma of the pancreas and biliary tract. Two different dose levels (1,000 mg/day and 1,500 mg/day) of lapatinib were evaluated. The combinations are well tolerated with infrequent nausea and diarrhea. Some significant responses were noted in patients with diffuse liver and peritoneal metastasis. The overall partial response rate was 25% (*69*).

5   Targeting HER-1 and -2 with Monoclonal Antibodies

In addition to small molecular inhibitors of HER-1 and -2, monoclonal antibodies that competitively inhibit ligand binding to the receptors have been developed. The antibodies are murine, chimeric, or humanized. Representative HER-1 and -2 targeted monoclonal antibodies that are in various stages of development are summarized in Table 36.1. Of all the available monoclonal antibodies, cetuximab (Erbitux™ Imclone Systems, Bristol-Myers Squibb, NY), a chimeric IgG1 anti HER-1 antibody is most extensively studied in pancreatic cancer. Effectiveness of cetuximab in pancreatic cancer alone or in combination with gemcitabine was demonstrated in an in vivo study using L3.6pl cells orthotopic pancreatic cancer model (*70*). Macroscopically visible tumors were observed in 50% fewer animals compared with the control, but in none of the animals treated with the combination of gemcitabine and cetuximab (*70*). In addition, none of the animals treated with gemcitabine and cetuximab developed liver metastasis, compared with 20% of those treated with cetuximab alone and 50% of control animals (*70*). In a multicenter phase II trial patients with locally advanced or metastatic pancreatic cancer who had HER-1 positive tumor, based on immunohistochemical analysis, were treated with gemcitabine and cetuximab (*71*). Gemcitabine was administered at 1,000 mg/m² weekly for 7 weeks, followed by a 1-week rest, and then cetuximab was administered at 400 mg/m² followed by 250 mg/m² weekly for 7 weeks (*71*). In subsequent cycles, cetuximab was administered weekly and gemcitabine was administered weekly for 3 weeks every 4 weeks (*71*). This regimen was well tolerated, with most common grade III/IV toxicity being neutropenia (39%). Of the 41 patients enrolled in the trial, five had a partial response (12%) and 26 (63%) had stable disease, resulting in an impressive 75% disease control rate (*71*). The median survival was 7.1 months and 1-year disease free survival, and overall survival rates were 12% and 31%, respectively. All were significantly better than would be expected with gemcitabine alone (*71*). These encouraging

Table 36.1 Strategies to inhibit HER signaling using monoclonal antibodies

Drug/agent	Type	Target	Company/ institution	Stage of development
Trastuzumab (Herceptin)	Humanized mAb	ErbB- 2	Genentech/Roche	Approved for ErbB-2 over expressing breast cancer
Cetuximab (Erbitux/ IMC-225)	Human-mouse Chimeric mAb	EGFR	ImClone/Merck KGaA Bristol-Myers Squibb	Approved for colorectal and head and neck cancers, Phase III trials ongoing for
Panitumumab (ABX-EGF)	Fully Human mAb	EGFR	Abgenix	and Approved for colorectal cancer
Pertuzumab (Omnitarg/2C4)	Humanized mAb	EGFR	Genentech	Phase II trials for ovarian cancer, breast cancer, prostate cancer and NSCLC
Matuzumab (EMD-72000)	Humanized mAb	EGFR	Merck KGaA	Phase II trials ongoing for gynaecological cancer, pancreatic cancer and esophageal cancer
Thera CIM (hR3)	Humanized mAb	EGFR	YM Biosciences/ CIM	Phase II trials for HNSCC
HuMab-Mouse (MDX-447)	Humanized mAb	EGFR	Medarex/Merck KGaA	Preclinical trials ongoing. Phase II trials ongoing for HNSCC
Mab 806	–	EGFR (del 2-7)/ EGFR vIII	Ludwig Institute	Preclinical trials ongoing.

EGFR, epidermal growth factor receptor, mAb, monoclonal antibody, NSCLC, non-small-cell lung cancer; HNSCC, head and neck squamous- cell cancer.

preclinical and clinical findings resulted in a phase III trial led by SWOG. In this trial Philip et al. randomized 736 patient with HER-1 expressing locally advanced and metastatic pancreatic cancer to the combined treatment of *cetuximab* and gemcitabine versus gemcitabine alone (72). They found no significant improvement in response rate, progression-free survival, or overall survival with the combination of cetuximab and gemcitabine compared with gemcitabine alone. The correlative studies are still waiting to better understand the benefit of adding cetuximab to gemcitabine therapy. A humanized IgG1 anti-HER-1 antibody *matuzumab* has also undergone a phase I trial in combination with gemcitabine in advanced pancreatic cancer (73). The study reported matuzumab to be well tolerated in combination with gemcitabine, and the major drug-related adverse

Table 36.2 Strategies to inhibit EGFRs signaling using small molecule tyrosine kinase inhibitors (TKIs)

Drug/agent	Molecular properties	Target selectivity	Clinical activity in cancer type	Company/Institution	Stage of development
Gefitinib (ZD 1839; Iressa)	Reversible TKI	EGFR inhibitor	NSCLC, HNSCC, colorectal cancer and breast cancer	AstraZeneca	Approved for NSCLC in 2003, ongoing Phase III Trials for other cancers
Erlotinib (OSI-774; Tarceva)	Reversible TKI	EGFR inhibitor	NSCLC, HNSCC, colorectal cancer and pancreatic cancer	Genentech/OSI pharmaceuticals	Approved for NSCLC in 2005, ongoing Phase III Trials for other cancers
Canertinib (CI-1033)/ (PD183805)	Irreversible TKI	EGFR/ErbB-2 inhibitor	NSCLC, HNSCC, Ovarian cancer, breast cancer	Pfizer	Phase II
Lapatinib (GW2016)	Reversible TKI	EGFR/ErbB-2 dual inhibitor	Breast cancer	Glaxo Smithkline	Phase III
EKB-569	Irreversible TKI	EGFR inhibitor	Colorectal cancer, breast cancer, HNSCC, and NSCLC	Wyeth- Ayerst	Phase II
AEE788	TKI	EGFR/ErbB-2/ VEGFR	Anti-proliferative effects in tumor cell lines and animal models of cancer	Novartis	Phase I
EXEL 7647/EXEL 0999	TKI	EGFR/ErbB-2/ VEGFR		EXELIXIS	Phase I
PKI-166	Reversible TKI	EGFR/ErbB-2	Thyroid, Renal, colorectal, HNSCC, and NSCLC	Novartis	Phase I
PD 168393	Irreversible TKI	EGFR	–	Calbiochem	Preclinical
AG-1478	Irreversible TKI	EGFR	–	Calbiochem	Preclinical
CGP-59326A	Reversible TKI	EGFR	–	Novartis/	Preclinical
BIBX 1382	TKI	EGFR	–	Boehringer/ Ingelheim	Preclinical

EGFR, epidemal growth factor receptor; TKI, tyrosine-kinase inhibitor; NSCLC, non-small-cell lung cancer; HNSCC, head and neck squamous-cell cancer; VEGFR, vasculoendothelial growth factor receptor.
List of selected EGFR TKIs, their manufactures and current status of their clinical development.

event was grade I and II skin rash (73). In patients treated with an 800 mg weekly dose, the disease control rate was 75%. No other anti-HER-1 antibodies are likely to undergo further development in combination with gemcitabine until correlative studies from SWOG 0205 are conducted to identify a subset of patients likely to benefit from such a therapy. Since HER-2 overexpression is also observed in a subset of pancreatic cancers, trastuzumab, a chimeric anti-HER-2 antibody has been evaluated in pancreatic cancer. Kimura et al. found 10/16 pancreatic cell lines to be 2+ by immunohistochemistry, but only 2/16 cell lines had 3+ expression (74). Trastuzumab inhibited tumor growth in a xenograft model only in pancreatic cells with 3+ HER-2 expression (74). The mechanism of growth inhibition was thought to be primarily due to antibody-dependent cell medicated cytotoxicity against high HER-2 (3+) expressing pancreatic cells. A phase II trial by Safran et al. (75) found HER-2 overexpression ($\geq$2+ as determined by IHC) in about 16% of patients who were treated with gemcitabine and Herceptin (4 mg/kg followed by 2 mg/kg weekly) until progression. Median survival in this group of patients was 7 months, and this combination resulted in a modest 6% partial response rate (75). It was concluded that due to infrequent HER-2 overexpression in pancreatic cancer, there are limitations in reaching a definitive conclusion about targeting HER-2 in this disease (75). However, it should be pointed out that only 12% of the patient had 3+ overexpression and since the benefit of trastuzumab was limited to 3+ overexpressing cells in in vivo studies, it does not definitively rule out any potential benefit of targeting HER-2 in a small subset of pancreatic cancer.

6 Predictive Factors for Response to Anti-HER-Targeted Therapies in Pancreatic Cancer

6.1 Receptor-Based Marker

The most common rationale provided for anti-HER-based therapy is overexpression of HER receptors and associated poor prognosis. Interestingly, the effectiveness of HER inhibitors does not seem to correlate with either degree of overexpression or gene amplification of HER-1 receptor. This observation is in contrast to anti HER-2-targeted therapy in breast cancer, in which degree of overexpression or gene amplification of HER-2 correlates with response (76, 77). Hence, there is a great interest in identifying predictors of response other than receptor expression for anti HER-1-targeted therapies. One such marker is mutation in tyrosine kinase domain (exon 18-22) of HER-1 receptor. The overall response rate of anti HER-1 tyrosine kinase inhibitors is <10% in advanced lung cancer patients (78). However, a subset of patients (about 10% of White and more than 50% of Asian patients) shows a marked response to erlotinib and gefitinib (*54, 55*). This is due to the presence of deletion and point mutation in exons 19 and 21, respectively, of the tyrosine kinase domain of HER-1, resulting in the constitutive activation of HER-1. Studies involving >200 patients with pancreatic cancer and 300 patients with colorectal cancers have failed to show the presence of such mutation in gastrointestinal cancers (*59, 79*).

6.2   Ligand Expression-Based Markers

Transcription profiling of pretreatment samples of 110 metastatic colorectal cancer patients treated with cetuximab identified expression of HER-1 ligands, epiregulin, and amphiregulin to be predictors of clinical outcome. Patients with tumors that had high expression of epiregulin or amphiregulin had significantly improved disease control and progression-free survival with cetuximab (*80*).

Schematic representation of ERRP (A); comparison of ERRP structure with EGFR (B) and hypothetical mechanism of action of ERRP (C)

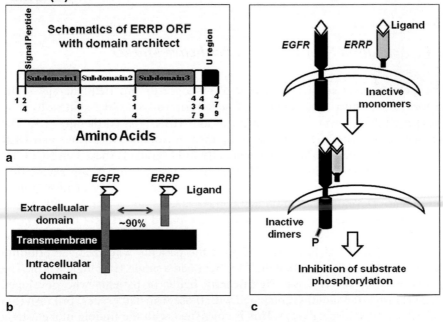

Fig. 36.3 Schematic representation of ERRP domain architecture (**A**), comparison of ERRP structure with EGFR (**B**), and hypothetical mechanism of action of ERRP (**C**). EGFR, epidermal growth factor receptor; ERRP, epidermal growth factor receptor-related protein.

In a preclinical study of pancreatic cancer cells, expression of yet another HER-1 ligand TGF-α, but not HER-1 receptor expression itself, correlated with the presence of constitutive HER-1 phosphorylation and growth inhibition with gefitinib (*81*). Hence, quantification of HER family ligand expression in a pretreatment specimen appears to be a promising predictive marker of response to HER inhibitors. This concept should be tested in a prospective fashion in clinical trials.

6.3   K-ras Mutation

K-ras is a small molecule GTPase, which signals downstream of HER receptors. Presence of exon 2 mutation in K-ras (found in 40% of colorectal cancers and >70% of pancreatic cancers) prevents GTP hydrolysis, locking ras in a constitutive ON switch resulting in increased proliferation, invasion, and metastasis. The presence of K-ras mutation in both lung and colon cancers seems to negatively correlate with response to erlotinib and cetuximab, respectively (*80, 82*). Analysis of K-ras mutation and response to erlotinib is being conducted in an NCIC trial in patients treated with a combination of erlotinib and gemcitabine.

6.4   Acneiform Skin Rash as a Predictive Marker

One potential and consistent marker of response to anti-HER therapy is the degree of skin rash. Development of acneiform (or acne-like skin rash) (Fig. 36.4) is an early event with treatment of anti-HER-1-based therapy (*83*). The majority of patients (68-100%) develop rash in response to various anti HER based targeted agents. The rash is generally mild (grade I) (based on NCI CTC 3.0 criteria) to moderate (grade II) and doses needed to develop severe rash (grade III or IV) are rarely used (*83*). However, the severity of rash is dose dependent. Development of grade II rash seems to correlate with tumor response to both antibody and tyrosine kinase-based anti HER-1 therapies (*59, 79, 84*).

In the NCIC CTG PA.3 trial, 72% of the patients who received erlotinib developed skin rash, and about half of them had a grade II or higher rash. The median overall survival was significantly better in patients who developed grade II rash (10.5 months) compared with those who had grade 0 or I rash (5.3 and 5.8 months, respectively). This is consistent with the finding in metastatic colorectal cancer, in which outcome in patient treated with cetuximab seems to correlate with a degree of acne-like rash (*59*). This concept is being tested in a phase I/II EVEREST trial, in which cetuximab will be dosed to develop a rash (*85*).

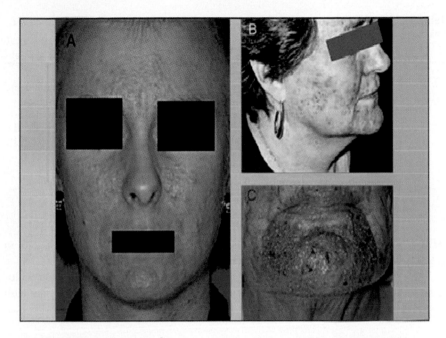

Fig. 36.4 A. Mild. **B.** Moderate. **C.** Severe acneiform rash associated with HER-1 inhibitor treatment. (Adapted from Pérez-Soler R, Delord JP, Halpern A, et al. HER1/EGFR inhibitor-associated rash: future directions for management and investigation outcomes from the HER1/EGFR inhibitor rash management forum. Oncologist 2005, 10(5):345–356).

6.5 Monoclonal Antibody- versus Tyrosine Kinase Inhibitor-Based Anti-HER Therapy

Monoclonal antibodies specifically bind to the extracellular ligand-binding domain of HER receptors and thereby competitively inhibit ligand binding and subsequent receptor dimerization, autophosphorylation, and activation. This results in specific inhibition of the HER receptor. In addition to inhibition of HER receptor activation, monoclonal antibodies exert their antitumor effect by at least two additional mechanisms, namely, receptor internalization with subsequent degradation and antibody-dependent cell-mediated cytotoxicity. In contrast, tyrosine kinase inhibitors of HER receptors are somewhat promiscuous in their specificity for the target and inhibit other tyrosine kinases to varying degrees. Their only mechanism of action is competitive inhibition of receptor phosphorylation and activation. There is also some non-overlapping cross-resistance between monoclonal antibodies and tyrosine kinase inhibitors directed at the same target. This fact is being exploited by combining cetuximab with erlotinib, which results in a greater inhibition of HER-1 phosphorylation as well as activation of downstream mediators such as AKT and MAPK compared with either agent alone (86). A phase I clinical trial is currently evaluating this concept of combining monoclonal antibody and tyrosine kinase inhibitor of

Table 36.3 Currently accruing/recently closed phase I/II trials evaluating various combination treatments with EGFR inhibitors

	Agent	Combinations	Type of Clinical Trial
1)	Erlotinib	Erlotinib + Cetuximab +/− Bevacizumab	Phase I/II
		Erlotinib + Bevacizumab	Phase II (second line)
		Erlotinib + Gemcitabine + Bevacizumab	Phase II (first line)
		Erlotinib + Gemcitabine + Genestine	Phase II (first line)
2)	Cetuximab	Cetuximab + Bevacizumab +/− Gemcitabine	Randomized phase II
		Gemcitabine + Bevacizumab + Erlotinib or cetuximab	Randomized phase II
		Gemcitabine +/− Cetuximab	III (closed)
3)	Gefitinib	Gefitinib + Docetaxel	II (second line)

HER-1 with or without the anti-VEGF monoclonal antibody bevacizumab in patients with advanced aerodigestive and gastrointestinal cancers (*87*).

Table 36.3 summarizes currently accruing/recently closed phase I/II trials evaluating various combinations utilizing chemotherapeutic and targeted biologics with EGFR inhibitors.

7 Novel HER-Based Approaches

Given the fact that ligand binding and subsequent homo- or heterodimerization of EGFRs are essential for activation, any intervention that affects these processes is likely to have a profound effect on the EGFR signal transduction pathways. Such a possibility was suggested, but not demonstrated, for the 2.7-kb truncated rat liver EGFR and the 1.8-kb alternate transcript for human EGFR, whose protein product is secreted (*88, 89*). However, studies from several laboratories have demonstrated that transfection of extracellular fragment of EGFR or kinase-negative dominant mutants of EGFR results in inhibition of EGFR phosphorylation and anchorage-dependent and/or independent growth (*90-93*). Wagner et al. (*90*) have demonstrated that transfection into pancreatic cancer cells (PANC-I) of a human EGFR cDNA fragment, generated by inserting a synthetic linker expressing only the extracellular domain of the receptor, resulted in a marked inhibition of EGF/TGF-α-induced EGFR tyrosine phosphorylation and anchorage-independent growth and increased sensitivity of cells to cisplatinum. In a similar study, Matsuda et al. (*94*) demonstrated that infection of four pancreatic cancer cell lines (ASPC-1, COLO-357, PANC-1, and T3M4) with an adenoviral vector encoding a truncated EGFR markedly attenuated EGF and HB-EGF-dependent cell growth, tyrosine phosphorylation of EGFR family, and phosphorylation of ERKs, JNKs, and p38, as well as activating transcription factor 2. In an analogous finding, Scott et al. (*95*) demonstrated that overexpression of a truncated HER2/Neu protein derived from a transcript (2.3 kb) present in different human breast cancer cell lines also affects proliferation. In evaluating the regulatory mechanism(s), Kashles et al. (93) demonstrated that, although the cells transfected with wild-type EGFR and mutant EGFR lacking the cytoplasmic domain, respond to EGF by forming homo- and heterodimers, only the homodimers of the wild-type EGFR underwent EGF-induced tyrosine autophosphorylation. The results suggest that although an EGFR mutant lacking the cytoplasmic domain can dimerize with wild-type EGFR in response to EGF, it does not induce the EGFR signaling process. Taken together, the data demonstrate that high levels of truncated EGFR generated by molecular biology manipulations modulate the EGFR-signaling process and play a role in regulating cellular growth.

7.1   EGF-Receptor Related Protein: A Novel Pan ErbB Inhibitor

Since most solid tumors express more than one ErbB member, it is imperative that strategies are developed to target multiple members of the EGFR family. EGFR related protein (ERRP), a 53-55 kDa protein that we isolated from the rat gastroduodenal mucosa, fits this scenario. ERRP is a truncated EGFR that contains three of the four extracellular subdomains of EGFR (Fig. 36.3A) (96). Subsequent studies have demonstrated that ERRP is a pan-ErbB inhibitor that targets multiple members of the EGFR family (97). ERRP possesses the extracellular domains of EGFR, which are responsible for the ligand binding, and subsequent homo/heterodimerization of various ErbB members. The ERRP cDNA shows 85-90% homology to the external domain of EGFR (see Fig. 36.3B) and 50-60% homology to ErbB-2, ErbB-3, and ErbB-4 (96). Although the human counterpart of the rat ERRP remains to be isolated, the rat ERRP shows approximately 85% homology to the extracellular domain of human EGFR. Nevertheless, immunohistologic analyses in conjunction with anti-rat ERRP polyclonal antibodies revealed that ERRP expression changes in various tissues (as discussed in the following) of the rat and human during carcinogenesis. These data suggest the presence of an ERRP-like molecule in humans.

Garrett et al. (98) reported that a truncated EGFR lacks the extracellular domain IV of the receptor that binds EGF and TGF-α with higher affinity than the full-length extracellular domain of EGFR. ERRP, which lacks most of the extracellular domain IV, also binds TGF-α and is expected to be effective in preferentially binding/sequestering other ligands of ErbBs. In addition, recent biochemical studies utilizing the EGFR mutant lacking exons 2-7 of the receptor extracellular domain demonstrated the intermolecular inhibitory function of EGFR extracellular domains (99). Such mutants dimerize with EGFR and cause phosphorylation of wild-type EGFR in the absence of ligands (98). In light of these findings and available experimental data, loss of such subdomains may be associated with constitutive activation of EGFR, whereas the truncated EGFRs containing only the extracellular domains serve as repressors of EGFR functions. Ectopic expression of recombinant ERRP causes increased binding/sequestration of EGFR ligand(s), resulting in decreased availability of the ligand(s) for binding to and activation of EGFR with a subsequent attenuation of EGFR signaling pathways. A schematic representation of this hypothesis is depicted in Fig. 36.3C. In support of this supposition, Marciniak et al. (*100*) demonstrated that that exposure of HCT-116 cells to recombinant ERRP and TGF-α results in the formation of heterodimers of EGFR and ERRP, with a molecular weight of about 220 kDa (*100*). TGF-α also induces the formation of a 340-kDa homodimer of EGFR (*100*). In addition, she demonstrated that the exposure of recombinant ERRP to prostate cancer PC cells leads to increased sequestration of EGFR ligands by ERRP, rendering them unavailable for binding to and activation of EGFRs (*101*).

7.2   ERRP in Carcinogenesis

In order to investigate the correlation between expression of ERRP protein and carcinogenesis, benign and neoplastic tissues from the pancreas, liver, and gastric and colonic mucosa were examined. Expression of ERRP was found to be high in benign human colonic and gastric mucosa as well as the liver and pancreas, but low in the respective carcinomas of these tissues (*100, 102-108*). It was further observed that expression of ERRP decreases progressively in colorectal and pancreatic cancers, with a decrease in differentiation (*103, 105*). In pancreatic adenocarcinoma, ERRP expression correlated well with patient survival (*103*). In the colon, ERRP expression became more attenuated in polyps with increasing grades of dysplasia (*105*). Expression of EGFR was found to be inversely related to ERRP in representative samples of normal and neoplastic colon (*105*). In light of these observations it is speculated that the loss of ERRP may be partly responsible for induction of EGFR, and may play a causative role in the development of carcinogenesis.

7.3   Therapeutic Potential of ERRP

Our hypothesis that ERRP could be a potential therapeutic agent for epithelial cancers came from the initial observation that transfection of ERRP cDNA into colon cancer cells inhibited proliferation in the matrix-dependent and -independent systems. This inhibition was associated with attenuation of tyrosine phosphorylation and tyrosine kinase activity of EGFR (*96*).

To further determine the therapeutic potential of ERRP, we generated recombinant ERRP using the *Drosophila* expression system (*100*). The affinity-purified recombinant protein was utilized to investigate its effects on the growth of colon and other epithelial cancer cells in vitro and in vivo. ERRP was reported to inhibit proliferation and stimulate apoptosis of colon, gastric, pancreas, prostate cancer cell lines in a dose-dependent manner (*97, 100, 101, 107, 110, 111*). These changes included inhibition of EGFR signaling and attenuation of downstream signaling involving activation of Akt, mitogen-activated protein kinase (MAPK) and nuclear factor-κB (NF-κB) (*100, 110, 111*). These effects were also observed in other studies involving breast cancer and cells that express varying levels of EGFR and/or its family members suggesting a pan-ErbB inhibitory role of ERRP (*97*). In vitro studies have further demonstrated that ERRP inhibits invasion of colon and pancreatic cells through matrigel and also interferes with tubule formation by endothelial cells (*112, 113*). These data suggest anti-angiogenic properties of ERRP. The results from efficacy trials using SCID mice xenograft models have further shown that ERRP inhibits growth of xenografts of colon or pancreatic cancer cells without any signs of toxicity (*100, 112, 113*). Immunohistochemical analysis of ERRP-treated tumors revealed that ERRP-induced inhibition resulted in a marked stimulation in expression of active caspase-3 and reductions in phosphorylated (activated) forms of Akt and ERKs as well as downregulation of NF-κB (*109, 111, 112*). This suggests that ERRP inhibits tumor growth, in part by inducing apoptosis, which was further supported by in vitro experiments (*43,111*). Additionally, it was demonstrated that ERRP treatment induces differentiation of tumor cells (*112*). Thus, ERRP, a novel pan-ErbB inhibitor, has a potential utility as a therapeutic agent for a wide variety of epithelial cancers, including pancreatic cancer.

8   Mechanisms of Resistance to Anti-HER Targeted Agents

Due to the complex interplay between receptor and non-receptor tyrosine kinases as well as the ability of tumors to acquire additional genetic mutations, there could be a failure of many targeted agents with limited specificity. Some of the common mechanisms leading to either primary or acquired resistance to HER-based therapy can be divided into the following categories.

8.1   Activation of Alternative Tyrosine Kinase Receptors That Bypass the HER-1 Pathway

The effects of activation of HER receptors are mediated by activation of certain downstream mediators that are common among various growth factor receptor signaling pathways, such as those involving insulin-like growth factor-1 receptor (IGF-1R) and hepatocyte growth factor receptor c-MET pathways. This redundancy in growth signaling might explain how receptors can mimic the function of one another (*114*). Expression of IGF-1R negatively correlates with response to HER tyrosine kinase inhibitor (*115*). This can be overcome by combining inhibitors of various growth factor receptors using agents that target more than one growth factor receptor (*116*). To this end, we have shown that curcumin (a yellow pigment found in Asian curry) can inhibit HER family receptors as well as IGF-1R, resulting in a significant growth inhibition of colon cancer cells when combined with oxali-platin or 5-fluorouracil (*117*).

Pancreatic cancer over-expresses not only HER-1, but other members of this family as well. To the best of our knowledge, no effective therapeutic strategy is currently available to target all HER family members. To this end we feel that ERRP, which we have shown to be a pan-HER inhibitor, will be an effective thera-peutic agent for pancreatic cancer.

8.2   Ligand-Independent Activation of HER Receptors

HER receptors, like other growth factor receptors, are activated upon ligand bind-ing, resulting in dimerization and autophosphorylation of the receptor and subse-quent activation of downstream mediators of the growth signaling pathway. In certain circumstances, HER receptors can be activated without the ligand, result-ing in constitutive activation and resistance to inhibition with HER inhibitors. In lung cancer cells resistant to erlotinib, Morgillo et al. (*118*) found a heterodimer of HER-1/IGF-1R causing increased expression of the receptors in surviving cells resulting in resistance to erlotinib therapy. In another study Jänne et al. (*119*) reported that lung cancer cells harboring HER-1 kinase mutation, when made resistant to erlotinib, demonstrated increased expression of c-MET receptor with formation of a HER-1/c-MET heterodimer. These cells were responsive to c-MET inhibitor treatment. Along a similar line of investigation, cetuximab-resist-ant cells generated from colon cancer cells initially sensitive to cetuximab showed increased activation of c-src with transactivation of the HER-1 receptor at the tyrosine 845 domain by passing the ligand-induced activation of HER-1 in the sensitive cells (*120*). These studies demonstrate the importance of identifica-tion of specific resistance mechanisms to HER inhibitors and employing strate-gies to overcome such resistance.

8.3   Constitutive Activation of Signaling Pathways Downstream of HER Receptors

One of the important downstream mediators of HER signaling is membrane-bound GTPase, K-ras, which is a target of genetic activation. Mutations in exon 2 of K-ras results in constitutive activation with subsequent downstream signaling. The presence of K-rass is a negative predictor of response to HER inhibitors. Hence inhibition of K-ras or its downstream signaling mediators might overcome resistance to HER inhibitors. One example of such an approach would be inhibition of the enzyme farnesyl transferase, the activity of which is required for membrane localization of K-ras and its activation by growth factor receptors (*121*). However, such an approach has not generated promising results in the treatment of pancreatic cancer (*122*). Another approach to overcome the growth stimulatory effect of K-ras mutation is to inhibit downstream signaling molecules such as B-RAF or MEK. In preclinical models sorafenib, an RAF kinase inhibitor, inhibited growth of both B-RAF and K-ras mutated colon and breast cancer xenografts (*123*). However, phase II trial of gemcitabine and sorafenib produced disappointing results with no objective responses with median progression-free and overall survival of 3.2 and 4 months, respectively (*124*). Hence better understating of the role of K-ras activation (the most common genetic abnormality in pancreatic cancer) is required to develop more effective therapy against this deadly disease.

8.4 Constitutively Increased Angiogenesis

A growing body of evidences suggests that the HER pathway is intimately involved in tumor angiogenesis by upregulating various proangiogenic molecules, including vascular endothelial growth factor (VEGF) (*125-127*). HER inhibitors have been shown to inhibit expression of VEGF in various preclinical models (*128*). However, colon cancer xenografts have been shown to develop resistance in response to chronic treatment of erlotinib with a five- to tenfold increased expression of VEGF (*129*). On the other hand, treatment of dual HER-1/VEGF inhibitor did not produce resistance in the xenograft model (*129*). This concept was clinically evaluated in a randomized phase II study in which patients with advanced pancreatic cancer were randomized to receive gemcitabine and bevacizumab with either cetuximab or erlotinib by Kindler et al. (*130*). Both regimens were well tolerated and demonstrated an encouraging 20% response rate and 59-67% disease stabilization.

9   Conclusion

Multiple signal transduction pathways become dysfunctional in most malignancies, including pancreatic cancer. Therefore, it is likely that the maximal and most durable therapeutic benefit against tumor growth could be achieved with combination therapies that will affect several targets. In particular, agents that will target growth factor receptors as well as non-receptor tyrosine kinases, such as c-Src, should be identified. Hence currently available HER inhibitors are unlikely to produce the desired therapeutic outcome. It is likely that combining agents with inhibitors of different signaling pathways will be an effective therapeutic strategy in combating pancreatic cancer. However, in the process of combining various targeted agents one should be mindful of incremental toxicities.

Acknowledgements A part of the work presented in this communication was supported by grants from the National Institute of Aging (5 RO1 AG14343) (APNM) and the Department of Veterans Affairs.

References

1. Bardeesy N, DePinho RA, 2002, Pancreatic cancer biology and genetics. Nat Rev Cancer 2(12):897–909.
2. Pellegata NS, Sessa F, Renault B, 1994, K-ras and p53 gene mutations in pancreatic cancer: ductal and nonductal tumors progress through different genetic lesions. Cancer Res 54(6):1556–1560.
3. Korc M, Chandrasekar B, Yamanaka Y, 1992, Overexpression of the epidermal growth factor receptor in human pancreatic cancer is associated with concomitant increases in the levels of epidermal growth factor and transforming growth factor alpha. J Clin Invest 90(4):1352–1360.
4. Hunter T, Cooper JA. 1985, Protein tyrosine kinases. Ann Rev Biochem 54:897–930.
5. Yarden Y, Ullrich A. 1987, Growth factor receptor tyrosine kinases. Ann Rev Biochem 57:443–487.
6. Candena DL, Gill GN. 1992, Receptor tyrosine kinases. FASEB J 6:2332–2337.
7. Glenney JR. 1992, Tyrosine-phosphorylated proteins: mediators of signal transduction from the tyrosine kinases. Biochim Biophys Acta 1134:113–127.
8. Joensuu HJ, Roberts PJ, Sarlomo-Rikala M, 2000, Effect of the tyrosine kinase inhibitor ST1571 in a patient with a metastatic gastrointestinal stromal tumor. N Engl J Med 344:1052–1056.
9. Reise DL, IIStern DF. 1998, Specificity within the EGF family/ErbB receptor family signaling network. Bioassays 20:41–48.
10. Carpenter G. 2000, The EGF receptor: a nexus for trafficking and signaling. Bioassays 22:697–707.
11. Downward J, Yarden Y, Mayes E, 1984, Close similarity of epidermal growth factor receptor and v-erbB oncogene protein sequences. Nature 307:521–527.
12. Sefton BM. 1987, Oncogenes encoding protein kinases. In: Bradshaw RA, Prentis S(eds.), oncogenes and growth factors. Elsevier Biomedixal Press, Amsterdam.
13. Betsholtz C, Heldin CH, Nister M, 1984, Co-expression of a PDGF-like growth factor and PDGF receptors in human osteosarcoma cell line: implications for autocrine receptor activation. Cell 39:447–457.
14. Sporn MB, Roberts AB. 1985, Autocrine growth factor and cancer. Nature 313:745–747.
15. Carpenter G. 2000, The EGF receptor: a nexus for trafficking and signaling. Bioessays 22:697–707.
16. Citri A, Yarden Y, 2006, EGF–ERBB signalling: towards the systems level. Nat Rev Mol Cell Biol 7(7):505–516.
17. Wang Q, Villeneuve G, Wang Z. 2005, Control of epidermal growth factor receptor endocytosis by receptor dimerization, rather than receptor kinase activation. EMBO Rep 6:942–948.
18. Rusnak DW, Affleck K, Cockerill SG, 2001, The characterization of novel, dual ErbB-2/EGFR, tyrosine kinase inhibitors: potential therapy for cancer. Cancer Res 61:7196 –7203.
19. Schaeffer L, Duclert N, Huchet-Dymanus M, 1998, Implication of a multisubunit Ets-related transcription factor in synaptic expression of the nicotinic acetylcholine receptor. EMBO J 17:3078–3090.
20. Massagué J, Pandiella A. 1993, Membrane-anchored growth factors. Annu Rev Biochem 62:515–541.
21. Yarden Y. 2001, The EGFR family and its ligands in human cancer. Signalling mechanisms and therapeutic opportunities. Eur J Cancer 37:S3–S8.
22. Zhang D, Sliwkowski MX, Mark M, 1997, Neuregulin-3 (NRG3):A novel neural tissue-enriched protein that binds and activates ErbB4. Proc Natl Acad Sci U S A 94:9562–9567.

23. Harari D, Tzahar E, Romano J, 1999, Neuregulin-4: a novel growth factor that acts through the ErbB-4 receptor tyrosine kinase. Oncogene 18:2681–2689.
24. Tzahar E, Waterman H, Chen X, 1996, A hierarchical network of inter-receptor interactions determines signal transduction by neu differentiation factor/neuregulin and epidermal growth factor. Mol Cell Biol 16:5276–5287.
25. Graus-Porta D, Beerli RR, Daly JM, 1997, ErbB-2, the preferred heterodimerization partner of all ErbB receptor, is a mediator of lateral signaling. EMBO J 16:1647–1655.
26. Beerli RR, Graus-Porta D, Woods-Cook K, 1995, Neu differentiation factor activation of ErbB-3 and ErbB-4 is cell specific and displays a differential requirement for ErbB-2. Mol Cell Biol 15:6496–6505.
27. Graus-Porta D, Beerli RR, Hynes NE. 1995, Single-chain antibody-mediated intracellular retention of ErbB-2 impairs neu differentiation factor and epidermal growth factor signaling. Mol Cell Biol 15:1182–1191.
28. Earp HS, Dawson TL, Li X, 1995, Heterodimerization and functional interaction between EGF receptor family members: a new signaling paradigm with implications for breast cancer research. Breast Cancer Res Treat 35:115–132.
29. Peles H, Levy RB, Or E, 1991, Oncogenic forms of the neu/HER2 tyrosine kinase are permanently coupled to phospholipase C gamma. Embo J 10:2077–2086.
30. Batzer AG, Rotin D, Urena JM, 1994, Hierarchy of binding sites for Grb2 and Shc on the epidermal growth factor receptor. Mol Cell Biol 14:5192–5201.
31. Fedi P, Pierce JH, Fiore PP, Di 1994, Efficient coupling with phosphatidylinositol 3-kinase, but not phospholipase C or GTPase-activating protein, distinguishes ErbB-3 signaling from that of other ErbB/EGFR family members. Mol Cell Biol 14:492–500.
32. Muthuswamy SK, Muller WJ. 1995, Direct and specific interaction of c-Src with Neu is involved in signaling by the epidermal growth factor receptor. Oncogene 11:271–279.
33. Ricci A, Lanfrancone L, Chiari R, 1995, Analysis of protein-protein interactions involved in the activation of the Shc/Grb-2 pathway by the ErbB-2 kinase. Oncogene 11:1519–1529.
34. Fiore PP, Di Segatto O, Taylor W, 1990, EGF receptor and erbB-2 tyrosine kinase domains confer cell specificity for mitogenic signaling. Science 248:79–83.
35. Olayioye MA, Neve RM, Lane HA, 2000, The ErbB signaling network:receptor heterodimerization in development and cancer. EMBO J 19:3159–3167.
36. Jorissen RN, Walker F, Pouliot N, 2003, Epidermal growth factor receptor: mechanisms of activation and signalling. Exp Cell Res 284:31–53.
37. Dankort D, Jeyabalan N, Jones N, 2001, Multiple ErbB-2/Neu phosphorylation sites mediate transformation through distinct effector proteins. J Biol Chem 276:38921–38928.
38. Kim HH, Vijapurkar U, Hellyer NJ, 1998, Signal transduction by epidermal growth factor and heregulin via the kinase-deficient ErbB3 protein. Biochem J 334:189–195.
39. Prigent SA, Gullick WJ. 1994, Identification of c-erbB-3 binding sites for phosphatidylinositol 3'-kinase and SHC using an EGF receptor/c-erbB-3 chimera. EMBO J 13:2831–2841.
40. Matsuda K, Idezawa T, You XJ, 2002, Multiple mitogenic pathways in pancreatic cancer cells are blocked by a truncated epidermal growth factor receptor. Cancer Res 62:5611–5617.
41. Murphy LO, Cluck MW, Lovas S, 2001, Pancreatic cancer cells require an EGF receptor-mediated autocrine pathway for proliferation in serum-free conditions. Br J Cancer 84:926–35.
42. Yamanaka Y, Friess H, Kobrin MS, 1993, Coexpression of epidermal growth factor receptor and ligands in human pancreatic cancer is associated with enhanced tumor aggressiveness. Anticancer Res 13:565–570.
43. Shirk AJ, Kuver R. 2005, Epidermal growth factor mediates detachment from and invasion through collagen I and Matrigel in Capan-1 pancreatic cancer cells. BMC Gastroenterol 5:12.
44. Friess H, Berberat P, Schilling M, 1996, Pancreatic cancer:the potential clinical relevance of alterations in growth factors and their receptors. J Mol Med 74(1):35–42.
45. Chen Y, Pan G, Hou X, 1990, Epidermal growth factor and its receptors in human pancreatic carcinoma. Pancreas 5:278–283.

630   B.B. Patel, A.P.N. Majumdar

46. Uegaki K, Nio Y, Inoue Y, 1997, Clinicopathological significance of epidermal growth factor and its receptor in human pancreatic cancer. Anticancer Res 17:3841–3847.
47. Yamanaka Y, Friess H, Kobrin MS, 1993, Coexpression of epidermal growth factor receptor and ligands in human pancreatic cancer is associated with enhanced tumor aggressiveness. Anticancer Res 13:565–570.
48. Kwak EL, Jankowski J, Thayer SP, 2006, Epidermal growth factor receptor kinase domain mutations in esophageal and pancreatic adenocarcinomas. Clin Cancer Res 12(14 Pt 1):4283–4287.
49. Slamon DJ, Godolphin W, Jones LA, 1989, Studies of the HER–2/neu proto–oncogene in human breast and ovarian cancer. Science 244:707–712.
50. Saxby AJ, Nielsen A, Scarlett CJ, 2005, Assessment of HER-2 status in pancreatic adenocarcinoma: correlation of immunohistochemistry, quantitative real-time RT-PCR, and FISH with aneuploidy and survival. Am J Surg Pathol 29(9):1125–1134.
51. Friess H, Yamanaka Y, Kobrin MS, 1995, Enhanced erbB-3 expression in human pancreatic cancer correlates with tumor progression. Clin Cancer Res 1(11):1413–1420.
52. Thybusch-Bernhardt A, Beckmann S, Juhl H, 2001, Comparative analysis of the EGF-receptor family in pancreatic cancer: expression of HER-4 correlates with a favourable tumor stage. Int J Surg Invest 2(5):393–400.
53. Laskin JJ, Sandler AB, 2004, Epidermal growth factor receptor: a promising target in solid tumours. Cancer Treatment Rev 30:1–17.
54. Lynch TJ, Bell DW, Sordella R, 2004, Activating mutations in epidermal growth factor receptor underlying responsiveness if non-small-cell lung cancer to gefitinib. N Engl J Med 350, 2129–2139.
55. Paez JG, Janne PA, Lee JC, 2004, EGFR mutations in lung cancer: correlation with clinical response to gefitinib therapy. Science 304:1497–1500.
56. Ng SS, Tsao MS, Nicklee T, 2002, Effects of the epidermal growth factor receptor inhibitor OSI-774, Tarceva, on downstream signaling pathways and apoptosis in human pancreatic adenocarcinoma. Mol Cancer Ther 1(10):777–783.
57. Li J, Kleeff J, Giese N, 2004, Gefitinib ('Iressa', ZD1839), a selective epidermal growth factor receptor tyrosine kinase inhibitor, inhibits pancreatic cancer cell growth, invasion, and colony formation. Int J Oncol 25(1):203–210.
58. Dragovich T, Huberman M, Hoff DD, Von. 2007, Erlotinib plus gemcitabine in patients with unresectable pancreatic cancer and other, solid tumors: phase IB trial. Cancer Chemother Pharmacol 60(2):295–303.
59. Moore MJ, Goldstein D, Hamm J, 2007, Erlotinib plus gemcitabine compared with gemcitabine alone in patients with advanced pancreatic cancer: a phase III trial of the National Cancer Institute of Canada Clinical Trials Group. J Clin Oncol 25(15):1960–1966.
60. Kulke MH, Blaszkowsky LS, Ryan DP, 2007, Capecitabine plus erlotinib in gemcitabine-refractory advanced pancreatic cancer. J Clin Oncol 25(30):4787–4792 .
61. Shadad F, Matin K, Evans TL, et al. Phase II study of gefitinib and docetaxel as salvage therapy in patients (pts) with advanced pancreatic adenocarcinoma (APC). J Clin Oncol 2006, 24(18S):Abst 4120.
62. Blaszkowsky LS, Ryan DP, Earle C, et al. A phase II study of docetaxel in combination with ZD1839 (gefitinib) in previously treated patients with metastatic pancreatic cancer. J Clin Oncol 2007, 25(18S):Abst 15080.
63. Ritter CA, Arteaga CL. 2003, The epidermal growth factor receptor-tyrosine kinase: a promising therapeutic target in solid tumors. Semin Oncol 30(Suppl 1):3–11.
64. Grunwald V, Hidalgo M. 2003, Developing inhibitors of the epidermal growth factor receptor for cancer treatment. J Natl Cancer Inst 95:851–867.
65. Kapitanovic S, Radosavic S, Kapitanovic M, 1997, The expression of p185 HER–2/neu correlates with the stage of disease and survival in colorectal cancer. Gastroenterology 112:1103–1113.
66. Allen LF, Lenehan PF, Eiseman IA, 2002, Potential benefits of the irreversible pan-erbB inhibitor, CI-1033, in the treatment of breast cancer. Semin Oncol 29(Suppl 11):11–21.
67. Rusnak DW, Affleck K, Cockerill SG, 2001, The characterization of novel, dual ErbB-2/EGFR, tyrosine kinase inhibitors: potential therapy for cancer. Cancer Res 61:7196–7203.

68. Baerman KM, Caskey LS, Dasi F, et al. EGFR/HER2 targeted therapy inhibits growth of pancreatic cancer cells. Gastroint Cancer Symp 2005, Abst 84.
69. Safran H, Iannitti D, Miner T, et al. GW572016/gemcitabine and GW572016/gemcitabine/oxaliplatin, a two-stage, phase I study for advanced pancreaticobiliary cancer. Gastrointest Cancers Symp 2006, Abst 124.
70. Bruns CJ, Harbison MT, Davis DW, 2000, Epidermal growth factor receptor blockade with C225 plus gemcitabine results in regression of human pancreatic carcinoma growing orthotopically in nude mice by antiangiogenic mechanisms. Clin Cancer Res 6(5):1936–1948.
71. Xiong HQ, Rosenberg A, LoBuglio A, 2004, Cetuximab, a monoclonal antibody targeting the epidermal growth factor receptor, in combination with gemcitabine for advanced pancreatic cancer: a multicenter phase II Trial. J Clin Oncol 22(13):2610–2616.
72. Philip PA, Benedetti J, Fenoglio-Preiser C, 2007, Phase III study of gemcitabine [G] plus cetuximab [C] versus gemcitabine in patients [pts] with locally advanced or metastatic pancreatic adenocarcinoma [PC]: SWOG S0205 study. J Clin Oncol 25 (18S)4509.
73. Graeven U, Kremer B, Südhoff T, 2006, Phase I study of the humanised anti–EGFR monoclonal antibody matuzumab (EMD 72000) combined with gemcitabine in advanced pancreatic cancer. Br J Cancer 94(9):1293–1299.
74. Kimura K, Sawada T, Komatsu M, 2006, Antitumor effect of trastuzumab for pancreatic cancer with high HER-2 expression and enhancement of effect by combined therapy with gemcitabine. Clin Cancer Res 12(16):4925–4932.
75. Safran H, Iannitti D, Ramanathan R, 2004, Herceptin and gemcitabine for metastatic pancreatic cancers that overexpress HER-2/neu. Cancer Invest 22(5):706–712.
76. Arteaga CL, 2003, Trastuzumab, an appropriate first-line single-agent therapy for HER-2 overexpressing metastatic breast cancer. Breast Cancer Res 5:96–100.
77. Vogel CL, Cobleigh MA, Tripathy D, 2002, Efficacy and safety of trastuzumab as a single–agent in first line treatment of HER-2 overexpressing metastatic breast cancer. J Clin Oncol 20:719–726.
78. Shepherd FA, Rodrigues Pereira J, 2005, Erlotinib in previously treated non-small-cell lung cancer. N Engl J Med 353:123–132.
79. Lenz HJ, Cutsem E, Van Khambata-Ford S, 2006, Multicenter phase II and translational study of cetuximab in metastatic colorectal carcinoma refractory to irinotecan, oxaliplatin, and fluoropyrimidines. J Clin Oncol. 24(30):4914–4921.
80. Khambata-Ford S, Garrett CR, Meropol NJ, 2007, Expression of epiregulin and amphiregulin and K-ras mutation status predict disease control in metastatic colorectal cancer patients treated with cetuximab. J Clin Oncol 25(22):3230–3237.
81. Pino MS, Shrader M, Baker CH, 2006, Transforming growth factor alpha expression drives constitutive epidermal growth factor receptor pathway activation and sensitivity to gefitinib (Iressa) in human pancreatic cancer cell lines. Cancer Res 66(7):3802–3812.
82. Tsao M, Zhu C, Sakurada A, 2006, An analysis of the prognostic and predictive importance of K-ras mutation status in the National Cancer Institute of Canada Clinical Trials Group BR.21 study of erlotinib versus placebo in the treatment of non–small cell lung cancer. J Clin Oncol 24(Suppl 18):365s.
83. Pérez-Soler R, Delord JP, Halpern A, 2005, HER1/EGFR inhibitor-associated rash:future directions for management and investigation outcomes from the HER1/EGFR inhibitor rash management forum. Oncologist 10(5):345–356.
84. Cunningham D, Humblet Y, Siena S, 2004, Cetuximab monotherapy and cetuximab plus irinotecan in irinotecan-refractory metastatic colorectal cancer. N Engl J Med 351(4):337–345.
85. Tejpar S, Peeters M, Humblet Y, 2006, Dose-escalation study using up to twice the standard dose of cetuximab in patients with metastatic colorectal cancer (mCRC) with no or slight skin reactions on cetuximab standard dose treatment (EVEREST study):Preliminary data. J Clin Oncol 24(18S):3554.
86. Huang S, Armstrong EA, Benavente S, 2004, Dual-agent molecular targeting of the epidermal growth factor receptor (EGFR): combining anti-EGFR antibody with tyrosine kinase inhibitor. Cancer Res 64(15):5355–5362.
87. http://clinicaltrials.gov/ct2/show/NCT00101348, last accessed 11/12/07.

88. Petch LA, Harris J, Raymond VW, 1990, A truncated, secreted form of the epidermal growth factor receptor is enclosed by an alternatively spliced transcript in normal rat tissue. Mol Cell Biol 6:2973–2982.
89. Reiter JL, Maihle N, 1996, A 1.8 alternative transcript from the human epidermal growth factor receptor gene encodes a truncated form of the receptor. Nucleic Acid Res 24:4050–4056.
90. Wagner M, Cao T, Lopez ME, 1996, Expression of a truncated EGF receptor is associated with inhibition of pancreatic cancer cell growth and enhanced sensitivity of cisplatinum. Int J Cancer 68:782–787.
91. Redemann N, Holtzmann B, Ruden T, Von, 1992, Anti-oncogenic activity of signaling-defective epidermal growth factor mutants. Mol Cell Biol 12:491–498.
92. Livneh E, 1986, Reconstruction of human epidermal growth factor receptors and its deletion mutants in cultured hamster cells. J Biol Chem 261:12490–12497.
93. Kashles O, Yarden Y, Fischer R, 1991, A dominant negative mutation suppresses the function of normal epidermal growth factor receptors by heterodimerization. Mol Cell Biol 11:1454–1463.
94. Matsuda K., Idezawa T, You XJ, 2002, Multiple mitogenic pathways in pancreatic cancer cells are blocked by a truncated epidermal growth factor receptor. Cancer Res 62:5611–5617.
95. Scott GK, Robles R, Park JW, 1993, A truncated intracellular HER2/neu receptor produced by alternative RNA processing affects growth of human carcinoma cells. Mol Cell Biol 13:2247–2257.
96. Yu Y, Rishi A, Turner J, 2001, Cloning of a novel EGFR related peptide: a putative negative regulator of EGFR. Am J Physiol 280:C1083–C1089.
97. Xu Hu, Yu Y, Marciniak D, 2005, Epidermal growth factor receptor (EGFR)–related protein inhibits multiple members of the EGFR family in colon and breast cancer cells. Mol Cancer Ther 4:435–442.
98. Garrett TP, McKern NM, Lou M, 2002, Crystal structure of a truncated epidermal growth factor receptor extracellular domain bound to transforming growth factor. α Cell 110:763–773.
99. Zhu H-J, Iaria J, Orchard S, 2003, Epidermal growth factor receptor: association of extracellular domain negatively regulates intracellular kinase activation in the absence of ligand. Growth Factors 21:15–30.
100. Marciniak DJ, Moragoda L, Mohammad R, 2003, Epidermal growth factor receptor related protein (ERRP): a potential therapeutic agent for colorectal cancer. Gastroenterology 124:1337–1347.
101. Marciniak DJ, Rishi AK, Sarkar FH, 2004, Epidermal growth factor receptor–related peptide inhibits growth of PC-3 prostate cancer cells. Mol Cancer Ther 3:1615–1621.
102. Majumdar APN. 2005, Therapeutic potential of EGFR-related protein, a universal EGFR family antagonist. Future Oncol 1:235–245.
103. Feng J, Adsay NV, Kruger M, 2002, Expression of ERRP in normal and neoplastic pancreata and its relationship to clinicopathological parameters in pancreatic adenocarcinoma. Pancreas 25:342–349.
104. Schmelz EM, Levi E, Du J, 2004, Loss of expression of EGF-receptor related peptide (ERRP) in the aging colon: a risk factor for colorectal cancer. Mech Ageing Dev 125:917–922.
105. Jaszewski R, Levi E, Sochacki P, 2004, Expression of epidermal growth factor-receptor related protein (ERRP) in human colorectal carcinogenesis. Cancer Letts 213:249–255.
106. Moon WS, Chang KJ, Majumdar APN, 2004, Reduced expression of epidermal growth factor receptor related protein in hepatocellular carcinoma: implications for cancer growth. Digestion 69:219–224.
107. Moon WS, Chai J, Yang JT, 2005, Reduction of epidermal growth factor receptor related protein expression in gastric cancer: a key to cancer growth and differentiation. Gut 54:201–206.
108. Majumdar APN, Du J, Hatfield J, 2003, Expression of EGR-receptor related protein (ERRP) decreases during aging and carcinogenesis. Dig Dis Sci 48:856–864.

109. Levi E, Mohammad R, Kodali U, 2004, EGF-receptor related protein causes cell cycle arrest and induces apoptosis of colon cancer cells in vitro and in vivo. Anticancer Res 24:2885–2892.
110. Zhang Y, Banerjee S, Wang Z-W, 2005, Epidermal growth factor receptor-related protein inhibits cell growth and induces apoptosis of BxPC3 pancreatic cells. Cancer Res 65:3877–3882.
111. Wang Z, Sengupta R, Banerjee S, 2006, Epidermal growth factor receptor-related protein inhibits cell growth and invasion in pancreatic cancer. Cancer Res 66:7653–7660.
112. Zhang Y, Banerjee S, Wang Z, 2006, Antitumor activity of epidermal growth factor-receptor–related protein is mediated by inactivation of erbB receptors and nuclear factor-κB in pancreatic cancer. Cancer Res 66:1025–1032.
113. Rishi AK, Parikh R, Wali A, 2006, EGF-receptor related protein (ERRP) inhibits invasion of colon cancer cells and tubule formation by endothelial cells in vitro. Anticancer Res 26:1029–1038.
114. Reinmuth N, Fan F, Liu W, 2002, Impact of insulin-like growth factor receptor-I function on angiogenesis, growth, and metastasis of colon cancer. Lab Invest 82:1377–1389 .
115. Kulik G, Klippel A, Weber MJ. 1997, Antiapoptotic signalling by the insulin–like growth factor I receptor, phosphatidylinositol 3-kinase, and Akt. Mol Cell Biol 17:1595–606.
116. Lu D, Zhang H, Ludwig D, 2004, Simultaneous blockade of both the epidermal growth factor receptor and the insulin-like growth factor receptor signaling pathways in cancer cells with a fully human recombinant bispecific antibody. J Biol Chem 279:2856–2865.
117. Patel BB, Sengupta R, Qazi S, 2007, Curcumin enhances the effects of 5-fluorouracil and oxaliplatin in mediating growth inhibition of colon cancer cells by modulating EGFR and IGF-1R. Int J Cancer 122(2):267–273.
118. Morgillo F, Woo JK, Kim ES, 2006, Heterodimerization of insulin-like growth factor receptor/epidermal growth factor receptor and induction of surviving expression counteract the antitumor action of erlotinib. Cancer Res 66(20):10100–10111.
119. Engelman JA, Zejnullahu K, Mitsudomi T, 2007, MET amplification leads to gefitinib resistance in lung cancer by activating ERBB3 signaling. Science 316(5827):1039–1043.
120. Lu Y, Li X, Liang K, 2007, Epidermal growth factor receptor (EGFR) ubiquitination as a mechanism of acquired resistance escaping treatment by the anti-EGFR monoclonal antibody cetuximab. Cancer Res 67(17):8240–8247.
121. Lobell RB, Omer CA, Abrams MT, 2001, Evaluation of farnesyl:protein transferase and geranylgeranyl: protein transferase inhibitor combinations in preclinical models. Cancer Res 61(24):8758–8768.
122. Macdonald JS, McCoy S, Whitehead RP, 2005, A phase II study of farnesyl transferase inhibitor R115777 in pancreatic cancer: a Southwest oncology group (SWOG 9924) study. Invest New Drugs 23(5):485–487.
123. Wilhelm SM, Carter C, Tang L, 2004, BAY 43-9006 exhibits broad oral antitumor activity and targets the RAF/MEK/ERK pathway and receptor tyrosine kinases involved in tumor progression and angiogenesis. Cancer Res 64:7099–7109.
124. Wallace JA, Locker G, Nattam S, 2007, Sorafenib (S) plus gemcitabine (G) for advanced pancreatic cancer (PC): a phase II trial of the University of Chicago Phase II Consortium. J Clin Oncol 25(918S):4608.
125. Bancroft CC, Chen Z, Yeh J, 2002, Effects of pharmacologic antagonists of epidermal growth factor receptor, PI3K and MEK signal kinases on NF- B and AP-1 activation and IL-8 and VEGF expression in human head and neck squamous cell carcinoma lines. Int J Cancer 99:538–548.
126. Goldman CK, Kim J, Wong WL, 1993, Epidermal growth factor stimulates vascular endothelial growth factor production by human malignant glioma cells: a model of glioblastoma multiforme pathophysiology. Mol Biol Cell 4:121–133.
127. Ravindranath N, Wion D, Brachet P, 2001, Epidermal growth factor modulates the expression of vascular endothelial growth factor in the human prostate. J Androl 22:432–443.
128. Ciardiello F, Bianco R, Damiano V, 2000, Antiangiogenic and antitumor activity of anti-epidermal growth factor receptor C225 monoclonal antibody in combination with vascular

endothelial growth factor antisense oligonucleotide in human GEO colon cancer cells. Clin Cancer Res 6:3739–3747.
129. Ciardiello F, Caputo R, Damiano V, 2003, Antitumor effects of ZD6474, a small molecule vascular endothelial growth factor receptor tyrosine kinase inhibitor, with additional activity against epidermal growth factor receptor tyrosine kinase. Clin Cancer Res 9:1546–1556.
130. Kindler HL, Bylow A, Hochster HS, 2006, A randomized phase II study of bevacizumab (B) and gemcitabine (G) plus cetuximab (C) or erlotinib (E) in patients (pts) with advanced pancreatic cancer (PC): a preliminary analysis. J Clin Oncol 24(18S):4040.

Chapter 37
GSK-3β Inhibition in Pancreatic Cancer

George P. Kim and Daniel D. Billadeau

1 Introduction

GSK-3 (glycogen synthase kinase-3) has emerged as a potential therapeutic target for the treatment of Alzheimer's disease, diabetes mellitus, and cancer. Although the prominent role of GSK-3 in the APC/β-catenin destruction complex implies that inhibition of GSK-3 could possibly lead to tumor promotion through the activation of the oncogene β-catenin, several studies contradict this concern. A greater understanding presently exists of the molecular mechanisms by which GSK-3β regulates tumor cell proliferation and survival in several human malignancies, including pancreatic cancer. In particular, GSK-3β has been discovered to be a critical regulator of NFκB nuclear activity, supporting the strategy of inhibiting GSK-3β specifically in cancers with constitutively active NFκB. This chapter reviews the current understanding of the role of GSK-3 in human cancer and its potential as a therapeutic target.

2 GSK-3 and Human Diseases

GSK-3 is a ubiquitously expressed cytoplasmic serine/threonine protein kinase that was first described as a component of the metabolic pathway for glycogen synthase regulation (1). There are two homologous mammalian isoforms encoded by different genes, GSK-3α and GSK-3β (2). These isoforms share substrate specificity in vitro and are involved in regulating cell fate determination and differentiation in a variety of organisms (3). GSK-3 kinases both positively and negatively regulate the activity of a broad range of substrates by phosphorylation (2). Recently, GSK-3 has emerged as a potential therapeutic target in various diseases, in which its overexpression is linked to multiple human pathologic processes (e.g., Alzheimer's disease and diabetes mellitus).

3 GSK-3 and Cancer: A Paradigm with a Controversial History

Inhibition of GSK-3 is theorized to result in neoplastic transformation and tumor development based on its role in the canonical Wnt/β-catenin signaling pathway. In Wnt signaling, GSK-3 is a critical component of the APC-β-catenin destruction

A.M. Lowy et al. (eds.) *Pancreatic Cancer*.
doi: 10.1007/978-0-387-69252-4, © Springer Science+Business Media, LLC 2008

complex (*4*). When β-catenin is phosphorylated by GSK-3, it becomes a target for ubiquitin-mediated proteosomal degradation, thereby limiting the amount of free β-catenin that can accumulate in the nucleus. This leads to the inhibition of the transcriptional coactivator function of β-catenin on TCF/Lef transcription factors, ultimately reducing expression of specific oncogenes (e.g., cyclin D1, MMP-7) involved in proliferation, differentiation, and survival (*4*). Interestingly, tissues from mice lacking GSK-3β do not accumulate β-catenin, even though total GSK-3 levels are reduced by 50% and no cellular GSK-3β is detected (*5*). Immunoprecipitation of the scaffolding protein, axis inhibition protein (axin), from these tissues reveals that GSK-3β can be replaced by GSK-3α (in wild-type cells, both GSK-3α and GSK-3β are found bound to axin), indicating that these two kinases substitute for each other in the regulation of β-catenin (*2*).

A critical aspect of GSK function in the Wnt pathway is that GSK-3 appears to be insulated from regulators of GSK-3 that lie outside of the Wnt pathway (*2*). For example, insulin/Akt signaling leads to inhibition of GSK-3 via serine phosphorylation (Ser21 in GSK-3α and Ser9 in GSK-3β), but this does not cause accumulation of β-catenin. Conversely, Wnt signaling does not affect insulin/Akt signaling and does not lead to serine phosphorylation of either GSK-3 isoform (*6*). How this insulation occurs is unclear, but it probably stems from the effective sequestration of a fraction of GSK-3 with axin in the destruction complex (*2*). It is of significant interest that embryonic stem cells lacking GSK-3 (α and β), but expressing a constitutive active version of GSK3α (S21A), can still regulate β-catenin nuclear accumulation in response to Wnt signaling (*7*). These data suggest that Wnt signaling does not inactivate GSK-3, but more likely disrupts the stability of the β-catenin destruction complex.

GSK-3 kinases control glucose metabolism through their phosphorylation and inactivation of glycogen synthase. This inhibitory activity is counteracted by insulin signaling through Akt-mediated phosphorylation and subsequent inactivation of GSK-3 (*8*). Akt is frequently activated in human cancer, including carcinomas, glioblastoma multiforme, and various hematologic malignancies (*9*). Activated Akt inhibits GSK-3 through the phosphorylation of GSK-3 at Ser21/Ser9 (the actual physiologic mechanism of insulin action), although this inactivation does not affect β-catenin levels and does not result in complete GSK-3 inhibition in human cancer cells. This is best exemplified in the two pancreatic cancer cell lines PANC1 and ASPC1, which exhibit 30- and 50-fold amplification of *AKT2*, respectively, and high levels of *AKT2* RNA and protein (*10*). However, using an in vitro kinase assay, it was shown that despite some inhibition by Akt-induced phosphorylation, GSK-3β remains highly active in these Akt overexpressing cell lines (*11*). Moreover, another study demonstrated high activity and increased expression level of GSK-3β in colon cancer cell lines and in human colorectal carcinomas by in vitro kinase assay and Western blotting (*12*). Significantly, this study demonstrated high levels of active phospho-Akt[Ser473] in 10 of 20 human colorectal carcinomas, yet low levels of inactive phospho-GSK-3β[Ser9] in 9 of these 10 high-expressing Akt cancers (*12*). Additionally, compared to normal tissue, GSK-3β was overexpressed in all colon cancer tumor samples (*12*). These studies suggest that Akt activation and GSK-3 inhibitory phosphorylation are not always correlated in human tumors in vivo and, irrespective of Akt activation, a pool of GSK-3 remains active in cancer cells. Thus, although GSK-3 has been shown to negatively regulate the stability and expression of cell-cycle regulators such as cyclin D1, cyclin E, c-Jun, and c-Myc, which are linked with tumorigenesis (*13*), GSK-3 may be involved in cancer cell proliferation and survival.

Taken together, one would predict that GSK-3 is a putative tumor suppressor protein since its inhibition is expected to mimic the activation of the Wnt-signaling pathway and stabilize oncogenic proteins. Thus, anti-GSK-3 therapy raises concerns that inhibition of GSK-3 could presumably lead to tumorigenesis. However, to date there have been no reports of GSK-3 mutations in human cancer, and in fact, Wnt signaling, cyclin D1 levels, and β-catenin nuclear accumulation are not perturbed in GSK-3β–deficient mice(*5*), presumably because GSK-3α is still present. Moreover, studies suggest that even in a colon cancer, in which β-catenin dysregulation is involved in the pathogenesis of the tumor, GSK-3β remains active and is even overexpressed in colon cancer cell lines and tumor specimens (*12*).

A potential reassurance that GSK inhibition is not tumorigenic is with the clinical example of treatment of psychiatric patients with lithium, a known potent inhibitor of GSK-3. Interestingly, it is reported that cancer risks in patients treated with lithium are lower than in the general population, and that an inverse relationship is observed between cancer morbidity and lithium dosage. Lithium inhibition of GSK-3 occurs at therapeutic concentrations (IC50 ~ 1 mM) (*14*). In preclinical models with APC mutant mice, 60 days of lithium exposure did not produce a significant increase in the number of tumors in these genetically predisposed mice (*11*). Lithium treatment was found to also decrease levels of cyclin E and PKB/Akt, and inhibit proliferation in hepatocellular carcinoma cell lines (*15*).

Thus, the role of GSK-3 in human cancer remains enigmatic and controversial. On the one hand, GSK-3 enzymes should function as tumor suppressors by regulating the activation of β-catenin signaling, but on the other hand, GSK-3 inhibition does not increase the incidence of cancer and seems to correlate with decreased tumor cell proliferation and survival. Further, in contrast to what would be predicted, overexpression of active GSK-3β has been found in human colon cancer tissues, which harbor constitutively active Akt, as well as β-catenin nuclear accumulation (*16*), suggesting that GSK-3β may participate in colon cancer tumorigenesis, independent of its effects on β-catenin. Additionally, GSK-3β is over-expressed in pancreatic cancer, showing increased expression in PanIN lesions, with increasing expression in frank adenocarcinoma and significant nuclear accumulation in the most poorly differentiated cancer specimens (*16*).

4   Inhibition of GSK-3β Suppresses Cancer Cell Proliferation and Survival by Abrogating NFκB Nuclear Activity

The activation of NFκB is needed for proper immune system function, however, inappropriate NFκB activation can mediate inflammation and tumorigenesis. In fact, constitutively active NFκB has been identified not only in cancer cell lines, but also in human tumor tissues derived from patients with multiple myeloma (*17*) and leukemia (*18–20*), as well as prostate, breast, and pancreatic cancers (*21–23*). A major consequence of tumors that have constitutive NFκB activity is their resistance to chemotherapy and radiation through the increased expression of survival genes (e.g., Bcl-2, Bcl-XL, XIAP). In fact, NFκB activation is part of the cancer cells' "autodefense" mechanism since most chemotherapeutic agents and radiation that induce apoptosis also activate NFκB (*24*), and thus hyperactive NFκB signaling can contribute to tumor chemoresistance and radioresistance (*25*). In addition, NFκB participates in tumor neovascularization, invasion, and metastasis through the up-regulation of VEGF and MMP-9 (*26, 27*). Consistent with these roles of NFκB in cancer, inhibition of NFκB activity in tumors *decreases* metastasis, causes cell cycle arrest, and leads to apoptosis (*26, 28*). In total, these studies highlight the crucial role of NFκB in tumorigenesis, revealing it to be a potential target in the treatment of cancer.

NFκB, p65/p50 heterodimers are generally found in a complex with IκBα in the cytosol of resting cells, in which IκBα sequesters p65/p50 by masking a nuclear localization signal sequence found on p65 (*28, 29*). Following receptor stimulation (e.g., TNFR), the IKK complex (IKKα, β, γ/Nemo) is activated, resulting in the phosphorylation of IκBα, leading to its ubiquitination and degradation. This exposes the nuclear localization signal sequence on p65, resulting in the nuclear translocation of p65/p50, and, following chromatin remodeling, transcriptional activation of NFκB target gene promoters (*28, 29*). It is currently unclear which molecular pathways are deregulated in pancreatic cancer, leading to constitutive activation of NFκB, but it may involve not only constitutive ligand/receptor signaling leading to IKK activation, but also the activation of other pathways, including those involved in chromatin remodeling, which cooperate with NFκB to drive expression of its target genes.

A link between NFκB and GSK-3β stems from observations that disruption of NFκB (p65 or IKKβ genes) or ablation of the murine GSK-3β gene both result in embryonic lethality with hepatocyte apoptosis and massive liver degeneration, due to an inability of the hepatocytes to respond to TNFα (*5, 30, 31*). Consistent with this notion, mouse embryonic fibroblasts (MEFs) derived from these animals are highly sensitive to TNFα-induced apoptosis (*5*). This knockout clearly identified a previously unexpected role for GSK-3β (but not GSK-3α) in the regulation of NFκB activation and identified GSK-3β as a potential therapeutic target. This is supported by studies with pharmacologic inhibition of GSK-3 or genetic depletion of GSK-3β by RNAi in which basal NFκB transcriptional activity of a subset of antiapoptotic (XIAP, Bcl-2) and proliferation (cyclin D1) genes is suppressed leading to decreased pancreatic cancer cell proliferation and survival (*11*). In addition, pharmacologic inhibition of GSK-3 suppresses NFκB transcriptional activity, arrests pancreatic tumor growth, and reduces survival in vivo and in established tumor xenografts. Moreover, GSK-3 inhibition reduces cancer cell proliferation and dramatically enhances TRAIL-induced apoptosis in prostate cancer cell lines (*32, 33*). Lastly, pharmacologic inhibition of GSK-3 or depletion of GSK-3β by RNAi induced apoptosis and attenuated proliferation of colon cancer cells (12). Thus, as demonstrated by these examples, inhibition of GSK-3 using small molecule inhibitors, or RNA interference to specifically deplete GSK-3β, results in decreased NFκB activity in cancer cells and induction of apoptosis.

The exact mechanism by which GSK-3β impacts NFκB activity is unknown. Using GSK-3β–deficient MEFs, it has been demonstrated that the early steps leading to NFκB activation following TNFα treatment (degradation of IκBα and translocation of NFκB to the nucleus) were unaffected by the loss of GSK-3β, indicating that NFκB is regulated by GSK-3β at the level of the transcriptional complex (5). Consistent with these observations, it has been shown that GSK-3β influences NFκB-mediated gene transcription in pancreatic cancer cells at a point distal to the Iκ kinase complex. Ectopic expression of the NFκB subunits p65/p50, but not an Iκ kinase β constitutively active mutant, can rescue the decreased cellular proliferation and survival associated with GSK-3β inhibition (11). These data exclude an effect of GSK-3β on the cascade of proteins that culminates in phosphorylation of IκBα and its degradation, and suggest that GSK-3β must be regulating the nuclear activity of NFκB p65/p50 (Fig. 37.1). It is of interest that GSK-3β is found co-localized with NFκB p65 in the nuclei of pancreatic cancer cell lines and samples from pancreatic cancer patients (34).

In light of observations that β-catenin can antagonize NFκB activity, the question is raised as to whether inhibition of GSK-3 (both GSK-3α and GSK-3β) affects NFκB activity through stabilization of transcriptionally inactive β-catenin/p65 complexes (35, 36). However, β-catenin levels are unaltered in GSK-3β null fibroblasts, providing an argument that GSK-3β regulation of NFκB is independent of β-catenin (5).

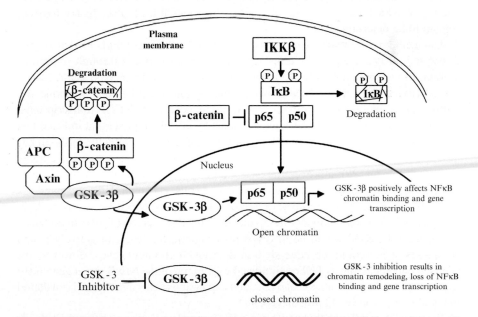

Fig. 37.1 GSK-3β is required for NFκB nuclear activity, independent of IκB degradation, and NFκB nuclear translocation. See text for details

Recently, it has been shown that ablation of GSK-3β in HCT116 p53$^{+/+}$ colon cancer cells, activates p53-dependent apoptosis and antagonizes xenograft tumor growth in vivo (37). In fact, NFκB is constitutively active in HCT116 colon cancer cells (38), and Twist, an NFκB regulated target gene, can inhibit p53-induced apoptosis through interference with the ARF/MDM pathway (39). NFκB itself can also up-regulate MDM2 and suppress p53 stabilization (40). Thus, depletion of GSK-3β may induce p53-dependent apoptosis through inhibition of basal NFκB activity in HCT116 p53$^{+/+}$ colon cancer cells, although other mechanisms cannot be excluded. In addition, several mutant p53 cancer cell lines (colon, SW480; pancreas, MIA-PaCa2, BXPC3) undergo apoptosis following incubation with GSK-3 inhibitors or depletion of GSK-3β by RNAi (11, 12). Thus, there may be p53-dependent, as well as -independent mechanisms controlling apoptosis following the inhibition of GSK-3. Further study is required to fully define the relationship among GSK-3, p53 status, and apoptosis.

The manner in which GSK-3β regulates NFκB has not completely been elucidated although a requirement is for GSK-3β to enter the cell nucleus. Although it does not harbor an identifiable nuclear localization signal sequence, GSK-3β shuttles in and out of the nucleus (41) in MEFs in response to TNFα stimulation (DDB, unpublished observation). Additionally, GSK-3β accumulates in the nucleus of pancreatic cancer cells (34) and CLL B-cells (42), two tumor types in which NFκB is known to accumulate in the nucleus and transactivate target genes involved in cell survival. Therefore, it is tempting to speculate that this nuclear accumulation of GSK-3β is required for optimal NFκB transcriptional activity in normal cell signaling, as well as in cancer, yet the molecular mechanisms by which receptor signaling leading to NFκB activation and the nuclear translocation of GSK-3β are tethered remain to be determined.

Upon entering the nucleus, it is possible that GSK-3β alters NFκB-mediated gene transcription by regulating its transcriptional binding partners through phosphorylation. In fact, although GSK-3β is known to positively influence NFκB transcriptional activity, GSK-3β has been shown to directly phosphorylate p65 on serine 468 within the transactivation domain, resulting in decreased NFκB transcriptional activation (43). However, this is argued against by conflicting data that indicate that serine 468 is phosphorylated by IKKβ, not GSK-3β (23). Additionally, GSK-3β has also been shown to phosphorylate p65 within another region encompassing the transactivation domain (29); however, the exact site of phosphorylation was not mapped. Lastly, it has been reported that GSK-3β in resting cells, phosphorylates and stabilizes p105, the precursor protein to p50 (a component of active NFκB p65/p50) while in response to TNFα stimulation, GSK-3β mediates the degradation of p105 to p50 (44). In this case, GSK-3β would be involved in regulating the levels of active p65/p50 complexes, which could subsequently transactivate NFκB target genes. However, this is not all encompassing as TNFα-stimulated expression of the NFκB target gene IκBα requires the binding of both p65 and p50, and expression of this target gene is unaltered in the absence of GSK-3β protein (28, 44).

Recently, it was shown that while p65/p50 accumulates in the nucleus of GSK-3β-deficient MEFs following TNFα stimulation, p65 was not able to interact with certain target gene promoters, as determined by chromatin immunoprecipitation (ChIP) (28). This suggests that either p65 does not have access to its target promoters, or once bound to the promoter, it is rapidly removed. Indeed, remodeling of the chromatin at NFκB target gene promoters occurs following TNFα stimulation and is a requisite event leading to binding of NFκB to the promoter and transcriptional activation (45). Thus, it remains possible that GSK-3β localizes to the nucleus in response to TNFα signaling in order to modulate proteins involved in chromatin remodeling leading to the formation of euchromatin at NFκB target gene promoters. This is interesting in light of a recent observation identifying that histone deacetylase 1 (HDAC1), but not HDAC2, HDAC3, or HDAC8, is specifically degraded following TNFα stimulation in an IKK-dependent manner (3). It is conceivable that GSK-3β works along with the IKK complex to target HDAC1 for degradation in response to TNFα stimulation, thereby permitting acetylation of histones at NFκB target promoters. This leads to the formation of euchromatin and ultimately, p65/p50 binding and transcriptional activation.

Furthermore, in pancreatic cancer cells, it is possible that constitutive signaling to NFκB and the nuclear accumulation of GSK-3β result in the maintenance of euchromatin at NFκB target gene promoters, thereby allowing high-level transcriptional activation. In fact, histone H3 at NFκB target gene promoters is hyperacetylated on K9 and K14 and, upon inhibition of GSK-3, their acetylation is lost and K9 and K14 become methylated (DDB, unpublished observation). This strongly supports the role of GSK-3 in maintaining the euchromatic state of NFκB target gene promoters in pancreatic cancer cells. Similar observations have been made in CLL B-cells; GSK-3 inhibition results in the hypermethylation of histone H3 (K9 and K27) within the XIAP and Bcl-2 promoters and loss of p65/p50 binding and transcriptional activation (46). Taken together, these data provide an intriguing hypothesis that GSK-3β regulates NFκB transcriptional activity by preventing the activity of HDACs or histone methyltransferases (HMTs) at target gene promoters (see Fig. 37.1). However, it is not yet clear if the epigenetic changes occurring within these promoters in response to GSK-3 inhibition are the due to the loss of p65/p50 binding or are the consequence of that loss. Thus, it can be summarized that GSK-3β may affect the regulation of NFκB at several levels and the exact mechanism(s) by which it exerts its effects on NFκB will require further study.

5 Expression and Localization of GSK-3β in Cancer Cells

Presently, GSK-3β protein over-expression has been reported in human ovarian (47), colon (12), and pancreatic (34) carcinomas. In addition, a mouse hepatic carcinogenesis model demonstrated higher levels of GSK-3β expression in liver tumors than in normal liver tissue (48). Although the cellular localization of GSK-3β has not been consistently reported in human cancers, one study found that cytoplasmic overexpression of GSK-3β was observed in most high-grade PanIN lesions and differentiated pancreatic adenocarcinomas, whereas nuclear accumulation of GSK-3β was significantly associated with poorly differentiated pancreatic adenocarcinomas (34). Although GSK-3β does not contain any identifiable nuclear localization or nuclear export signal sequences, it is known to translocate from the cytoplasm to the nucleus, where it is thought to participate in the regulation of gene transcription through the phosphorylation of transcription factors (e.g., NFAT, c-Jun, c-myc) (49, 50). Although the GSK-3β interacting protein Frat1 has been suggested to bind to GSK-3β in the nucleus and shuttle it to the cytoplasm, the mechanism by which GSK-3β is transported into the nucleus is not clear. However, a recent report has identified the TNF-like family member TWEAK (TNF weak inducer of apoptosis) as a molecule that interacts with GSK-3β (51). It was found that a membrane cleaved form of TWEAK (sTWEAK), could enter cells that lacks its known receptor (Fn14) and promote the nuclear accumulation of GSK-3β and subsequently NFκB-mediated gene transcription. This provides a possible link between GSK-3β nuclear accumulation and the regulation of nuclear NFκB activation (51). It is of interest that many tumor cell lines and tumors express TWEAK. However, the role of TWEAK in the pathogenesis of human malignancies is controversial, since TWEAK can have both proliferative and antiproliferative effects on cancer cell lines. Further work is needed to definitively determine if TWEAK participates in the nuclear accumulation of GSK-3β in cancer cells allowing it to regulate NFκB activity.

6   Inhibition of GSK-3β by CDK (Cyclin-Dependent Kinase) Inhibitors

As demonstrated in numerous publications, CDK inhibitors suppress the proliferation and survival of a broad range of cancer cell lines in vitro and in vivo (52). In fact, CDK inhibitors induce cell cycle arrest and apoptosis in cell lines that lack p53 and retinoblastoma (Rb), where normal cell cycle checkpoints are not in place. Presently, the mechanism by which CDK inhibitors induce apoptosis in cancer cells is unknown, but several studies have convincingly suggested that CDK inhibitors act on targets other than CDKs to induce apoptosis (52). CDK inhibitors target a variety of kinases and of interest, most reported CDK inhibitors are also powerful GSK-3 inhibitors (53). For example, staurosporine, its derivative UCN-01 (7-hydroxystaurosporine) and flavopiridol inhibit GSK-3 with an IC50 of 15, 70, and 450 nM, respectively (53). Indeed, flavopiridol inhibits TNFα-mediated NFκB activation and induces apoptosis in small cell lung cancer cell lines, but the reason for this effect of flavopiridol is unknown (54). Yet, the potential explanation could be found in another study showing that inhibition of GSK-3 suppressed NFκB activity and sensitized hepatocytes toward TNFα-mediated apoptosis (55). Moreover, similar to genetic depletion of GSK-3β by RNAi (14), CDK inhibitors down-regulate expression of NFκB target genes cyclin D1, Bcl-2, and XIAP in cancer cells (56, 57). Thus, it is possible that CDK inhibitors induce apoptosis through inhibition of GSK-3 resulting in decreased NFκB transcriptional activity in cancer cells.

Another question is how CDK inhibitors could be effective in the treatment of cancer cells (small cell lung cancer, SCLC) that are nearly universally Rb mutated (*58*). Staurosporine suppresses proliferation and survival of SCLC cancer cells (*59*), which support possible "off-targeting" of CDK inhibitors. Again, this effect could be explained by inhibition of GSK-3 with subsequent inactivation of NFκB-mediated transcription resulting in decreased cancer cell proliferation and survival in SCLC. In fact, this has been demonstrated to occur with GSK-3 inhibition (*11*, 34, 60). In addition, similarity was observed in induction of TRAIL-mediated apoptosis using either flavopiridol (*54*) or GSK-3 inhibitors (*32*) in cancer cells. Of course, although these suggestions are speculative, previously published papers on the cellular effects of CDK inhibitors need to be re-examined in the context of GSK-3 inhibition and its effects on cancer cell proliferation and survival.

7   GSK-3β Inhibition in the Clinic

Over the past several years, GSK inhibitors have been in development for medical conditions such as Alzheimer's disease and diabetes. In general, both direct and indirect inhibitors are being evaluated; the former include lithium, small molecule, and peptide inhibitors. The small molecule inhibitors include paullones (benzazepiones, known CDK inhibitors), maleimides (ATP binding site blockers), aminopyrimidine (Bcr-Abl inhibitors), indirubin (active ingredient of a Chinese herbal remedy), thiazoles, and thiadiazolidinones. Indirect inhibitors increase N-terminal phosphorylation of GSK-3, thereby inhibiting its activity and include valproic acid, and some cholinergic and serotonergic agents.

Another potential GSK inhibitor that is already being tested in pancreatic cancer is enzastaurin, an acyclic bisindolylmaleimide, which was initially developed as a selective inhibitor of protein kinase C β (IC50 ~ 6 nM). Additional screening revealed that enzastaurin is also a potent inhibitor of GSK-3β (IC50 ~ 24 nM). In support of this, treatment of pancreatic cancer cell lines with enzastaurin leads to a significant reduction in the phosphorylation of glycogen synthase, a well-known target of GSK-3 kinases. A randomized, phase II study in untreated, advanced pancreatic cancer patients is ongoing comparing gemcitabine in combination with enzastaurin versus gemcitabine alone. Preliminary data from the trial reveal the combination to be tolerable with a lack of significant toxicities. There is an early suggestion of added benefit with the combination treatment as measured by several clinical endpoints. The doses and schedule of enzastaurin in the trial were empirically selected and currently it is not known whether enzastaurin clinical activity is a result of GSK-3β targeting.

8   Future Perspective

With an increasing understanding of the function and regulation of GSK-3 in cancer, the potential benefits of inhibiting this specific kinase to treat malignancies is evident. Future studies are required to fully comprehend the multiple mechanisms by which GSK-3 contributes to the pathogenesis of human cancers. The important regulators of GSK-3 function and the other cellular targets of GSK-3 that contribute to proliferation and survival in cancer cells need further examination. The inhibition of GSK-3 suppresses tumor growth supporting the use of GSK-3 inhibitors as monotherapy in cancers with constitutively active NFκB. In addition, GSK-3 inhibition may be optimized when combined with chemotherapeutic drugs, such as gemcitabine, and radiotherapy, that inadvertently activate NFκB. This strategy may help overcome NFκB-induced drug resistance and apoptosis inhibition. In view of its effects in pancreatic cancer, therapeutic inhibition of GSK-3 is intriguing and, with more than 50 inhibitors already identified, clinical trials targeting GSK-3 will provide proof-of-principle that this approach is valid.

References

1. Plyte Se, Hughes K, Nikolakaki E, et al. 1992, Glycogen synthase kinase-3: functions in oncogenesis and development. Biochim Biophys Acta 1114(2–3):147–162.
2. Doble BW, Woodgett Jr. 2003, GSK-3: tricks of the trade for a multi-tasking kinase. J Cell Sci 116(Pt 7):1175–1186.
3. Woodgett Jr. 1990, Molecular cloning and expression of glycogen synthase kinase-3/factor A. Embo J 9(8):2431–2438.
4. Polakis P. 2000, Wnt signaling and cancer. Genes Dev 14(15):1837–1851.
5. Hoeflich KP, Luo J, Rubie EA, et al. 2000, Requirement for glycogen synthase kinase-3beta in cell survival and NF-kappaB activation. Nature 406(6791):86–90.
6. Ding VW, Chen R, McCormick F. 2000, Differential regulation of glycogen synthase kinase 3beta by insulin and Wnt signaling. J Biol Chem 275(42):32475–32481.
7. Patel S, Doble BW Jr. 2004, Glycogen synthase kinase-3 in insulin and Wnt signalling: a double-edged sword? Biochem Soc Trans 32(Pt 5):803–808.
8. Cross DA, Alessi DR, Cohen P, et al. 1995, Inhibition of glycogen synthase kinase-3 by insulin mediated by protein kinase B. Nature 378(6559):785–789.
9. Altomare DA, Testa JR. 2005, Perturbations of the AKT signaling pathway in human cancer. Oncogene 24(50):7455–7464.
10. Cheng JQ, Ruggeri B, Klein WM, et al. 1996, Amplification of AKT2 in human pancreatic cells and inhibition of AKT2 expression and tumorigenicity by antisense RNA. Proc Natl Acad Sci U S A 93(8):3636–3641.
11. Ougolkov AV, Fernandez-Zapico ME, Savoy DN, et al. 2005, Glycogen synthase kinase-3beta participates in nuclear factor kappaB-mediated gene transcription and cell survival in pancreatic cancer cells. Cancer Res 65(6):2076–2081.
12. Shakoori A, Ougolkov A, Yu ZW, et al. 2005, Deregulated GSK3beta activity in colorectal cancer: its association with tumor cell survival and proliferation. Biochem Biophys Res Commun 334(4):1365–1373.
13. Ryves WJ, Harwood AJ. 2003, The interaction of glycogen synthase kinase-3 (GSK-3) with the cell cycle. Prog Cell Cycle Res 5:489–495.
14. Cohen Y, Chetrit A, Cohen Y, et al. 1998, Cancer morbidity in psychiatric patients: influence of lithium carbonate treatment. Med Oncol 15(1):32–36.
15. Erdal E, Ozturk N, Cagatay T, et al. 2005, Lithium-mediated downregulation of PKB/Akt and cyclin E with growth inhibition in hepatocellular carcinoma cells. Int J Cancer 115(6):903–910.
16. Hezel AF, Kimmelman AC, Stanger BZ, et al. 2006, Genetics and biology of pancreatic ductal adenocarcinoma. Genes Dev 20(10):1218–1249.

17. Feinman R, Koury J, Thames M, et al. 1999, Role of NF-kappaB in the rescue of multiple myeloma cells from glucocorticoid-induced apoptosis by bcl-2. Blood 93(9):3044–3052.

18. Baron F, Turhan AG, Giron-Michel J, et al. 2002, Leukemic target susceptibility to natural killer cytotoxicity: relationship with BCR-ABL expression. Blood 99(6):2107–2113.

19. Griffin JD. 2001, Leukemia stem cells and constitutive activation of NF-kappaB. Blood 98(8):2291.

20. Kordes U, Krappmann D, Heissmeyer V, et al. 2000, Transcription factor NF-kappaB is constitutively activated in acute lymphoblastic leukemia cells. Leukemia 14(3):399–402.

21. Nakshatri H, Bhat-Nakshatri P, Martin DA, et al. 1997, Constitutive activation of NF-kappaB during progression of breast cancer to hormone-independent growth. Mol Cell Biol 17(7):3629–3639.

22. Palayoor ST, Youmell MY, Calderwood SK, et al. 1999, Constitutive activation of IkappaB kinase alpha and NF-kappaB in prostate cancer cells is inhibited by ibuprofen. Oncogene 18(51):7389–7394.

23. Wang W, Abbruzzese JL, Evans DB, et al. 1999, The nuclear factor-kappa B RelA transcription factor is constitutively activated in human pancreatic adenocarcinoma cells. Clin Cancer Res 5(1):119–127.

24. Beg AA, Baltimore D. 1996, An essential role for NF-kappaB in preventing TNF-alpha-induced cell death. Science 274(5288):782–784.

25. Wang CY, Cusack JC Jr, Liu RB Jr.1999, Control of inducible chemoresistance: enhanced antitumor therapy through increased apoptosis by inhibition of NF-kappaB. Nat Med 5(4):412–417.

26. Andela VB, Schwarz EM, Puzas JE, et al. 2000, Tumor metastasis and the reciprocal regulation of prometastatic and antimetastatic factors by nuclear factor kappaB. Cancer Res 60(23):6557–6562.

27. Pahl HL. 1999, Activators and target genes of Rel/NF-kappaB transcription factors. Oncogene 18(49):6853–6866.

28. Aggarwal BB. 2004, Nuclear factor-kappaB: the enemy within. Cancer Cell 6(3):203–208.

29. Karin M, Cao Y, Greten FL, et al. 2002, NF-kappaB in cancer: from innocent bystander to major culprit. Nat Rev Cancer 2(4):301–310.

30. Beg AA, Sha WC, Bronson RT, et al. 1995, Embryonic lethality and liver degeneration in mice lacking the RelA component of NF-kappa B. Nature 376(6536):167–170.

31. Li Q, Van Antwerp D, Mercurio F, et al. 1999, Severe liver degeneration in mice lacking the IkappaB kinase 2 gene. Science 284(5412):321–325.

32. Liao X, Zhang L, Thrasher JB, et al. 2003, Glycogen synthase kinase-3beta suppression eliminates tumor necrosis factor-related apoptosis-inducing ligand resistance in prostate cancer. Mol Cancer Ther 2(11):1215–1222.

33. Mazor M, Kawano Y, Zhu H, et al. 2004, Inhibition of glycogen synthase kinase-3 represses androgen receptor activity and prostate cancer cell growth. Oncogene 23(47):7882–7892.

34. Ougolkov AV, Fernandez-Zapico ME, Bilim VN, et al. 2006, Aberrant nuclear accumulation of glycogen synthase kinase-3beta in human pancreatic cancer: association with kinase activity and tumor dedifferentiation. Clin Cancer Res 12(17):5074–5081.

35. Deng J, Miller SA, Wang HY, et al. 2002, Beta-catenin interacts with and inhibits NF-kappa B in human colon and breast cancer. Cancer Cell 2(4):323–334.

36. Deng J, Xia W, Miller SA, et al. 2004, Cross-regulation of NF-kappaB by the APC/GSK-3beta/beta-catenin pathway. Mol Carcinog 39(3):139–146.

37. Ghosh JC, Altieri DC. 2005, Activation of p53-dependent apoptosis by acute ablation of glycogen synthase kinase-3beta in colorectal cancer cells. Clin Cancer Res 11(12):4580–4588.

38. Collett GP, Campbell FC. 2004, Curcumin induces c-jun N-terminal kinase-dependent apoptosis in HCT116 human colon cancer cells. Carcinogenesis 25(11):2183–2189.

39. Thisse C, Perrin-Schmitt F, Stoetzel C, et al. 1991, Sequence-specific transactivation of the Drosophila twist gene by the dorsal gene product. Cell 65(7):1191–1201.

40. Tergaonkar V, Pando M, Vafa O, et al. 2002, p53 Stabilization is decreased upon NFkappaB activation: a role for NFkappaB in acquisition of resistance to chemotherapy. Cancer Cell 1(5):493–503.

41. Beals CR, Sheridan CM, Turck CW, et al. 1997, Nuclear export of NF-ATc enhanced by glycogen synthase kinase-3. Science 275(5308):1930–1934.
42. Ougolkov AV, Bone ND, Fernandez-Zapico ME, et al. 2007, Inhibition of glycogen synthase kinase-3 activity leads to epigenetic silencing of nuclear factor {kappa}B target genes and induction of apoptosis in chronic lymphocytic leukemia B cells. Blood 110(2):735–742.
43. Kern SE. 2000, Molecular genetic alterations in ductal pancreatic adenocarcinomas. Med Clin North Am 84(3):691–695, xi.
44. Arlt A, Gehrz A, Muerkoster S, et al. 2003, Role of NF-kappaB and Akt/PI3K in the resistance of pancreatic carcinoma cell lines against gemcitabine-induced cell death. Oncogene 22(21):3243–3251.
45. Demarchi F, Bertoli C, Sandy P, et al. 2003, Glycogen synthase kinase-3 beta regulates NF-kappa B1/p105 stability. J Biol Chem 278(41):39583–39590.
46. Maitra A, Kern SE, Hruban RH. 2006, Molecular pathogenesis of pancreatic cancer. Best Pract Res Clin Gastroenterol 20(2):211–226.
47. Rask K, Nilsson A, Brannstrom M, et al. 2003, Wnt-signalling pathway in ovarian epithelial tumours: increased expression of beta-catenin and GSK3beta. Br J Cancer 89(7):1298–1304.
48. Gotoh JObata M, Yoshie M, et al. 2003, Cyclin D1 over-expression correlates with beta-catenin activation, but not with H-ras mutations, and phosphorylation of Akt, GSK3 beta and ERK1/2 in mouse hepatic carcinogenesis. Carcinogenesis 24(3):435–442.
49. Beals CR, Sheridan CM, Turck CW, et al. 1997, Nuclear export of NF-ATc enhanced by glycogen synthase kinase-3. Science 275(5308):1930–1934.
50. Wei W, Jin J, Schlisio S, et al. 2005, The v-Jun point mutation allows c-Jun to escape GSK3-dependent recognition and destruction by the Fbw7 ubiquitin ligase. Cancer Cell 8(1):25–33.
51. De Ketelaere A, Vermeulen L, Vialard J, et al. 2004, Involvement of GSK-3beta in TWEAK-mediated NF-kappaB activation. FEBS Lett 566(1–3):60–64.
52. Senderowicz AM. 2003, Novel small molecule cyclin-dependent kinases modulators in human clinical trials. Cancer Biol Ther 2(4 Suppl 1):S84–95.
53. Leclerc S, Garnier M, Hoessel R, et al. 2001, Indirubins inhibit glycogen synthase kinase-3 beta and CDK5/p25, two protein kinases involved in abnormal tau phosphorylation in Alzheimer's disease. A property common to most cyclin-dependent kinase inhibitors? J Biol Chem 276(1):251–260.
54. Kim DM, Koo SY, Jeon K, et al. 2003, Rapid induction of apoptosis by combination of flavopiridol and tumor necrosis factor (TNF)-alpha or TNF-related apoptosis-inducing ligand in human cancer cell lines. Cancer Res 63(3):621–626.
55. Schwabe RF, Brenner DA. 2002, Role of glycogen synthase kinase-3 in TNF-alpha-induced NF-kappaB activation and apoptosis in hepatocytes. Am J Physiol Gastrointest Liver Physiol 283(1):G204–211.
56. Kitada S, Zapata JM, Andreeff M, et al. 2000, Protein kinase inhibitors flavopiridol and 7-hydroxy-staurosporine down-regulate antiapoptosis proteins in B-cell chronic lymphocytic leukemia. Blood 96(2):393–397.
57. Wittmann S, Bali P, Donapaty S, et al. 2003, Flavopiridol down-regulates antiapoptotic proteins and sensitizes human breast cancer cells to epothilone B-induced apoptosis. Cancer Res 63(1):93–99.
58. Salgia R, Skarin AT. 1998, Molecular abnormalities in lung cancer. J Clin Oncol 16(3):1207–1217.
59. Joseph B, Marchetti P, Formstecher P, et al. 2002, Mitochondrial dysfunction is an essential step for killing of non-small cell lung carcinomas resistant to conventional treatment. Oncogene 21(1):65–77.
60. Ougolkov AV, Bone ND, Fernandez-Zapico ME, et al. 2007, Inhibition of glycogen synthase kinase-3 activity leads to epigenetic silencing of nuclear factor kappaB target genes and induction of apoptosis in chronic lymphocytic leukemia B cells. Blood 110(2):735–742.
61. Arlt A, Vorndamm J, Breitenbroich M, et al. 2001, Inhibition of NF-kappaB sensitizes human pancreatic carcinoma cells to apoptosis induced by etoposide (VP16) or doxorubicin. Oncogene 20(7):859–868.

Chapter 38
Inactivation of NF-κB

Fazlul H. Sarkar and Yiwei Li

1 Introduction

Pancreatic cancer is the fourth leading cause of cancer-related deaths among adults in the United States, with an estimated 37,170 new cases and 33,370 deaths in 2007 (*1*). Only 5% of all patients with pancreatic cancer survive 5 years after diagnosis (*1*). Even for those patients diagnosed with local disease, the 5-year survival rate is only 20%. The presence of occult or clinical metastases at the time of diagnosis together with the lack of effective chemotherapies contributes to the high mortality in patients with pancreatic cancer. Cancer cells' resistance to chemotherapeutic agents is also a major cause of treatment failure in most solid tumors, especially for pancreatic cancer. The major culprits involved in the drug resistance include multidrug resistance gene (MDR), NF-κB, and Akt. Among them, NF-κB is an important molecule and is considered to be the master switch that promotes cell survival and protects cells from apoptotic cell death (*2, 3*).

2 NF-κB Pathway

The NF-κB signaling pathway plays important roles in the control of cell growth, differentiation, apoptosis, inflammation, stress response, and many other physiologic processes in cellular signaling. Within the cellular signaling pathway, NF-κB is the key protein and important transcription factor that has been described as a major culprit and a therapeutic target in cancer (*4–6*). The NF-κB family is composed of five proteins: RelA (p65), RelB, Rel, NF-κB1 (p50), and NF–κB2 (p52), each of which may form homo- or heterodimers. In human cells without specific extracellular signal, NF-κB is sequestered in the cytoplasm through tight association with its inhibitors: IκBα, which acts as an NF-κB inhibitor, and p100 proteins, which serves as both an inhibitor and precursor of NF-κB DNA-binding subunits. NF-κB can be activated by many types of stimuli, including TNF-α, UV radiation, free radicals, etc. The activation of NF-κB occurs through phosphorylation of IκBα by IKKβ and/or phosphorylation of p100 by IKKα, leading to the degradation of IκBα

A.M. Lowy et al. (eds.) *Pancreatic Cancer*.
doi: 10.1007/978-0-387-69252-4, © Springer Science+Business Media, LLC 2008

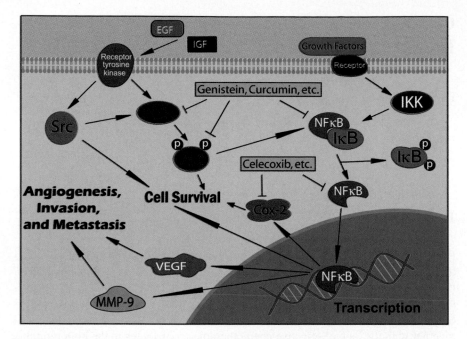

Fig. 38.1 Regulation of NF-κB cellular signaling by natural and synthetic NF-κB inhibitors

and/or the processing of p100 into small form (p52). This process allows two forms of NF-κB (p50-p65 and p52-RelB) to become free, resulting in the translocation of active NF-κB into the nucleus (Fig. 38.1) for binding to NF-κB-specific DNA-binding sites and, in turn, regulating gene transcription (7, 8).

By binding to the promoters of target genes, NF-κB controls the expression of many genes that are involved in cell survival and apoptosis. It has been reported that over-expression of NF-κB protects cells from apoptosis, whereas inhibition or absence of NF-κB induces apoptosis or sensitizes cells to apoptosis-inducing agents, including TNF-α, ionizing radiation, and cancer therapeutic agents, etc. (9, 10). NF-κB can also bind to the promoters and enhancers of some genes (i.e., MMP-9, uPA, VEGF, etc.) that control cancer cell invasion, metastasis, and angiogenesis (see Fig. 38.1), suggesting that NF-κB is a critical factor for carcinogenesis and cancer progression.

3 Activation of NF-κB in Pancreatic Cancers

NF-κB is constitutively activated in most human pancreatic cancer tissues (Fig. 38.2) and cell lines but not in normal pancreatic tissues and immortalized pancreatic ductal epithelial cells (11–13), suggesting that the activation of NF-κB

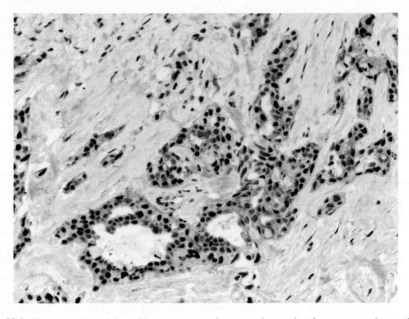

Fig. 38.2 Phospho-p65 staining of human pancreatic cancer tissues showing strong nuclear activity of NF-κB p65

is involved in the carcinogenesis of pancreatic cancers. It has been shown that NF-κB is activated in pancreatic cancers through constitutive activation of IκB kinase (IKK) and degradation of IκBα. Inhibition of NF-κB by a super-inhibitor of NF-κB (delta-N-IκBα) results in impaired proliferation and induction of apoptosis (*12*), suggesting the important role of NF-κB in pancreatic tumorigenesis.

Moreover, evidence has shown that NF-κB participates in the process of pancreatic cancer metastasis (*14*). It was found that inhibition of constitutive NF-κB activity by a mutant IκBα (S32A, S36A) completely suppressed the liver metastasis of the pancreatic cancer cell line ASPC-1. The inhibition of NF-κB activity also inhibited the tumorigenic phenotype of a nonmetastatic pancreatic cancer cell line, PANC-1, suggesting that constitutive NF-κB activity plays a key role in pancreatic cancer metastasis and tumor progression (*14, 15*). An experimental study also demonstrated that urokinase-type plasminogen activator (uPA), one of the critical proteases involved in tumor invasion and metastasis, is over-expressed in pancreatic cancer cells, and its over-expression is induced by constitutive NF-κB activity (*16*). These results suggest that constitutively activated NF-κB is tightly related to the invasion and metastasis, which is frequently observed in pancreatic cancers.

De novo and acquired resistance to chemotherapeutic agents is a major cause of treatment failure in pancreatic cancer. Moreover, it has been found that chemotherapeutic agents can activate NF-κB in pancreatic and other cancer cells, leading to cancer cell resistance to chemotherapy (*17–20*). Experimental studies have also demonstrated that other molecules (i.e., IL-1, E3-ubiquitin ligase receptor subunit βTRCP1, etc.) could induce constitutive NF-κB activation and lead to chemoresistance in human pancreatic cancer cell lines, suggesting that NF-κB plays important roles in the development of chemoresistance in pancreatic cancers (*21, 22*). In addition, NF-κB could be activated by multiple growth factor signaling pathways, e.g., EGFR, Akt, etc. (see Fig. 38.1), suggesting its key regulatory effects on cancer cell growth (*17, 23, 24*). Therefore, the strategies targeting the NF-κB pathway could be a novel approach for better cancer cell killing in designing therapeutic strategies for pancreatic cancer.

4 Inactivation of NF-κB Enhances Cancer Therapeutic Efficacy

Conventional cancer therapies have a limited role in the treatment of pancreatic cancers. Research strategies for pancreatic cancer treatment using inhibition of NF-κB appear to be promising, which may be translated into better survival in patients. The natural antioxidant compounds and the synthetic compounds, which exert inhibitory effects on molecular pathways of NF-κB activation and lead to the inhibition of its activity, could be useful in combination therapies for pancreatic cancers (*25–27*). The following sections summarize our knowledge of different agents that are known to inactivate NF-κB signaling, which could be useful for pancreatic cancer prevention and therapy.

5 Inhibition of NF-κB by Natural Antioxidants

In recent years, an increasing number of dietary anti-oxidant compounds, i.e. isoflavone genistein, indole-3-carbinol (I3C), 3,3′-diindolylmethane (DIM), curcumin, (-)-epigallocatechin-3-gallate (EGCG), resveratrol, etc., have been recognized as cancer chemopreventive agents because of their anticarcinogenic activities (*25, 28*). Importantly, these natural compounds also exert antitumor effects through regulation of NF-κB signaling pathway without toxic effects on normal cells. Therefore, chemotherapy combined with these dietary compounds may have enhanced antitumor activity through synergistic action, reduced chemoresistance, or compensation of inverse properties.

5.1 Isoflavone Genistein

Genistein is the main isoflavone found in a relatively high concentration in soybeans and most soy protein products. Experimental studies have revealed that genistein inhibits carcinogenesis and cancer progression through inhibition of oxidative stress and NF-κB activation (see Fig. 38.1). In preclinical systems genistein can enhance antitumor activity of cytotoxic agents in several types of cancers, including pancreatic cancer.

Our laboratory has investigated whether genistein modulated NF-κB DNA binding activity in prostate, breast, and pancreatic cancer cells. We found that 50 μM genistein treatment for 24–72 hours significantly inhibited NF-κB DNA-binding activity in cell lines tested (29). We also found that genistein could block NF-κB induction by oxidative stress inducers, H_2O_2, and TNF-α (29). These results demonstrated that genistein not only reduced NF-κB DNA binding activity in non-stimulated conditions, but also inhibited NF-κB activation in cells under oxidative stress condition.

We have also investigated the effect of isoflavone supplementation, which mainly contains genistein, on NF-κB activation *in vivo* in human volunteers (30). We found that when human volunteers received the soy isoflavone supplements, TNF-α failed to activate NF-κB activity in lymphocytes harvested from these volunteers, whereas lymphocytes collected prior to soy isoflavone intervention showed activation of NF-κB DNA binding activity upon TNF-α treatment *ex vivo* (30). We also tested the effects of genistein on NF-κB DNA binding activity in animal models of pancreatic and prostate cancers. We found that genistein significantly inhibited cancer cell growth in animal models, which was partly contributed by inactivation of NF-κB activity (17, 19).

The *in vitro* and *in vivo* studies from our laboratory and others have demonstrated that the antitumor effects of chemotherapeutic agents could be enhanced by combination treatment with genistein through the inhibition of NF-κB DNA binding activity. We have reported that genistein *in vitro* and *in vivo* potentiated growth inhibition and apoptotic cell death caused by cisplatin, docetaxel, doxorubicin, and gemcitabine in prostate, breast, pancreatic, and lung cancers (17, 19, 31). By *in vitro* and *in vivo* studies, we also found that NF-κB activity was significantly increased by cisplatin, docetaxel, doxorubicin, and gemcitabine treatment and that the NF-κB inducing activity of these agents was completely abrogated by genistein pretreatment in pancreatic, prostate, breast, and lung cancer cells, suggesting that genistein pretreatment inactivates NF-κB and may contribute to increased growth inhibition and apoptosis induced by these agents (17, 19, 31). Other investigators have reported similar observations demonstrating that the antitumor effects of chemotherapeutics could be enhanced by genistein (32–34).

We are currently conducting a phase II study of combination treatment with isoflavone (Novasoy®), gemcitabine, and erlotinib in locally advanced or metastatic pancreatic cancer in our institute (Karmanos Cancer Institute) in collaboration with the MD Anderson Cancer Center. Patients are receiving gemcitabine 1,000 mg/m² on days 1, 8, and 15, and erlotinib 150 mg once daily on day 1 to day 28. Isoflavone (Novasoy® containing genistein, daidzein, and glycitein) is administered at a dose of 177 mg twice daily starting day 7 until day 28. Cycle is repeated every 28 days. Preliminary data are encouraging, especially because isoflavone can be safely administered in combination with gemcitabine and erlotinib and further results await the completion of the study. Several phase I and II clinical trials using isoflavone as a single agent supplementation in the treatment of prostate, breast, and bladder cancers have also been or are being conducted (*35*) (www.clinicaltrials.gov) and thus it is hoped that these studies are likely to yield fruits in the near future.

5.2   Curcumin

Curcumin is a compound from *Curcuma longa* (tumeric). *Curcuma longa* is a plant widely cultivated in tropical regions of Asia and Central America. Curcumin has recently received considerable attention due to its pronounced anti-inflammatory, antioxidative, immunomodulating, antiatherogenic, and anticarcinogenic activities (*36–38*). It has been found that curcumin inhibited IKK, suppressed both constitutive and inducible NF-κB activation, and potentiated TNF-induced apoptosis (*39*). Curcumin also showed strong antioxidant and anticancer properties through regulating the expression of genes that require the activation of NF-κB (*40*), suggesting that curcumin is a strong inhibitor of NF-κB (see Fig. 38.1). In pancreatic cancer, NF-κB and IKK are constitutively active and their down-regulation by curcumin is associated with the suppression of proliferation and the induction of apoptosis (*11*).

It has been believed that curcumin could enhance cancer therapeutic efficacy by inhibition of NF-κB. Indeed, curcumin has been found to significantly inhibit chemotherapeutic agent doxorubicin- and paclitaxel-induced NF-κB activation (*41, 42*), suggesting its effect on reducing drug resistance and sensitizing cancer cell to chemotherapeutic agents. Lev-Ari et al. reported that curcumin and celecoxib synergistically inhibited cell growth and induced apoptosis in pancreatic cancer cells (*43*). This effect of curcumin could be mediated through inhibition of NF-κB because curcumin has been found to suppress NF-κB DNA binding activity and decrease the expression of NF-κB–regulated gene products including Cox-2, prostaglandin E2, and IL-8 in pancreatic cancers (*11*). Curcumin also potentiated antitumor activity of gemcitabine in an orthotopic model of pancreatic cancer through suppression of proliferation, angiogenesis, and inhibition of NF-κB–regulated gene products (*44*). In addition, curcumin enhanced the antitumor activities of cisplatin, doxorubicin, and paclitaxel through inhibition of NF-κB in different type of cancers (*45–47*). These results suggest that curcumin is a potent agent in enhancing therapeutic efficacy of multiple chemotherapeutic agents in pancreatic cancer by inactivation of NF-κB DNA binding activity and the down-regulation of NF-κB downstream genes.

Two phase I trials using curcumin have been conducted to test the safety, biomarkers, and activity of curcumin. The results demonstrated that PGE2 production in blood and target tissue could indicate the biological activity of curcumin (*48*) and that curcumin showed its biological effect on the chemoprevention of cancer (*49*). A phase III clinical trial using combination of gemcitabine, curcumin, and Celebrex in patients with advance or inoperable pancreatic cancer is being conducted (www.

clinicaltrials.gov). This trial will demonstrate whether the combination effect is correlated with synergistic augmentation of apoptosis, which may involve down-regulation of COX-2 protein. Another ongoing phase II trial is investigating whether curcumin improve the efficacy of gemcitabine in patients with advanced pancreatic cancer (www.clinicaltrials.gov).

5.3   Indole-3-Carbinol and 3,3'-Diindolylmethane

Indole-3-carbinol (I3C) is produced from naturally occurring glucosinolates contained in a wide variety of plants including members of the family Brassica. I3C is biologically active and is easily converted *in vivo* to its dimeric product 3,3'-diindolylmethane (DIM), which is known to be biologically active. I3C and DIM have been shown to reduce oxidative stress and stimulate antioxidant response element-driven gene expression as antioxidants (50–52).

We and other investigators have found that I3C and DIM inhibit oncogenesis and cancer cell growth, and induce apoptosis in various cancer cells (53–55), suggesting that I3C and DIM may serve as potent agents for the prevention and/or treatment of cancers. We have also found that I3C and DIM significantly inhibited NF-κB DNA binding activity in cancer cells, corresponding with the inhibition of cell proliferation and the induction of apoptosis by I3C and DIM (54, 55). Importantly, it has been found that the combinations of I3C and cisplatin or tamoxifen cooperate to inhibit the growth of PC-3 prostate and MCF-7 breast cancer cells more effectively than either agent alone (56, 57), suggesting that inhibition of NF-κB activity by I3C and DIM may contribute to the enhanced anti-tumor activity of chemotherapeutic agents.

Several clinical trials using I3C and DIM in the treatment of various cancers have been or are being conducted (58, 59) (www.clinicaltrials.gov). Our institute is also conducting a phase I clinical trial using a proprietary formulation of DIM (BioResponse DIM obtained from BioResponse, Inc.) in hormone refractory nonmetastatic prostate cancer patients with rising PSA for assessing the pharmacokinetics and determining the dose limited toxicity (LTD) and maximum tolerated dose (MTD) for further recommendation of the phase II dose for future clinical trials (www.clinicaltrials.gov).

5.4   Epigallocatechin-3-Gallate

Epigallocatechin-3-gallate (EGCG) is a compound from green tea. Green tea contains several catechins, including epicatechin (EC), epigallocatechin (EGC), epicatechin-3-gallate (ECG), and EGCG. However, EGCG has been believed to be the most potent for the inhibition of oncogenesis and reduction of oxidative stress among these catechins (60).

EGCG has been shown to have strong antioxidant and anti–NF-κB activity. It has been reported that EGCG treatment resulted in a significant dose- and time-dependent inhibition of activation and translocation of NF-κB to the nucleus by suppressing the degradation of IκBα in the cytoplasm (61, 62). EGCG has also been shown to inhibit activation of IKK and phosphorylation of IκBα, corresponding with the inhibition of NF-κB activation (63, 64). These results demonstrate that EGCG is a potent inhibitor of NF-κB.

EGCG has been found to inhibit the growth of pancreatic cancer cells (65, 66). It has been reported that EGCG and tamoxifen synergistically induced apoptosis and growth inhibition in cancer cells (67) and this effect of EGCG could be mediated through inhibition of NF-κB. EGCG could also sensitize chemoresistant tumor cells to doxorubicin through an increase in the accumulation of doxorubicin in the tumors of human carcinoma xenograft model (68).

An NCI sponsored phase I/II trial of decaffeinated green tea extracts for patients with asymptomatic, early stage of chronic lymphocytic leukemia has opened at Mayo Clinic to define the optimal dosing, schedule, toxicities, and clinical efficacy (69). Several phase II trials using green tea in preventing breast, prostate, lung, cervical, and esophageal cancers are being conducted (www.clinicaltrials.gov). A phase II trial of erlotinib and green tea extract in preventing cancer recurrence in former smokers who have undergone surgery for bladder cancer are also being conducted.

5.5   *Resveratrol*

Resveratrol (3,5,4′-trihydroxystilbene) is a phytoalexin present in a wide variety of plant species, including grapes, mulberries, and peanuts. Relatively high quantities of resveratrol are found in grapes. Resveratrol has been shown to have beneficial effects on the reduction of oxidative stress and the prevention of heart diseases, degenerative diseases, and cancers (70).

Experimental studies have shown that resveratrol inhibits the growth of various cancer cells, including pancreatic cancer cells, and induces apoptotic cell death (71–73). The induction of apoptosis by resveratrol has been believed to be mediated through NF-κB, p53, Src, or Stat3 signaling pathway (74, 75), all of which are known to cross-talk in carcinogenesis. Resveratrol shows its inhibitory effects on the activation of NF-κB (74), suggesting its role as NF-κB inhibitor contributing to the inhibition of cancer cell growth and the chemosensitization of cancer cells to chemotherapeutic agents. Indeed, resveratrol could sensitize TRAIL-induced apoptosis in pancreatic cancer cells (76); thus, the chemotherapeutic strategy combined with resveratrol may be a novel approach to enhance the efficacy of chemotherapy for pancreatic cancers.

Phase I and II clinical trials using resveratrol in preventing colorectal cancer and follicular lymphoma are currently being conducted.

5.6   Other Natural Antioxidants

Other natural antioxidants including lycopene and vitamins E and C could be beneficial for the prevention and treatment of pancreatic cancer. The consumption of tomatoes and tomato products containing lycopene have been shown to be associated with decreased risk of pancreatic cancer (77). Because lycopene is an inhibitor of NF-κB, it is believed that lycopene could inhibit the growth of pancreatic cancer similar to those that we have observed in clinical trial showing that lycopene supplements reduce tumor size in localized prostate cancers (78). Vitamin C and E also inhibit NF-κB activation and cell proliferation (79, 80). Therefore, vitamin C and E could be used for enhancing efficacy of cancer therapy in pancreatic cancer through inhibition of NF-κB activation in future studies.

6   Inhibition of NF-κB by Synthetic NF-κB Inhibitors

6.1   Dehydroxymethylepoxyquinomicin

Dehydroxymethylepoxyquinomicin (DHMEQ) is a novel synthesized NF-κB inhibitor. It has been found that DHMEQ inhibited NF-κB p65 translocation to the nucleus and induced apoptotic cell death DHMEQ inhibited the growth and infiltration of cancer cells transplanted in SCID mice *in vitro* (81) and *in vivo* (81, 82). More importantly, DHMEQ could inhibit constitutively activated NF-κB and exhibit synergistically inhibitory effect on cell growth with cisplatin (83). In cancer cells, DHMEQ decreased the level of activated nuclear NF-κB in a dose-dependent manner and attenuated NF-κB activation induced by cisplatin. The combination of DHMEQ with cisplatin also decreased the levels of IL-6 and Bcl-xL mRNA, suggesting that DHMEQ could inhibit activation of NF-κB and expression of NF-κB target genes (83). The effect of DHMEQ combined with TNF-α was evaluated in PK-8 pancreatic cancer cells (84). NF-κB was activated by TNF-α; however, the administration of DHMEQ abrogated its transcriptional activity. The addition of DHMEQ to TNF-α markedly induced apoptosis with down-regulation of anti-apoptotic c-FLIP and surviving in PK-8 cells (84). These findings suggest that DHMEQ in combination with chemotherapeutic agents may be a promising strategy for the treatment of pancreatic cancer.

6.2   Cyclooxygenase-2 Inhibitors

Recently, aspirin has been considered as a cancer prevention drug because of its ability to down-regulate COX-2 signaling. Experimental studies have shown that aspirin inhibited constitutive NF-κB activity and, in turn, decreased the expression of the NF-κB downstream gene, COX-2, in pancreatic cancer cells (85). Another COX-2 inhibitor, SC236, has been shown to suppress NF-κB DNA binding activity and NF-κB–mediated gene transcription (86). However, this effect was regulated through a mechanism independent of cyclooxygenase activity and prostaglandin synthesis. Unlike aspirin, SC236 affects neither the phosphorylation and degradation, nor expression of IκBα, suggesting that the effects of SC236 are also independent of IKK and IκBα activities. It is believed that SC236 directly targets proteins that facilitate the nuclear translocation of NF-κB, resulting in the suppression of the nuclear translocation of NF-κB (86).

We have found that celecoxib, one of the COX-2 inhibitors, significantly inhibited NF-κB activation and COX-2 expression in pancreatic cancer cells (87, 88). Other investigators also reported that tumor growth inhibition by celecoxib was associated with increased rate of apoptosis and that a dose-dependent effect on tumor growth inhibition by celecoxib was associated with reduced expression of NF-κB p65 and COX-2 (89). It has been recognized that the COX-2 mediated production of PGE2 could activate EGFR signaling (90), suggesting that the inhibition of NF-κB, COX-2, and EGFR could be synergistic in killing cancer cells. We and others have found that celecoxib combined with erlotinib (EGFR blocker) or curcumin synergistically potentiate the growth inhibitory and pro-apoptotic effects in pancreatic cancer cells (43, 87), suggesting that celecoxib could be a potent agent for combination treatment of pancreatic cancers together with inhibitors of NF-κB and EGFR (see Fig. 38.1).

A phase II trial of celecoxib, gemcitabine, and cisplatin in advanced pancreatic cancer has been conducted in our institute. However, the results showed that the addition of celecoxib to gemcitabine and cisplatin did not appear to increase the efficacy of the chemotherapy doublet in patients with advanced pancreatic cancer. Celecoxib alone may not be sufficient to sensitize pancreatic cancer to the effects of conventional cytotoxic therapy (91). Currently, several phase II and III clinical trials using celecoxib in combination with other conventional therapeutic agents for the treatment of pancreatic, prostate, lung, and colon cancers are being conducted.

6.3   Parthenolide

Parthenolide is a synthesized small molecule which has been shown to suppress NF-κB activation and sensitize cancer cells to TNF-α–induced apoptosis in human cancer cells (92). In pancreatic cancer cell lines (BxPC-3, PANC-1, and MIA PaCa-2), parthenolide treatment dose dependently increased the amount of IκBα and decreased NF-κB DNA binding activity (93). To determine whether inhibition of the NF-κB pathway by parthenolide could sensitize pancreatic cancer cells to NSAID, BxPC-3, PANC-1, and MIA PaCa-2 cells were treated with parthenolide and NSAID sulindac, either alone or in combination. The combination treatment with parthenolide and NSAID sulindac synergistically inhibited cell growth, induced apoptosis, increased levels of IκBα, and decreased NF-κB DNA-binding activity, suggesting that a chemotherapeutic approach, including NF-κB inhibitors and NSAIDs could be a novel strategy for the treatment of pancreatic cancer (*93*); however, further clinical trials must be designed for proving the benefit of this combination in the future.

6.4   Sulfasalazine

Sulfasalazine is commonly used as an anti-inflammatory agent and is known as a potent inhibitor of NF-κB. Muerkoster et al. have investigated whether blockade of NF-κB activity with sulfasalazine is suitable for overcoming NF-κB activation induced chemoresistance *in vivo* in a mouse model of pancreatic cancer (*94*). They found that treatment with chemotherapeutic agent etoposide alone moderately reduced tumor size (32–35% reduction), as compared with untreated tumors. Sulfasalazine alone only temporarily decreased tumor sizes. However, sulfasalazine in combination with etoposide significantly reduced tumor size (80% reduction) in all experiments. TUNEL-staining showed higher numbers of apoptotic cells in tumors from the combination group. Immunohistochemical staining of the activated p65 subunit showed that sulfasalazine treatment abolished the basal NF-κB activity in tumor xenografts, suggesting that anti-inflammatory drug sulfasalazine sensitizes pancreatic cancer cells to chemotherapeutic agents by inhibition of NF-κB (*94*).

6.5   Proteasome Inhibitor: PS-341 and MG-132

Proteasome inhibitors PS-341 (Bortezomib, Velcade) and MG-132 have been found to block intracellular degradation of IκBα proteins and, in turn, inhibit activation of NF-κB. In pancreatic cancer cell lines (AsPc-1, MDAPanc-28, Capan-1, and Panc-1), NF-κB is constitutively activated and Bcl-xL, one of the NF-κB downstream target genes, is highly expressed. Dong et al. found that PS-341 completely abolished NF-κB DNA binding activity through inhibition of IκBα degradation and inhibited expression of Bcl-xL in these pancreatic cancer cell lines (*95*). Moreover, they found that PS-341 sensitized pancreatic cancer cells to apoptosis induced by paclitaxel. It has been known that paclitaxel can reactivate NF-κB through phosphorylation and degradation of IκBα and induce expression of Bcl-xL through NF-κB activation. Sensitization of pancreatic cancer cell to paclitaxel could be mediated through the inhibition of IκBα degradation by PS-341 (*95*). In addition to PS-341, MG-132 has also been found to inhibit NF-κB activation by down regulation of IκBα degradation. It was found that MG-132 down-regulated expression of MMP-9, one of the NF-κB downstream target genes, through inhibition of NF-κB (*96*). More importantly, MG-132 has been found to sensitize cancer

658 F.H. Sarkar, Y. Li

cells to Fas-mediated apoptosis and radiation therapy (97, 98). These findings suggest that combination treatment with proteasome inhibitors could enhance the efficacy of cancer therapies.

A phase II clinical trial of PS-341 (Bortezomib) in combination with carboplatin in patients with metastatic pancreatic cancer is being conducted at the MD Anderson Cancer Center, Houston, TX.

6.6 BAY 11-7082

BAY 11-7082 is a synthetic NF-κB inhibitor that down-regulates IκBα phosphorylation and leads to the inhibition of NF-κB activation. It has been found that BAY 11-7082 inhibits constitutive NF-κB activity, leading to cell cycle arrest in G_1 phase and rapid induction of apoptosis in multidrug-resistant cancers (99–101). BAY 11-7082 also down-regulates NF-κB-inducible genes such as IL-10, IL-15, Bcl-xL, TNF-α, and TGF-β (100). BAY 11-7082 induced apoptosis was associated with the down-regulation of cyclin D1, XIAP and c-FLIP, the induction of cleavage of caspase-8 and poly(ADP-ribose) polymerase, and the release of cytochrome c from the mitochondria (101). These data suggest that suppression of constitutive NF-κB activity by BAY 11-7082 could be a useful treatment strategy for multidrug-resistant cancers, such as pancreatic cancer. Moreover, BAY 11-7082 has been found to sensitize cancer cells to TPA-induced growth inhibition and apoptosis through inhibition of NF-κB activation induced by TPA (102), suggesting that BAY 11-7082 could be useful for enhancing the efficacy of chemotherapy in combination treatment.

6.7 Other Synthetic NF-κB Inhibitors

IMD-0354 is a new IKKβ inhibitor. It has been reported that treatment with IMD-0354 abolished NF-κB activity, arrested cancer cells at the G_0-G_1 phase, and induced apoptosis (103). In addition to the specific inhibitors of NF-κB or its regulators, recent studies have shown that SAHA, one of the histone deacetylase (HDAC) inhibitors, also suppresses NF-κB activation induced by TNF, IL-1β, okadaic acid, doxorubicin, lipopolysaccharide, H_2O_2, phorbol myristate acetate, and cigarette smoke (104, 105). It has been reported that the NF-κB inactivation by SAHA was mediated through sequential inhibition of IKK, IκBα phosphorylation, IκBα ubiquitination, IκBα degradation, p65 phosphorylation, and p65 nuclear translocation (104). However, other investigators found that SAHA could increase NF-κB activity (106, 107). Therefore, further studies are required in resolving this controversy for assessing the role of SAHA or other HDAC inhibitors in the regulation of NF-κB DNA binding activity.

7 Conclusion and Perspective

The *in vitro* and *in vivo* studies reviewed above all suggest that the strategies to reduce the activity of NF-κB by natural or synthetic NF-κB inhibitors may be novel and potent approaches for enhancing the therapeutic efficacy of chemotherapy for the treatment of human pancreatic cancers. However, further in-depth mechanistic studies, *in vivo* animal experiments, and clinical trials are needed to bring this concept into practice to fully appreciate the value of NF-κB inhibitors in combination therapy of human pancreatic cancers.

Acknowledgment The authors' work cited in this review was funded by grants from the National Cancer Institute, NIH (2R01CA083695, 5R01CA101870, and 5R01CA108535 awarded to FHS), a subcontract award to FHS from the University of Texas MD Anderson Cancer Center through a SPORE grant (5P20-CA101936) on pancreatic cancer awarded to James Abbruzzese, and a grant from the Department of Defense (DOD Prostate Cancer Research Program DAMD17-03-1-0042 awarded to FHS).

References

1. Jemal A, Siegel R, Ward E, 2007, Cancer statistics, 2007. CA Cancer J Clin 57:43–66.
2. Wang CY, Mayo MW, Korneluk RG, 1998, NF-kappaB antiapoptosis: induction of TRAF1 and TRAF2 and c-IAP1 and c-IAP2 to suppress caspase-8 activation. Science 281:1680–1683.
3. Karin M, 2006, Nuclear factor-kappaB in cancer development and progression. Nature 441:431–436.
4. Karin M, 2006, NF-kappaB and cancer: mechanisms and targets. Mol Carcinog 45:355–361.
5. Haefner B, 2002, NF-kappaB: arresting a major culprit in cancer. Drug Discov Today 7:653–663.
6. Orlowski RZ, Baldwin AS, 2002, NF-kappaB as a therapeutic target in cancer. Trends Mol Med 8:385–389.
7. Ghosh G, Duyne G, van Ghosh S, 1995, Structure of NF-kappa B p50 homodimer bound to a kappa B site. Nature 373:303–310.
8. Karin M, Greten FR, 2005, NF-kappaB: linking inflammation and immunity to cancer development and progression. Nat Rev Immunol 5:749–759.
9. Wu M, Lee H, Bellas RE, 1996, Inhibition of NF-kappaB/Rel induces apoptosis of murine B cells. EMBO J 15:4682–4690.
10. Antwerp DJ, Van Martin SJ, Kafri T, 1996, Suppression of TNF-alpha-induced apoptosis by NF-kappaB. Science 274:787–789.
11. Li L, Aggarwal BB, Shishodia S, 2004, Nuclear factor-kappaB and IkappaB kinase are constitutively active in human pancreatic cells, and their down-regulation by curcumin (diferuloylmethane) is associated with the suppression of proliferation and the induction of apoptosis. Cancer 101:2351–2362.
12. Liptay S, Weber CK, Ludwig L, 2003, Mitogenic and antiapoptotic role of constitutive NF-kappaB/Rel activity in pancreatic cancer. Int J Cancer 105:735–746.
13. Wang W, Abbruzzese JL, Evans DB, 1999, The nuclear factor-kappa B RelA transcription factor is constitutively activated in human pancreatic adenocarcinoma cells. Clin Cancer Res 5:119–127.

14. Fujioka S, Sclabas GM, Schmidt C, 2003, Function of nuclear factor kappaB in pancreatic cancer metastasis. Clin Cancer Res 9:346–354.
15. Fujioka S, Sclabas GM, Schmidt C, 2003, Inhibition of constitutive NF-kappa B activity by I kappa B alpha M suppresses tumorigenesis. Oncogene 22:1365–1370.
16. Wang W, Abbruzzese JL, Evans DB, 1999, Overexpression of urokinase-type plasminogen activator in pancreatic adenocarcinoma is regulated by constitutively activated RelA. Oncogene 18:4554–4563.
17. Banerjee S, Zhang Y, Ali S, 2005, Molecular evidence for increased antitumor activity of gemcitabine by genistein in vitro and in vivo using an orthotopic model of pancreatic cancer. Cancer Res 65:9064–9072.
18. Fahy BN, Schlieman MG, Virudachalam S, 2004, Inhibition of AKT abrogates chemotherapy-induced NF-kappaB survival mechanisms: implications for therapy in pancreatic cancer. J Am Coll Surg 198:591–599.
19. Li Y, Ahmed F, Ali S, 2005, Inactivation of nuclear factor kappaB by soy isoflavone genistein contributes to increased apoptosis induced by chemotherapeutic agents in human cancer cells. Cancer Res 65:6934–6942.
20. Chuang SE, Yeh PY, Lu YS, 2002, Basal levels and patterns of anticancer drug-induced activation of nuclear factor-kappaB (NF-kappaB), and its attenuation by tamoxifen, dexamethasone, and curcumin in carcinoma cells. Biochem Pharmacol 63:1709–1716.
21. Arlt A, Vorndamm J, Muerkoster S, 2002, Autocrine production of interleukin 1beta confers constitutive nuclear factor kappaB activity and chemoresistance in pancreatic carcinoma cell lines. Cancer Res 62:910–916.
22. Muerkoster S, Arlt A, Sipos B, 2005, Increased expression of the E3-ubiquitin ligase receptor subunit betaTRCP1 relates to constitutive nuclear factor-kappaB activation and chemoresistance in pancreatic carcinoma cells. Cancer Res 65:1316–1324.
23. Li Y, Sarkar FH, 2002, Inhibition of nuclear factor kappaB activation in PC3 cells by genistein is mediated via Akt signaling pathway. Clin Cancer Res 8:2369–2377.
24. Zhang Y, Banerjee S, Wang Z, 2006, Antitumor activity of epidermal growth factor receptor-related protein is mediated by inactivation of ErbB receptors and nuclear factor-kappaB in pancreatic cancer. Cancer Res 66:1025–1032.
25. Kelloff GJ, Lippman SM, Dannenberg AJ, et al. Progress in chemoprevention drug development: the promise of molecular biomarkers for prevention of Intraepithelial neoplasia and cancer—a plan to move forward. Clin Cancer Res 2006, 1078–1432.
26. Sarkar FH, Li Y, 2006, Using chemopreventive agents to enhance the efficacy of cancer therapy. Cancer Res 66:3347–3350.
27. Aggarwal BB, Shishodia S. 2006, Molecular targets of dietary agents for prevention and therapy of cancer. Biochem Pharmacol 71:1397–1421.
28. Surh YJ. 2003, Cancer chemoprevention with dietary phytochemicals. Nat Rev Cancer 3:768–780.
29. Davis JN, Kucuk O, Sarkar FH, 1999, Genistein inhibits NF-kappa B activation in prostate cancer cells. Nutr Cancer 35:167–174.
30. Davis JN, Kucuk O, Djuric Z, 2001, Soy isoflavone supplementation in healthy men prevents NF-kappa B activation by TNF-alpha in blood lymphocytes. Free Radic Biol Med 30:1293–1302.
31. Li Y, Ellis KL, Ali S, 2001, Apoptosis-inducing effect of chemotherapeutic agents is potentiated by soy isoflavone genistein, a natural inhibitor of NF-kappaB in BxPC-3 pancreatic cancer cell line. Pancreas 28:e90–e95.
32. Hwang JT, Ha J, Park OJ, 2005, Combination of 5-fluorouracil and genistein induces apoptosis synergistically in chemo-resistant cancer cells through the modulation of AMPK and COX-2 signaling pathways. Biochem Biophys Res Commun 332:433–440.
33. Satoh H, Nishikawa K, Suzuki K, 2003, Genistein, a soy isoflavone, enhances necrotic-like cell death in a breast cancer cell treated with a chemotherapeutic agent. Res Commun Mol Pathol Pharmacol 113–114:149–158.
34. Tanos V, Brzezinski A, Drize O, 2002, Synergistic inhibitory effects of genistein and tamoxifen on human dysplastic and malignant epithelial breast cells in vitro. Eur J Obstet Gynecol Reprod Biol 102:188–194.

35. Takimoto CH, Glover K, Huang X, 2003, Phase I pharmacokinetic and pharmacodynamic analysis of unconjugated soy isoflavones administered to individuals with cancer. Cancer Epidemiol Biomarkers Prev 12:1213–1221.

36. Miquel J, Bernd A, Sempere JM, 2002, The curcuma antioxidants: pharmacological effects and prospects for future clinical use. Arch Gerontol Geriatr 34:37–46A review. .

37. Banerjee M, Tripathi LM, Srivastava VM, 2003, Modulation of inflammatory mediators by ibuprofen and curcumin treatment during chronic inflammation in rat. Immunopharmacol Immunotoxicol 25:213–224.

38. Rao CV, Rivenson A, Simi B, 1995, Chemoprevention of colon carcinogenesis by dietary curcumin, a naturally occurring plant phenolic compound. Cancer Res 55:259–266.

39. Bharti AC, Donato N, Singh S, 2003, Curcumin (diferuloylmethane) down-regulates the constitutive activation of nuclear factor-kappa B and IkappaBalpha kinase in human multiple myeloma cells, leading to suppression of proliferation and induction of apoptosis. Blood 101:1053–1062.

40. Duvoix A, Morceau F, Delhalle S, 2003, Induction of apoptosis by curcumin: mediation by glutathione S-transferase P1-1 inhibition. Biochem Pharmacol 66:1475–1483.

41. Chuang SE, Yeh PY, Lu YS, 2002, Basal levels and patterns of anticancer drug-induced activation of nuclear factor-kappaB (NF-kappaB), and its attenuation by tamoxifen, dexamethasone, and curcumin in carcinoma cells. Biochem Pharmacol 63:1709–1716.

42. Aggarwal BB, Shishodia S, Takada Y, 2005, Curcumin suppresses the paclitaxel-induced nuclear factor-kappaB pathway in breast cancer cells and inhibits lung metastasis of human breast cancer in nude mice. Clin Cancer Res 11:7490–7498.

43. Lev-Ari S, Zinger H, Kazanov D, 2005, Curcumin synergistically potentiates the growth inhibitory and pro-apoptotic effects of celecoxib in pancreatic adenocarcinoma cells. Biomed Pharmacother 59(Suppl 2):S276–S280.

44. Kunnumakkara AB, Guha S, Krishnan S, 2007, Curcumin potentiates antitumor activity of gemcitabine in an orthotopic model of pancreatic cancer through suppression of proliferation, angiogenesis, and inhibition of nuclear factor-kappaB-regulated gene products. Cancer Res 67:3853–3861.

45. Notarbartolo M, Poma P, Perri D, 2005, Antitumor effects of curcumin, alone or in combination with cisplatin or doxorubicin, on human hepatic cancer cells. Analysis of their possible relationship to changes in NF-kB activation levels and in IAP gene expression. Cancer Lett 224:53–65.

46. Bava SV, Puliappadamba VT, Deepti A, 2005, Sensitization of taxol-induced apoptosis by curcumin involves down-regulation of nuclear factor-kappaB and the serine/threonine kinase Akt and is independent of tubulin polymerization. J Biol Chem 280:6301–6308.

47. Venkatraman M, Anto RJ, Nair A, 2005, Biological and chemical inhibitors of NF-kappaB sensitize SiHa cells to cisplatin-induced apoptosis. Mol Carcinog 44:51–59.

48. Sharma RA, Euden SA, Platton SL, 2004, Phase I clinical trial of oral curcumin: biomarkers of systemic activity and compliance. Clin Cancer Res 10:6847–6854.

49. Cheng AL, Hsu CH, Lin JK, 2001, Phase I clinical trial of curcumin, a chemopreventive agent, in patients with high-risk or pre-malignant lesions. Anticancer Res 21:2895–2900.

50. Nho CW, Jeffery E, 2004, Crambene, a bioactive nitrile derived from glucosinolate hydrolysis, acts via the antioxidant response element to upregulate quinone reductase alone or synergistically with indole-3-carbinol. Toxicol Appl Pharmacol 198:40–48.

51. Benabadji SH, Wen R, Zheng JB, 2004, Anticarcinogenic and antioxidant activity of diindolylmethane derivatives. Acta Pharmacol Sin 25:666–671.

52. Aggarwal BB, Ichikawa H. 2005, Molecular targets and anticancer potential of indole-3-carbinol and its derivatives. Cell Cycle 4:1201–1215.

53. Firestone GL, Bjeldanes LF, 2003, Indole-3-carbinol and 3-3Î-diindolylmethane antiproliferative signaling pathways control cell-cycle gene transcription in human breast cancer cells by regulating promoter-Sp1 transcription factor interactions. J Nutr 133:2448S–2455S.

54. Li Y, Chinni SR, Sarkar FH, 2005, Selective growth regulatory and pro-apoptotic effects of DIM is mediated by AKT and NF-kappaB pathways in prostate cancer cells. Front Biosci 10:236–243.

55. Rahman KW, Sarkar FH, 2005, Inhibition of nuclear translocation of nuclear factor-{kappa}B contributes to 3,3'-diindolylmethane-induced apoptosis in breast cancer cells. Cancer Res 65:364–371.
56. Cover CM, Hsieh SJ, Cram EJ, 1999, Indole-3-carbinol and tamoxifen cooperate to arrest the cell cycle of MCF-7 human breast cancer cells. Cancer Res 59:1244–1251.
57. Sarkar FH, Li Y. 2004, Indole-3-carbinol and prostate cancer. J Nutr 134:3493S–3498S.
58. Naik R, Nixon S, Lopes A, 2006, A randomized phase II trial of indole-3-carbinol in the treatment of vulvar intraepithelial neoplasia. Int J Gynecol Cancer 16:786–790.
59. Reed GA, Peterson KS, Smith HJ, 2005, A phase I study of indole-3-carbinol in women: tolerability and effects. Cancer Epidemiol Biomarkers Prev 14:1953–1960.
60. Mukhtar H, Ahmad N. 1999, Green tea in chemoprevention of cancer. Toxicol Sci 52:111–117.
61. Afaq F, Adhami VM, Ahmad N, 2003, Inhibition of ultraviolet B-mediated activation of nuclear factor kappaB in normal human epidermal keratinocytes by green tea Constituent (-)-epigallocatechin-3-gallate. Oncogene 22:1035–1044.
62. Ahmad N, Gupta S, Mukhtar H. 2000, Green tea polyphenol epigallocatechin-3-gallate differentially modulates nuclear factor kappaB in cancer cells versus normal cells. Arch Biochem Biophys 376:338–346.
63. Chen PC, Wheeler DS, Malhotra V, 2002, A green tea-derived polyphenol, epigallocatechin-3-gallate, inhibits IkappaB kinase activation and IL-8 gene expression in respiratory epithelium. Inflammation 26:233–241.
64. Yang F, Oz HS, Barve S, 2001, The green tea polyphenol (-)-epigallocatechin-3-gallate blocks nuclear factor-kappa B activation by inhibiting I kappa B kinase activity in the intestinal epithelial cell line IEC-6. Mol Pharmacol 60:528–533.
65. Takada M, Nakamura Y, Koizumi T, 2002, Suppression of human pancreatic carcinoma cell growth and invasion by epigallocatechin-3-gallate. Pancreas 25:45–48.
66. Lyn-Cook BD, Rogers T, Yan Y, 1999, Chemopreventive effects of tea extracts and various components on human pancreatic and prostate tumor cells in vitro. Nutr Cancer 35:80–86.
67. Zhang Q, Wei D, Liu J, 2004, In vivo reversal of doxorubicin resistance by (-)-epigallocatechin gallate in a solid human carcinoma xenograft. Cancer Lett 208:179–186.
68. Fremont L. 2000, Biological effects of resveratrol. Life Sci 66:663–673.
69. Shanafelt TD, Lee YK, Call TG, 2006, Clinical effects of oral green tea extracts in four patients with low grade B-cell malignancies. Leuk Res 30:707–712.
70. Olas B, Wachowicz B, Saluk-Juszczak J, 2002, Effect of resveratrol, a natural polyphenolic compound, on platelet activation induced by endotoxin or thrombin. Thromb Res 107:141–145.
71. Scarlatti F, Sala G, Somenzi G, 2003, Resveratrol induces growth inhibition and apoptosis in metastatic breast cancer cells via de novo ceramide signaling. FASEB J 17:2339–2341.
72. Delmas D, Rebe C, Lacour S, 2003, Resveratrol-induced apoptosis is associated with Fas redistribution in the rafts and the formation of a death-inducing signaling complex in colon cancer cells. J Biol Chem 278:41482–41490.
73. Ding XZ, Adrian TE. 2002, Resveratrol inhibits proliferation and induces apoptosis in human pancreatic cancer cells. Pancreas 25:e71–e76.
74. Estrov Z, Shishodia S, Faderl S, 2003, Resveratrol blocks interleukin-1beta-induced activation of the nuclear transcription factor NF-kappaB, inhibits proliferation, causes S-phase arrest, and induces apoptosis of acute myeloid leukemia cells. Blood 102:987–995.
75. Kotha A, Sekharam M, Cilenti L, 2006, Resveratrol inhibits Src and Stat3 signaling and induces the apoptosis of malignant cells containing activated Stat3 protein. Mol Cancer Ther 5:621–629.
76. Fulda S, Debatin KM, 2004, Sensitization for tumor necrosis factor-related apoptosis-inducing ligand-induced apoptosis by the chemopreventive agent resveratrol. Cancer Res 64:337–346.
77. Nkondjock A, Ghadirian P, Johnson KC, 2005, Dietary intake of lycopene is associated with reduced pancreatic cancer risk. J Nutr 135:592–597.
78. Kucuk O, Sarkar FH, Djuric Z, 2002, Effects of lycopene supplementation in patients with localized prostate cancer. Exp Biol Med (Maywood) 227:881–885.

79. Calfee-Mason KG, Spear BT, Glauert HP, 2002, Vitamin E inhibits hepatic NF-kappaB activation in rats administered the hepatic tumor promoter, phenobarbital. J Nutr 132:3178–3185.
80. Carcamo JM, Pedraza A, Borquez-Ojeda O, 2002, Vitamin C suppresses TNF alpha-induced NF kappa B activation by inhibiting I kappa B alpha phosphorylation. Biochemistry 41:12995–13002.
81. Ohsugi T, Kumasaka T, Ishida A, 2006, In vitro and in vivo antitumor activity of the NF-kappaB inhibitor DHMEQ in the human T-cell leukemia virus type I-infected cell line, HUT-102. Leuk Res 30:90–97.
82. Watanabe M, Ohsugi T, Shoda M, 2005, Dual targeting of transformed and untransformed HTLV-1-infected T cells by DHMEQ, a potent and selective inhibitor of NF-kappaB, as a strategy for chemoprevention and therapy of adult T-cell leukemia. Blood 106:2462–2471.
83. Poma P, Notarbartolo M, Labbozzetta M, 2006, Antitumor effects of the novel NF-kappaB inhibitor dehydroxymethyl-epoxyquinomicin on human hepatic cancer cells: analysis of synergy with cisplatin and of possible correlation with inhibition of pro-survival genes and IL-6 production. Int J Oncol 28:923–930.
84. Matsumoto G, Muta M, Umezawa K, 2005, Enhancement of the caspase-independent apoptotic sensitivity of pancreatic cancer cells by DHMEQ, an NF-kappaB inhibitor. Int J Oncol 27:1247–1255.
85. Sclabas GM, Uwagawa T, Schmidt C, 2005, Nuclear factor kappa B activation is a potential target for preventing pancreatic carcinoma by aspirin. Cancer 103:2485–2490.
86. Wong BC, Jiang X, Fan XM, 2003, Suppression of RelA/p65 nuclear translocation independent of IkappaB-alpha degradation by cyclooxygenase-2 inhibitor in gastric cancer. Oncogene 22:1189–1197.
87. Ali S, El-Rayes BF, Sarkar FH, 2005, Simultaneous targeting of the epidermal growth factor receptor and cyclooxygenase-2 pathways for pancreatic cancer therapy. Mol Cancer Ther 4:1943–1951.
88. El-Rayes BF, Ali S, Sarkar FH, 2004, Cyclooxygenase-2-dependent and -independent effects of celecoxib in pancreatic cancer cell lines. Mol Cancer Ther 3:1421–1426.
89. Narayanan BA, Narayanan NK, Pttman B, 2006, Adenocarcinoma of the mouse prostate growth inhibition by celecoxib: downregulation of transcription factors involved in COX-2 inhibition. Prostate 66:257–265.
90. Han C, Wu T, 2005, Cyclooxygenase-2-derived prostaglandin E2 promotes human cholangiocarcinoma cell growth and invasion through EP1 receptor-mediated activation of the epidermal growth factor receptor and Akt. J Biol Chem 280:24053–24063.
91. El-Rayes BF, Zalupski MM, Shields AF, 2005, A phase II study of celecoxib, gemcitabine, and cisplatin in advanced pancreatic cancer. Invest New Drugs 23:583–590.
92. Zhang S, Lin ZN, Yang CF, 2004, Suppressed NF-kappaB and sustained JNK activation contribute to the sensitization effect of parthenolide to TNF-alpha-induced apoptosis in human cancer cells. Carcinogenesis 25:2191–2199.
93. Yip-Schneider MT, Nakshatri H, Sweeney CJ, 2005, Parthenolide and sulindac cooperate to mediate growth suppression and inhibit the nuclear factor-kappa B pathway in pancreatic carcinoma cells. Mol Cancer Ther 4:587–594.
94. Muerkoster S, Arlt A, Witt M, 2003, Usage of the NF-kappaB inhibitor sulfasalazine as sensitizing agent in combined chemotherapy of pancreatic cancer. Int J Cancer 104:469–476.
95. Dong QG, Sclabas GM, Fujioka S, 2002, The function of multiple IkappaB : NF-kappaB complexes in the resistance of cancer cells to Taxol-induced apoptosis. Oncogene 21:6510–6519.
96. Lu Y, Wahl LM. 2005, Production of matrix metalloproteinase-9 by activated human monocytes involves a phosphatidylinositol-3 kinase/Akt/IKKalpha/NF-kappaB pathway. J Leukoc Biol 78:259–265.
97. Meli M, D'Alessandro N, Tolomeo M, 2003, NF-kappaB inhibition restores sensitivity to Fas-mediated apoptosis in lymphoma cell lines. Ann N Y Acad Sci 1010:232–236.
98. Munshi A, Kurland JF, Nishikawa T, 2004, Inhibition of constitutively activated nuclear factor-kappaB radiosensitizes human melanoma cells. Mol Cancer Ther 3:985–992.

99. Garcia MG, Alaniz L, Lopes EC, 2005, Inhibition of NF-kappaB activity by BAY 11-7082 increases apoptosis in multidrug resistant leukemic T-cell lines. Leuk Res 29:1425–1434.

100. Kim K, Ryu K, Ko Y, 2005, Effects of nuclear factor-kappaB inhibitors and its implication on natural killer T-cell lymphoma cells. Br J Haematol 131:59–66.

101. Pham LV, Tamayo AT, Yoshimura LC, 2003, Inhibition of constitutive NF-kappa B activation in mantle cell lymphoma B cells leads to induction of cell cycle arrest and apoptosis. J Immunol 171:88–95.

102. Hansson A, Marin YE, Suh J, 2005, Enhancement of TPA-induced growth inhibition and apoptosis in myeloid leukemia cells by BAY 11-7082, an NF-kappaB inhibitor. Int J Oncol 27:941–948.

103. Tanaka A, Muto S, Konno M, 2006, A new IkappaB kinase beta inhibitor prevents human breast cancer progression through negative regulation of cell cycle transition. Cancer Res 66:419–426.

104. Takada Y, Gillenwater A, Ichikawa H, 2006, Suberoylanilide hydroxamic acid potentiates apoptosis, inhibits invasion, and abolishes osteoclastogenesis by suppressing nuclear factor-kappaB activation. J Biol Chem 281:5612–5622.

105. Imre G, Gekeler V, Leja A, 2006, Histone deacetylase inhibitors suppress the inducibility of nuclear factor-kappaB by tumor necrosis factor-alpha receptor-1 down-regulation. Cancer Res 66:5409–5418.

106. Gao N, Dai Y, Rahmani M, 2004, Contribution of disruption of the nuclear factor-kappaB pathway to induction of apoptosis in human leukemia cells by histone deacetylase inhibitors and flavopiridol. Mol Pharmacol 66:956–963.

107. Rundall BK, Denlinger CE, Jones DR. 2004, Combined histone deacetylase and NF-kappaB inhibition sensitizes non-small cell lung cancer to cell death. Surgery 136:416–425.

Chapter 39
Novel Targets for the Treatment of Pancreatic Cancer I: Insulin-like Growth Factor Receptor

Chris H. Takimoto

1   Introduction

The field of oncology drug development is undergoing radical change. The development of molecular targeted therapies is altering previously established paradigms for drug discovery. Instead of simplistic searches for toxic cellular poisons, modern drug discovery is now a sophisticated, rationally designed, scientifically driven process employing high throughput, mechanism-based screening strategies. Fueling this change is the rapid growth in our understanding of cancer at the molecular level. Advances in biomedical research, such as the sequencing of the human genome, are accelerating this process. Unlike classic chemotherapy, the newer targeted treatments for cancer specifically exploit fundamental differences between normal and malignant cells. A prime example is the Bcr-Abl fusion protein, an abnormal constitutively activated tyrosine kinase that is responsible for the development of chronic myelogenous leukemia (CML) (1). A rationally designed and thoughtfully implemented effort to discover specific inhibitors of this abnormal kinase ultimately led to the discovery of imatinib (Gleevec™). This small molecule kinase inhibitor subsequently demonstrated impressive anticancer activity in phase I clinical trials in CML patients. Surprisingly, it also demonstrated impressive activity in gastrointestinal stromal cell tumors (GIST), largely because of its ability to inhibit the c-Kit kinase, another constitutively active signaling protein found in GIST. Thus, our growing understanding of the molecular basis for cancer is changing our approach to drug discovery across the globe.

Despite these impressive advances, substantial progress in the treatment of some solid tumors, such as adenocarcinoma of the pancreas, remains elusive. Conventional chemotherapy with gemcitabine alone has limited activity in this disease (2). Furthermore, targeted therapies, such as the FDA-approved agent, erlotinib—a small molecule inhibitor of the epidermal growth factor receptor (EGFR)—only modestly improves gemcitabine chemotherapy (3). From one perspective, this minimal impact of targeted therapies in pancreatic cancer is surprising, given the large number of genetic alterations that have been identified in this disease (4). The high incidence of well-characterized genetic changes, such as K-ras mutations, in pancreatic tumors has raised the expecta-

A.M. Lowy et al. (eds.) *Pancreatic Cancer*.
doi: 10.1007/978-0-387-69252-4, © Springer Science+Business Media, LLC 2008

tion that therapies designed to selectively target these altered pathways will yield great clinical benefits. Pancreatic tumors are also characterized by the over-expression of a number of different growth factors and/or their receptors, including transforming growth factor-β (5) and hepatocyte growth factor (6). Despite our growing understanding of the molecular changes driving pancreatic tumors, translation of this knowledge into improved therapeutics for this deadly disease has not been forthcoming.

Currently, most ongoing clinical research on targeted therapies for this disease is focusing on the VEGF and EGFR signaling pathways using agents such as bevacizumab (Avastin™) or cetuximab (Erbitux™), often in combination with established chemotherapeutic agents. These strategies are largely based upon the success of this approach in the treatment of other gastrointestinal malignancies, such as colorectal cancer. This and the next chapter attempt to anticipate further into the future by focusing on some novel targets for pancreatic cancer that are just entering into clinical development. These include targeting the insulin-like growth factor receptor and the Hedgehog cancer stem cell signaling pathways. At this relatively early stage of clinical development, it is impossible to predict precisely how successful these specific strategies will be. It is both exciting and exhilarating to hypothesize that these highly promising areas of scientific research may provide the foundation for tomorrow's great therapeutic advances in the treatment of this devastating disease.

2 Insulin-Like Growth Factor Receptor Signaling Pathway

2.1 IGF Biology

The insulin-like growth factor (IGF) pathway is a complex signal transduction system involved in the regulation of cell proliferation and survival (7l, 8–15) (Fig. 39.1). Components of this pathway include the ligands, IGF-I and IGF-II, the cell surface receptor molecules, IGF-1R and IGF-2R, the family of IGF binding proteins (IGFBP1 through IGFBP6), and a number of IGFBP proteases. The IGF receptors are related to the insulin receptor and are found in a diverse range of normal and malignant tissues. A growing body of evidence has implicated IGF signaling as an important stimulus for cancer cell growth and invasion. IGF-1R activation in tumors can occur through the release of stimulatory ligands acting via an endocrine, paracrine, or autocrine fashion. Thus, inhibition of the IGF pathway represents a promising target for developmental therapeutics in oncology. Currently, a number of strategies for targeting IGF signaling are in early clinical development for treatment of solid tumors, such as pancreatic cancer. Two IGF receptor ligands have been well characterized: IGF-I and IGF-II. Both are single chain polypeptides with homology to proinsulin. Expression of IGF-I in liver and other tissues is regulated by growth hormone and other nutritional factors. IGF-I is a major mediator

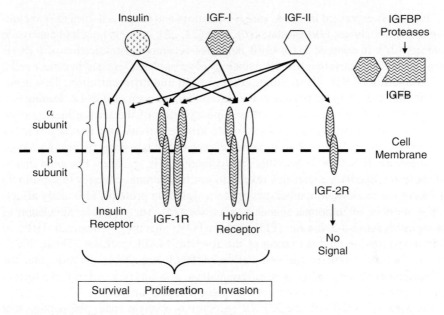

Fig. 39.1 Insulin-like growth factor pathway. IGF-I, insulin-like growth factor-I; IGF-II, insulin-like growth factor-II; IGFBP, insulin-like growth factor binding protein; IGF-1R, insulin-like growth factor receptor-1; IGF-2R, insulin-like growth factor receptor-2

of growth hormone action (9). IGF-I is a 70 amino acid protein with a basic pH, and >90% of it circulates bound to plasma proteins, such as IGF binding protein-3 (IGFBP-3). Hormones, such as estrogen and tamoxifen, can decrease IGF-1 levels, possibly by blocking hepatic IGF-1 production (9). IGF-I can bind to IGF-1R and to the insulin receptor (subtype A), as well as to hybrid receptors composed of subunits from both receptors.

In contrast, IGF-II is an acidic protein composed of 67 amino acid residues. IGF-II is also produced in the liver and extrahepatic tissues, but less is known about its regulation and control compared with IGF-I. In normal cells, only a single IGF-II allele is expressed (genomic imprinting); however, in colorectal cancer, expression of both IGF-II alleles (loss of genomic imprinting) is a common finding (16). IGF-II can bind to IGF-1R, IGF-2R, and the insulin receptor.

Two major IGF receptor subtypes have been identified: IGF-1R and IGF-2R. IGF-1R is a transmembrane glycoprotein with tyrosine kinase activity localized to its intracellular domain. It is composed of four subunits, two extracellular α subunits, and two intracellular β subunits, linked by inter- and intra-subunit disulfide bonds (see Fig. 39.1). IGF-1R is synthesized from a single pre-proreceptor precursor composed of 1,367 amino acids. This precursor polypeptide contains an α and β sequence, plus a 30 amino acid signal peptide domain all arising from a single mRNA molecule (7). Subsequent proteolytic processing of two precursor polypeptides ultimately generates a mature heterotetramer receptor molecule.

IGF-1R is expressed in a wide variety of tumors and tumor cell lines (*17*), including colon (*18*), breast (*19*), prostate (*20*), lung (*21, 22*), sarcoma (*23*), and pancreatic cancers (*24*). In contrast to the ErbB family of receptors, amplification of IGF-1R gene is rare and activating IGF-1R mutations have not been reported in cancer cells.

Activation of IGF-1R stimulates cell growth and differentiation. This process is initiated by ligand binding to the extracellular domain of IGF-1R, leading to a conformational change causing autophosphorylation of the intracellular portion of the receptor. This enhances its tyrosine kinase activity and results in further phosphorylation of IGF-1R–associated adaptor proteins such as the insulin receptor substrate (IRS-1) or the Src homology/collagen (SHC) proteins. Phosphorylation of these intermediary molecules results in conformational changes that promote docking interactions with other downstream signaling proteins, ultimately affecting a number of important signaling processes (*15*). These include stimulation of phosphatidylinositol-3′-kinase (PI3K)/Akt/mTOR signaling, enhanced HIF1-α/ VEGF expression, and activation of the Ras/Raf/MAPK pathway. These downstream actions result in the stimulation of RNA and DNA synthesis, and the enhancement of cell proliferation, differentiation, and survival. All of these factors can contribute to the expression of the malignant phenotype.

In contrast to IGF-1R, the IGF-2R receptor is a single chain polypeptide that lacks any kinase activity and is structurally similar to the mannose-6 phosphate receptor. The IGF-2R is thought to function as a ligand clearance receptor by binding and sequestering IGF-II, thereby blocking its growth-enhancing effects. In some systems, IGF-2R acts like a tumor suppressor gene, because decreased expression can promote cell proliferation. Down-regulation of IGF-2R has been observed in various tumor types, including some colorectal cancers (*14*).

The IGF signaling pathway can be affected directly by the presence of IGF-binding proteins. This diverse group of secreted proteins contains cysteine-rich N-terminal domains that can bind to circulating IGFs and modulate their function. Some of these binding proteins may also have intrinsic biological effects independent of IGF. At least six different IGF binding proteins (IGFBP1–IGFBP6) have been characterized and five of these (IGFBP1–IGFBP5) have preferential affinity for IGF-I over IGF-II. In contrast, the sixth, IGFBP6, has 100-fold greater affinity for IGF-II (*14*). IGFBP1 is produced in the liver and its expression is enhanced by insulin. It can enhance or inhibit IGF activity depending on the experimental system studied. IGFBP1 can also independently bind to α5β1 integrin to promote endothelial cell adhesion. The most common IGFBP circulating in serum is IGFBP3. It is produced in the liver and its production is enhanced by growth hormone stimulation. Overexpression of IGFBP3 slows cancer growth and enhances apoptosis in some tumor models by decreasing the availability of active, unbound IGF-I. IGFBP3 can also promote TGF-β1–induced growth proliferation and it may also increase p53-dependent apoptosis. Thus, enhanced expression of IGFBP3 can interfere with cancer cell growth via a variety of mechanisms.

Finally, IGF signaling can be modulated by a series of specific and nonspecific IGFBP proteases that can enhance the levels of circulating biologically active IGF. Metalloproteinases, caspases, and prostate-specific antigen all can degrade various

IGF-binding proteins, resulting in an enhancement of IGF-1R signaling (9). Under normal conditions, IGFBP3 proteolytic activity in serum is minimal, but it can increase in certain disease states, such as colorectal cancer (25), and it is enhanced in rapidly proliferating cells (14).

The IGF-1R protein is 85% homologous to the insulin receptor (26); although in terms of ligand binding, IGF-I does not bind to the insulin receptor, whereas IGF-II binds to both IGF receptors subtypes and the insulin receptor (15). In some pancreatic cancer cell lines, stimulation of the insulin receptor leads to activation of the PI-3 kinase and MAPK signaling pathways (27). Thus, the insulin receptor may function as a growth stimulatory pathway in some tumors. This functional overlap raises the possibility that IGF-1R inhibition could also affect glucose metabolism, thereby complicating anticancer therapy. Finally, some cells express IGF-1R and insulin receptor hybrids that can bind IGF-I and IGF-II, thereby increasing the potential for interaction and cross-talk.

In humans, homozygous deletions of IGF-I are not lethal, but are associated with intrauterine growth retardation, deafness, impaired development, and mild cognitive deficits (28). Patients with the autosomal recessive condition of Laron dwarfism and insensitivity to growth hormone also have low levels of circulating IGF-I (29). In knockout mice deficient in either IGF-I or IGF-II, growth retardation is observed at birth; however, postnatal growth impairment is only seen in IGF-I deficient animals. Thus, IGF-I is postulated to have important functions in regulating postnatal growth, whereas IGF-II is involved in regulating embryonic and fetal cell growth. Receptor mutations in the IGF-1R gene are associated with impaired growth and development in humans (30). In mice, IGF-1R knockouts animals are severely growth retarded and die shortly after birth from respiratory failure (31). Thus, the IGF signaling pathway has major physiologic functions in regulating growth in the pre- and postnatal period.

2.2 Rationale for Targeting IGF-1R in Pancreatic Cancer

In laboratory studies, the enhanced expression of IGF-1R can cause malignant transformation of fibroblasts and is associated with an increase in cell proliferation, survival, and invasive potential (32). In mice lacking hepatic production of IGF-I, human colorectal cancer xenograft growth is substantially impaired (33). Furthermore, down-regulation of IGF-1R in breast and other cancer cells can interfere with their metastatic potential (34). Thus, in some solid tumors, the IGF pathway is an important regulator of the malignant phenotype.

Clinical epidemiologic studies also provide further evidence for the importance of IGF signaling in carcinogenesis. Elevated systemic levels of IGF-I are associated with an increased risk of developing breast, colon, and prostate cancers (35). One hypothesis supporting the pivotal role of IGF-I signaling in solid tumor carcinogenesis suggests that endocrine effects of systemically secreted IGF-1 may lead to premalignant cell proliferation. The development of additional genetic mutations in these premalignant cells could result in the paracrine or autocrine production of IGF growth factors, ultimately leading to full malignant transformation. In epidemiologic studies in pancreatic cancer patients, baseline levels of IGFBP3 and IGF-I are associated with increased risk of cancer-related death (*10*). This observation is not explained by an association between cigarette smoking and IGF-I levels.

A specific role for IGF-1R signaling in pancreatic cancer was suggested by Bergmann and colleagues (*24*). In vitro growth of the pancreatic cell lines, COLO-357 and ASPC-1, was stimulated by nanomolar concentrations of IGF-I, and this effect was selectively blocked by anti–IGF-1R antibodies (*24*). Direct down-regulation of IGF-1R using antisense molecules also interfered with the growth of these pancreatic cell lines. These human pancreatic cancer cell lines did not express substantial amounts of IGF-1 mRNA, but remained exquisitely sensitive to IGF-1 growth stimulation (*24*). This suggests that a paracrine growth mechanism involving IGF-1 secretion from nearby tumor stromal tissues may be driving tumor cell proliferation. A paracrine stimulus arising from IGF-1 production in the liver may explain, in part, the propensity of pancreatic cancers to form hepatic metastases.

In a direct analysis of clinical pancreatic tumor specimens, IGF-I ligand mRNA was found in eight of 12 pancreatic tumors by Northern blot analysis (*24*). These tumoral levels were substantially higher than those seen in the normal pancreas. The receptor IGF-1R mRNA expression was detected in seven of eight normal pancreatic tissues and in seven of seven pancreatic tumors. The common association of both IGF-I ligand mRNA and IGF-1R receptor mRNA over-expression in the same pancreatic tumors raises the possibility that an autocrine growth loop can drive the growth of some pancreatic tumors. IGF-1R over-expression has also been detected in clinically resected pancreatic tumors using immunohistochemical assays (*36*). Collectively, these data strongly support the inhibition of IGF signaling as a treatment strategy for pancreatic tumors.

Recent studies have highlighted the interactive role of IGF signaling with other important signaling pathways. Enhanced IGF-1R activation can confer resistance to agents that block ErbB2 signaling (*37*), which provides a strong rationale for combining IGF-1R inhibitors with other targeted agents, such as trastuzumab. In pancreatic tumors, inhibition of IGF-1R by expression of a dominant negative mutant blocks Erk activation and decreases the expression of HIF1-α and VEGF (*38*). In ASPC-1 pancreatic cancer cells, IGF-1R activation is required for VEGF expression (*39*) and the downstream activation of Src was associated with cell proliferation. IGF-1R mediated cell invasion was associated with downstream activation of both Ras and Src (*39*). Thus, the diverse cellular effects resulting from IGF-1R activation, such as angiogenesis, proliferation, and metastatic potential, may be mediated by different signaling pathways, all triggered by the same upstream signal. Because selective inhibitors of VEGF, ErbB1 (EGFR), ErbB2, and Src are FDA approved, the strategy of combining targeted therapies with IGF-1R inhibitors is very promising. Recent in vivo studies demonstrating that IGF-1R inhibition increases radiation- and chemotherapy-induced apoptosis in pancreatic cancers suggests that other therapeutic combination may also have clinical benefits (*40*). Collectively, these data strongly support the use of combination regimens for treating human malignancies.

2.3   Status of anti-IGF1R Agents in Clinical Development

Given the growing body of evidence of the importance of IGF-1R signaling in cancer, a number of therapeutic strategies are currently being explored to inhibit this signaling pathway (12). One approach is to develop antibodies that directly target the IGF-1R receptor. Another immunotherapy strategy is to sequester the ligands using anti-IGF-I or anti–IGF-II neutralizing antibodies. These antibodies can interfere with endocrine and paracrine IGF receptor stimulation and can block cancer cell growth in laboratory models (41). Small molecule tyrosine kinase inhibitors can also be utilized to block IGF receptor signaling (11). However, if such inhibitors are not highly specific for IGF-1R, theoretically they could also interfere with insulin receptor function. Finally, gene therapy approaches have also been proposed as a mechanism to down-regulate IGF-1R expression.

The complexity of the IGF signaling pathway also suggests that a number of alternative strategies might be employed to target the IGF pathway in tumor cells. For example, inhibition of human growth hormone function can block IGF-1 production in the liver. This approach can be initiated by administering growth hormone-releasing hormone antagonists or specific direct inhibitors of growth hormone action. Alternatively, administration or enhancement of binding protein expression, such as IGFBP1, can increase the sequestration of IGF-I and can inhibit breast cancer proliferation in vitro (42). Unfortunately, the short half-life of IGFBP1 limits its clinical effectiveness, although strategies to prolong its systemic circulation using PEGylated binding proteins have been proposed (43). Other strategies include administration of soluble IGF-1R receptors to block pancreatic cancer growth in vitro or in vivo (40).

Antibodies designed to directly target the IGF receptor have been studied extensively in preclinical models, and a number of these antibodies have entered into clinical testing. One of the furthest along is IMC-A12, a fully human IgG1 antibody that is being developed by ImClone. It binds to IGF-1R with high affinity (kDa of 0.04 nM), and it can cross-react with mouse, monkey, and human IGF-1R (44). Binding to this receptor prevents its interaction with ligands, IGF-I, and IGF-II; however, IMC-A12 does not recognize the insulin receptor. In preclinical studies, IMC-A12 blocks IGF-1R autophosphorylation and results in receptor degradation, thereby inhibiting further downstream signaling. As an IgG1 antibody, it has the potential to induce antibody-dependent cellular cytotoxicity, although the importance of this property is unclear. In preclinical studies, IMC-A12 inhibits the growth of human tumor xenografts, including BxPC3 pancreatic tumors (45). Antitumor activity has also been reported in laboratory models of human breast, prostate, colon, myeloma, renal, and lung cancers. Additive antitumor activity has been reported in combination with a wide range of chemotherapeutic agents, including paclitaxel, irinotecan, 5-fluorouracil, and cisplatin. In preliminary phase I trials, weekly IV infusions of IMC-A12 in patients with advanced solid tumors was generally well tolerated, with mild drug-related toxicities consisting of anemia, skin rash, and hyperglycemia (46) At higher dose levels, dose-limiting hyperglycemia was observed. Additional clinical studies of this agent are ongoing.

Several other anti-IGF-1R antibodies are also in early clinical development. These include EMI164, a humanized antibody being developed by Sanofi-Aventis (*11, 15, 47*), CP-751,871, a fully human antibody IgG2 from Pfizer with nanomolar potency against monkey and human IGF-1R (*48*), and h7C10, a humanized IgG1 from Merck (*49*). Other anti-IGF-1R antibodies in clinical development include Schering Plough's fully human antibody, 19D12, Amgen's AMG 479, and Roche's RO4858696. Thus, the field is crowded with a growing number of competing antibodies targeting this important pathway. All are in early phase I clinical testing and preliminary clinical data are forthcoming.

Small molecule IGF-1R tyrosine kinase inhibitors are less far along in clinical development (*11, 15*). As mentioned, a substantial challenge to this approach is to avoid cross-reactivity with the insulin receptor. One of these small molecule tyrosine kinase inhibitors, INSM-18, is an orally bioavailable agent that can block both IGF-1 and HER2 signaling (*11*). This agent is in phase I clinical trials. The pyrrol pyrimidines NVP-AEW541 and NVP-AD742 purportedly have selective IGF-1R kinase inhibitory activity and are both active in preclinical models (*50, 51*). Other small molecules in preclinical development are BMS-536924 (*52*) and BMS-554417 (*53*). Clinical programs studying these very interesting small molecule IGF-1R inhibitors are just being initiated.

Targeting the IGF signaling pathway has great promise for the treatment of solid tumors, and pancreatic cancer specifically. However, major hurdles still exist; most important will be to identify the spectrum of clinical toxicities associated with these approaches. As mentioned, concerns about cross-reactivity and the interplay between the IGF-1R and insulin receptor raise the specter of unwanted metabolic effects, such as type II diabetes. Even though monoclonal antibodies are highly specific, because of the potential to form hybrid receptors in tissues that express both IGF-1R and insulin receptors, specific anti–IGF-1R antibodies could affect both pathways. Furthermore, the high expression of IGF-1R in tissues such as the heart, bone, and central nervous system raises the concern about hitting the target pathway in these normal tissues. In addition, there is the potential to develop long-term treatment-related adverse effects that mimic those seen in growth hormone deficiency, such as osteoporosis, hyperlipidemia, adiposity, and psychological problems. For small molecule tyrosine kinase inhibitors, the lack of specificity may not be a major hindrance given the success of multitargeted kinases such as sunitinib and sorafenib in treating solid tumors. However, a broad spectrum of action increases the risk of toxic off-target effects.

2.4   SWOG S0727 Trial

An important clinical evaluation of IGF-1R targeting in pancreatic cancer will be the Southwest Oncology Group's S0727 clinical trial. This study is a phase I/randomized phase II study of gemcitabine and erlotinib plus or minus the anti–IGF-1R antibody, IMC-A12. The initial phase I part of this study will determine the maximally tolerated dose (MTD) of this three-agent combination regimen in previously

S0727: Randomized Phase II
Study Design

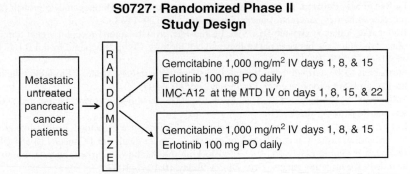

Cycles repeated every 28 days

Fig. 39.2 Schematic for the Southwest Oncology Group's S0727 study evaluating the anti IGF-1R antibody, IMC-A12, in patients with metastatic pancreatic cancer

untreated patients with metastatic pancreatic cancer. In the phase II part of the trial, metastatic pancreatic cancer patients will be randomized to gemcitabine, erlotinib, and IMC-A12 at the MTD or to gemcitabine and erlotinib alone (Fig. 39.2). Endpoints for the randomized Phase II portion of the study will include progression-free survival, overall survival, and the probability of objective responses.

The S0727 trial will also include pilot correlative laboratory assessments of the tumor expression levels of genes involved in the EGFR, IGF-1R, and gemcitabine pathways, including VEGF, IL-8, cyclin D, IGF-1R, IGFII, cda, cdk, and RRM1 and RRM2. The presence of germline DNA polymorphisms of these genes will also be evaluated. Finally, the relevance of mutations in the Ras and PI3K oncogenes in tumor tissues to clinical outcomes in patients treated with this regimen will also be analyzed. This trial will be the first to evaluate an IGF-1R targeting strategy in pancreatic cancer.

References

1. Druker BJ, 2004, Imatinib as a paradigm of targeted therapies. Adv Cancer Res 91:1–30.
2. Burris HA, 3rd., Moore MJ, Andersen J, 1997, Improvements in survival and clinical benefit with gemcitabine as first-line therapy for patients with advanced pancreas cancer: a randomized trial. J Clin Oncol 15:2403–2413.
3. Moore MJ, Goldstein D, Hamm J, et al. Erlotinib plus gemcitabine compared with gemcitabine alone in patients with advanced pancreatic cancer: a Phase III trial of the National Cancer Institute of Canada Clinical Trials Group. J Clin Oncol 2007.
4. Giovannetti E, Mey V, Nannizzi S, 2006, Pharmacogenetics of anticancer drug sensitivity in pancreatic cancer. Mol Cancer Ther 5:1387–1395.
5. Rane SG, Lee JH, Lin HM, 2006, Transforming growth factor-beta pathway: role in pancreas development and pancreatic disease. Cytokine Growth Factor Rev 17:107–119.

6. Di Renzo MF, Poulsom R, Olivero M, 1995, Expression of the Met/hepatocyte growth factor receptor in human pancreatic cancer. Cancer Res 55:1129–1138.
7. Butler AA, Yakar S, Gewolb IH, 1998, Insulin-like growth factor-I receptor signal transduction: at the interface between physiology and cell biology. Comp Biochem Physiol B Biochem Mol Biol 121:19–26.
8. Surmacz E. 2003, Growth factor receptors as therapeutic targets: strategies to inhibit the insulin-like growth factor I receptor. Oncogene 22:6589–6597.
9. Pollak MN, Schernhammer ES, Hankinson SE, 2004, Insulin-like growth factors and neoplasia. Nat Rev Cancer 4:505–518.
10. Lin Y, Tamakoshi A, Kikuchi S, 2004, Serum insulin-like growth factor-I, insulin-like growth factor binding protein-3, and the risk of pancreatic cancer death. Int J Cancer 110:584–588.
11. Hofmann F, Garcia-Echeverria C. 2005, Blocking the insulin-like growth factor-I receptor as a strategy for targeting cancer. Drug Discov Today 10:1041–1047.
12. Miller BS, Yee D, 2005, Type I insulin-like growth factor receptor as a therapeutic target in cancer. Cancer Res 65:10123–10127.
13. Larsson O, Girnita A, Girnita L, 2005, Role of insulin-like growth factor 1 receptor signalling in cancer. Br J Cancer 92:2097–2101.
14. Durai R, Yang W, Gupta S, 2005, The role of the insulin-like growth factor system in colorectal cancer: review of current knowledge. Int J Colorectal Dis 20:203–220.
15. Sachdev D, Yee D. 2007, Disrupting insulin-like growth factor signaling as a potential cancer therapy. Mol Cancer Ther 6:1–12.
16. Cui H, Cruz-Correa M, Giardiello FM, 2003, Loss of IGF2 imprinting: a potential marker of colorectal cancer risk. Science 299:1753–1755.
17. Ouban A, Muraca P, Yeatman T, 2003, Expression and distribution of insulin-like growth factor-1 receptor in human carcinomas. Hum Pathol 34:803–808.
18. Weber MM, Fottner C, Liu SB, 2002, Overexpression of the insulin-like growth factor I receptor in human colon carcinomas. Cancer 95:2086–2095.
19. Happerfield LC, Miles DW, Barnes DM, 1997, The localization of the insulin-like growth factor receptor 1 (IGFR-1) in benign and malignant breast tissue. J Pathol 183:412–417.
20. Hellawell GO, Turner GD, Davies DR, 2002, Expression of the type 1 insulin-like growth factor receptor is up-regulated in primary prostate cancer and commonly persists in metastatic disease. Cancer Res 62:2942–2950.
21. Cappuzzo F, Toschi L, Tallini G, 2006, Insulin-like growth factor receptor 1 (IGFR-1) is significantly associated with longer survival in non-small-cell lung cancer patients treated with gefitinib. Ann Oncol 17:1120–1127.
22. Shigematsu K, Kataoka Y, Kamio T, 1990, Partial characterization of insulin-like growth factor I in primary human lung cancers using immunohistochemical and receptor autoradiographic techniques. Cancer Res 50:2481–2484.
23. Xie Y, Skytting B, Nilsson G, 1999, Expression of insulin-like growth factor-1 receptor in synovial sarcoma: association with an aggressive phenotype. Cancer Res 59:3588–3591.
24. Bergmann U, Funatomi H, Yokoyama M, 1995, Insulin-like growth factor I overexpression in human pancreatic cancer: evidence for autocrine and paracrine roles. Cancer Res 55:2007–2011.
25. Baciuchka M, Remacle-Bonnet M, Garrouste F, 1998, Insulin-like growth factor (IGF)-binding protein-3 (IGFBP-3) proteolysis in patients with colorectal cancer: possible association with the metastatic potential of the tumor. Int J Cancer 79:460–467.
26. Meyts P, De Wallach B, Christoffersen CT, 1994, The insulin-like growth factor-I receptor. Structure, ligand-binding mechanism and signal transduction. Horm Res 42:152–169.
27. Nair PN, Armond DT, De Adamo ML, 2001, Aberrant expression and activation of insulin-like growth factor-1 receptor (IGF-1R) are mediated by an induction of IGF-1R promoter activity and stabilization of IGF-1R mRNA and contributes to growth factor independence and increased survival of the pancreatic cancer cell line MIA PaCa-2. Oncogene 20:8203–8214.
28. Woods KA, Camacho-Hubner C, Savage MO, 1996, Intrauterine growth retardation and postnatal growth failure associated with deletion of the insulin-like growth factor I gene. N Engl J Med 335:1363–1367.

29. Laron Z, Klinger B, Erster B, 1988, Effect of acute administration of insulin-like growth factor I in patients with Laron-type dwarfism. Lancet 2:1170–1172.
30. Abuzzahab MJ, Schneider A, Goddard A, 2003, IGF-I receptor mutations resulting in intrauterine and postnatal growth retardation. N Engl J Med 349:2211–2222.
31. Liu JP, Baker J, Perkins AS, 1993, Mice carrying null mutations of the genes encoding insulin-like growth factor I (Igf-1) and type 1 IGF receptor (Igf1r). Cell 75:59–72.
32. Kaleko M, Rutter WJ, Miller AD. 1990, Overexpression of the human insulinlike growth factor I receptor promotes ligand-dependent neoplastic transformation. Mol Cell Biol 10:464–473.
33. Wu Y, Yakar S, Zhao L, 2002, Circulating insulin-like growth factor-I levels regulate colon cancer growth and metastasis. Cancer Res 62:1030–1035.
34. Sachdev D, Hartell JS, Lee AV, 2004, A dominant negative type I insulin-like growth factor receptor inhibits metastasis of human cancer cells. J Biol Chem 279:5017–5024.
35. Yu H, Rohan T. 2000, Role of the insulin-like growth factor family in cancer development and progression. J Natl Cancer Inst 92:1472–1489.
36. Ueda S, Hatsuse K, Tsuda H, 2006, Potential crosstalk between insulin-like growth factor receptor type 1 and epidermal growth factor receptor in progression and metastasis of pancreatic cancer. Mod Pathol 19:788–796.
37. Lu Y, Zi X, Zhao Y, 2001, Insulin-like growth factor-I receptor signaling and resistance to trastuzumab (Herceptin). J Natl Cancer Inst 93:1852–1857.
38. Stoeltzing O, Liu W, Reinmuth N, 2003, Regulation of hypoxia-inducible factor-1alpha, vascular endothelial growth factor, and angiogenesis by an insulin-like growth factor-I receptor autocrine loop in human pancreatic cancer. Am J Pathol 163:1001–1011.
39. Zeng H, Datta K, Neid M, 2003, Requirement of different signaling pathways mediated by insulin-like growth factor-I receptor for proliferation, invasion, and VPF/VEGF expression in a pancreatic carcinoma cell line. Biochem Biophys Res Commun 302:46–55.
40. Min Y, Adachi Y, Yamamoto H, 2003, Genetic blockade of the insulin-like growth factor-I receptor: a promising strategy for human pancreatic cancer. Cancer Res 63:6432–6441.
41. Goya M, Miyamoto S, Nagai K, 2004, Growth inhibition of human prostate cancer cells in human adult bone implanted into nonobese diabetic/severe combined immunodeficient mice by a ligand-specific antibody to human insulin-like growth factors. Cancer Res 64:6252–6258.
42. Yee D, Jackson JG, Kozelsky TW, 1994, Insulin-like growth factor binding protein 1 expression inhibits insulin-like growth factor I action in MCF-7 breast cancer cells. Cell Growth Differ 5:73–77.
43. den Berg CL, Van Cox GN, Stroh CA, 1997, Polyethylene glycol conjugated insulin-like growth factor binding protein-1 (IGFBP-1) inhibits growth of breast cancer in athymic mice. Eur J Cancer 33:1108–1113.
44. Lu D, Zhang H, Koo H, 2005, A fully human recombinant IgG-like bispecific antibody to both the epidermal growth factor receptor and the insulin-like growth factor receptor for enhanced antitumor activity. J Biol Chem 280:19665–19672.
45. Burtrum D, Zhu Z, Lu D, 2003, A fully human monoclonal antibody to the insulin-like growth factor I receptor blocks ligand-dependent signaling and inhibits human tumor growth in vivo. Cancer Res 63:8912–8921.
46. Higano CS, Yu Y, Whiting SH, et al. A phase I, first in man study of weekly IMC-A12, a fully human insulin like growth factor-I receptor IgG1 monoclonal antibody, in patients with advanced solid tumors. 2007 Prostate Cancer Symposium 2007, 269.
47. Maloney EK, McLaughlin JL, Dagdigian NE, 2003, An anti-insulin-like growth factor I receptor antibody that is a potent inhibitor of cancer cell proliferation. Cancer Res 63:5073–5083.
48. Cohen BD, Baker DA, Soderstrom C, 2005, Combination therapy enhances the inhibition of tumor growth with the fully human anti-type 1 insulin-like growth factor receptor monoclonal antibody CP-751,871. Clin Cancer Res 11:2063–2073.
49. Goetsch L, Gonzalez A, Leger O, 2005, A recombinant humanized anti-insulin-like growth factor receptor type I antibody (h7C10) enhances the antitumor activity of vinorelbine and

anti-epidermal growth factor receptor therapy against human cancer xenografts. Int J Cancer 113:316–328.

50. Garcia-Echeverria C, Pearson MA, Marti A, 2004, In vivo antitumor activity of NVP-AEW541-A novel, potent, and selective inhibitor of the IGF-IR kinase. Cancer Cell 5:231–239.

51. Warshamana-Greene GS, Litz J, Buchdunger E, 2005, The insulin-like growth factor-I receptor kinase inhibitor, NVP-ADW742, sensitizes small cell lung cancer cell lines to the effects of chemotherapy. Clin Cancer Res 11:1563–1571.

52. Wittman M, Carboni J, Attar R, 2005, Discovery of a (1H-benzoimidazol-2-yl)-1H-pyridin-2-one (BMS-536924) inhibitor of insulin-like growth factor I receptor kinase with in vivo antitumor activity. J Med Chem 48:5639–5643.

53. Haluska P, Carboni JM, Loegering DA, 2006, In vitro and in vivo antitumor effects of the dual insulin-like growth factor-I/insulin receptor inhibitor, BMS-554417. Cancer Res 66:362–371.

Chapter 40
Novel Targets for the Treatment of Pancreatic Cancer II: The Hedgehog Signaling Pathway

Chris H. Takimoto

1 Hedgehog Signaling Pathway

Another very promising target for the treatment of pancreatic cancer is the Hedgehog signaling pathway. Currently, a large body of research is focused on modulating solid tumor stem cells as a means to selectively target malignant disease. This strategy is dependent upon the hypothesis that a small, discrete population of stem cells is present in solid tumors that posses an immortal self-renewal capacity with the potential for diverse differentiation. Regulation of cancer stem cells is modulated by a group of signaling molecules with important functions in embryonic development; these include Hedgehog, Notch, Wnt, and bone morphogenic protein/transforming growth factor-β (BMP/TGF-β). Altered regulation of these proteins may occur in a variety of cancer types. One target with particular promise for treating pancreatic cancer is the Hedgehog (Hh) signaling pathway (*1, 2*).

The Hedgehog signaling pathway is comprised of three creatively named secretory proteins, Sonic Hedgehog (SHH), Indian Hedgehog (IHH), and Desert Hedgehog (DHH). All can modulate cell-cell signaling and are involved in the control of tissue formation or "patterning" during normal embryonic development (*2*). In some systems, activation of Hh signaling promotes cell proliferation, whereas in others it can induce differentiation. In tumor cells, aberrant Hh signaling may contribute to the expression of an aggressive malignant phenotype. Recently, it has been a focus for new therapeutic strategies for treating various cancers, including pancreatic tumors (*3*).

1.2 Hedgehog Biology

Because of its importance in embryonic development, Hh signaling modulates cellular proliferation and differentiation in a highly coordinated fashion. Defective Hh signaling results in major aberrations in human fetal development, including a condition called *holoprosencephaly,* which is characterized by the failure of the central nervous system hemispheres to properly separate, and *cyclopia,* the development of a single centrally placed eye (*4*). The importance of Hh signaling in cancer and its potential as a therapeutic target is just starting to emerge (*1*).

A.M. Lowy et al. (eds.) *Pancreatic Cancer.*
doi: 10.1007/978-0-387-69252-4, © Springer Science+Business Media, LLC 2008

Hedgehog signaling proteins were first characterized in *Drosophila,* although their function is well conserved across diverse types of species (*2*). They are hydrophobic secretory proteins that can form tissue gradients through diffusion to guide embryonic tissue development. Thus, they are thought to act in a paracrine fashion, with Hh secretion occurring in cells distinct from target cells. In humans there are three Hh homologues—Sonic, Indian, and Desert Hedgehog proteins (SHH, IHH, and DHH, respectively). They differ in potency (*5*), as well as temporal and tissue distribution (*6*); however, they share a high degree of homology and can trigger the same downstream signaling pathway. The biological activity of Hh is affected by Hh-binding proteins, such as Hh-interaction protein (Hip). Low levels of Hip expression in some tumor lines is associated with enhanced Hh signaling (*7*).

Hh proteins bind to the Patched 1 (PTCH1) protein in humans, which corresponds to Ptc in *Drosophila* (*1*). PTCH1 is a complex transmembrane protein located on the surface of Hh-responsive cells. (Fig. 40.1) It acts to inhibit the activity of another transmembrane protein, Smoothened (SMOH), by interfering with the translocation of SMOH to the cell surface. Normally, SMOH proteins are sequestered intracellularly within endosomes, and in the presence of active, unbound PTCH1, SMOH is blocked from reaching the cell's plasma membrane. However, when Hh proteins bind to PTCH1, the inhibition of SMOH translocation is lost, and SMOH accumulates on the cell membrane mostly localizing in non-motile cilia structures. These events trigger a signaling cascade that ultimately results in the activation of a number of zinc finger transcriptional factors, called glioma-associated (GLi) proteins—GLi1, GLi2, and GLi3. These transcriptional factors promote Hh-responsive gene expression. The precise mechanism by which

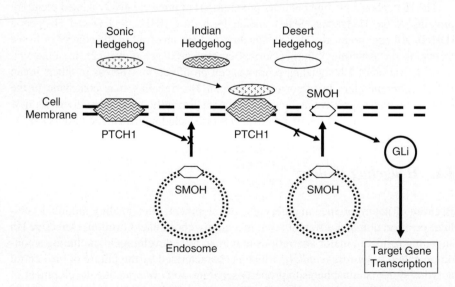

Fig. 40.1 Hedgehog signaling pathway. GLi, Glioma-associated proteins; PTCH1, patched 1; SMOH, smoothened

SMOH activates GLi1 is not well understood. However, in the absence of Hh sign-aling, the GLi proteins undergo phosphorylation and proteosomal degradation to release an inhibitory N-terminal fragment that blocks Hh-mediated gene expres-sion. Thus, in the presence of Hh binding to PTCH1, SMOH-mediated cleavage of GLi does not occur, and gene transcription proceeds in an unencumbered fashion.

In mammalian cells, the Hh signal triggers the activation of a large number of genes, including *Wnt, Bmps, FOXM, IGF-2, PTCH,* and *MYCN,* to name only a few (*3*). Ultimately, this Hh-induced gene expression cascade activates cyclins and cyclin-dependent kinases to promote cell proliferation. Changes in cell differentia-tion also occur, most likely due to the involvement of other intermediary transcrip-tional activators. In the adult organism, Hh signaling is less common than in embryonic tissues; however, certain cells, such as gut epithelial and CNS neural stem cells, have active Hh signaling pathways. In most quiescent tissues, activated Hh signaling occurs only after tissue damage during the initiation of tissue repair.

1.3   Rationale for Targeting Hedgehog Signaling Pathway in Pancreatic Cancer

The role of Hh signaling in human tumorogenesis was recognized by the discovery of a genetic disorder called Gorlin syndrome, which is associated with PTCH1 mutations (*8*). This rare condition results in the development of numerous basal cell skin cancers and it increases the risk of developing other tumors, such as medulloblastomas and rhabomyosarcomas. Many spontaneously arising basal cell tumors activate Hh signaling through the over-expression of GLI1 and PTCH1 target genes, or because of PTCH1 and SMOH mutations (*9*). Similar mutations have also been identified in sporadic medullob-lastomas. Mice with heterozygous PTCH1 mutations (analogous to Gorlin syndrome) are larger than wild-type animals and also develop skin cancers and medulloblastomas (*10*).

The role of Hh in other solid tumor types is less well characterized. However, over-expression of SHH has been observed in central nervous system tumors, and IHH is found in bone and cartilage sarcomas (*6*). In some small cell lung cancers (SCLC), high SHH and GLI1 expression and sensitivity to Hh inhibitory agents has been observed (*11*). The best characterized experimental inhibitor of Hh signaling is cyclopamine, a naturally occurring small molecule SMOH inhibitor. Cyclopamine inhibits the in vivo growth of human SCLC xenografts (*12*). Interestingly, Hh path-way activation is common in a number of gastrointestinal tumors, including esophageal, gastric, biliary, and pancreatic cancers, but it is less frequent in color-ectal tumors. Furthermore, the responsiveness of some gastrointestinal cancer cell lines to anti-Hh neutralizing antibodies in vivo supports the importance of this pathway in driving malignant cell growth. In clinical study of resected tumors, PTCH1 mRNA was 129- and 448-fold higher in gastric and pancreatic tumors, respectively, compared with the corresponding adjacent normal tissues (*13*).

In the pancreas, Hh signaling is active during embryonic development (*3, 14*). Increased PTC1 expression by immunohistochemical assay is seen in premalignant and malignant pancreatic lesions, but not in normal pancreatic epithelium. Some pancreatic cancer cell lines demonstrate suppressed expression of Hh-binding protein, Hip, resulting in enhanced Hh signaling (7). A large number of pancreatic cell lines are sensitive to treatment with Hh pathway inhibitor, cyclopamine (15). For example, orthotopically implanted E3LZ10.7 pancreatic tumors treated with cyclopamine resulted in a modest inhibition of primary tumor growth, but tumor metastases was significantly reduced. Tumor growth inhibition was even more effective when combined with gemcitabine. Collectively, this evidence supports the use of Hh inhibitors in pancreatic tumors as a promising experimental strategy for cancer therapeutics.

Hedgehog signaling pathways may also interact with other important proliferation signals in solid tumors. Ji and colleagues reported that K-ras signaling, which is extremely common in pancreatic cancer, activates Hedgehog signaling via stimulation of the Raf-MAPK pathway, independent of ligand activation (16). This association was independent of Akt/mTOR signaling; however, Hh pathway inhibitors blocked the oncogenic effects of K-ras expression. This lends further support for targeting Hh signaling in pancreatic cancers, possibly in combination with other targeted therapies.

1.4 Status of Clinical Agents in Development

Curis Pharmaceuticals has developed Cur-61414, an aminoproline Hh signaling inhibitor with tremendous activity in preclinical models of basal cell carcinoma (17). Topical preparations of Cur-61414 have been tested in phase I clinical studies and a systemic formulation is just entering clinical testing. This very interesting cancer therapeutic is under joint development by Curis and Genentech. No other Hh targeting therapy agent has entered clinical testing, although preclinical research in this area is being vigorously pursued.

Clearly more research and development work must be done; however, the expectations for targeting Hedgehog and other tumor stem cell signaling pathways in cancer therapeutics are great. In particular, Hh targeting has special promise in the treatment of medulloblastoma, basal cell, small cell lung, and pancreatic cancers. However, the range of systemic toxicities associated with Hh inhibition in mature tissues must still be defined. Although relatively few mature tissues require constitutive Hh activation, the effects of such approaches on the nervous system, gut, and other tissues must be monitored closely. Wound repair and healing is another area that may be altered by Hh inhibition. Finally, the applicability of this strategy in targeting a wider range of common solid tumors, such as non-small cell lung, breast, prostate, and other tumors, much still be defined.

2 Conclusions

The Hedgehog signaling pathway discussed here and the insulin-like growth factor receptor (IGF-1R) pathway described in the previous chapter are promising targets for cancer therapy. However, our clinical experience in this area is just beginning and much hard work must still be done to define the safety, toxicity, and therapeutic potential of these approaches. Another major challenge in the development of these therapeutics is the identification of appropriate biomarkers for predicting sensitivity and resistance. At present, validated assays for predicting response to IGF or Hh inhibition have not been identified, although much research is ongoing on this important topic. Overall in clinical oncology to date, the development of clinically useful biomarker tests for predicting who will respond to specific targeted therapies has been problematic, with the sole exception of ErbB2 targeting with trastuzumab. Given the multiplicity of important downstream effects arising from IGF-1R or Hh inhibition, the clinical situation is likely to be just as complex for these new signaling pathways.

Targeting difficult to treat diseases, such as pancreatic cancer, by inhibiting IGF receptor or Hh signaling pathways offers great hope for the development of new therapeutic advances based upon sound science rationales. Although the utility of these targets in pancreatic cancer must still be established, these strategies represent exciting areas of scientific research with tremendous potential. They provide outstanding examples of how major advances in molecular oncology can fuel drug discovery and development. Thus, even if these specific approaches do not meet our high expectations, there is little doubt that with time and much effort, similarly rigorous scientific strategies will ultimately improve upon our existing therapies for pancreatic cancer.

References

1. Evangelista M, Tian H, de Sauvage FJ. The hedgehog signaling pathway in cancer. Clin Cancer Res 2006, 12:5924–8.
2. Rubin LL, de Sauvage FJ, 2006, Targeting the Hedgehog pathway in cancer. Nat Rev Drug Discov 5:1026–1033.
3. Kayed H, Kleeff J, Osman T, 2006, Hedgehog signaling in the normal and diseased pancreas. Pancreas 32:119–129.
4. Roessler E, Belloni E, Gaudenz K, 1997, Mutations in the C-terminal domain of Sonic Hedgehog cause holoprosencephaly. Hum Mol Genet 6:1847–1853.
5. Pathi S, Pagan-Westphal S, Baker DP, 2001, Comparative biological responses to human Sonic, Indian, and Desert hedgehog. Mech Dev 106:107–117.
6. Sacedon R, Varas A, Hernandez-Lopez C, 2003, Expression of hedgehog proteins in the human thymus. J Histochem Cytochem 51:1557–1566.
7. Kayed H, Kleeff J, Esposito I, 2005, Localization of the human hedgehog-interacting protein (Hip) in the normal and diseased pancreas. Mol Carcinog 42:183–192.
8. Gorlin RJ, 2004, Nevoid basal cell carcinoma (Gorlin) syndrome. Genet Med 6:530–539.
9. Lindstrom E, Shimokawa T, Toftgard R, 2006, PTCH mutations: distribution and analyses. Hum Mutat 27:215–219.
10. Adolphe C, Hetherington R, Ellis T, 2006, Patched1 functions as a gatekeeper by promoting cell cycle progression. Cancer Res 66:2081–2088.
11. Watkins DN, Berman DM, Baylin SB, 2003, Hedgehog signaling: progenitor phenotype in small-cell lung cancer. Cell Cycle 2:196–198.
12. Watkins DN, Berman DM, Burkholder SG, 2003, Hedgehog signalling within airway epithelial progenitors and in small-cell lung cancer. Nature 422:313–317.
13. Berman DM, Karhadkar SS, Maitra A, 2003, Widespread requirement for Hedgehog ligand stimulation in growth of digestive tract tumours. Nature 425:846–851.

14. Pasca di Magliano M, Sekine S, Ermilov A, 2006, Hedgehog/Ras interactions regulate early stages of pancreatic cancer. Genes Dev 20:3161–3173.
15. Feldmann G, Dhara S, Fendrich V, 2007, Blockade of hedgehog signaling inhibits pancreatic cancer invasion and metastases: a new paradigm for combination therapy in solid cancers. Cancer Res 67:2187–2196.
16. Ji Z, Mei FC, Xie J, 2007, Oncogenic kras suppresses GLI1 degradation and activates hedgehog signaling pathway in pancreatic cancer cells. J Biol Chem 278:38254–38259.
17. Williams JA, Guicherit OM, Zaharian BI, 2003, Identification of a small molecule inhibitor of the hedgehog signaling pathway: effects on basal cell carcinoma-like lesions. Proc Natl Acad Sci U S A 100:4616–4121.

Chapter 41
Development of Vaccine Therapy for Pancreas Cancer

Dung Le, Elizabeth M. Jaffee, and Dan Laheru

1 Introduction

Despite recent advances in drug therapies for cancer, pancreatic cancer remains one of the most difficult cancers to treat at any stage. As with many solid tumors, the only opportunity for cure is complete resection. Unfortunately, only 20–30% of patients are eligible for resection, and even for resected patients the 5-year survival is 15–20% (*1–3*). For a majority of the 33,000 patients diagnosed each year, this disease is fatal and prolonged survival is rare (*4, 5*). Although other cancers are increasingly being viewed as chronic in nature, this is not the case for pancreatic cancer. The median survival for patients with metastatic disease is 3–6 months and current treatments provide marginal survival benefits.

The mainstay of therapy for pancreatic cancer has been surgery, radiation, and chemotherapy. Newer studies are integrating targeted agents with some incremental benefits (*6*). Conventional therapies have not been effective in the treatment of pancreatic cancer and innovative approaches are necessary to make an impact in this disease.

2 Antitumor Immune Therapies

Since the nineteenth century, physicians have recognized the capacity of the immune system to target tumors. In the 1890s, surgeon William Coley treated patients with extracts from bacteria after observing that some patients who developed infections subsequently experienced tumor regressions as a result of immune activation (*7*). In the mid-twentieth century, Thomas proposed the concept of immune surveillance and Burnet further elaborated by suggesting that the immune system eliminated tumors based on its ability to recognize tumor-associated antigens (*8, 9*). More recently, it has become increasingly evident that virus-associated malignancies often arise in the immunodeficient host. As an example, Epstein-Barr virus is associated with lymphomas in human immunodeficiency virus (HIV)–infected patients (*10*).

A.M. Lowy et al. (eds.) *Pancreatic Cancer*.
doi: 10.1007/978-0-387-69252-4, © Springer Science+Business Media, LLC 2008

There are successful examples of immunotherapy currently available to practicing clinicians. Among these treatments is rituximab (Rituxan), an antibody targeted to CD20 on the surface of B cells, for the treatment of lymphomas (11–13). High-dose interleukin-2 induces durable remissions in a small subset of metastatic melanoma patients (14). Another example is the use of immune-modulating agents such as thalidomide and its analogs in hematologic malignancies (15, 16). Finally, some malignancies are susceptible to the allogeneic effects of bone marrow transplantation (17–20). In general, malignancies that have been susceptible to these approaches are considered to be more immunogenic in nature.

The ideal cancer therapy would specifically target neoplastic cells while sparing normal tissues. The adaptive immune system is extraordinary in its capacity to recognize a multitude of antigens in an exquisitely specific manner. The benefit of this specificity is its ability to discriminate self versus non-self in its effort to control foreign invasion such as bacterial infections without destruction to host tissues.

Clinically, the most success has been achieved with passive immunotherapy utilizing monoclonal antibodies. The advantages of antibody therapies are that they have antigen specificity, are reasonable to produce and administer, and have relatively low toxicity profiles. Distinct disadvantages include the absence of T-cell activation and memory induction. Whereas antibodies have access to mostly cell surface antigens, T cells can target antigen from intracellular compartments. T-cell–mediated therapies have the potential to mediate tumor regressions. This is supported by the use of allogeneic bone marrow transplantation and donor lymphocyte infusion for hematologic malignancies (18, 19). Additionally, melanoma-specific tumor infiltrating lymphocytes have been expanded ex vivo and subsequently transferred into patients, resulting in objective tumor regressions (21).

Traditionally, vaccines have been designed for infectious disease prevention. This differs significantly from the paradigm of treatment for malignancy. First, the targeted population for prevention is generally healthy with an intact immune system. Second, vaccines targeted at microorganisms often generate a more potent humoral immune response rather than a T-cell–mediated response (22). Finally, tolerance is not a major barrier with foreign antigens but provides a formidable barrier to inducing T cells directed at progressing cancers.

3 Mechanisms of Immune Tolerance

3.1 Systemic Mechanisms

As immune targets, tumors pose some challenging obstacles (Fig. 41.1). Tumors have a survival advantage over microbial pathogens because they have evolved from normal cells in the body to which the immune system is normally tolerant. Pancreatic tumor cells have acquired multiple genetic mutations, which are essentially altered self proteins, including mutations in oncogenes (K-ras) and tumor

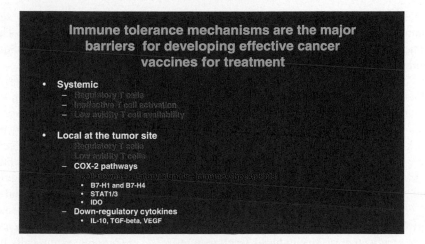

Fig. 41.1 Immune tolerance mechanisms are the major barriers for developing effective cancer vaccine treatments. These tolerance mechanisms occur at both the systemic level and in the local tumor environment. Studies using patient samples and preclinical models have begun to dissect this complex interaction between tumors and the immune system. There is increasing knowledge about the role of T regulatory cells in the modulation of tumor-specific T-cell responses. Ongoing research aims to characterize the available tumor-specific T-cell repertoires. In addition to systemic tolerance mechanisms, immunologic checkpoints also exist in the tumor microenvironment. *STAT3* activation in tumors and immune infiltrating cells results in multiple downstream immune inhibitory effects including the release of down-regulatory cytokines. Furthermore, tumors can express cell surface molecules, such as B7-H1 and B7-H4 that inhibit T-cell activation

suppressor genes *(TP53, CDKN2A, DPC4, BRCA2, ERBB2)* (*1, 23, 23–30*). By necessity, the immune system has evolved to be tolerant of self antigens in order to prevent a state of autoimmunity. Tolerance induction to self antigens has been postulated to occur through several mechanisms, including deletion of autoreactive T cells and suppression of T cells by regulatory cells. A T cell can also enter a state of ignorance in which it is unaware of the presence of its antigen, or a state of anergy in which it is unable to react to an antigen. The premise of vaccine therapy is that tumor-specific T cells have not been deleted and can be effectively recruited to promote tumor regression. However, vaccines will have to be engineered to overcome the hurdle of ineffective activation of existing tumor-specific T cells, which as a result of the T-cell selection process, may be of low avidity (*31*). In addition, vaccines will likely have to be combined with agents that bypass one or more immune tolerance mechanisms to achieve optimal effectiveness in cancer patients.

Tumors secrete a host of cytokines that have both local and systemic immunosuppressive effects, including interleukin-6 (IL-6), IL-10, and transforming growth factor-beta (TGF-β) (*32–34*). These cytokines have also been implicated in the cachexia syndrome associated with pancreatic adenocarcinoma characterized by weight loss, fatigue, and immune deficiency (*32, 33*). Contributing to this concept of general immune suppression is the observation that T cells from patients with metastatic pancreatic adenocarcinoma had reduced expression of the TCR zeta chain, a T-cell receptor (TCR)-associated signal transduction molecule. This reduced expression often correlates with decreased T cell activation and cytokine production (34, 35).

There has also been a growing list of cancers, including pancreatic cancer, in which a role for CD4$^+$CD25$^+$ regulatory T cells (T$_{regs}$) has been suggested in the suppression of activated T cells (36–38). Although the concept of suppressor T cells was first described in the 1970s, interest in the population was renewed by the work of Sakaguchi in the 1990s showing that thymically derived CD4$^+$CD25$^+$ cells were important in the control of autoreactive T cells (39, 40). Subsequently, FOXP3, a member of the forkhead/winged-helix family of transcriptional regulators, was discovered to be the master regulator in the development and function of T$_{regs}$ (41, 42). This subset of T cells plays an important role in the maintenance of peripheral tolerance and manipulation of this population may be necessary to promote an effective vaccine induced T-cell response. T$_{regs}$ are present systemically but also have been demonstrated to accumulate at tumor sites. Ovarian carcinomas have been shown to produce the chemokine CCL22, which binds to the CCR4 receptor on T$_{regs}$ contributing to this local accumulation (37).

3.2   Local Mechanisms in the Tumor and Its Microenvironment

Tumors have developed the capacity to alter themselves and their microenvironment to become invisible to the effector cells of the immune system. In particular, T cells recognize their target antigens in the context of major histocompatibility complex (MHC) molecules. Tumors may impair T-cell recognition by down-regulation of genes involved in antigen presentation, including TAP (transporter associated with antigen presentation) genes, subunits of the proteasome (LMP-2, LMP-7), and MHC class I molecules and its components (43–48). The loss of tumor-associated antigens has also been purported to be a mechanism of immune escape (49, 50).

In addition to adapting cell surface molecules to impair T-cell recognition, tumors have evolved mechanisms that have direct immunosuppressive effects in the surrounding microenvironment and beyond. STAT-3 is constitutively activated in many tumor types and induces cell cycle regulatory genes and anti-apoptotic genes such as CYCLIN D1 and BCL-X$_L$ (51). STAT-3 activation results in the suppression of proinflammatory mediators and the release of factors such as vascular endothelial growth factor (VEGF) and IL-10 that result in downstream inhibitory effects on hematopoietic elements. STAT-3 is also up-regulated in dendritic cells, NK cells, and neutrophils in the tumor contributing to an immune-tolerant microenvironment (52–54).

As investigators dissect tumor microenvironments, the list of vital components continues to grow. In addition to the secretion of immunosuppressive cytokines, tumors secrete local cyclo-oxygenase 2, which has been shown to inhibit dendritic cell function (55). Furthermore, other cell types have been identified to play a role in the tolerogenic environment. In addition to the presence of T_{regs}, immature myeloid cells and myeloid suppressor cells contribute to the inhibition of tumor reactive T cells through the production of reactive oxygen and nitrogen species (56–60). Indoleamine 2,3-dioxygenase (IDO) production by plasmacytoid dendritic cells contributes to the hostile environment against T cells by locally depleting the amino acid tryptophan, and survival of activated T cells is particularly dependent on tryptophan utilization (61–63).

4 Scientific Progress Toward Vaccine Development

Despite significant barriers to effective therapeutic vaccines, the elucidation of mechanisms of immune tolerance and regulation will provide insight to help develop the next generation of immunotherapy strategies. Molecular tools available today such as gene expression analysis allows for the identification of new pancreatic cancer antigen targets. An ideal tumor antigen would be unique to and overexpressed in pancreatic cancer cells, presented on the cell-surface, and essential for cell survival. Additionally, it should be immunogenic and produce a robust tumor specific response. Among the first identified tumor antigens identified for pancreatic cancer were carcinoembryonic antigen (CEA), mutated K-ras, mucin-1 (MUC1), and gastrin (23, 24, 30, 64, 64–66). These were identified based on their overexpression or altered expression in pancreatic tumors but not necessarily based on immunogenicity.

Two common methods are being employed to identify more relevant immune targets for immunotherapy. The first method, serologic analysis of recombinant tumor cDNA expression libraries (SEREX), uses patient serum to screen libraries prepared from tumor cells. This method was used to identify coactosin-like protein as a potential pancreatic cancer antigen, recognized both by antibodies and T cells from pancreatic cancer patients (67). A second method that has identified some melanoma-specific T cells is the screening of autologous tumor libraries using tumor reactive T cells from cancer patients (68, 69). This method is limited by the need for pairs of autologous tumors and isolated and cultured tumor-specific T-cell clones. A newer method of immune relevant antigen discovery involves that use of patient's lymphocytes after whole cell vaccination to evaluate responses to proteins found to be differentially expressed by tumors (25). This method does not require autologous tumor or T-cell clones. The candidate tumor antigens are determined by serial analysis of gene expression (SAGE), which uses differential gene-display technology to identify genes that are more strongly expressed by tumor cells relative to normal cells (70, 71). Enzyme-linked immunosorbent spot (ELISPOT) readout is a sensitive method used to quantify antigen-specific T-cell responses from peripheral blood lymphocytes from the vaccinated patients.

Mesothelin and prostate stem cell antigen (PSCA) are two tumor antigens discovered by the use of SAGE (70, 71). Mesothelin, a differentiation antigen, is a promising candidate for a tumor antigen as its expression in normal tissues is limited to mesothelial cells and is highly expressed on several tumor types, including mesothelioma and ovarian and pancreatic adenocarcinoma (70, 72, 73). Mesothelin targeted antibodies are currently undergoing early phase clinical trials. In addition, SS1(dsFV)PE38 (SS1P), a recombinant anti-mesothelin immunotoxin, is undergoing evaluation in mesothelin-expressing tumors (74). PSCA mRNA is overexpressed in 60% of human pancreatic cancer tissues and is present on the cell surface of pancreatic cancer cell lines. Treatment with an antibody to PSCA significantly reduced tumor growth initiation in a pancreatic cancer xenograft model (75). PSCA is a potential target for therapy in prostate and pancreatic cancer (76).

There is evidence that both mesothelin and PSCA are potentially immunogenic. In a Phase I trial evaluating an irradiated, allogeneic, GM-CSF secreting tumor cell line in patients with resected pancreatic cancer, there was evidence of both mesothelin-specific T-cell responses and PSCA-specific T-cell responses (Jaffee, unpublished) only in the three long-term survivors (77).

In addition to new antigen discovery methods, immune monitoring assays are facilitating the correlation of in vivo immunologic responses with clinical responses. These antigen-specific analyses include ELISPOT and tetramer analysis. Furthermore, relevant animal models of immune tolerance are now available. These models, such as the *Her2/neu* mammary cancer model and the TRAMP prostate cancer model, consist of transgenic mice in which tolerance induction to tumor antigens can be followed during the spontaneous formation of tumors (78, 79). The analysis and manipulation of these models provides a system to characterize and subsequently activate latent tumor reactive T cells. Preclinical models specific to pancreatic cancer have also been developed that recapitulate the tumorigenesis process from early preinvasive genetic changes following K-ras activation to more invasive lesions that have subsequent inactivation of tumor suppressor genes (80). These preclinical models facilitate vaccine development by providing efficient and meaningful tools for hypothesis testing.

5   The Dendritic Cell at the Center of Vaccine Design

Although there are a myriad of vaccine strategies currently being employed, at the center of all of these strategies is the dendritic cell (DC) and its capacity to adequately present tumor associated antigens in the context of an MHC (signal 1) and express appropriate costimulatory signals (signal 2) that will result in T-cell activation (Fig. 41.2). DCs respond to stimuli such as cytokines, chemokines, and bacterial and fungal products by undergoing a maturation process (22). If an immature DC presents antigen to a T cell without the proper costimulation, this can result in a state of tolerance. DCs respond to stimuli through various receptors including toll-like receptors (TLR), which bind chemical moieties from pathogens, and via the tumor necrosis factor (TNF) receptor family, which bind to endogenous ligands such as TNF-α and CD40L (81–84). Once DCs start to mature, they migrate to draining lymph nodes where they present antigen and costimulatory signals to T cells. Costimulatory

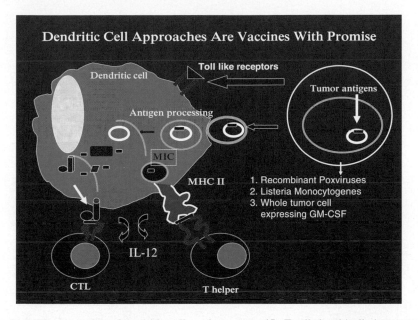

Fig. 41.2 The interaction of dendritic cells and tumor-specific T cells is critically important to the design of effective vaccine strategies. T-cell activation is dependent on the signal delivered through the T-cell receptor after engagement with a peptide–MHC complex on an antigen-presenting cell. Importantly, costimulation is also required to promote T-cell activation rather than T-cell tolerance. Costimulatory signals occur in the form of cell surface molecules, including B7 and TNF family molecules or stimulatory cytokines such as IL-12. Furthermore, DCs must be of the proper maturation status to promote activation. In addition to promoting the proper interaction between DCs and T cells, effective vaccine strategies should enhance antigen presentation in both the MHC class I and II pathways

signals include the release of IL-12 and the expression of cell surface molecules such as the B7 family members (*81, 84*). Additionally, T cells receive costimulation through TNF family receptors including 4–1BBL and OX40-L22 (*85–87*).

In general, vaccine design has centered on enhancing this interaction of mature DCs and tumor specific T cells. From pure peptide vaccines to genetically modified tumor cells, the goal is to enhance the presentation of tumor specific antigens in the context of costimulation to promote T-cell activation. Selected pancreatic cancer vaccine trials are discussed further and a summary can be found in Table 41.1.

5.1 Peptide-Based Vaccines

With the discovery of several proteins specifically overexpressed in pancreatic cancer cells, the administration of tumor-associated proteins and peptides was among the first techniques to manipulate dendritic cell function. These proteins included

Table 41.1 Selected pancreatic cancer vaccine clinical trials

Vaccine class	Protocol regimen	Stage	Phase	Results
Peptide	HSPPC-96 (autologous peptides complexed with heat shock protein 96)	Adjuvant	I	Completed. Feasible in 10 patients. 3 of 10 patients alive at 2.5, 2.7, and 5 years of follow-up. No observed correlation between immune responses and prognosis. (Maki)
	Ras peptide + GM-CSF	Adjuvant and advanced	I/II	Completed. Immune response in 25 of 43 subjects. Subjects with advanced cancer with an immune response showed prolonged survival compared to non-responders (median survival 148 days vs 61 days). (Gjertsen)
	Muc1 peptide + SB-AS2 (adjuvant)	Adjuvant and advanced	I	Completed. Induction of immune responses including humoral responses in 5 of 16. (Ramanathan)
	CAP1–6D (CEA agonist peptide)	Adjuvant and advanced	II	Enrolling. www.clinicaltrials.gov
	Personalized peptide + gemcitabine	Advanced	I	Completed. 11 of 13 had a response by reduction in tumor or tumor markers. Augmentation of peptide-specific T cells observed at each dose level. (Yanagimoto)
	Survivin peptide	Advanced pancreatic, melanoma, colon, cervical	I/II	Enrolling. www.clinicaltrials.gov
	GV1001 (telomerase peptide) + gemcitabine	Advanced	II/III	Phase II completed. Immune responses in 7 of 12 subjects. Phase III enrolling. (Nava-Parada review)
	GV1001 (telomerase peptide) + imiquimod (TLR agonist)	Advanced	I/II	Phase I completed. Immune responses in 5 of 13 subjects. (Nava-Parada review)
	GV1001 (telomerase peptide) + gemcitabine + capecitabine	Advanced	III	Enrolling. www.clinicaltrials.gov
Dendritic cell	Intratumoral DCs + GEM + stereotactic radiosurgery	Advanced	I/II	Enrolling. www.clinicaltrials.gov

Category	Vaccine	Setting	Phase	Status/Results
	Autologous, tumor-lysate pulsed DCs	Recurrence after surgery	I/II	Ongoing. 10 patients vaccinated. 1 PR, 1SD. Both had immunologic response. (Bauer) www.clinicaltrials.gov
Whole cell	Pancreatic tumor cells modified to introduce foreign carbohydrates.	Adjuvant	I/II	Completed. Data not available. http://www.newlinkgenetics.com/
	GM-CSF modified allogeneic pancreatic cancer cells	Adjuvant + chemoradiation	I/II	Completed. Phase I: 3 of 14 long term survivors with DTH and mesothelin-specific T cell responses. Phase II: 60 patients. 2 year survival 76%. Survival correlates with mesothelin-specific T cell responses. (Jaffee)
	GM-CSF modified allogeneic pancreatic cancer cells	Adjuvant after completion of standard therapies	II	Enrolling. www.clinicaltrials.gov http://immunology.onc.jhmi.edu
	GM-CSF modified allogeneic pancreatic cancer cells + CY	Advanced	II	Completed. Vaccine alone median survival 2.3 months vs CY + vaccine 4.7 months. Patients had received multiple lines of therapy. (Laheru)
	GM-CSF modified allogeneic pancreatic cancer cells + CY + Cetuximab	Advanced pancreatic cancer	II	Enrolling. www.clinicaltrials.gov http://immunology.onc.jhmi.edu
Micro-organism vectors	Recombinant *Saccharomyces cerevisiae* expressing mutant ras + gemcitabine	Adjuvant	II	Enrolling. http://www.globeimmune.com
	PANVAC (poxviral-based vaccine targeting CEA and MUC1)	Advanced	III	Completed. No survival benefit. Study in locally advanced pancreatic cancer with chemoradiation being designed. (Madan review)
	CRS-207 (mesothelin-modified *Listeria monocytogenes*)	Advanced pancreatic, ovarian, NSCLC and mesothelioma	I	Enrolling. www.ceruscorp.com

CEA, mutated K-ras, MUC1, and gastrin (*64, 65, 88–92*). Vaccines and antibodies targeted at these antigens have been tested in early phase clinical trials alone and with immune modulating agents such as GM-CSF and IL-2. Mutated K-ras vaccines have been administered to patients with resected and advanced pancreatic adenocarcinoma. In a trial in which the peptide vaccine was combined with GM-CSF, a positive delayed-type hypersensitivity (DTH) response was observed in 21/43 patients and a K-ras–specific T-cell response in 17/43 patients. The median survival in the group that demonstrated an immune response was 148 days versus 61 days in the group without an immune response (*88*). MUC1 and CEA peptides have also elicited peptide-specific immune responses (*90, 91*). Although several studies demonstrate a post-vaccination peptide-specific T-cell response, objective clinical remissions are limited. Factors that may limit peptide strategies include the selection of ideal peptides, immune tolerance mechanisms, especially in advanced cancer cases, lack of adequate costimulation, and the inability for the peptides to reach the dendritic cell target.

Another DC-based approach is the modification of tumor antigens to enhance antigen presentation. One method used for this strategy is the complexing of antigens to heat shock proteins with the expectation that this would target the antigens to DCs and MHC processing pathways (*22, 93, 94*). This strategy has been studied as an adjuvant treatment of pancreatic cancer. Clinical responses did not correlate with immune responses in this 10 patient study (*95*). Another technique used to modify the antigen is the use of agonist peptides such as CAP1–6D, which is a modified CAP1, an immunodominant epitope of CEA. This peptide is modified at position 6 replacing an asparagine with an aspartic acid and has been shown to enhance T-cell activation (*96, 97*). CAP1–6D administered in the adjuvant mixture of Montanide/GM-CSF is currently being studied in patients with locally advanced or resected pancreatic adenocarcinoma. Additionally, this peptide is being studied in the adjuvant setting after the administration of traditional adjuvant therapies. Agonist mesothelin epitopes have also been reported (*98*).

In addition to antigen modification, newer tumor antigens applicable to multiple cancer types are also being targeted in pancreatic cancer. Among these antigens are survivin and telomerase. Survivin is an anti-apoptotic gene differentially expressed in tumors and tumor vasculature (*99–101*). Telomerase is important for the maintenance of chromosome integrity (*102*). A telomerase peptide vaccine plus gemcitabine is currently undergoing evaluation in a phase III trial in advanced pancreatic cancer.

5.2 Dendritic Cell Vaccines

To improve the targeting of peptides to dendritic cells, investigators have attempted ex vivo expansion and antigen loading of dendritic cells. This process continues to undergo refinement to overcome the technical difficulties of isolating individual patient dendritic cells and ensuring an appropriate maturation status to promote activation rather than tolerance. Various techniques have been employed to enhance antigen presentation by dendritic cells, including transduction of DCs with genes or purified RNA encoding tumor antigens and fusion of dendritic cells with tumor. To enhance stimulation, DCs have been loaded with antigen and transduced with GM-CSF and CD40L. Ex vivo generated dendritic cells modified with a recombinant fowlpox vector is currently under development for CEA-producing tumors and is being combined with denileukin diftitox, an agent targeted at T_{regs} (*103*). Denileukin diftitox is a fusion protein consisting of IL-2 and diphtheria toxin, which targets CD25+ (IL-2 R alpha chain) cells (*104*). The effectiveness of inhibiting T_{regs} with this agent in cancer patients has not yet been determined.

Studies utilizing dendritic cells in patients with pancreatic cancer are still early relative to studies of DC vaccines in melanoma. An ongoing study was reported at ASCO 2007 of 10 patients vaccinated with autologous, tumor-lysate pulsed DCs with concomitant gemcitabine. One patient had a partial response and a second patient had stable disease. Both patients had an immunologic response (*105*). The correlation of an immunologic response with clinical response will have to be confirmed as more patients are enrolled.

5.3 Whole Tumor Cell Vaccines

Alternatively, in vivo manipulation of DCs is an approach used by the administration of GM-CSF gene modified allogeneic pancreatic tumor cells. The use of whole-cell vaccines is promising because it delivers a range of peptide antigens without the need for specific knowledge of the relevant target antigens. Preclinical studies show that among tumor cells genetically modified to express various cytokines, GM-CSF is the cytokine most effective in inducing antitumor immunity (*106*). GM-CSF is an important growth and differentiation factor for DCs and its local secretion serves to recruit endogenous DCs to the site of vaccination. This method of GM-CSF delivery is unique in that it provides local and sustained levels of GM-CSF required for adequate priming. The use of allogeneic tumor cells for vaccine development over autologous tumor cells is attractive for several reasons. Autologous tumor cells are not always available and the production of an autologous vaccine is technically difficult, costly, and inefficient. Supporting the use of allogeneic tumor cells is the characterization of tumor-associated antigens in melanoma, which revealed that regardless of HLA type, 50% of tumors share common antigens (*107*, *108*). In addition, both preclinical and human data support that the antigen-presenting cells important in GM-CSF based vaccination are host derived, suggesting that the vaccine cells and the host do not have to be HLA compatible (*44*, *77*).

In a phase I study of 14 patients with resected pancreatic adenocarcinoma, the allogeneic vaccine was combined with chemoradiation (*109*). Systemic GM-CSF levels were detectable for up to 96 hours after vaccination. More importantly, the only three long-term survivors were in the two highest dose cohorts and all three developed post-vaccination DTH responses and mesothelin-specific T-cell responses. These immune responses were not seen in the patients who ultimately progressed. Interestingly, the HLA restriction correlated with the HLA type of the host not the vaccine that supports the concept of cross-presentation (77). A 60-patient phase II trial of the vaccine has recently been completed. The preliminary analysis shows a 1-year survival of 88% in 56 evaluable patients and a 2-year survival of 76% in 36 evaluable patients (110). This vaccine has also been integrated with immune modulating doses of cyclophosphamide, as a T_{reg} inhibitor, in the metastatic setting. This study demonstrated that mesothelin-specific T cell responses can also be detected in advanced disease and may correlate with time to progression and overall survival (111).

A phase I/II trial of adjuvant treatment with killed pancreatic tumor cells genetically modified to introduce a foreign pattern of carbohydrate structures to antigens on the cell surface has been completed. The results of this trial are not yet available. Humans naturally produce antibodies to alphaGal epitopes. In a mouse model, anti-alphaGal antibodies targeted to cells expressing alphaGal trigger a complement-mediated hyperacute rejection of target cells (B16alphaGal). The mice subsequently rejected B16null tumor challenges, suggesting that exposure to the alphaGal-modified tumor cells boosted the immune response to other tumor associated antigens present in alphaGal-negative B16 melanoma cells (112, 113).

5.4 Recombinant Microorganism-Based Vaccines

Recombinant viral- and bacterial-vector delivery systems are also undergoing clinical development. These vectors are advantageous because they naturally enhance cell-mediated immunity and their intracellular nature can increase assess to class I pathways. They can be genetically manipulated to express tumor antigens and modify their virulence. In particular, recombinant avian poxviruses have been tested in several clinical trials and potent cellular immunity has been demonstrated. PANVAC is a cancer vaccine therapy that consists of a recombinant vaccinia vector and a recombinant fowlpox vector that are given sequentially. Both vectors contain transgenes for *MUC1* and *CEA*. The vector also contains transgenes for three T-cell costimulatory molecules (TRICOM). A phase III trial in patients who had failed gemcitabine showed no survival benefit in the PANVAC arm (114). A study in locally advanced pancreatic cancer with chemoradiation is currently under development.

Vaccine strategies using other microorganisms include intracellular bacteria and recombinant yeast. *Listeria monocytogenes* is an interesting intracellular bacterial vector that is in its early stages of clinical development. The *Listeria* vaccine platform aims to induce innate and adaptive immunity (115, 116). Clinical protocols utilizing the *Listeria* platform to express mesothelin are currently being developed and will target mesothelin producing tumors, such as pancreatic and ovarian adenocarcinomas (117). Other investigators are evaluating inactivated recombinant

Saccharomyces cerevisiae expressing mutant *ras* protein in combination with gemcitabine in the adjuvant treatment of pancreatic cancer (*118, 119*).

5.5 Other T-Cell–Mediated Approaches

Allogeneic nonmyeloablative haploidentical stem cell transplantation has become increasingly popular as a strategy to obtain an immune mediated graft-versus-tumor effect, mostly in hematologic malignancies. The premise of this strategy does not rely on the chemotherapeutic effects of the conditioning regimen; rather, it limits upfront mortality by using a reduced-intensity regimen designed to promote engraftment of the donor cells. The donors can be haploidentical, which substantially increases the pool of patients with eligible donors. In a study performed in Japan, seven patients with unresectable pancreatic cancer were treated using this strategy (*120*). Two patients had objective responses, with an additional patient who responded after donor lymphocyte infusion. This further supports the concept of T-cell–mediated therapies in the treatment of pancreatic cancer.

6 Combinatorial Strategies Driving Future Directions

Emerging knowledge about T_{regs} and other immunologic checkpoints is driving the next generation of cancer immunotherapy (Fig. 41.3). These checkpoints exist to appropriately down-regulate immune responses either to maintain self-tolerance or control pathogen-specific responses. Strategies combining vaccines and agents targeted at the tumor microenvironment, such as COX-2 inhibitors and anti-VEGF, are effective in preclinical models (*121, 122*). Synergistic approaches combining the activation of tumor-specific responses and blocking of immunologic checkpoints are being employed to enhance anti-tumor immunity. T_{reg} inhibitory agents, such as low-dose Cy and denileukin diftitox, are already being integrated into vaccine strategies.

Additionally, a range of B7–family member interactions are being targeted. These ligands interact with co-stimulatory and counter-regulatory inhibitory receptors on T cells. CD28 is a co-stimulatory receptor expressed on naïve T cells, which binds to B7.1/B7.2 on antigen presenting cells. Cytotoxic T-lymphocyte–associated protein 4 (CTLA-4) is expressed by T cells once they are activated. Additionally, it is constitutively expressed on T_{regs}. CTLA4 binds to B7.1/B7.2 with a 20-fold higher affinity than CD28 resulting in down-modulation of T cell responses (*123–127*). CTLA4 blocking antibodies are currently in various stages of development, including phase III trials in melanoma. Interestingly, CTLA-4 blockade does result in autoimmune-like events that correlate with disease responses (*128*). Anti-CTLA4 is being evaluated as a single agent in advanced pancreatic cancer and trials are currently being designed to integrate it with a GM-CSF–based allogeneic pancreatic cancer vaccine.

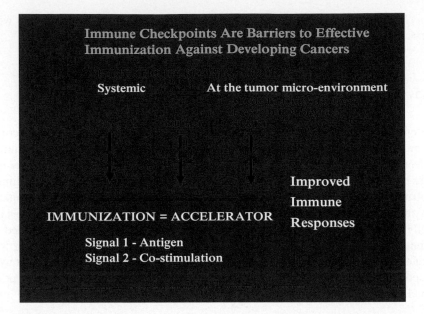

Fig. 41.3 Strategies combining vaccines and agents targeting immune checkpoints are currently under development. Vaccine strategies promote T-cell activation by optimizing antigen-presentation and costimulation. However, the amplitude of these responses is reduced by inhibitory immunologic checkpoints, which exist on multiple levels. Inhibition of T-regulatory cells as well as blockade of counter-regulatory molecules improves immune responses in multiple preclinical models. These strategies are increasingly being translated into clinical trials

With the advances in monoclonal antibody production, antibodies are increasingly being used as tools to manipulate their targets. Antibodies directed at other B7 family members, B7-H1 and B7-H4, are in development (*129, 130*). B7-H1 (PD-L1) is up-regulated on activated T cells. Its ligand, PD-1, is expressed on inactivated or suppressed T cells. Both B7-H1 and B7-H4 are expressed on various tumor types, including pancreatic cancer and may play a role in T-cell suppression (*131*). An antagonist antibody is about to be tested in metastatic pancreatic cancer patients with PD-1 expressing T cells. In addition to blocking antibodies, agonist antibodies directed at TNFR family molecules on T cells are being developed to enhance T-cell activation. Anti-4–1BB improves anti-tumor immunity in animal models and will soon be integrated into clinical trials (*85*).

7 A Multimodality Treatment Approach

The scheduling of vaccines with traditional therapies has to be thoughtfully considered. Historically, integrating chemotherapy and radiation with immunotherapy was strategically designed to minimize the immune suppressive effects of these modalities. However, these modalities are increasingly being exploited for their immune stimulatory capacities. The mechanisms for this phenomenon range from cyclophosphamide-induced inhibition of regulatory T cells to gemcitabine-induced cross presentation of tumor antigens by DCs and sensitization of tumor cells to T-cell–mediated killing. Interestingly, chemotherapy may not only be synergistic when given concurrently with immunotherapy, there is increasing evidence that chemotherapy given after progression during vaccine treatments may actually be more effective. This has been observed after a plasmid/microparticle vaccine directed against cytochrome P4501B1 and an adeno-p53 vaccine (*132*). Mechanisms proposed for this phenomenon include suppression of regulatory cells after a previous induction of tumor-specific T cells, direct stimulatory capacity on these tumor-specific T cells, treatment-associated tumor cell death, and the promotion of cross-presentation, and increasing tumor susceptibility by up-regulating tumor-associated antigens, fas, adhesion molecules, and apoptotic genes (*133*). Similarly, low dose radiation may also have these local effects.

There are a multitude of clinical trials in pancreatic cancer studying vaccines in combination with both chemotherapy and radiation. There is a phase III trial in pancreatic patients with advanced disease evaluating the concurrent administration of a telomerase peptide vaccine and a commonly used regimen of gemcitabine and Xeloda or the sequential use of these agents. Additionally, a phase III trial is also currently under development in the adjuvant setting that will test the GM-CSF modified allogeneic pancreatic tumor immunotherapy in combination with two acceptable adjuvant approaches, which include single-agent gemcitabine or chemoradiation. A study using a personalized peptide vaccination in combination with GEM has suggested that immune responses can be induced despite full doses of GEM (*134*). GI-4000 (inactivated recombinant saccharomyces cerevisiae expressing mutant Ras protein) in combination with gemcitabine is also being compared with gemcitabine alone in patients with resected pancreatic cancer. After completion of adjuvant therapy, a majority of patients still recur and this is another setting in which vaccines may be applied. One trial using the modified CEA (CAP1–6D) and another trial using the GM-CSF allogeneic immunotherapy are being conducted in this setting. Another interesting multimodality approach being studied at Stanford University is the combination of intratumoral autologous dendritic cells in combination with gemcitabine and stereotactic radiosurgery in patients with advanced disease. The direct delivery of DCs to a tumor microenvironment that has been manipulated to secrete pro-inflammatory cytokines and release a multitude of tumor antigens has been shown in animal models to promote regression of tumors at distant sites (*135*). Understanding the complex interplay of the immune regulatory processes and the tumor microenvironment will allow investigators to integrate traditional therapies in such a way that rather than hindering immune responses, these therapies can actually enhance antitumor activity.

8   Conclusion

Although immunotherapy is a novel approach to the management of pancreatic cancer, the induction of immune tolerance remains a major obstacle to an effective therapeutic vaccine strategy. Induction of T-cell responses to tumor-associated antigens has been demonstrated in early phase clinical trials. However, the translation of these responses to clear clinical benefit remains to be proved. Although new treatment strategies are often tested in patients with metastatic disease, vaccine-based therapies are most likely to make the most impact in the adjuvant setting, where there is minimal residual disease and a presumably less immune tolerant state. Additionally, the patient's immune system has not been subjected to multiple lines of immunosuppressive chemotherapies. Taking this a step further, investigators are testing vaccines in preclinical systems that model the pancreatic cancer tumorigenesis process from preinvasive lesions to frank cancer (*80*). Interestingly, an increasing number of T_{regs} are also found in precursor lesions (*136*). These findings will have to be considered when vaccines are eventually targeted in the prevention of pancreatic cancer in high-risk populations.

With the growing knowledge of T-cell regulation and the elucidation of immune checkpoints, a trend toward combinatorial strategies is emerging. Utilizing modern biotechnology and drawing from scientific concepts derived from more relevant preclinical models is crucial to the effective translation of these advances to clinical vaccine development.

Acknowledgments This work was supported by a gift from the Sol Goldman Pancreatic Cancer Center, grant U19CA72108 from the National Cooperative Drug Discovery Group, Grant 1K23CA098409 from the National Institutes of Health (NIH), grant P50CA62924 from the Gastrointestinal Diseases Specialized Program of Research Excellence, grant M070733 from the Broad Foundation, and grant 5-T32-CA009071–25 from the NIH National Research Service Award Institutional Research Training Grant (T32). Elizabeth Jaffee is the first recipient of the Dana and Albert Broccoli Professorship at the Sidney Kimmel Comprehensive Cancer Center at Johns Hopkins.

References

1. Li D, Xie K, Wolff R, Abbruzzese JL. Pancreatic cancer. Lancet 2004, 363(9414):1049–1057.
2. Sohn TA, Yeo CJ, Cameron JL, 2000, Resected adenocarcinoma of the pancreas–616 patients: Results, outcomes, and prognostic indicators. J Gastrointest Surg 4(6):567–579.
3. Yeo CJ, Pluth-Yeo T, Hruban R, et al. Cancer of the pancreas. In: Devita VT (ed.) Principles and practice of oncology, 7th ed. Philadelphia, Lippincott, 2005, 945.
4. American Cancer Society. Cancer facts and figures 2006. Atlanta, American Cancer Society, 2006.
5. DeVita VT, Hellman S, Rosenberg SA. 2005, Cancer: principles & practice of oncology, Lippincott Williams & Wilkins, Philadelphia, 7th ed..
6. Moore MJ, Hamm J, Kotecha J, et al. Erlotinib improves survival when added to gemcitabine in patients with advanced pancreatic cancer. A Phase III Trial of the NCI of Canada Clinical Trials Group. Am Soc Clin Oncol. 2005, Abstract 77.
7. Coley WB. The treatment of malignant tumors by repeated inoculations of erysipelas. with a report of ten original cases. 1893. Clin Orthop Relat Res 1991, (262):3–11.
8. Lawrence HS (ed). 1959, Discussion of cellular and humoral aspects of the hypersensitive states. Hoeber-Harper, New York, .
9. Burnet FM. 1970, The concept of immunological surveillance. Prog Exp Tumor Res 13:1–27.

10. Gaidano G, Dalla-Favera R. 1992, Biologic aspects of human immunodeficiency virus-related lymphoma. Curr Opin Oncol 4(5):900–906.
11. Coiffier B, Lepage E, Briere J, 2002, CHOP chemotherapy plus rituximab compared with CHOP alone in elderly patients with diffuse large-B-cell lymphoma. N Engl J Med 346(4):235–242.
12. Held G, Poschel V, Pfreundschuh M. 2006, Rituximab for the treatment of diffuse large B-cell lymphomas. Expert Rev Anticancer Ther 6(8):1175–1186.
13. Pfreundschuh M, Trumper L, Osterborg A, 2006, CHOP-like chemotherapy plus rituximab versus CHOP-like chemotherapy alone in young patients with good-prognosis diffuse large-B-cell lymphoma: a randomised controlled trial by the MabThera international trial (MInT) group. Lancet Oncol 7(5):379–391.
14. Atkins MB, Lotze MT, Dutcher JP, 1999, High-dose recombinant interleukin 2 therapy for patients with metastatic melanoma: analysis of 270 patients treated between 1985 and 1993. J Clin Oncol 17(7):2105–2116.
15. Chang DH, Liu N, Klimek V, 2006, Enhancement of ligand-dependent activation of human natural killer T cells by lenalidomide: Therapeutic implications. Blood 108(2):618–621.
16. Teo SK. 2005, Properties of thalidomide and its analogues: Implications for anticancer therapy. AAPS J 7(1):E14–19.
17. Biggs JC, Szer J, Crilley P, 1992, Treatment of chronic myeloid leukemia with allogeneic bone marrow transplantation after preparation with BuCy2. Blood 80(5):1352–1357.
18. Cummins M, Cwynarski K, Marktel S, 2005, Management of chronic myeloid leukaemia in relapse following donor lymphocyte infusion induced remission: a retrospective study of the clinical trials committee of the british society of blood & marrow transplantation (BSBMT). Bone Marrow Transplant 36(12):1065–1069.
19. Weisser M, Tischer J, Schnittger S, 2006, A comparison of donor lymphocyte infusions or imatinib mesylate for patients with chronic myelogenous leukemia who have relapsed after allogeneic stem cell transplantation. Haematologica 91(5):663–666.
20. Wu CJ, Biernacki M, Kutok JL, 2005, Graft-versus-leukemia target antigens in chronic myelogenous leukemia are expressed on myeloid progenitor cells. Clin Cancer Res 11(12):4504–4511.
21. Dudley ME, Wunderlich JR, Yang JC, 2005, Adoptive cell transfer therapy following non-myeloablative but lymphodepleting chemotherapy for the treatment of patients with refractory metastatic melanoma. J Clin Oncol 23(10):2346–2357.
22. Abeloff MD (ed). 2004Clinical oncology, 3Elsevier Churchill Livingstone, Philadelphia, rd ed. .
23. Hruban RH, Offerhaus GJ, Kern SE, 1998, Tumor-suppressor genes in pancreatic cancer. J Hepatobiliary Pancreat Surg 5(4):383–391.
24. Hruban RH, Mansfeld AD, van Offerhaus GJ, 1993, K-Ras oncogene activation in adenocarcinoma of the human pancreas. A study of 82 carcinomas using a combination of mutant-enriched polymerase chain reaction analysis and allele-specific oligonucleotide hybridization. Am J Pathol 143(2):545–554.
25. Laheru D, Jaffee EM. 2005, Immunotherapy for pancreatic cancer—science driving clinical progress. Nat Rev Cancer 5(6):459–467.
26. Laheru D, Biedrzycki B, Jaffee EM. 2001, Immunologic approaches to the management of pancreatic cancer. Cancer J 7(4):324–337.
27. Hruban RH, Goggins M, Parsons J, 2000, Progression model for pancreatic cancer. Clin Cancer Res 6(8):2969–2972.
28. Sohn TA, Yeo CJ. 2000, The molecular genetics of pancreatic ductal carcinoma: A review. Surg Oncol 9(3):95–101.
29. Wilentz RE, Su GH, Dai JL, 2000, Immunohistochemical labeling for dpc4 mirrors genetic status in pancreatic adenocarcinomas: a new marker of DPC4 inactivation. Am J Pathol 156(1):37–43.
30. Bos JL. 1989, Ras oncogenes in human cancer: a review. Cancer Res 49(17):4682–4689.
31. Zehn D, Bevan MJ. 2006, T cells with low avidity for a tissue-restricted antigen routinely evade central and peripheral tolerance and cause autoimmunity. Immunity 25(2):261–270.

32. Martignoni ME, Kunze P, Hildebrandt W, 2005, Role of mononuclear cells and inflammatory cytokines in pancreatic cancer-related cachexia. Clin Cancer Res 11(16):5802–5808.

33. Shibata M, Nezu T, Kanou H, 2002, Decreased production of interleukin-12 and type 2 immune responses are marked in cachectic patients with colorectal and gastric cancer. J Clin Gastroenterol 34(4):416–420.

34. Bernstorff W, von Voss M, Freichel S, 2001, Systemic and local immunosuppression in pancreatic cancer patients. Clin Cancer Res 7(3 Suppl):925s–932s.

35. Schmielau J, Nalesnik MA, Finn OJ. 2001, Suppressed T-cell receptor zeta chain expression and cytokine production in pancreatic cancer patients. Clin Cancer Res 7(3 Suppl):933s–939s.

36. Wolf AM, Wolf D, Steurer M, 2003, Increase of regulatory T cells in the peripheral blood of cancer patients. Clin Cancer Res 9(2):606–612.

37. Curiel TJ, Coukos G, Zou L, 2004, Specific recruitment of regulatory T cells in ovarian carcinoma fosters immune privilege and predicts reduced survival. Nat Med 10(9):942–949.

38. Liyanage UK, Moore TT, Joo HG, 2002, Prevalence of regulatory T cells is increased in peripheral blood and tumor microenvironment of patients with pancreas or breast adenocarcinoma. J Immunol 169(5):2756–2761.

39. Berendt MJ, North RJ. 1980, T-cell-mediated suppression of anti-tumor immunity. an explanation for progressive growth of an immunogenic tumor. J Exp Med 151(1):69–80.

40. Sakaguchi S, Sakaguchi N, Shimizu J, 2001, Immunologic tolerance maintained by CD25+ CD4+ regulatory T cells: their common role in controlling autoimmunity, tumor immunity, and transplantation tolerance. Immunol Rev 182:18–32.

41. Hori S, Nomura T, Sakaguchi S. 2003, Control of regulatory T cell development by the transcription factor Foxp3. Science 299(5609):1057–1061.

42. Fontenot JD, Gavin MA, Rudensky AY. 2003, Foxp3 programs the development and function of CD4+CD25+ regulatory T cells. Nat Immunol 4(4):330–336.

43. Alpan RS, Zhang M, Pardee AB. 1996, Cell cycle-dependent expression of TAP1, TAP2, and HLA-B27 messenger RNAs in a human breast cancer cell line. Cancer Res 56(19):4358–4361.

44. Huang AY, Bruce AT, Pardoll DM, 1996, In vivo cross-priming of MHC class I-restricted antigens requires the TAP transporter. Immunity 4(4):349–355.

45. Seliger B, Hohne A, Knuth A, 1996, Reduced membrane major histocompatibility complex class I density and stability in a subset of human renal cell carcinomas with low TAP and LMP expression. Clin Cancer Res 2(8):1427–1433.

46. Restifo NP, Kawakami Y, Marincola F, 1993, Molecular mechanisms used by tumors to escape immune recognition: immunogenetherapy and the cell biology of major histocompatibility complex class I. J Immunother 14(3):182–190.

47. Wang Z, Cao Y, Albino AP, 1993, Lack of HLA class I antigen expression by melanoma cells SK-MEL-33 caused by a reading frameshift in beta 2-microglobulin messenger RNA. J Clin Invest 91(2):684–692.

48. Ferrone S, Marincola FM. 1995, Loss of HLA class I antigens by melanoma cells: molecular mechanisms, functional significance and clinical relevance. Immunol Today 16(10):487–494.

49. Yee C, Thompson JA, Byrd D, 2002, Adoptive T cell therapy using antigen-specific CD8+ T cell clones for the treatment of patients with metastatic melanoma: In vivo persistence, migration, and antitumor effect of transferred T cells. Proc Natl Acad Sci U S A 99(25):16168–16173.

50. Uyttenhove C, Maryanski J, Boon T. 1983, Escape of mouse mastocytoma P815 after nearly complete rejection is due to antigen-loss variants rather than immunosuppression. J Exp Med 157(3):1040–1052.

51. Bromberg JF, Wrzeszczynska MH, Devgan G, 1999, Stat3 as an oncogene. Cell 98(3):295–303.

52. Kortylewski M, Kujawski M, Wang T, 2005, Inhibiting Stat3 signaling in the hematopoietic system elicits multicomponent antitumor immunity. Nat Med 11(12):1314–1321.

53. Wang T, Niu G, Kortylewski M, 2004, Regulation of the innate and adaptive immune responses by stat-3 signaling in tumor cells. Nat Med 10(1):48–54.
54. Cheng F, Wang HW, Cuenca A, 2003, A critical role for Stat3 signaling in immune tolerance. Immunity 19(3):425–436.
55. Sharma S, Stolina M, Yang SC, 2003, Tumor cyclooxygenase 2-dependent suppression of dendritic cell function. Clin Cancer Res 9(3):961–968.
56. Drake CG, Jaffee E, Pardoll DM. 2006, Mechanisms of immune evasion by tumors. Adv Immunol 90:51–81.
57. Apolloni E, Bronte V, Mazzoni A, 2000, Immortalized myeloid suppressor cells trigger apoptosis in antigen-activated T lymphocytes. J Immunol 165(12):6723–6730.
58. Bronte V, Apolloni E, Cabrelle A, 2000, Identification of a CD11b(+)/Gr-1(+)/CD31(+) myeloid progenitor capable of activating or suppressing CD8(+) T cells. Blood 96(12):3838–3846.
59. Kusmartsev S, Gabrilovich DI. 2006, Role of immature myeloid cells in mechanisms of immune evasion in cancer. Cancer Immunol Immunother 55(3):237–245.
60. Kusmartsev S, Nefedova Y, Yoder D, 2004, Antigen-specific inhibition of CD8+ T cell response by immature myeloid cells in cancer is mediated by reactive oxygen species. J Immunol 172(2):989–999.
61. Muller AJ, DuHadaway JB, Donover PS, Sutanto-Ward E, Prendergast GC. 2005, Inhibition of indoleamine 2,3-dioxygenase, an immunoregulatory target of the cancer suppression gene Bin1, potentiates cancer chemotherapy. Nat Med 11(3):312–319.
62. Munn DH, Sharma MD, Hou D, 2004, Expression of indoleamine 2,3-dioxygenase by plasmacytoid dendritic cells in tumor-draining lymph nodes. J Clin Invest 114(2):280–290.
63. Uyttenhove C, Pilotte L, Theate I, 2003, Evidence for a tumoral immune resistance mechanism based on tryptophan degradation by indoleamine 2,3-dioxygenase. Nat Med 9(10):1269–1274.
64. Apostolopoulos V, McKenzie IF. 1994, Cellular mucins: targets for immunotherapy. Crit Rev Immunol 14(3–4):293–309.
65. Hammarstrom S. 1999, The carcinoembryonic antigen (CEA) family: structures, suggested functions and expression in normal and malignant tissues. Semin Cancer Biol 9(2):67–81.
66. Harris JC, Gilliam AD, McKenzie AJ, 2004, The biological and therapeutic importance of gastrin gene expression in pancreatic adenocarcinomas. Cancer Res 64(16):5624–5631.
67. Nakatsura T, Senju S, Ito M, 2002, Cellular and humoral immune responses to a human pancreatic cancer antigen, coactosin-like protein, originally defined by the SEREX method. Eur J Immunol 32(3):826–836.
68. Rosenberg SA. 2001, Progress in human tumour immunology and immunotherapy. Nature 411(6835):380–384.
69. Boon T, Cerottini JC, den Eynde B, Van 1994, Tumor antigens recognized by T lymphocytes. Annu Rev Immunol 12:337–365.
70. Argani P, Iacobuzio-Donahue C, Ryu B, 2001, Mesothelin is overexpressed in the vast majority of ductal adenocarcinomas of the pancreas: identification of a new pancreatic cancer marker by serial analysis of gene expression (SAGE). Clin Cancer Res 7(12):3862–3868.
71. Argani P, Rosty C, Reiter RE, 2001, Discovery of new markers of cancer through serial analysis of gene expression: prostate stem cell antigen is overexpressed in pancreatic adenocarcinoma. Cancer Res 61(11):4320–4324.
72. Hassan R, Remaley AT, Sampson ML, 2006, Detection and quantitation of serum mesothelin, a tumor marker for patients with mesothelioma and ovarian cancer. Clin Cancer Res 12(2):447–453.
73. Hassan R, Bera T, Pastan I. 2004, Mesothelin: a new target for immunotherapy. Clin Cancer Res 10(12 Pt 1):3937–3942.
74. Hassan R, Williams-Gould J, Steinberg SM, 2006, Tumor-directed radiation and the immunotoxin SS1P in the treatment of mesothelin-expressing tumor xenografts. Clin Cancer Res 12(16):4983–4988.
75. Wente MN, Jain A, Kono E, 2005, Prostate stem cell antigen is a putative target for immunotherapy in pancreatic cancer. Pancreas 31(2):119–125.

76. Dannull J, Diener PA, Prikler L, 2000, Prostate stem cell antigen is a promising candidate for immunotherapy of advanced prostate cancer. Cancer Res 60(19):5522–5528.
77. Thomas AM, Santarsiero LM, Lutz ER, 2004, Mesothelin-specific CD8(+) T cell responses provide evidence of in vivo cross-priming by antigen-presenting cells in vaccinated pancreatic cancer patients. J Exp Med 200(3):297–306.
78. Guy CT, Webster MA, Schaller M, 1992, Expression of the neu protooncogene in the mammary epithelium of transgenic mice induces metastatic disease. Proc Natl Acad Sci U S A. 89(22):10578–10582.
79. Greenberg NM, DeMayo F, Finegold MJ, 1995, Prostate cancer in a transgenic mouse. Proc Natl Acad Sci U S A 92(8):3439–3443.
80. Hingorani SR, Petricoin EF, Maitra A, 2003, Preinvasive and invasive ductal pancreatic cancer and its early detection in the mouse. Cancer Cell 4(6):437–450.
81. Schnare M, Barton GM, Holt AC, 2001, Toll-like receptors control activation of adaptive immune responses. Nat Immunol 2(10):947–950.
82. Sallusto F, Lanzavecchia A. 1994, Efficient presentation of soluble antigen by cultured human dendritic cells is maintained by granulocyte/macrophage colony-stimulating factor plus interleukin 4 and downregulated by tumor necrosis factor alpha. J Exp Med 179(4):1109–1118.
83. Caux C, Massacrier C, Vanbervliet B, 1994, Activation of human dendritic cells through CD40 cross-linking. J Exp Med 180(4):1263–1272.
84. Cella M, Scheidegger D, Palmer-Lehmann K, 1996, Ligation of CD40 on dendritic cells triggers production of high levels of interleukin-12 and enhances T cell stimulatory capacity: T-T help via APC activation. J Exp Med 184(2):747–752.
85. Melero I, Shuford WW, Newby SA, 1997, Monoclonal antibodies against the 4-1BB T-cell activation molecule eradicate established tumors. Nat Med 3(6):682–685.
86. Weinberg AD, Rivera MM, Prell R, 2000, Engagement of the OX-40 receptor in vivo enhances antitumor immunity. J Immunol 164(4):2160–2169.
87. Bansal-Pakala P, Jember AG, Croft M. 2001, Signaling through OX40 (CD134) breaks peripheral T-cell tolerance. Nat Med 7(8):907–912.
88. Gjertsen MK, Buanes T, Rosseland AR, 2001, Intradermal ras peptide vaccination with granulocyte-macrophage colony-stimulating factor as adjuvant: Clinical and immunological responses in patients with pancreatic adenocarcinoma. Int J Cancer 92(3):441–450.
89. Gjertsen MK, Bakka A, Breivik J, 1995, Vaccination with mutant ras peptides and induction of T-cell responsiveness in pancreatic carcinoma patients carrying the corresponding RAS mutation. Lancet 346(8987):1399–1400.
90. Finn OJ, Jerome KR, Henderson RA, 1995, MUC-1 epithelial tumor mucin-based immunity and cancer vaccines. Immunol Rev 145:61–89.
91. Ramanathan RK, Lee KM, McKolanis J, 2005, Phase I study of a MUC1 vaccine composed of different doses of MUC1 peptide with SB-AS2 adjuvant in resected and locally advanced pancreatic cancer. Cancer Immunol Immunother 54(3):254–264.
92. Gilliam AD, Topuzov A, Garin AM, 2004, Randomised, double blind, placebo-controlled, multi-centre, group-sequential trial of G17DT for patients with advanced pancreatic cancer unsuitable or unwilling to take chemotherapy. Proc Am Soc Clin Oncol 23:A2511.
93. Chen CH, Wang TL, Hung CF, 2000, Enhancement of DNA vaccine potency by linkage of antigen gene to an HSP70 gene. Cancer Res 60(4):1035–1042.
94. Hoos A, Levey DL, Lewis JJ. 2004, Autologous heat shock protein-peptide complexes for vaccination against cancer: from bench to bedside. Dev Biol (Basel) 116:109–115; discussion 133–143.
95. Maki RG, Livingston PO, Lewis JJ, 2007, A phase I pilot study of autologous heat shock protein vaccine HSPPC-96 in patients with resected pancreatic adenocarcinoma. Dig Dis Sci 52(8):1964–1972.
96. Zaremba S, Barzaga E, Zhu M, 1997, Identification of an enhancer agonist cytotoxic T lymphocyte peptide from human carcinoembryonic antigen. Cancer Res 57(20):4570–4577.

97. Salazar E, Zaremba S, Arlen PM, 2000, Agonist peptide from a cytotoxic t-lymphocyte epitope of human carcinoembryonic antigen stimulates production of tc1-type cytokines and increases tyrosine phosphorylation more efficiently than cognate peptide. Int J Cancer 85(6):829–838.

98. Yokokawa J, Palena C, Arlen P, 2005, Identification of novel human CTL epitopes and their agonist epitopes of mesothelin. Clin Cancer Res 11(17):6342–6351.

99. Bhanot U, Heydrich R, Moller P, 2006, Survivin expression in pancreatic intraepithelial neoplasia (PanIN): steady increase along the developmental stages of pancreatic ductal adenocarcinoma. Am J Surg Pathol 30(6):754–759.

100. Wobser M, Keikavoussi P, Kunzmann V, 2006, Complete remission of liver metastasis of pancreatic cancer under vaccination with a HLA-A2 restricted peptide derived from the universal tumor antigen survivin. Cancer Immunol Immunother 55(10):1294–1298.

101. Lee MA, Park GS, Lee HJ, 2005, Survivin expression and its clinical significance in pancreatic cancer. BMC Cancer 5:127.

102. Bernhardt SL, Gjertsen MK, Trachsel S, et al. Telomerase peptide vaccination of patients with non-resectable pancreatic cancer: a dose escalating phase I/II study. Br J Cancer 2006.

103. Morse MA, Clay TM, Hobeika AC, 2005, Phase I study of immunization with dendritic cells modified with fowlpox encoding carcinoembryonic antigen and costimulatory molecules. Clin Cancer Res 11(8):3017–3024.

104. Dannull J, Su Z, Rizzieri D, 2005, Enhancement of vaccine-mediated antitumor immunity in cancer patients after depletion of regulatory T cells. J Clin Invest 115(12):3623–3633.

105. Bauer C, Dauer M, Saraj S, et al. Immunological and clinical response after vaccination therapy of pancreatic carcinoma patients with autologous, tumor-lysate pulsed dendritic cells: results of a phase ii study. ASCO Annual Meeting 2007.

106. Dranoff G, Jaffee E, Lazenby A, 1993, Vaccination with irradiated tumor cells engineered to secrete murine granulocyte-macrophage colony-stimulating factor stimulates potent, specific, and long-lasting anti-tumor immunity. Proc Natl Acad Sci U S A 90(8):3539–3543.

107. Cox AL, Skipper J, Chen Y, 1994, Identification of a peptide recognized by five melanoma-specific human cytotoxic T cell lines. Science 264(5159):716–719.

108. Kawakami Y, Eliyahu S, Delgado CH, 1994, Cloning of the gene coding for a shared human melanoma antigen recognized by autologous T cells infiltrating into tumor. Proc Natl Acad Sci U S A 91(9):3515–3519.

109. Jaffee EM, Hruban RH, Biedrzycki B, 2001, Novel allogeneic granulocyte-macrophage colony-stimulating factor-secreting tumor vaccine for pancreatic cancer: A phase I trial of safety and immune activation. J Clin Oncol 19(1):145–156.

110. Laheru DA, Yeo C, Biedrzycki B, et al. A safety and efficacy trial of lethally irradiated allogeneic pancreatic tumor cells transfected with the GM-CSF gene in combination with adjuvant chemoradiotherapy for the treatment of adenocarcinoma of the pancreas. Proc AACR/NCI/EORTC 2005, (C28):204.

111. Laheru D, Burke J, Biedrzycki B, et al. Allogeneic GM-CSF secreting tumor vaccine (GVAX) alone or in sequence with cyclophosphamide for metastatic pancreatic cancer: a pilot study of safety, feasibility and immune activation. Manuscript in preparation.

112. Rossi GR, Mautino MR, Unfer RC, 2005, Effective treatment of preexisting melanoma with whole cell vaccines expressing alpha(1,3)-galactosyl epitopes. Cancer Res 65(22):10555–10561.

113. Rossi GR, Unfer RC, Seregina T, 2005, Complete protection against melanoma in absence of autoimmune depigmentation after rejection of melanoma cells expressing alpha(1,3)galactosyl epitopes. Cancer Immunol Immunother 54(10):999–1009.

114. Madan RA, Arlen PM, Gulley JL. 2007, PANVAC-VF: Poxviral-based vaccine therapy targeting CEA and MUC1 in carcinoma. Expert Opin Biol Ther 7(4):543–554.

115. Brockstedt DG, Giedlin MA, Leong ML, 2004, Listeria-based cancer vaccines that segregate immunogenicity from toxicity. Proc Natl Acad Sci U S A 101(38):13832–13837.

116. Dietrich G, Spreng S, Favre D, 2003, Live attenuated bacteria as vectors to deliver plasmid DNA vaccines. Curr Opin Mol Ther 5(1):10–19.
117. Brockstedt DG, Leong ML, Luckett W, et al. Recombinant Listeria monocytogenes-based immunotherapy targeting mesothelin for the treatment of pancreatic and ovarian cancer. Proc AACR 2005, 46:Abstract 6028.
118. Franzusoff A, Duke RC, King TH, 2005, Yeasts encoding tumour antigens in cancer immunotherapy. Expert Opin Biol Ther 5(4):565–575.
119. Lu Y, Bellgrau D, Dwyer-Nield LD, 2004, Mutation-selective tumor remission with ras-targeted, whole yeast-based immunotherapy. Cancer Res 64(15):5084–5088.
120. Kanda Y, Komatsu Y, Akahane M, 2005, Graft-versus-tumor effect against advanced pancreatic cancer after allogeneic reduced-intensity stem cell transplantation. Transplantation 79(7):821–827.
121. Haas AR, Sun J, Vachani A, 2006, Cycloxygenase-2 inhibition augments the efficacy of a cancer vaccine. Clin Cancer Res 12(1):214–222.
122. Pedersen AE, Buus S, Claesson MH. 2006, Treatment of transplanted CT26 tumour with dendritic cell vaccine in combination with blockade of vascular endothelial growth factor receptor 2 and CTLA-4. Cancer Lett 235(2):229–238.
123. Lenschow DJ, Walunas TL, Bluestone JA. 1996, CD28/B7 system of T cell costimulation. Annu Rev Immunol 14:233–258.
124. Walunas TL, Lenschow DJ, Bakker CY, 1994, CTLA-4 can function as a negative regulator of T cell activation. Immunity 1(5):405–413.
125. Chen L, Ashe S, Brady WA, 1992, Costimulation of antitumor immunity by the B7 counter-receptor for the T lymphocyte molecules CD28 and CTLA-4. Cell 71(7):1093–1102.
126. Krummel MF, Sullivan TJ, Allison JP. 1996, Superantigen responses and co-stimulation: CD28 and CTLA-4 have opposing effects on T cell expansion in vitro and in vivo. Int Immunol 8(4):519–523.
127. Krummel MF, Allison JP. 1995, CD28 and CTLA-4 have opposing effects on the response of T cells to stimulation. J Exp Med 182(2):459–465.
128. Attia P, Phan GQ, Maker AV, 2005, Autoimmunity correlates with tumor regression in patients with metastatic melanoma treated with anti-cytotoxic T-lymphocyte antigen-4. J Clin Oncol 23(25):6043–6053.
129. Hirano F, Kaneko K, Tamura H, 2005, Blockade of B7-H1 and PD-1 by monoclonal antibodies potentiates cancer therapeutic immunity. Cancer Res 65(3):1089–1096.
130. Strome SE, Dong H, Tamura H, 2003, B7-H1 blockade augments adoptive T-cell immunotherapy for squamous cell carcinoma. Cancer Res 63(19):6501–6505.
131. Dong H, Strome SE, Salomao DR, 2002, Tumor-associated B7-H1 promotes T-cell apoptosis: a potential mechanism of immune evasion. Nat Med 8(8):793–800.
132. Gribben JG, Ryan DP, Boyajian R, 2005, Unexpected association between induction of immunity to the universal tumor antigen CYP1B1 and response to next therapy. Clin Cancer Res 11(12):4430–4436.
133. Schlom J, Arlen PM, Gulley JL. 2007, Cancer vaccines: moving beyond current paradigms. Clin Cancer Res 13(13):3776–3782.
134. Yanagimoto H, Mine T, Yamamoto K, 2007, Immunological evaluation of personalized peptide vaccination with gemcitabine for pancreatic cancer. Cancer Sci 98(4):605–611.
135. Saji H, Song W, Furumoto K, 2006, Systemic antitumor effect of intratumoral injection of dendritic cells in combination with local photodynamic therapy. Clin Cancer Res 12(8):2568–2574.
136. Hiraoka N, Onozato K, Kosuge T, 2006, Prevalence of FOXP3+ regulatory T cells increases during the progression of pancreatic ductal adenocarcinoma and its premalignant lesions. Clin Cancer Res 12(18):5423–5434.

Chapter 42
Novel Approaches in Chemoradiation for Localized Pancreas Cancer

Christopher H. Crane

1 Introduction

Attempts to improve results of chemoradiotherapy in patients with pancreatic cancer by either increasing the total dose of radiation or chemotherapy or by changing cytotoxic drugs have not been very successful. Additionally, some combinations have been associated with a high rate of unacceptable treatment-related morbidity, underscoring the need for new treatment strategies to combine with radiation to improve the therapeutic ratio of such treatment. Gemcitabine has stood the test of time as a systemic agent in advanced and early disease but was not widely adopted as a radiosensitizer in pancreatic cancer. Single-arm clinical trials that initially explored gemcitabine as a radiosensitizer in locally advanced pancreatic cancer demonstrated the potential for significant toxicity without dramatic improvements in efficacy. Subsequent studies showed marked improvement in patient tolerance with the refinements of delivery of radiation. Recent strategies include radiosensitization by the incorporation of targeted agents and continued improvement in delivery of radiation through novel means such as steriotactic radiotherapy. This chapter focuses on data evaluating the incorporation of targeted agents with radiation therapy in the context of a multidisciplinary approach for the treatment of localized pancreatic cancer.

2 Incorporation of Molecular Targeted Therapy with Radiation in Pancreatic Cancer

Aberrant signal transduction pathways, involving oncogenes and their normal counterparts the proto-oncogenes lead to the phenotype of cellular radioresistance. These findings are potentially useful in developing new strategies to improve the therapeutic ratio of radiation therapy in pancreatic cancer. Despite the significant improvements in knowledge of cellular mechanisms that affect radiosensitivity, we still cannot account for most of the clinically observed heterogeneity of normal tissue and tumor responses to radiotherapy; nor can we accurately predict which

A.M. Lowy et al. (eds.) *Pancreatic Cancer.*
doi: 10.1007/978-0-387-69252-4, © Springer Science+Business Media, LLC 2008

individual tumors will be locally controlled and which patients will develop more severe normal tissue damage after radiotherapy.

3   K-ras Oncogene

The development of pancreatic cancer is a result of the accumulation of multiple genetic mutations. The Ras oncogene, when activated, results in enhanced radioresistance. Its inactivation renders cells with activated Ras more radiosensitive (1). The progress in targeting the K-ras pathway in clinical studies has been hampered by the lack of effective agents that selectively target this oncoprotein. The phosphoinositide-3-kinase (PI3 kinase) may be a critical component of a downstream pathway resulting in the radioresistance. Epidermal growth factor receptor (EGFR) activation, which is upstream of PI3 kinase, may also mediate resistance through a common pathway. In addition to EGFR and Ras, PTEN can also regulate the PI3 kinase pathway. Identifying a common signal for EGFR, Ras, and PTEN that results in radiation resistance may uncover targets for developing molecular-based radiosensitization protocols for tumors resistant to radiation and thus lead to improvement of local control (2).

4   Vascular Endothelial Growth Factor

Randomized trials demonstrated the efficacy of bevacizumab, a humanized anti-vascular endothelial growth factor (VEGF) monoclonal antibody in several cancers including advanced colorectal cancer (3, 4). Most investigations of these and other drugs have focused on their benefits as components of systemic therapy in patients with advanced disease, although investigations of their benefits in the adjuvant setting are now underway in colon cancer.

The possible mechanisms of radiosensitization with bevacizumab are not clear, but could include enhanced lethality of the endothelial cell (5), the tumor cell (6), or the improvement in vascular physiology leading to a reduction in tumor hypoxia (7). The role of bevacizumab in the concurrent chemoradiation of rectal cancer is currently under investigation. Willett et al. have performed a phase I trial on bevacizumab and 5-FU with concurrent preoperative radiotherapy (8, 9). Bevacizumab was well tolerated with protracted venous infusion 5-fluorouracil (5-FU) and radiotherapy at a dose of 5 mg/kg ($n = 6$), but there were two grade III gastrointestinal adverse events at the dose of 10 mg/kg, leading authors to recommend the 5 m/kg dose level. A complement of correlative studies showed that bevacizumab decreased tumor perfusion, interstitial pressure, and microvascular density in rectal cancers (8). Interestingly, 10 out 11 patients had clinical complete responses. Eight patients had microscopic residual disease and two had complete histologic responses. Compared with historical controls, there appear to be fewer patients with gross residual disease and approximately the same number of complete histologic responses as with 5-FU–based chemoradiation (*10*).

A study of bevacizumab in combination with radiation as a phase I dose escalation study in patients with locally advanced, unresectable pancreatic cancer was conducted at M. D. Anderson Cancer Center. Forty-seven patients received capecitabine (650–825 mg/m^2 twice daily) and bevacizumab in combination with radiation (50.4 Gy) to the gross tumor alone (*11*). The study demonstrated that bevacizumab is generally safe when combined with chemoradiation in patients with locally advanced pancreatic cancer. The acute toxicity was minimal and easily managed with dose adjustments of capecitabine, without interruption or attenuation of either the bevacizumab or radiation dose. Bevacizumab did not appear to enhance acute toxicity; however, tumors with invasion of the duodenum appeared to be at higher risk for bleeding or perforation. Among the first 30 patients enrolled, three bleeding events were associated with tumor invasion of the duodenum. After this was recognized, such patients were excluded from protocol entry and there were no further bleeding events among the final 16 patients enrolled. Overall, the tumors in nine (20%) of 46 evaluable patients had an objective partial response to initial therapy. This included six of 12 tumors treated at a dose of 5 mg/kg of bevacizumab. Based on that trial, the recommended dose of bevacizumab for further study was 5 mg/kg every 2 weeks with radiotherapy (50.4 Gray in 28 fractions) and concurrent capecitabine (825 mg/m^2 twice daily Monday through Friday).

The Radiation Therapy Oncology Group (RTOG) has completed accrual to a phase II trial evaluating capecitabine-based chemoradiation with bevacizumab followed by systemic therapy with concurrent gemcitabine and bevacizumab (RTOG PA04-11). Ninety-four patients were treated, and preliminary analysis indicates that the treatment was generally well tolerated in comparison with previous RTOG phase II studies with similar inclusion criteria. Specific exclusion of patients with tumor invasion of the duodenum seemed to have avoided significant problems with bleeding thus far. Initial safety analysis of 50 patients has revealed that there have been no tumor-associated duodenal bleeding, illustrating the importance of excluding these patients.

5   Epidermal Growth Factor Receptor

Increasing evidence suggests that epidermal growth factor family receptors (HERs) play a significant role in radiation response. EGFR expression levels and activation by ligand correlate with radioresistance, and exogenous HER2 expression modulates radiation response. The EGFR inhibitors are among the most commonly studied targeted agents in nonhematologic malignancies. Whether EGFR inhibitors influence response to radiation directly, or whether the improved response is a result of additive antiproliferative/proapoptotic effects of the two modalities remains to be determined. However, cell-cycle arrest, endothelial cell sensitivity, and apoptotic potential are all important factors in radiation response of epithelial tumors. Furthermore, less-studied effects of EGFR inhibitors on DNA repair suggest that modulation of DNA damage response to cytotoxic injury might result in radio- or chemosensitization. Preclinical studies of anti-EGFR anti-HER2 antibodies, and kinase inhibitors that inhibit EGFR, both EGFR and HER2, or all four family members show potential for clinical radiosensitization (*12–14*). The mechanisms(s) of radiation response modulation by HERs appear complex and diverse. Signal transduction initiated by receptor activation promotes survival and proliferation after ionizing radiation, and HER inhibitors affect cellular responses to radiation in diverse ways, including inducing apoptosis, cell cycle arrest, and impeding DNA repair. HER signaling and inhibition also affect tumor–stroma interactions, particularly angiogenesis and endothelial survival after radiation. Recent data also suggest that a dual EGFR and HER2/neu targeting may have potential for radiosensitization in tumors in which both of these pathways are active (*15*).

5.1 Anti-EGFR Monoclonal Antibodies

Preclinical work with cetuximab demonstrated an important role in radiosensitization in vivo (*12*). Earlier work also indicated a relationship between EGFR expression and the treatment outcome with cetuximab and radiation. However, the EGFR expression levels have shown no influence on response to EGFR blockers in general when used as systemic therapies alone or in combination with cytotoxic therapy. Cetuximab is also the only targeted agent that has been shown to improve local tumor control and overall survival outcome as a radiosensitizer and is also the only chemotherapeutic agent to be approved by the FDA for use specifically as a radiosensitizer based on a phase III trial in patients with locally advanced head and neck cancer (*16*). There have been two studies incorporating cetuximab with neoadjuvant chemoradiation regimens in locally advanced rectal cancer patients. Both single-arm studies have been presented in abstract form and have included locally advanced rectal cancer patients and delivered standard doses of pelvic radiation (50.4 Gy), in combination with capecitabine (650–825 mg/m^2) (*17*) or protracted infusional 5-FU (225 mg/m^2/day) (*18*) and have evaluated cetuximab (400 mg/m^2 D1, then 250 mg/m^2 weekly) (*17, 18*). Both studies showed a pathologic complete response rate of approximately 12%. Given the fact that neoadjuvant 5-FU–based chemoradiation produces a pathologic complete rate of 10–20 percent, there does not appear to be a strong efficacy signal using that endpoint as a surrogate for local treatment effect.

5.2 EGFR-Related Receptor Tyrosine Kinase Inhibition

There have also been studies evaluating receptor tyrosine kinase inhibition in combination with radiotherapy in patients with localized gastrointestinal malignancies. Preclinical studies demonstrated marked radiosensitization with use of tyrosine kinase inhibitors gefitinib and erlotinib in human cancer cell lines (*13, 14*) A phase I dose escalation study has recently been published from Brown University combining gemcitabine, 75 mg/m^2, and paclitaxel, 40 mg/m^2 weekly and daily erlotinib with 50.4 Gy to the primary tumor and regional lymphatics. The maximum tolerated dose of erlotinib was 50 mg/m^2. The median survival was 14.0 months and 6/13 (46%) of locally advanced patients had a partial response, indicating that erlotinib-based chemoradiation regimens are possibly worthy of further study in pancreatic cancer (*19*). There was a significant amount of high-grade diarrhea, which limited the inability to give full-dose erlotinib. Toxicity could have been due to the concurrent gemcitabine and paclitaxel, the use of regional nodal irradiation, or the combination of radiotherapy and erlotinib. Another phase I study is ongoing at Memorial Sloan Kettering evaluating gemcitabine-based chemotherapy in combination with erlotinib. A phase I study at Duke University has been conducted evaluating concurrent gefitinib (250 mg daily), capecitabine (650–825 mg/m^2 BID, 7 days/week) and radiotherapy in locally advanced pancreatic and rectal cancers. Patients were treated to a dose of 50.4 Gy (45 Gy in 25 fractions to the regional lymphatics followed by an additional 5.4 Gy in three fractions to the primary tumor). Dose-limiting toxicity (DLT) was seen in two of six patients with rectal cancer and six of 10 patients with pancreatic cancer. Diarrhea as well as nausea and vomiting with dehydration were common (*20*). A recommended dose was not established due to these toxicities. These data do not suggest that gefitinib should be further studied with radiotherapy in gastrointestinal malignancies. None of the currently available EGFR inhibitors (erlotinib, gefitinib, and cetuximab) have been evaluated in completed multi-institutional trials in combination with radiation in locally advanced pancreatic cancer.

6 Cyclo-oxygenase-2

Cyclo-oxygenase-2 (COX-2) enzyme may promote tumor cell survival and is responsible for tumor resistance to proapoptotic agents, and hence may serve as potential targets for augmentation of radio response (*21*). COX-2 is often over-expressed in cancers, including pancreatic cancer. Preclinical studies provided solid evidence that inhibition of this enzyme with selective COX-2 inhibitors prevents carcinogenesis, slows the growth of established tumors, and enhances tumor response to radiation without appreciably affecting normal tissue radioresponse. The mechanisms of enhancement of tumor radioresponse involve direct actions on tumor cells and indirect actions, primarily on tumor vasculature. COX-2 inhibitors also improve tumor response to cytotoxic drugs. COX-2 blockade as a therapeutic strategy is not being pursued in clinical trials because of concerns about efficacy and safety from the accumulated clinical experience in treating cancers, including pancreatic cancer. However, these studies were undertaken in the absence of molecularly guided patient selection for COX-2. In animal models, selective inhibition of COX-2 activity is associated with the enhanced radiation sensitivity of tumors without appreciably increasing the effects of radiation on normal tissue, and preclinical evidence suggests that the principal mechanism of radiation potentiation through selective COX-2 inhibition is the direct increase in cellular radiation sensitivity and the direct inhibition of tumor neovascularization. Results of current early-phase studies of non-small cell lung, esophageal, cervical, and brain cancers will determine whether therapies that combine COX-2 inhibitors and radiation will enter randomized clinical trials (22).

7 Intensity Modulated Radiotherapy or Stereotactic Radiation Therapy

Intensity Modulated Radiotherapy (IMRT) and steriotactic radiation therapy are relatively recent technical innovations in radiotherapy. Both techniques are capable of very precise delivery of radiation. If that target is not near a radiosensitive structure, it is possible that the dose could safely be escalated, which may or may not improve outcome. Pancreatic tumors move considerably with respiration and are virtually always surrounded by the duodenum, which is a radiosensitive structure. Finally, dose escalation of radiotherapy beyond 50.4 Gy has never been demonstrated to convincingly improve outcome. We abandoned the investigation of IMRT after our phase I trial failed to reduce the toxicity of gemcitabine-based chemoradiation in spite of improved dose precision at the target (23). Stereotactic radiation therapy using the Cyberknife® system with very careful correction for organ motion using implanted metallic markers at the time of laparoscopy, laparotomy, or percutaneously under CT guidance, has been evaluated in a phase I dose escalation trial using a single fraction of radiation therapy at Stanford University (24). The final dose of 25 Gy was well tolerated and has been recommended for further study. The median time to progression was 2 months and there have been no objective responses among an updated experience of 80 patients (Koong, personal communication). The follow-up study used 45 Gy in 25 fractions with IMRT and concurrent 5-FU, followed by 25 Gy in one fraction as a steriotactic boost. Although the treatment was reasonably well tolerated, the median survival was an extremely disappointing 7.6 months (24). These studies were conducted at a center with very specialized capabilities that are not yet ready for use outside the setting of a clinical trial. Even so, the authors acknowledge that it was "impossible to avoid treating" the duodenum to a high dose in the majority of cases (25). Given the lack of any convincing prospective data, the constraints of organ motion, and the lack of any evidence that dose escalation in pancreatic cancer improves outcome in any meaningful way, there is no role for either IMRT or steriotactic radiation to be used outside the setting of a clinical trial in pancreatic cancer patients. As discussed, treatment of locally advanced pancreatic cancer is very well tolerated, and a modest median survival benefit is seen when the treatment volumes are confined to the gross tumor and clinically enlarged lymph nodes. This can be accomplished with a standard four-field conformal plan. The dose to the spinal cord, kidneys, and liver can very easily be kept within tolerance using this straight-forward approach.

8 Conclusions

Pancreatic cancer is an extremely challenging disease to treat. Even when the disease is localized and treated with chemoradiation, there are very high rates of both distant and local failure. Although chemoradiation appears to prolong median survival in the adjuvant and possibly locally advanced disease settings, current regimens utilizing cytotoxic drugs given concurrently with radiation have significant limitations. The study of targeted therapies in pancreatic cancer could lead to improvement in local disease control. Current clinical interest is focused on evaluating EGFR and VEGF as targets to modulate radioresistance. Additional studies are needed to establish the safety and efficacy of such approaches. These studies are complicated by uncertainty on the best experimental endpoint to reliably capture enhanced radiosensitization. With the limited number of patients with localized pancreatic cancer that go on clinical trials it is unlikely that we will see large rand-omized trials using targeted approaches in the foreseeable future unless a strong signal of efficacy is captured in pilot trials. Despite initial interest in targeting COX-2 clinical research, activity has waned with the concerns of developing COX-2 targeting agents in the clinic given their potential toxicities. At this time it is unclear what, if any, role more precise targeting of radiation therapy will have in the future in pancreatic cancer.

Acknowledgments The author received research support by Genentech and Bristol Meyers Squibb and honoraria from Roche. This chapter was supported in part by grants CA06294 and CA16672 from the National Cancer Institute, Department of Health and Human Services.

References

1. Kim IA, Bae SS, Fernandes A, 2005, Selective inhibition of Ras, phosphoinositide 3 kinase, and Akt isoforms increases the radiosensitivity of human carcinoma cell lines. Cancer Res 65(17):7902–7910.
2. McKenna WG, Muschel RJ, 2003, Targeting tumor cells by enhancing radiation sensitivity. Genes Chromosomes Cancer 38(4):330–338.
3. Hurwitz H, Fehrenbacher L, Novotny W, 2004, Bevacizumab plus irinotecan, fluorouracil, and leucovorin for metastatic colorectal cancer. N Engl J Med 350:2335–2342 [see comment].
4. Kabbinavar FF, Hambleton J, Mass RD, 2005, Combined analysis of efficacy: the addition of bevacizumab to fluorouracil/leucovorin improves survival for patients with metastatic color-ectal cancer. J Clin Oncol 23:3706–3712.
5. Gorski DH, Beckett MA, Jaskowiak NT, 1999, Blockage of the vascular endothelial growth factor stress response increases the antitumor effects of ionizing radiation. Cancer Res 59:3374–3378.

6. Wey J, Fan F, Gray M, 2005, Vascular endothelial growth factor receptor-1 promotes migration and invasion in pancreatic carcinoma cell lines. Cancer 104:427–438.
7. Jain RK. 2005, Normalization of tumor vasculature: an emerging concept in antiangiogenic therapy. Science 307:58–62.
8. Willett CG, Boucher Y, di Tomaso E, 2004, Direct evidence that the VEGF-specific antibody bevacizumab has antivascular effects in human rectal cancer. Nat Med 10:145–147 [see comment] [erratum appears in Nat Med 2004, 10(6):649].
9. Willett CG, Boucher Y, Duda DG, 2005, Surrogate markers for antiangiogenic therapy and dose-limiting toxicities for bevacizumab with radiation and chemotherapy: continued experience of a phase I trial in rectal cancer patients. J Clin Oncol 23:8136–8139.
10. Bonnen M, Crane C, Vauthey J-N, 2004, Long-term results using local excision after preoperative chemoradiation among selected T3 rectal cancer patients. Int J Radiat Oncol Biol Phys 60:1098–1105.
11. Crane CH, Ellis LM, Abbruzzese JL, 2006, Phase I trial evaluating the safety of bevacizumab with concurrent radiotherapy and capecitabine in locally advanced pancreatic cancer. J Clin Oncol 24:1145–1151.
12. Milas L, Fan Z, Andratschke NH, 2004, Epidermal growth factor receptor and tumor response to radiation: in vivo preclinical studies. Int J Radiat Oncol Biol Phys 58(3):966–971.
13. Solomon B, Hagekyriakou J, Trivett MK, 2003, EGFR blockade with ZD1839 ("Iressa") potentiates the antitumor effects of single and multiple fractions of ionizing radiation in human A431 squamous cell carcinoma. Epidermal growth factor receptor. Int J Radiat Oncol Biol Phys. 55(3):713–723.
14. Chinnaiyan P, Huang S, Vallabhaneni G, 2005, Mechanisms of enhanced radiation response following epidermal growth factor receptor signaling inhibition by erlotinib (Tarceva). Cancer Res 65:3328–3335.
15. Fukutome M, Maebayashi K, Nasu S, 2006, Enhancement of radiosensitivity by dual inhibition of the HER family with ZD1839 ("Iressa") and trastuzumab ("Herceptin"). Int J Radiat Oncol Biol Phys 66(2):528–536.
16. Bonner JA, Harari PM, Giralt J, 2006, Radiotherapy plus cetuximab for squamous-cell carcinoma of the head and neck. N Engl J Med 354:567–578.
17. Machiels J, Sempoux C, Scalliet P, et al. Phase I study of preoperative cetuximab, capecitabine, and external beam radiotherapy in patients with rectal cancer. J Clin Oncol 2006, 24(18S) Abstract 3552.
18. Chung K, Minsky B, Schrag D, et al. Phase I trial of preoperative cetuximab with concurrent continuous infusion 5-fluorouracil and pelvic radiation in patients with local-regionally advanced rectal cancer. J Clin Oncol 2006, 24(18S):Abstract 3560.
19. Iannitti DMD, Dipetrillo TMD, Akerman PMD, 2005, Erlotinib and chemoradiation followed by maintenance erlotinib for locally advanced pancreatic cancer: a phase I study. Am J Clin Oncol 28:570–575.
20. Czito BG, Willett CG, Bendell JC, 2006, Increased toxicity with gefitinib, capecitabine, and radiation therapy in pancreatic and rectal cancer: phase I trial results J Clin Oncol 24:656–662.
21. Milas L, Mason KA, Crane CH, 2003, Improvement of radiotherapy or chemoradiotherapy by targeting COX-2 enzyme. Oncology 17(5 Suppl 5):15–24.
22. Choi H, Milas L. 2003, Enhancing radiotherapy with cyclooxygenase-2 enzyme inhibitors: a rational advance? J Natl Cancer Inst 95(19):1440–1452.
23. Crane CH, Antolak JA, Rosen II, 2001, Phase I study of concomitant gemcitabine and IMRT for patients with unresectable adenocarcinoma of the pancreatic head. Int J Gastrointest Cancer 30:123–132.
24. Koong AC, Christofferson E, Le Q-T, 2005, Phase II study to assess the efficacy of conventionally fractionated radiotherapy followed by a stereotactic radiosurgery boost in patients with locally advanced pancreatic cancer. Int J Radiat Oncol Biol Phys 63:320–323.
25. Koong AC, Le QT, Ho A, 2004, Phase I study of stereotactic radiosurgery in patients with locally advanced pancreatic cancer. Int J Radiat Oncol Biol Phys 58:1017–1021.

Chapter 43
Incorporation of Genomics and Proteomics in Drug and Biomarker Development

David G. Heidt, David Misek, David M. Lubman, and Diane M. Simeone

1 Introduction

Pancreatic cancer is resistant to standard surgical and non-selective antimetabolite therapy, with median survival of patients with resectable disease and adjuvant therapy remaining around 20 months and those with unresectable disease at <6 months with the most effective currently available therapy (*1, 2*). Innovations in genomics and proteomics have led to the identification of numerous potential targets for the development of novel antineoplastic agents and early detection biomarkers. This chapter looks at the history of targeted approaches to drug design, recent developments in the fields of genomics and proteomics, and the potential application of these approaches to pancreatic cancer treatment and early detection.

Molecular targeting by pharmaceuticals was made possible in the middle of the last century by the discovery of specific biochemical pathways. Early examples of targeted drugs included propranolol, allopurinol, and cimetidine. Black, Hutchings, and Elion received the Nobel Prize in 1988 for their work on developing these compounds (*3, 4*). Identification of similarly specific targets in cancer has noticeably lagged behind, with the exception of antimetabolites. Only recently have targeted therapies such as trastuzumab (anti-HER2 neu antibody effective against breast cancer) and imatinib mesylate (a BCR-ABL tyrosine kinase inhibitor for treatment of chronic myeloid leukemia and gastrointestinal stromal tumors) become available. For pancreatic cancer, bevacizumab (Avastin), a recombinant humanized antivascular endothelial growth factor (VEGF) monoclonal antibody, showed promising results in phase II trials (*5*), but was subsequently shown to provide no survival benefit (*6*). The push to identify specific molecular targets for the rational design of antineoplastics (in particular cancer cell signaling molecules and molecules that can affect the cancer cell microenvironment) has led to rapid development of techniques in genomics and proteomics. These techniques hold promise in identifying novel and effective targets for the treatment of pancreatic cancer.

A.M. Lowy et al. (eds.) *Pancreatic Cancer.*
doi: 10.1007/978-0-387-69252-4, © Springer Science+Business Media, LLC 2008

2 Developments in Genomics

The early 1990s saw the development of differential display by Liang and Pardee (7), which combined the reverse transcription polymerase chain reaction and gel electrophoresis to identify unique mRNAs in small samples. Using this method, which employed random primers for mRNA amplification, novel mRNAs could be identified without reference to the genome. These developments and others allowed for the identification of specific genetic alterations in pancreatic cancer, including p16, DPC-4, and K-ras (8–10). Identification of expressed mRNA allowed for the development of cDNA microarrays (11) and GeneChip arrays (12), where spotted cDNAs or oligos are affixed to a plate and read out using fluorescent tags. More recently, with completion of the human genome project, complex arrays with thousands of known genes have been constructed. These profiling studies generate a great deal of information and require sophisticated data analysis. In addition, great care must be taken in sample collection, especially in a heterogeneous tumor such as pancreatic adenocarcinoma, which is composed of neoplastic cells in a densely fibrotic stroma with infiltrating inflammatory cells (13).

Several studies were initially undertaken that identified differentially expressed genes in pancreatic carcinoma compared with normal pancreas (14–18). However, these studies failed to take into account the profound desmoplastic stromal reaction induced by pancreatic adenocarcinoma, with the neoplastic epithelium making up only a small proportion of the tissue mass. Differences in the levels of specific mRNAs in different tissue samples may be caused by these variations in cellular composition as well as changes in gene expression levels. Laser capture microdissection allows for the isolation of neoplastic epithelium from the surrounding desmoplastic stromal tissue, and thus provides a more accurate characterization of the unique gene expression profile of pancreatic adenocarcinoma. It should be noted that any study of differential gene expression in pancreatic adenocarcinoma should include samples of chronic pancreatitis as a control due to the profound desmoplastic response associated with pancreatic adenocarcinoma (19, 20).

Gene profiling has yielded a large number of differentially expressed genes in human pancreatic cancer. A useful resource to examine all published gene array data for pancreatic cancer is the cancer profiling database Oncomine (www.oncomine.com), a website for examining published gene expression data sets in many different types of human cancer. A search of the Oncomine database reveals a number of differentially expressed genes in pancreatic cancer, including S100P, 14-3-3σ, S100A6, β4-Integrin, UHRF1, ATP7A, and aldehyde oxidase-1, among many others (19, 20). S100P, a gene expressed in high levels in the majority of pancreatic cancers, has been found to promote cell proliferation, survival, migration, and invasion in pancreatic cancer cell lines. This regulatory protein is also expressed in other human cancers, including breast, colon, prostate, and lung cancers. S100P has been shown to confer resistance to chemotherapeutic agents such as 5-FU. In breast cancer cell lines, S100P levels were associated with cellular immortalization (21). In colon cancer cell lines, its expression level was correlated with resistance to chemotherapy (22).

In lung cancer, S100P expression correlated with decreased patient survival (23). Direct inhibition of S100P as well as inhibition of S100P binding with its down stream target receptor for activated glycosylation end-products (RAGE) resulted in attenuation of pancreatic cancer cell lines' malignant behavior (19). Further work by Arumugam and colleagues found that cromolyn, a commonly used antiallergy compound, binds S100P, prevents activation of RAGE, and inhibits tumor growth and increases the effectiveness of gemcitabine in experimental models (24). Identification of therapeutic agents with the ability to block these targets as well as other downstream targets holds great promise for the future.

The field of genomics has also led to inroads in the identification of potential serum biomarkers for the early detection of pancreatic cancer. Several recent reports have described aberrantly expressed proteins in the serum of pancreatic cancer patients which were originally identified in genomic studies of pancreatic cancer samples. In one report, Koopmann and co-workers evaluated osteopontin as a serum biomarker of pancreatic adenocarcinoma (25). Although osteopontin expression was not observed in pancreatic cancer cells, in normal pancreata or in macrophages distant from the infiltrating cancer, a strong osteopontin mRNA signal was observed in tumor-infiltrating macrophages in 8/14 pancreatic adenocarcinomas. Elevated levels of serum osteopontin was observed in the sera of 50 patients with resectable pancreatic adenocarcinoma (482 + 170 ng/ml), as compared to serum from 22 healthy subjects (204 + 65 ng/ml). However, these authors did not evaluate serum osteopontin levels in patients with inflammatory diseases of the pancreas (i.e., chronic pancreatitis). Thus, it is unknown whether the increased serum osteopontin levels are cancer specific, or instead due to the associated extensive desmoplastic response seen in pancreatic adenocarcinoma.

Serum macrophage inhibitory cytokine 1 (MIC-1) has been shown to have potential utility as a serum biomarker of pancreatic cancer (25, 26). Serum MIC-1 levels were found to be significantly higher in patients with PDAC and those with ampullary and cholangiocellular carcinomas than in those with benign pancreatic neoplasms, chronic pancreatitis, or in healthy controls by ELISA assay. It has been shown that serum MIC-1 outperforms other candidate biomarkers, including CA19-9, in the differentiation of patients with resectable pancreatic cancer from controls.

Serum levels of phosphoglycerate kinase 1 (PGK1) have also been shown to have potential utility as a serum biomarker of pancreatic cancer. Hwang and co-workers identified PGK1 as being over-expressed in PDAC, as compared to adjacent nontumor pancreata. They subsequently found that serum levels of PGK1 were significantly elevated in PDAC patients, compared with normal controls and to other cancer types (27).

In a recent study, Simeone and co-workers observed PDAC-specific over-expression of CEACAM1, a member of the human carcinoembryonic antigen family (28). They subsequently measured CEACAM1 serum levels in patients with PDAC, chronic pancreatitis, and in normal subjects by a double determinant ELISA. CEACAM1 was found to be expressed in the sera of 91% (74/81) PDAC patients, in 24% (15/61) of normal subjects, and in 66% (35/53) of patients with chronic pancreatitis, with a sensitivity and specificity superior to CA19-9. Unfortunately, however, none of these protein biomarkers (osteopontin, MIC1, PGK1, and CEACAM1) has the requisite sensitivity/specificity to have utility individually as a biomarker for the early detection of pancreatic cancer, but may have utility within a panel of protein biomarkers.

3   Developments in Proteomics

Proteomics is the combination of protein separation and identification technologies used to define the proteome, or differential expression of proteins by organisms. A thorough elucidation of the proteome would provide a much more biologically relevant description of pancreatic cancer on a molecular basis than genomic analysis alone, as it captures the changes associated with transcriptional, translational, and posttranslational modification of the proteins encoded by the genome. The roots of proteomics as applied to cancer lie in the discovery of the tumor-suppressor gene p53 in 1979 with the use of the one-dimensional protein gel. p53 was seen to be upregulated in cells infected by the DNA tumor virus SV40 (29). Refinements in gel technology led O' Farrell to develop 2D electrophoresis, which allowed further characterization of the proteome (30). Using the 2-D gel electrophoresis technique to compare wild-type and transformed BALB/c-3T3 cells, Croy and Pardee found that very few of the thousands of proteins identified by 2D electrophoresis were differentially expressed between wild-type and transformed cells, indicating that malignancy was the result of changes in specific biochemical pathways (31). Limitations in this technique were clearly apparent, as the proteome was known to include tens of thousands of molecules. In addition, the small amount of protein recovered made further characterization beyond molecular weight difficult. Recent developments have enabled high throughput processing of samples, resulting in the ability to both identify and quantify proteins with very low amounts of starting material.

Current techniques include laser capture microdissection of tissues to allow identification of proteins from a single tissue type (32); protein microarrays, similar to RNA microarrays, which have either protein libraries or known antibodies embedded in nitrocellulose, allowing the screening of the tumor lysate for known proteins; and matrix-assisted laser desorption and ionization with time-of-flight detection and mass spectrometry (MALDI-TOF, MS) (which can be used for the identification of proteins <20 kDa) and surface-enhanced laser desorption and ionization with time-of-flight detection (SELDI-TOF), both of which use the charge to mass ratio (μ/z) to separate proteins of interest and generate hundreds of thousands of data points (33). The large amount of data generated requires bioinformatics technologies to recognize the protein signature of various disease states in tumor lysates (34).

The information obtained using these analytical methods has the promise of resulting not only in the identification of potential therapeutic targets, but also the identification of serum profiles for early detection of malignancy. Several groups have been working on establishing profiles on ovarian, breast, and prostate cancer as well as pancreatic cancer. Serum samples must first be depleted of high-abundance, high molecular weight proteins by affinity columns, acetonitrile precipitation, or immunoprecipitation (*35, 36*). Koopman et al. identified four differentially expressed protein peaks in the sera of patients with resectable or unresectable pancreatic cancer, or pancreatitis (*25*). The identity of the specific proteins representing these peaks was not determined. These peaks demonstrated an area under the curve (AUC) of the receiver operating characteristics of 0.97, which represents superior sensitivity and specificity when compared with CA19-9, with an AUC of 0.85. The test has a specificity of 97%; however, the sensitivity required for a positive predictive value of 10% in the general population is >99% (*37*). Other groups are currently applying proteomic techniques to the characterization of pancreatic cyst fluid aspirate, in hopes of developing a means of reliably identifying malignant, premalignant, and benign cystic lesions. This approach is attractive because the cyst fluid contains proteins directly secreted by the neoplastic cells, undiluted by the high-abundance proteins present in serum.

An important emerging area for early cancer detection and identification of drug targets is the field of glycoproteomics. Glycoproteins are proteins with complex carbohydrate groups known as glycans attached in specific positions and are often involved in cell-cell signaling and cell recognition processes. Glycan variants of glycoproteins on the cell surface and in plasma have been shown to correlate with the progression of cancer and other diseases (*38*). Serum glycoproteins may be secreted (or released) into the blood and changes in glycosylation patterns have been associated with prostate cancer (*38, 39*), colorectal cancer (*40*), and breast cancer (*41*). There have been several efforts to detect changes in glycan structure in serum during cancer progression using lectins, which are natural agents that respond to different carbohydrate structures. In recent work, an approach using a glycoprotein microarray printed from glycoproteins extracted from serum and probed with a variety of lectins was used to screen glycosylation patterns in sera from normal, chronic pancreatitis, and pancreatic cancer patients (*42*). Data analysis showed that normal and chronic pancreatitis sera were found to cluster close together, although in two distinct groups, whereas pancreatic cancer sera were significantly different from the other two groups (Fig. 43.1). Both sialylation and fucosylation increased as a function of cancer on several proteins, including hemopexin, kininogen-1, antithrombin-III, and haptoglobin-related protein, whereas decreased sialylation was detected on plasma protease C1 inhibitor. Target alterations on glycosylations were verified by lectin blotting experiments and are currently undergoing large-scale validation. These altered glycan structures may have utility for the differential diagnosis of pancreatic cancer and chronic pancreatitis and may be important targets for drug therapy.

Protein analysis has important implications for the validation of drug targets identified by genomic methods. A novel agent is validated only after it has been demonstrated that a given therapeutic agent is clinically effective and acts through the target against which it was designed (*43*). Proteomic tools can also be used to assess the safety of potential drugs. Animal safety studies remain the standard for preclinical toxicity studies, but numerous examples of the failure of these tests to predict human toxicity have occurred. Identification of protein signatures of early

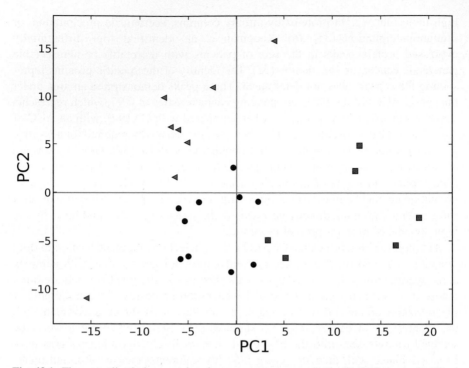

Fig. 43.1 The normalized glycoprotein microarray responses to the lectin AAL were visualized by principal component analysis (PCA). 24 serum samples (10 normal, 8 chronic pancreatitis and 6 pancreatic cancers) were studied. Blue circles represent samples of normal sera, orange squares represent samples of pancreatic cancer sera and yellow triangles represent samples of chronic pancreatitis sera

toxicity in vitro would theoretically keep potentially lethal agents from making it to phase I trials. The field of toxoproteomics uses global protein expression techniques to identify key proteins and pathways in biological systems that change in response to novel chemical entities. Early in vitro work has been promising. Gao et al. (*44*) utilized multidimensional high performance liquid chromatography coupled to tandem mass spectrometry to analyze proteomic changes in immortalized human hepatocytes which overexpressed cytochrome P450 3A4. These cells were treated with several known hepatotoxic and non-hepatotoxic compounds (PPAR γ agonists and HIV protease inhibitors). There was early up-regulation of two secreted proteins (BMS-PTX-265 and BMS-PTX-837) by the cells treated with hepatotoxic agents. Using immunoassays specific for these proteins, an expanded study was performed with a total of 20 compounds, consisting of known hepatotoxic and non-hepatotoxic agents. Of the 20 compounds tested, 19 out of 20 compounds were classified correctly. Similar results have been obtained in vivo. A group from Merck reported using two-dimensional difference gel electrophoresis (2D-DIGE) and mass spectrometry to analyze changes in serum protein expression as early as 6 hours following administration of known hepatotoxic compounds (*45*).

The investigators found upregulation of pyruvate dehydrogenase, phenylalanine hydroxylase and 2-oxoisovalerate dehydrogenase and downregulation of sulfite oxidase (an enzyme that may play a role in triglyceride accumulation) and glucose-regulated protein 78 (a chaperone and stress-related protein). These changes were consistent with development of steatosis, and occurred earlier than traditional biochemical markers or histopathological changes. The ability to prospectively identify potentially toxic agents more effectively in vivo and in vitro holds the promise to increase patient safety and streamline phase I trials.

4 Summary

The use of genomics and proteomics is likely to have a great impact on our ability to more effectively diagnose and treat pancreatic cancer. It is clear that novel approaches are needed outside of our standard regimens of chemotherapy and radiation therapy to make an impact on this terrible disease. Advances in proteomics and genomics have led to the elucidation of pathways critical to the development of the malignant phenotype of pancreatic cancer. The identification of these critical pathways in pancreatic cancer development and propagation has led to an increase in research activity in developing novel therapeutic agents that might enable more effective targeted treatment of pancreatic cancer. Additionally, although biomarker discovery for early detection remains in the discovery phase, it is likely that multiple approaches utilizing genomic and proteomic research tools will aid into transitioning this work from the discovery to the validation phase, with ultimate utility in the clinical setting.

References

1. Burris HA, 3rdMoore MJ, Andersen J, 1997, Improvement in survival and clinical benefit with gemcitabine as first-line therapy for patients with advanced pancreatic cancer: A randomized trial. J Clin Oncol 15:2403–2413.
2. et al. Resected adenocarcinoma of the pancreas-616 patients: results, outcomes, and prognostic indicators. J Gastrointest Surg 2000, 4:567–79.
3. Black JW, Duncan WAM, Durant CJ, 1972, Definition and antagonism of H2-receptors. Nature 236:385–390.
4. Rundles RW, Wyngaarden JB, Hitchings GH, 1969, Drugs and uric acid. Rev Ann Pharmacol 9:345–362.
5. Kindler HL, Friberg G Singh DA, 2005, Phase II trial of bevacizumab plus gemcitabine in patients with advanced pancreatic cancer. J Clin Oncol 23(31):8033–8040.
6. Kindler HL, Niedzwiecki D, Hollis D, 2007, A double-blind, placebo-controlled, randomized phase III trial of gemcitabine (G) plus bevacizumab (B) versus gemcitabine plus placebo (P) in patients (pts) with advanced pancreatic cancer (PC): A preliminary analysis of Cancer and Leukemia Group B (CALGB). J Clin Oncol 25(18S): 4508.
7. Liang P, Pardee AB. 1992, Differential display of eukaryotic mRNA by means of the polymerase chain reaction. Science 257:967–971.

8. Caldas C, Hahn SA, Costa LT, da 1994, Frequent somatic mutations and homozygous deletions of the p16 (MTS1) gene in pancreatic adenocarcinoma. Nat Genet 8:27–32.
9. Hahn SA, Schutte M, Hoque AT, 1996, DPC4, a candidate tumor suppressor gene at human chromosome 18q21.1. Science 271:350–353.
10. Cerny WL, Mangold KA, Scarpelli DG. 1992, K-ras mutation is an early event in pancreatic duct carcinogenesis in the Syrian golden hamster. Cancer Res 15:4507–4513.
11. Schena M, Shalon D, Davis RW, 1995, Quantitative monitoring of gene expression patterns with a complementary DNA microarray. Science 270:467–470.
12. Chee M, Yang R, Hubbell E, 1996, Accessing genetic information with high-density DNA arrays. Science 274:610–614.
13. Misek DE, Kuick R, Hanash SM, 1997, Oligonucleotide-directed microarray gene profiling of pancreatic adenocarcinoma. In: Su G (ed.) Methods in molecular medicine, vol. 103. Pancreatic cancer: methods and protocols. NJ. Humana Press, Totowa, 175–188.
14. Aragani P, Rosty C, Reiter RE, 2001, Discovery of new markers of cancer through serial analysis of gene expression: prostate stem cell antigen is overexpressed in pancreatic adenocarcinoma. Cancer Res 61:4320–4324.
15. Iacobuzio-Donahue CA, Ryu B, Hruban RH, 2002, Exploring the host desmoplastic response to pancreatic adenocarcinoma: gene expression of stromal and neoplastic cells at the site of primary invasion. Am J Pathol 160:91–99.
16. Zhang L, Zhou W, Velculescu VE, 1997, Gene expression profiles normal and cancer cells. Science 276:1268–1272.
17. Zhou W, Sokoll LJ, Bruzek DJ, 1998, Identifying markers for pancreatic cancer by gene expression analysis, Cancer Epidemiol Biomark Prev 7:109–112.
18. Gress TM Muller-Pillasch F, Geng M, 1998, A pancreatic cancer-specific expression profile. Oncogene 13:1819–1830.
19. Logsdon CD, Simeone DM, Binkley C, 2003, Molecular profiling of pancreatic adenocarcinoma and chronic pancreatitis identifies multiple genes differentially regulated in pancreatic cancer. Cancer Res 63:2649–2657.
20. Crnogorac-Jurcevic T, Gangeswaran R, Bhakta V, 2005, Proteomic analysis of chronic pancreatitis and pancreatic adenocarcinoma. Gastroenterology 129:1454–1463.
21. Guerreiro DS, Hu YF, Russo IH, 2000, S100P calcium-binding protein overexpression is associated with immortalization of human breast epithelial cells in vitro and early stages of breast cancer development in vivo. Int J Oncol 16:231–240.
22. Bertram J, Palfner K, Hiddemann W, 1998, Elevated expression of S100P, CAPL and MAGE 3 in doxorubicin-resistant cell lines: comparison of mRNA differential display reverse transcription-polymerase chain reaction and subtractive suppressive hybridization for the analysis of differential gene expression. Anticancer Drugs 9:311–317.
23. Beer DG, Kardia SL, Huang CC, 2002, Gene-expression profiles predict survival of patients with lung adenocarcinoma. Nat Med 8:816–824.
24. Arumugam T, Ramachandran V, Logsdon CD. 2006, Effect of cromolyn on S100P interactions with RAGE and pancreatic cancer growth and invasion in mouse models. J Natl Cancer Inst 98:1806–1818.
25. Koopman J, Zhang Z, White N, 2004, Serum diagnosis of pancreatic adenocarcinoma using surface-enhanced laser desorption and ionization mass spectrometry. Clin. Cancer Res 10:860–868.
26. Koopmann J, Rosenzweig NW, Zhang Z, 2006, Serum markers in patients with resectable pancreatic adenocarcinoma: macrophage inhibitory cytokine 1 versus CA19-9. Clin Can Res 12:442–446.
27. Hwang TL, Liang Y, Chien KY, 2006, Overexpression and elevated serum levels of phosphoglycerate kinase 1 in pancreatic ductal adenocarcinoma. Proteomics 6:2259–2272.
28. Simeone DM, Ji B, Banerjee M, 2007, CEACAM1, a novel serum biomarker for pancreatic cancer. Pancreas 34:436–443.
29. Linzer DI, Levine AJ. 1979, Characterization of a 54K Dalton cellular SV40 tumor antigen present in SV40-transformed cells and uninfected embryonal carcinoma cells. Cell 17:43–52.

30. O'Farrell PH. 1975, High-resolution two-dimensional electrophoresis of proteins. J Biol Chem 250:4007–4021.
31. Croy RG, Pardee AB. 1983, Enhanced synthesis and stabilization of Mr 68,000 protein in transformed BALB/c-3T3cells: candidate for restriction point control of cell growth. Proc Natl Acad Sci U S A 80:4699–4703.
32. Emmert-Buck MR, Bonner RF, Smith PD, 1996, Laser capture microdissection. Science 274:998–1001.
33. O'Neil KA, Miller FR, Lubman DM. 2003, Profiling the progression of cancer: the separation of microsomal proteins in MCF10 breast epithelial cell lines using nonporous chromatophoresis, MALDI-TOF-MS and MALDI-QTOF-MS-MS. Proteomics 3:1256–1269.
34. Petricoin EF, Ornstein DK, Paweletz CP, 2002, Serum proteomic patterns for detection of prostate cancer. J Natl Cancer Inst 94:1576–1578.
35. Merrill K, Southwick K, Graves SW, 2004, Analysis of low-abundance, low-molecular weight serum proteins using mass spectrometry. J Biomol Tech 15:238–248.
36. Zhang H, Yi EC, Li XJ, 2005, High throughput quantitative analysis of serum proteins using glycopeptide capture and liquid chromatography mass spectrometry. Mol Cell Proteomics 4:144–155.
37. Jacobs IJ, Skates SJ, MacDonald N, 2002, Screening for ovarian cancer: a pilot randomised controlled trial. Lancet 359:572–577.
38. Peracaula R, Royle L, Tabares G, 2003, Glycosylation of human pancreatic ribonuclease: differences between normal and tumor states. Glycobiology 13:227–244.
39. Drake RR, Schwegler EE, Malik G, 2006, Lectin capture strategies combined with mass spectrometry for the discovery of serum glycoprotein biomarkers. Mol Cell Proteomics 5:1957–1967.
40. Kasbaoui L, Harb J, Bernard S, 1989, Differences in glycosylation state of fibronectin from two rat colon carcinoma cell lines in relation to tumoral progressiveness. Cancer Res 49:5317–5322.
41. Ng RC, Roberts AN, Wilson RG, 1987, Analyses of protein extracts of human breast cancers: changes in glycoprotein content linked to the malignant phenotype. Br J Cancer 55:249–254.
42. Zhao J, Patwa TH, Qiu W, et al. Glycoprotein microarrays with multi-lectin detection: unique lectin binding patterns as a tool for classifying normal, chronic pancreatitits and pancreatic cancer sera. J Proteome Res, in press.
43. Benson JD, Chen YP, Cornell-Kennon SA, 2004, Identification of in vitro protein biomarkers of idiosyncratic liver toxicity. Toxicol In Vitro 18:533–541.
45. Meneses-Lorente G, Guest PC, Lawrence J, N. 2004, A proteomic investigation of drug-induced steatosis in rat liver. Chem Res Toxicol 17:605–612.
Arumugam T, Simeone DM, Golen K, Van 2005, S100P promotes pancreatic cancer growth, survival, and invasion. Clin Cancer Res 11:5356–5364.
Elrick MM, Walgren JL, Mitchell MD, 2006, Proteomics: recent applications and new technologies. Basic Clin Pharmacol Toxicol 98:432–441.
Koopmann J, Fedarko NS, Jain A, 2004, Evaluation of osteopontin as biomarker for pancreatic adenocarcinoma. Cancer Epidemiol Biomarkers Prev 13:487–491.
Koopmann J, Buckhaults P, Brown DA, 2004, Serum macrophage inhibitory cytokine 1 as a marker of pancreatic and other periampullary cancers. Clin Can Res 10:2386–2392.
Saif MW. 2006, Anti-angiogenesis therapy in pancreatic carcinoma. JOP 9:163–173.

Chapter 44
Pitfalls in Clinical Trials and Future Directions

Philip A. Philip, Lance K. Heilbrun, and Judith Abrams

1 Introduction

Out of every 100 patients with newly diagnosed pancreatic cancer, only a handful is considered to be cured of the disease. The median survival of patients with advanced pancreatic cancer remains at <6 months. This highlights the significance of overt and micrometastases in this disease. Improvements in the survival of patients with pancreatic cancer depends on future advances in systemic therapies. Unfortunately, therapy of pancreatic cancer has not made the major headway seen with the treatment of other nonhematologic cancers, such as breast and colon. This is not to dismiss the relentless research efforts over the past decade or so that involved a large number of phase II trials and over a dozen well-conducted phase III trials. Clinical trials during the 1990s and early 2000s focused on the addition of newer agents to gemcitabine. Drugs tested included different classes of cytotoxics and more recently biological agents. Despite some interesting results in phase II settings, the translation of benefit to phase III testing was absent with one or two exceptions.

There is growing pressure from within and without pancreas research groups to improve the efficacy of clinical drug development in pancreatic cancer. This chapter discusses some of the issues related to existing experimental designs and challenges to clinical and translational research in this disease. The discussion points are partly generic in that they also pertain to research in other nonhematologic cancers.

2 Drug Targets

With the advent of the biological therapy era selectivity of drugs to cellular targets generated much enthusiasm to test these agents in the clinic. Most newly developed drugs appear to be predominantly linked to a single cellular molecule or pathway for its predominant antitumor effect. Examples include the antiepidermal growth factor receptor (anti-EGFR) agents and drugs that bind to the vascular endothelial growth factor (VEGF) that have successfully affected the outcome of advanced colorectal

A.M. Lowy et al. (eds.) *Pancreatic Cancer.*
doi: 10.1007/978-0-387-69252-4, © Springer Science+Business Media, LLC 2008

cancer. Some drugs may have more than one targeted molecule, for example sorafenib, which has anti-Raf kinase activity and also an inhibitory effect on VEGF receptors. The presence of multiple rather than one predominant gene mutation in cancers such as that of the pancreas makes a single gene target approach a strategy less likely to succeed in the treatment of pancreatic cancer (*1*). K-ras mutations, for example, although very prevalent in pancreatic cancer (*2, 3*), are not sufficient for the progression and maintenance of the malignant process in the absence of additional gene mutations. By targeting K-ras alone, one may not expect a major impact on the disease. Unfortunately, we were never able to test the hypothesis adequately in the clinic because of the lack of agents that effectively targeted the Ras oncoprotein.

Target validation is a crucial part of developing any new therapy for pancreatic cancer. The EGFR pathway targeting illustrates how an incomplete validation process may influence the outcome of subsequent clinical trials. More than 1,000 patients with advanced pancreatic cancer were included in studies testing anti-EGFR strategies. To date we have neither a definite answer for our central research question nor the ability to build on the findings of these trials. These studies were rationalized by the fact that EGFR pathway activation was prevalent in patients with pancreatic cancer. However, this was based on the immunohistochemical detection of EGFR protein in tumor samples and was wrongly assumed to represent activation of the pathway. The efficacy of anti-EGFR strategy was tested in only a few preclinical models that did not represent the range and complexity of genetic abnormalities in human pancreatic cancer (*4, 5*).

Investigators have combined targeted drugs with gemcitabine in an effort to show an improvement over gemcitabine. The rationale was to provide selective tumor sensitization to gemcitabine and/or an additive antitumor effect. These studies that include phase III trials were discussed in detail in several of the chapters in this book. With one exception (*6*), none showed a statistically and clinically important difference in survival with the addition of the new agent. The targets tested thus far included matrix metalloproteinases, farnesyl transferase, EGFR, and VEGF. It is noteworthy that none of these studies selected participants with respect to the target molecule.

3 Multitargeted Approaches

Anticancer drug development is full of attempts to test drug combinations. Early successes in treating lymphoid malignancies and testicular cancers laid the foundations for combination therapy to maximize antitumor effect. Interestingly, those combinations were largely based on empiricism provided that there were no major overlapping toxicities.

The multiplicity of genetic mutations and their complexity in pancreatic cancer necessitates a multitargeted approach to therapy. We now have a much better opportunity to develop new therapies developed on a scientific basis and we have better tools to accomplish this. However, we are somewhat limited by the availability of preclinical models of pancreatic cancer that faithfully mimic human disease.

Multitargeted approaches may be achieved by single drugs that can target more than one molecule (e.g., sorafenib, lapatinib). More commonly, two or more drugs are used to hit several cellular targets. Successful developments of drug combinations face certain challenges. Pharmacokinetic and pharmacodynamic interactions between drugs may limit their individual antitumor activities and/or increase toxicities. Logistics of working with multiple drug sponsors may significantly slow the process of drug development. The increased cost of multiple drugs must be balanced against the gains in efficacy and toxicity. However, the major hurdle is the ability to effectively translate preclinical data into the clinic by developing appropriate tumor models that would guide the choice of agents to be tested in clinical trials.

4 The Cytotoxic Platform

In the targeted therapy era we continue to view newer drugs as a means to enhance the poor antitumor activity of conventional cytotoxic drugs in patients with pancreatic cancer. Gemcitabine remains the only cytotoxic platform to test targeted agents in pancreatic cancer. It is noteworthy that preclinical studies have generally shown additive activity of targeted agents when combined with gemcitabine rather than synergy. Gemcitabine, a cell-cycle–specific agent, may interfere with the activity of certain targeted agents or vice versa. The combination of erlotinib with cytotoxics in patients with advanced non-small cell lung cancer showed no additive benefit (7). However, in a similar population of patients, erlotinib demonstrated anti-tumor activity when used as a single agent (8).

Alternative cytotoxics to gemcitabine are capecitabine, oxaliplatin (with a fluoropyrimidine), S1, or ixabepilone. No randomized trial has compared the activity of any of those agents to that of gemcitabine in the phase III setting. Consideration should also be given to designing studies without a cytotoxic platform given the very small benefit of those drugs in treating pancreatic cancer.

5 Clinical Trial Design

The relatively high failure rates of phase III trials in advanced pancreatic cancer raised major issues regarding the interpretation of phase II trial results in the transition to phase III testing of new regimes. Several of the combinations evaluated in phase II setting demonstrated activity that was superior to activity of standard agents in historical controls. These phase II studies were single arm trials and patient heterogeneity and selection may have contributed to the false-positivity of the results. Interestingly, the only phase III trial of a targeted agent to demonstrate a statistically significant benefit was that of erlotinib, which was never preceded by any phase II studies. Early phase clinical trials that are well controlled are increasingly viewed as necessary step to screen for effectiveness of new regimens (9). The reliance on historical controls is considered to increase the risk of false-positivity that would lead to an unnecessary phase III trial. The recent example of gemcitabine plus bevacizumab well illustrates this fact.

5.1 Experimental Endpoints in Pilot Studies

Objective response rates were traditionally used in phase II studies in the past as a surrogate endpoint to assess efficacy of new regimens. However, the difficulties in determining response based on WHO or the more recent response evaluation criteria in solid tumors (RECIST) (*10*) in localized and metastatic pancreatic cancer raised questions about the validity of this endpoint. In pancreatic cancer difficulties arise from radiologic abnormalities relating to chronic pancreatic disease and fibrosis associated with the cancer. Progression-free survival is another potential surrogate endpoint that may be more meaningful from the clinical standpoint. However, the accurate identification of the time of progression is very challenging and subject to multiple biases and errors in single-arm studies (*11*), leading to proposals to improve its use (*12*). Recently the concept of an endpoint that is the continuous change in tumor size was revisited. This takes into consideration disease stabilization as a major mechanism of tumor control in targeted therapies (*13*). This approach requires further study and validation before its adoption in clinical trials. There is also discussion of using both progression-free survival and objective tumor response as dual primary endpoints. At this time survival remains the preferred primary endpoint.

5.2 Statistical Designs

In an effort to minimize the number of failures in phase III trials of advanced pancreatic cancer there is tremendous pressure to perform better-designed pilot phase II trials in this disease. Single-arm phase II studies are now increasingly replaced by randomized phase II studies to account for the uncertainties of comparisons to historical controls (*14, 15*). A screening design uses a control arm of gemcitabine or gemcitabine plus erlotinib. Although such a design requires a large sample size will not allow formal statistical tests for comparisons of experimental versus control arms it improves the ability to interpret the results of the study (*16*). For example, a retrospective evaluation of the single arm phase II trial that led to the phase III trial of gemcitabine plus bevacizumab revealed patient exclusion based on history of venous clotting and tumors adjacent to major vessels (*17*). The efficacy was of much interest to proceed to a phase III trial that did not demonstrate any benefit for bevacizumab when added to gemcitabine (*18*). A control arm of gemcitabine alone in the initial phase II trial may have influenced the interpretation of the results in favor of not proceeding to a phase III trial.

An alternative phase II design is the selection design that will have two or more experimental arms without provision for direct comparison of the two arms. Such a selection design allows the investigator to choose for further testing the regimen that is more likely to have a better efficacy and toxicity profile. The marked de novo resistance to therapy in pancreatic cancer makes it likely that investigators will have to accept the possibility that none of the regimens tested would be further developed. It is therefore much preferable to perform randomized phase II studies to select a regimen when the regimens have a reasonable chance of showing activity. A major concern for randomized phase II trial design is also the rate of false positivity (19). Other statistical designs have been proposed such as the randomized discontinuation design (20) that remains to be validated in pancreatic cancer.

5.3 Single-Agent Activity

Testing of new drugs as single agents in treatment naïve patients is challenged by the fact that gemcitabine is the only active drug available. Delaying the start of gemcitabine may be unethical and unacceptable by patients and/or oncologists. The practice of testing targeted agents in combination with gemcitabine deprives investigators of valuable information on single-agent activity of a drug. For example, the FDA approved erlotinib for therapy in advanced pancreatic cancer on the basis of combination with gemcitabine. To date there is no information on what to expect with single-agent erlotinib in advanced pancreatic cancer because the phase III trial did not include testing erlotinib by itself. Lack of knowledge on single agent activity limits the ability to design trials in which magnitude of treatment effect needs to be more accurately predicted. Recent attempts have included the study of gemcitabine-refractory patients to determine single agent activity of targeted agents. However, only 30–40% of patients undergoing therapy with gemcitabine will be able to receive a subsequent treatment because of the rapid decline in performance status and short survival.

6 Patient Selection

A principle of clinical trials was the delivery of maximum anti-tumor activity to the broadest population of patients with a given cancer. The majority of conventional anticancer drugs were considered to be nonselective cytotoxics, although one may challenge this notion today. As a result, combinations of cytotoxics were used at or near their maximum tolerated doses with lesser emphasis to tailor therapies based on patient variables. In the era of targeted therapies patient selection becomes an increasingly important factor for the success of any therapy.

6.1 Clinical Factors

Studies have shown that factors such as performance status, tumor burden, and pathologic features such as grade and mucinous histology determine a patient's outcome. Despite this, patients with locally advanced, metastatic, and those with end-stage disease were studied as one group. As many as 30% of patients on phase III trials had localized disease, which carries a survival approximately double that of metastatic disease. In contrast, patients with end-stage disease have very short survival, weeks to a few months, that are not impacted by any therapy. Patients with poor performance status are included not infrequently in clinical trials despite restrictions of eligibility to performance status of 2 or less (*21*). These variables account for the difficulties in interpreting results of phase II studies when no control arm is included.

6.2   Molecular Markers

Targeted drugs are assumed to benefit only patients whose tumors have the target molecule that is the underlying abnormality to maintain the malignant status. Predictive biomarkers are lacking for all drug classes at this time. Given the expected low frequency of occurrence of those activating mutations in pancreatic cancer, with the exception of mutated K-ras, minimal activity for those agents may be seen in a nonselected population. The targeting of EGFR represents an excellent example of outcome in the absence of patient selection. The use of immunohistochemistry (IHC) to select patients for anti-EGFR treatment was unsuccessful in colon and lung cancers, in which these drugs were largely studied. It is conceivable that a significant benefit may have accrued in a subgroup of those patients not currently identified.

Experience from other cancers indicates that in diseases with multiple and complex genetic mutations, a single-agent activity of a drug may be seen in up to 10% of patients. This relatively low level of activity can be amplified severalfold if the population was enriched for the presence of a predictive biomarker. Patient selection will also allow the inclusion of fewer patients in clinical trials for a large magnitude of benefit.

7   Predictive Biomarkers

Predictive biomarkers function as single or multiple molecular signatures that define and characterize a patient's cancer with respect to its responsiveness to a given anticancer treatment (*22*). This should be distinguished from prognostic biomarkers that may help decide on therapy purely for prognostic reasons but without the ability to predict the probability for a given treatment to succeed. The field of biomarkers and their validation is rapidly evolving with improvements in techniques to study gene expression profiles and protein expression patterns. The following represent major challenges for the clinical trials to validate predictive markers.

1. The paucity of biological material is the major limitation to perform assays to characterize pancreatic cancer molecularly. The majority of diagnostic tumor samples are performed using small needles. This contributes to the poor quality of biological specimens in approximately half of the samples. Performing a biopsy procedure solely for research purposes is unlikely to be accepted by patients and institutional review boards because of the associated risks and costs. However, small samples obtained by diagnostic fine-needle aspirates may still be analyzable by IHC and PCR based DNA and RNA assays (*23*). Use of surrogate tissues such as peripheral blood mononuclear cells, although very convenient, lacks the ability to predict tumor biology unless one is interested in studying germline mutations or polymorphisms.
2. The molecular abnormalities may be different between primary and secondary tumor deposits. The latter is often obtained during diagnostic tissue sampling and hence may be the source of profiling a patient's cancer.
3. The genetic changes in advanced human pancreatic cancer differ substantially from those in preclinical models. This eventually limits the ability to develop predictive biomarkers based on those models.
4. Data on biomarkers are often based on small data sets from nonrandomized trials. Therefore any such information must be prospectively validated in larger studies.
5. The usefulness of a biomarker may be limited by lack of knowledge of the full spectrum of mechanism of action of a drug. This is especially true for kinase inhibitors, which may affect multiple targets. The development of sorafenib is an example of improvements in target definition during the drug development path.
6. Ancillary studies to discover and validate biomarkers increase cost of clinical trials and require extra funding.

8 Future Directions

It is clear from the previous discussions that major challenges lie ahead in the design and execution of clinical studies in pancreatic cancer. However, with the availability of targeted drugs and improvements in preclinical models, one would expect major opportunities for research in this disease. Undoubtedly a close collaboration between basic and clinical scientists is crucial for new drug development. Major points with respect to performing pilot trials are summarized in the following.

- Developing animal models of pancreatic cancer that are more predictive of human biology and response to therapy
- Testing of hypotheses to prove efficacy in patients selected by validated biomarkers

- Rational designing of multitargeted approaches instead of empirically chosen drugs
- Developing clinical trial endpoints to best answer scientific question(s) and determine the advancement to phase III testing
- Developing innovative strategies for the testing of drugs in the clinical setting including computer simulations and mathematical modeling prior to embarking on phase II and III trials
- Enrolling newly diagnosed patients with pancreatic cancer in clinical trials and increasing public awareness of the benefit of clinical research

References

1. Braiteh F, Kurzrock R, 2007, Uncommon tumors and exceptional therapies: paradox or paradigm? Mol Cancer Ther 6:1175–1179.
2. Deramaudt T, Rustgi AK, 2005, Mutant K-ras in the initiation of pancreatic cancer. Biochim Biophys Acta 1756:97–101.
3. Furukawa T, Sunamura M, Horii A, 2006, Molecular mechanisms of pancreatic carcinogenesis. Cancer Sci 97:1–7.
4. Overholser JP, Prewett MC, Hooper AT, 2000, Epidermal growth factor receptor blockade by antibody IMC-C225 inhibits growth of a human pancreatic carcinoma xenograft in nude mice. Cancer 89:74–82.
5. Bruns CJ, Harbison MT, Davis DW, 2000, Epidermal growth factor receptor blockade with C225 plus gemcitabine results in regression of human pancreatic carcinoma growing orthotopically in nude mice by antiangiogenic mechanisms. Clin Cancer Res 6:1936–1948.
6. Moore MJ, Goldstein D, Hamm J, 2007, Erlotinib plus gemcitabine compared with gemcitabine alone in patients with advanced pancreatic cancer: a phase III trial of the National Cancer Institute of Canada Clinical Trials Group. J Clin Oncol 25:1960–1966.
7. Herbst RS, Prager D, Hermann R, 2005, TRIBUTE: a phase III trial of erlotinib hydrochloride (OSI-774) combined with carboplatin and paclitaxel chemotherapy in advanced non-small-cell lung cancer. J Clin Oncol 23:5892–5899.
8. Shepherd FA, Rodrigues PJ, 2005, Erlotinib in previously treated non-small-cell lung cancer. N Engl J Med 353:123–132.
9. Roberts TG, Jr., Lynch TJ, Jr., Chabner BA, 2003, The phase III trial in the era of targeted therapy: unraveling the "go or no go" decision. J Clin Oncol 21:3683–3695.
10. Therasse P, Arbuck SG, Eisenhauer EA, 2000, New guidelines to evaluate the response to treatment in solid tumors. J Natl Cancer Inst 92:205–216.
11. Schilsky RL. 2002, End points in cancer clinical trials and the drug approval process. Clinical Cancer Res 8:935–938.
12. Freidlin B, Korn EL, Hunsberger S, 2007, Proposal for the use of progression-free survival in unblinded randomized trials. J Clin Oncol 25:2122–2126.
13. Karrison TG, Maitland ML, Stadler WM, 2007, Design of phase II cancer trials using a continuous endpoint of change in tumor size: application to a study of sorafenib and erlotinib in non-small-cell lung cancer. J Natl Cancer Inst 99:1455–1461.
14. Taylor JMG, Braun TM, Li Z, 2006, Comparing an experimental agent to a standard agent: relative merits of a one-arm or randomized two-arm Phase II design. Clin Trials 3:335–348.
15. Stone A, Wheeler C, Barge A, 2007, Improving the design of phase II trials of cytostatic anticancer agents. Contemp Clin Trials 28:138–145.
16. Rubinstein LV, Korn EL, Freidlin B, 2005, Design issues of randomized phase II trials and a proposal for phase II screening trials. J Clin Oncol 23:7199–7206.

17. Kindler HL, Friberg G, Singh DA, 2005, Phase II trial of bevacizumab plus gemcitabine in patients with advanced pancreatic cancer. J Clin Oncol 23:8033–8040.
18. Kindler HL, Niedzwiecki D, Hollis D, 2007, A double-blind, placebo-controlled, randomized phase III trial of gemcitabine (G) plus bevacizumab (B) versus gemcitabine plus placebo (P) in patients (pts) with advanced pancreatic cancer (PC): A preliminary analysis of Cancer and Leukemia Group B (CALGB). ASCO Meeting Abstracts 25:4508.
19. Liu PY, LeBlanc M, Desai M, 1999, False positive rates of randomized phase II designs. Control Clin Trials 20:343–352.
20. Rosner GL, Stadler W, Ratain MJ, Randomized discontinuation design: application to cytostatic antineoplastic agents. 2002, 20:4478–4484.
21. Boeck S, Hinke A, Wilkowski R, 2007, Importance of performance status for treatment outcome I advanced pancreatic cancer. World J Gastroenterol 13:224–227.
22. Sargent DJ, Conley BA, Alegra C, 2005, Clinical trial designs for predictive marker validation in cancer treatment trials. J Clin Oncol 23:2020–2027.
23. Mishra G, 2006, DNA analysis of cells obtained from endoscopic ultrasound-fine needle aspiration in pancreatic adenocarcinoma: fool's gold, Pandora's box, or holy grail? Am J Gastroenterol 101:2501–2503.

Index